# ACSM's Resources for the Personal Trainer

FIFTH EDITION

# ACSM's
# Resources for the
# Personal Trainer

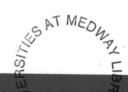

## FIFTH EDITION

### SENIOR EDITOR

**Rebecca A. Battista, PhD, FACSM**

Associate Professor
Department of Health and Exercise Science
Appalachian State University
Boone, North Carolina

*See Appendix A for a list of editors for the previous two editions.

### ASSOCIATE EDITORS

**Mindy Mayol, MS, ACSM EP-C**

Assistant Professor
Department of Kinesiology
University of Indianapolis
Indianapolis, Indiana

**Trent Hargens, PhD, FACSM, ACSM CEP, ACSM EIM3**

Associate Professor
Department of Kinesiology
James Madison University
Harrisonburg, Virginia

**Kenneth Lee Everett, PhD**

Assistant Professor
Department of Kinesiology
University of Indianapolis
Indianapolis, Indiana

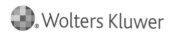 Wolters Kluwer

Philadelphia · Baltimore · New York · London
Buenos Aires · Hong Kong · Sydney · Tokyo

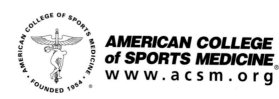

**AMERICAN COLLEGE
of SPORTS MEDICINE**
w w w . a c s m . o r g

*Executive Editor*: Michael Nobel
*Senior Product Development Editor*: Amy Millholen
*Editorial Coordinator*: Lindsay Ries
*Marketing Manager*: Shauna Kelley
*Production Project Manager*: Kim Cox
*Design Coordinator*: Stephen Druding
*Manufacturing Coordinator*: Margie Orzech
*Compositor*: Absolute Service, Inc.
*ACSM Committee on Certification and Registry Boards Chair*: William Simpson, PhD, FACSM
*ACSM Publications Committee Chair*: Jeffrey Potteiger, PhD, FACSM
*ACSM Group Publisher*: Katie Feltman
*ACSM Development Editor*: Angela Chastain

Fifth Edition

9  8  7  6  5  4  3  2  1

Printed in China

**Library of Congress Cataloging-in-Publication Data**

Names: Battista, Rebecca, editor. | Everett, Kenneth Lee, editor. | Hargens,
    Trent, editor. | Mayol, Mindy, editor. | American College of Sports
    Medicine, issuing body.
Title: ACSM's resources for the personal trainer / senior editor, Rebecca
    Battista ; associate editors, Kenneth Lee Everett, Trent Hargens, Mindy
    Mayol.
Other titles: Resources for the personal trainer | American College of Sports
    Medicine's resources for the personal trainer
Description: Fifth edition. | Philadelphia : Wolters Kluwer, [2018] |
    Includes bibliographical references and index.
Identifiers: LCCN 2017023354 | ISBN 9781496322890
Subjects: | MESH: Physical Education and Training | Exercise—physiology
Classification: LCC GV428.7 | NLM QT 255 | DDC 613.7/1—dc23 LC record available at
    https://lccn.loc.gov/2017023354

DISCLAIMER

Care has been taken to confirm the accuracy of the information present and to describe generally accepted practices. However, the authors, editors, and publisher are not responsible for errors or omissions or for any consequences from application of the information in this publication and make no warranty, expressed or implied, with respect to the currency, completeness, or accuracy of the contents of the publication. Application of this information in a particular situation remains the professional responsibility of the practitioner; the clinical treatments described and recommended may not be considered absolute and universal recommendations.

The authors, editors, and publisher have exerted every effort to ensure that drug selection and dosage set forth in this text are in accordance with the current recommendations and practice at the time of publication. However, in view of ongoing research, changes in government regulations, and the constant flow of information relating to drug therapy and drug reactions, the reader is urged to check the package insert for each drug for any change in indications and dosage and for added warnings and precautions. This is particularly important when the recommended agent is a new or infrequently employed drug.

Some drugs and medical devices presented in this publication have Food and Drug Administration (FDA) clearance for limited use in restricted research settings. It is the responsibility of the health care provider to ascertain the FDA status of each drug or device planned for use in their clinical practice.

# Preface

## Additional Resources

This fifth edition of *ACSM's Resources for the Personal Trainer* represents another step forward from the previous edition and is based on *ACSM's Guidelines for Exercise Testing and Prescription, 10th edition*. In this fifth edition, the editors and contributors have continued to respond to the needs of practicing Personal Trainers. This edition has expanded upon the fourth edition in that content was updated with the latest scientific evidence, preparticipation screening recommendations were revised to reflect new guidelines for participating in physical activity, and a new chapter on functional movement was added.

## Overview

*ACSM's Resources for the Personal Trainer, 5th edition*, continues to recognize the Personal Trainer as a professional in the continuum of creating healthy lifestyles. This text provides the Personal Trainer with both the tools and scientific evidence to help build safe and effective exercise programs for a variety of clients. The book is divided into six distinctly different parts, ranging from an introduction to the profession of personal training to considerations of how to run your own business. In between are chapters dedicated to the foundations of exercise science which include anatomy, exercise physiology, biomechanics, behavior modification, and nutrition. The science- and evidence-based approach provides a way for the transfer of knowledge from the Personal Trainer to the client, allowing for the opportunity for success from a business standpoint, as well as for the individual clients. The middle chapters include establishing goals and objectives for clients and a "how-to" manual for preparticipation screening guidelines as well as assessing body composition, cardiovascular fitness, muscular fitness, and flexibility. The last sections of chapters are dedicated to developing various training programs, addressing special populations and advanced training program options, and providing the basics on business and legal concerns facing Personal Trainers.

## Organization

The chapters are divided into six parts designed for ease of navigation throughout the text. Using this approach, usefulness will be maximized for every Personal Trainer.

**Part I: Introduction to the Field and Profession of Personal Training.** Two introductory chapters are designed to introduce the new and aspiring Personal Trainer to the profession. Chapter 1 provides insight into why the health and fitness professions are some of the fastest growing industries in the world and how the Personal Trainer can capitalize on this growth. Chapter 2 provides a career track for the Personal Trainer, helping prospective Personal Trainers to examine their own interest in personal training and how to make personal training a viable career.

**Part II: The Science of Personal Training.** In Part II, Chapters 3–6 provide the scientific foundations for personal training. Every Personal Trainer, regardless of experience, will find these chapters helpful. For the Personal Trainer just starting out, these chapters introduce the scientific basis for physical activity. For the advanced Personal Trainer, these chapters serve as a foundational resource for specific lifestyle modification programs. These four chapters include anatomy and kinesiology, applied biomechanics, exercise physiology, and nutrition.

**Part III: Behavior Modification.** The next section of this book is dedicated to learning how and why people are either willing or unwilling to change their behavior. One of the most frustrating aspects of personal training is when a client refuses to change a deleterious habit or even "cheats" between training sessions. Chapters 7–9 include discussions of the concept of "coaching"—a new way of looking at and creating your relationship with a client. These chapters will forever change your approach to personal training.

**Part IV: Initial Client Screening.** Part IV comprises Chapters 10, 11, and 12 and walks the Personal Trainer through the first client meeting to a comprehensive health-related physical fitness assessment. Capitalizing on the learning objectives of Part III, this section establishes a framework for developing client-centered goals and objectives. Though certainly not an exhaustive list of physical fitness assessments, Chapter 12 provides critical techniques to evaluate a client both in the field and in the laboratory. This section includes many tables, figures, and case studies that will assist with placing clients into various fitness categories.

**Part V: Developing the Exercise Program.** Chapter 13 introduces the concept of developing a comprehensive exercise program. On the basis of the goals established by the client and the Personal Trainer, Chapters 14–16 (resistance training, cardiorespiratory, and flexibility programs, respectively) are specific "how-to" manuals. New to this book, Chapter 17 presents information regarding functional movement assessments and programming. Chapter 18 is dedicated to the proper sequencing of exercises within a given personal training session, whereas Chapter 19 has been written for the Personal Trainer who works with individuals who desire more advanced training options. Finally, Chapter 20 provides expanded coverage about working with clients with special health or medical conditions. As more people decide that being active is a good thing, Personal Trainers will encounter these special populations. This chapter also discusses the scope of a Personal Trainer's knowledge, skills, and abilities when it comes to working with these "special populations."

**Part VI: The Business of Personal Training.** Although seeing clients improve is rewarding, one goal of a successful business is to be profitable financially. Chapters 21 and 22 introduce the professional Personal Trainer to common business practices and provide information about how to avoid some of the common mistakes beginners typically make in the development of their practices. Chapter 22 deals specifically with legal issues. Written by a practicing attorney with years of experience litigating court cases, this chapter encourages each Personal Trainer to take their responsibility seriously by getting the necessary training and experience.

## Features

Specific elements within the chapters will appeal to the Personal Trainer. A list of objectives precedes each chapter. **Key points** highlight important concepts addressed in the text and boxes expand on material presented. **Case Studies** present common scenarios that allow for application of concepts covered within the chapters. **Icons** are provided in selected chapters directing the reader to valuable videos found at thepoint.lww.com/ACSMRPT5e. Numerous four-color tables, figures, and photographs will help the Personal Trainer understand the written material. A **chapter summary** concisely wraps up the content, and **references** are provided at the conclusion of each chapter for easy access to the evidence.

## Additional Resources

*ACSM's Resources for the Personal Trainer, Fifth Edition*, includes additional resources for students and instructors that are available on the book's companion website at http://thepoint.lww.com/activate. See the inside front cover of this text for more details, including the passcode you will need to gain access to the website. Any updates made in this edition of the book prior to the publication of the next edition can be accessed at http://certification.acsm.org/updates.

## Students

- Video clips

## Instructors

Approved adopting instructors will be given access to the following additional resources:

- Brownstone test generator
- PowerPoint presentations
- Image bank
- Lesson plans
- Moodle/Angel/Blackboard-ready cartridges

# Acknowledgments

The fifth edition of *ACSM's Resources for the Personal Trainer* continues to build on previous editions to make it an all-encompassing resource for Personal Trainers. As with the previous editions of this text, without the many volunteer contributors who wrote the chapters, this text would not be the resource it has become. Additionally, the editors would like to thank the many dedicated reviewers who also volunteered their time to carefully review each chapter to ensure the content was current and established guidelines were accurately presented. This text is a true team effort of volunteer editors, contributors, and reviewers.

Thank you to the staff at the American College of Sports Medicine (ACSM), specifically the Editorial Services, Publications, and Marketing departments for their support and assistance. The staff at ACSM work tirelessly to make projects like this happen and ensure consistency among all ACSM-related publications.

Personally, I would like to thank Angie Chastain and Katie Feltman for the understanding, constant support, and encouragement they have provided for the past 3 years, this year in particular. Thank you to the associate editors that contributed hours of their time to improving this edition.

And last, but certainly not least, thank you to the many dedicated Personal Trainers that make this work so rewarding. We wish you continued success in a career that has such a direct influence on the health of others.

Rebecca A. Battista
Mindy Mayol
Trent Hargens
Kenneth Lee Everett

# Contributors*

**Brent A. Alvar, PhD, FACSM**
Rocky Mountain University of Health Professions
Provo, Utah
*Chapter 14*

**Dan Benardot, PhD, DHC, RD, FACSM**
Georgia State University
Atlanta, Georgia
*Chapter 6*

**Barbara A. Bushman, PhD, FACSM, ACSM PD, ACSM CEP, ACSM EP-C, ACSM CPT**
Missouri State University
Springfield, Missouri
*Chapter 13*

**Kathy Campbell, EdD, FACSM**
Arizona State University
Phoenix, Arizona
*Chapter 15*

**Marissa E. Carraway, PhD**
East Carolina University
Greenville, North Carolina
*Chapter 7*

**Carol N. Cole, MS, ACSM HFD, ACSM EIM2**
Sinclair Community College
Dayton, Ohio
*Chapter 21*

**Lance Dalleck, PhD**
The University of Auckland
Auckland, New Zealand
*Chapter 20*

**Emily K. Di Natale, PhD**
Sinclair Community College
Dayton, Ohio
*Chapter 7*

**Danae Dinkel, PhD**
University of Nebraska Medical Center
Omaha, Nebraska
*Chapter 8*

**Ayla Donlin, EdD, ACSM CPT, ACSM EIM1**
California State University, Long Beach
Long Beach, California
*Chapter 16*

**Julie J. Downing, PhD, FACSM, ACSM HFD, ACSM CPT**
Central Oregon Community College
Bend, Oregon
*Chapter 1*

**Gregory Dwyer, PhD, FACSM, ACSM PD, ACSM RCEP, ACSM CEP, ACSM ETT, ACSM EIM3**
East Stroudsburg University
East Stroudsburg, Pennsylvania
*Chapter 11*

**Diane Ehlers, PhD**
University of Illinois at Urbana Champaign
Urbana, Illinois
*Chapter 8*

**Yuri Feito, PhD, MPH, ACSM RCEP, ACSM CEP**
Kennesaw State University
Kennesaw, Georgia
*Chapter 5*

**Brian Goslin, PhD**
Oakland University
Rochester, Michigan
*Chapter 5*

*See Appendix B for a list of contributors for the previous two editions.

**Anita M. Gust, PhD**
Concordia College
Moorhead, Minnesota
*Chapter 1*

**Trent Hargens, PhD, FACSM, ACSM CEP, ACSM EIM3**
James Madison University
Harrisonburg, Virginia
*Chapter 12*

**Andy Hayes, MS**
Atlas Fitness Evolved, LLC
St. Louis, Missouri
*Chapter 13*

**Jennifer Huberty, PhD**
Arizona State University
Phoenix, Arizona
*Chapter 8*

**Jeffrey M. Janot, PhD**
University of Wisconsin-Eau Claire
Eau Claire, Wisconsin
*Chapter 20*

**Alexandra Jurasin, MS**
Plus One/Optum
San Francisco, California
*Chapter 10*

**NiCole R. Keith, PhD, FACSM**
Indiana University-Purdue University Indianapolis
Indianapolis, Indiana
*Chapter 9*

**Jim Lewis, PT, DPT, ATC**
Brenau University
Gainesville, Georgia
*Chapter 3*

**Lesley Lutes, PhD**
East Carolina University
Greenville, North Carolina
*Chapter 7*

**Peter Magyari, PhD, FACSM, ACSM EP-C**
University of North Florida
Jacksonville, Florida
*Chapter 11*

**Mike Motta, MS**
Net Positive Coaching
New York, New York
*Chapter 2*

**Nicole Nelson, MHS, LMT, ACSM EP-C**
University of North Florida
Jacksonville, Florida
*Chapter 17*

**Nicholas Ratamess, Jr., PhD**
The College of New Jersey
Ewing, New Jersey
*Chapter 19*

**Jan Schroeder, PhD**
California State University, Long Beach
Long Beach, California
*Chapter 16*

**Deon L. Thompson, PhD, ACSM PD**
Georgia State University
Atlanta, Georgia
*Chapter 3*

**Walter R. Thompson, PhD, FACSM, ACSM PD, ACSM RCEP**
Georgia State University
Atlanta, Georgia
*Chapter 6*

**Jacquelyn Wesson, JD, RN**
Wesson & Wesson, LLC
Warrior, Alabama
*Chapter 22*

**Daniel Wilson, PhD**
Missouri State University
Springfield, Missouri
*Chapter 4*

**Mary Yoke, MA, FACSM**
Indiana University
Bloomington, Indiana
*Chapter 18*

# Reviewers

Jessica N. Ascenzo, ACSM CPT
Georgia Gwinnett College
Alpharetta, Georgia

Lorie Beardsley-Heyn, ACSM CPT
Training Made Personal
Milan, Michigan

Nicholas A. Burke, ACSM CPT
Burke Fitness, LLC
Columbus, Ohio

Daniel P. Connaughton, EdD, ACSM EP-C
University of Florida
Gainesville, Florida

Michael Hemmer, ACSM CPT
MetroHealth's Aamoth Family Pediatric Wellness Center
Cleveland, Ohio

Jonathan T. Keown, ACSM CPT
University of South Carolina
Columbia, South Carolina

Denise Murray, ACSM CPT, ACSM EP-C
EcoPlexus, Inc.
Lake Orian, Michigan

Colleen E. Oakes, ACSM CPT
Ivy Rehab Physical Therapy
Highland Park, Illinois

Janet T. Peterson, DrPH, FACSM, ACSM EP-C, ACSM RCEP
Linfield College
McMinnville, Oregon

Amy Jo Sutterluety, PhD, FACSM, ACSM CEP, ACSM EIM3
Baldwin-Wallace College
Berea, Ohio

Jessica Tax, ACSM CPT, ACSM/ACS CET
Move Up Health and Fitness
Sacramento, California

Sara L. Townley, ACSM CPT
NRH Centre
North Richland Hills, Texas

Kristin A. Traskie, MPH, ACSM CPT
Michigan State University
East Lansing, Michigan

# Contents

# Introduction to the Field and Profession of Personal Training

# 1

# Importance of the Field and Profession of Personal Training

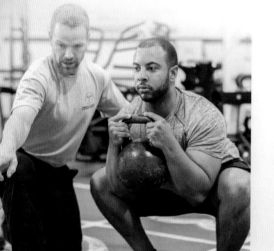

## OBJECTIVES

**Personal Trainers should be able to:**

- Recognize the need for a Personal Trainer.

- Describe the scope of practice of a Personal Trainer, including the background and experience needed to become a Personal Trainer.

- Discuss professional career environments and other educational opportunities for Personal Trainers.

- Identify future trends that will affect the fitness industry and personal training.

## INTRODUCTION

Personal training (practiced by one referred to in this book as the "Personal Trainer" but often described as a "fitness trainer," "personal fitness trainer," "fitness professional," or "weight trainer") continues to be a fast growing professions in the United States. According to the U.S. Department of Labor, Bureau of Labor Statistics, the job outlook for this profession is projected to grow "faster than the average" for all occupations between 2014 and 2024, which is further defined as an increase of 8.4% during this decade (6). The increased emphasis on health and fitness, diverse clientele interested in and in need of health and fitness, and recent links between sedentary activities and all-cause mortality provide multiple opportunities for Personal Trainers.

Consider some groups for whom personal training may be of increased interest. Baby boomers (approximately 78 million Americans born from 1946 to 1964) are the first generation in the United States that grew up exercising, and they are now reaching retirement age; they have the time and desire to begin or continue exercising in their 70s and beyond (16). Life expectancy has also increased to an average age of 79.68 years (9). In addition, an increasing number of businesses are recognizing the many cost-related benefits that health and fitness programs provide for their employees (6). The recent emphasis and reliance on technology in the office and home has led to an increased time spent in sedentary-type activities (*e.g.*, sitting and working at a computer). This increased sedentary time is associated with obesity, diabetes, and cardiovascular disease (11).

Older adults and working adults are not the only potential clients for Personal Trainers. A growing concern about childhood obesity and the reduction of physical education programs in schools will also contribute to the increased demand for fitness professionals. Personal Trainers are increasingly being hired to work with children in nonschool settings, such as health and fitness facilities. Because of the increased concern for fitness, the number of weight-training centers for children and health and fitness center membership among young adults is expected to continue to grow steadily (13,14).

## The Fitness Industry: An Overview of the Landscape

Interestingly, although the population may be more physically inactive than ever, the health and fitness center industry has never been in better "shape." Consider the following information reported by the United States from the International Health, Racquet and Sportsclub Association (IHRSA), a trade association serving the health and fitness facilities industry (13) and the U.S. Department of Labor, Bureau of Labor Statistics (6):

| | |
|---|---|
| 36,180 | Number of U.S. health clubs |
| 55.3 million | Number of U.S. health club members |
| $25.8 billion | Total U.S. fitness industry revenues for 2015 |
| | California, Texas, Florida, New York, and Illinois have the most fitness clubs |
| 22% | Increase in total health club members since 2009 |
| 279,100 | Number of U.S. fitness trainers/aerobics instructors |

According to the U.S. Department of Labor, Bureau of Labor Statistics, the job outlook for this profession is projected to grow "faster than the average" for all occupations between 2014 and 2024.

Although these numbers may seem impressive, consider how many people actually live in the United States compared to the number that are health club members. It is likely that only 15% of the population has a membership to a fitness center. Although there are certainly a variety of avenues to engage in physical activity, data suggest adults are not meeting the recommendations for physical activity. According to the Centers for Disease Control and Prevention (CDC), 24% of adults perform no leisure time activity (Fig. 1.1) (7). Additionally, the southeastern part of the United States not only has low leisure time activity but also reports the highest rates of obesity and diabetes (Figs. 1.2 and 1.3).

A large proportion of the population could benefit from involvement in some type of regular physical activity as part of a healthy lifestyle, whether as a member of a health/fitness facility or on their own. Personal Trainers are well positioned to influence the greater scope of public health in this regard. As the health and fitness facility industry continues to grow, so too will the demand for highly qualified and certified fitness professionals to serve the needs of their members (17).

Despite the growth of the fitness industry and emerging opportunities for physical fitness, high inactivity rates among Americans remain, with only 1 in 5 adults meeting the recommended amounts of physical activity and fewer than 3 in 10 high school students achieve at least 60 minutes of physical activity every day (7). Public schools continue to cut back or eliminate physical education. In fact, at the elementary school level, six states require schools to follow the

## 2008 Physical Activity Guidelines for Americans

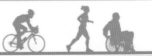

| | | | | | | | | |
|---|---|---|---|---|---|---|---|---|
| **Trends in Meeting the 2008 Physical Activity Guidelines, 2008—2015** <br> **Percentage (95% Confidence Interval)** | | | | | | | | |
| **2008** | **2009** | **2010** | **2011** | **2012** | **2013** | **2014** | **2015** | **Percentage Point Change*** |
| Adults engaging in no leisure-time physical activity | | | | | | | | |
| 36.2 <br> (35.0-37.4) | 32.3 <br> (31.3-33.3) | 32.4 <br> (31.5-33.3) | 31.6 <br> (30.7-32.5) | 29.6 <br> (28.8-30.5) | 30.3 <br> (29.5-31.1) | 30.0 <br> (29.1-30.9) | 30.0 <br> (29.2-30.9) | Decrease 2008—2012 (-1.3 / year) <br> **No change 2012—2015** |
| Adults meeting minimum aerobic physical activity guideline—Moderate-intensity for ≥ 150 minutes/week, or vigorous-intensity for ≥ 75 minutes/week, or an equivalent combination | | | | | | | | |
| 43.5 <br> (42.4-44.6) | 47.2 <br> (46.2-48.2) | 47.1 <br> (46.2-48.0) | 48.8 <br> (47.9-49.7) | 50.0 <br> (49.1-50.8) | 49.9 <br> (49.1-50.8) | 49.9 <br> (49.0-50.8) | 49.8 <br> (48.9-50.6) | Increase 2008—2012 (1.4 / year) <br> **No change 2012—2015** |
| Adults meeting high aerobic physical activity guideline—Moderate-intensity for > 300 minutes/week, or vigorous-intensity for > 150 minutes/week, or an equivalent combination | | | | | | | | |
| 28.4 <br> (27.5-29.4) | 31.2 <br> (30.4-32.1) | 31.7 <br> (30.9-32.5) | 33.1 <br> (32.4-34.0) | 34.3 <br> (33.5-35.1) | 34.3 <br> (33.5-35.2) | 34.0 <br> (33.2-34.9) | 33.6 <br> (32.7-34.4) | Increase 2008—2012 (1.4 / year) <br> **No change 2012—2015** |
| Adults meeting muscle-strengthening guideline—Muscle-strengthening activities ≥ 2 days/week | | | | | | | | |
| 21.9 <br> (21.2-22.7) | 22.6 <br> (21.8-23.3) | 24.2 <br> (23.4-24.9) | 24.2 <br> (23.5-24.9) | 23.9 <br> (23.2-24.5) | 24.1 <br> (23.4-24.9) | 24.4 <br> (23.7-25.2) | 24.8 <br> (24.2-25.5) | Increase 2008—2010 (1.1 / year) <br> **No change 2010—2015** |
| Adults meeting guidelines for aerobic physical activity and muscle-strengthening activity | | | | | | | | |
| 18.2 <br> (17.5-19.0) | 19.0 <br> (18.3-19.7) | 20.6 <br> (19.9-21.3) | 20.8 <br> (20.2-21.5) | 20.6 <br> (20.0-21.2) | 20.8 <br> (20.1-21.4) | 21.3 <br> (20.6-22.0) | 21.4 <br> (20.8-22.1) | Increase 2008—2010 (1.2 / year) <br> Increase 2010—2015 (0.2 / year) |
| Adolescents meeting aerobic physical activity guideline—Physically active ≥ 60 minutes per day on 7 days/week | | | | | | | | |
| - | - | - | 28.7 <br> (27.1-30.3) | - | 27.1 <br> (25.5-28.8) | - | 27.1 <br> (25.4-28.7) | **No change 2010—2015** |
| Adolescents meeting guideline for muscle-strengthening activity—Muscle-strengthening activities on ≥ 3 days/week | | | | | | | | |
| - | - | - | 55.6 <br> (53.6-57.5) | - | 51.7 <br> (49.6-53.8) | - | 53.4 <br> (51.2-55.6) | **No change 2010—2015** |
| Adolescents meeting guidelines for aerobic physical activity and muscle-strengthening activity | | | | | | | | |
| - | - | - | 21.9 <br> (20.0-23.9) | - | 21.6 <br> (19.6-23.7) | - | 20.5 <br> (18.4-22.7) | **No change 2010—2015** |

Adult estimates (18+ years) are based on data from the National Health Interview Survey (NHIS). Participation in moderate-intensity aerobic activity includes light- or moderate-intensity activities. Adult estimates are age adjusted to the projected 2000 US standard population using 5 age groups: 18–24, 25–34, 35–44, 45–64, and ≥65 years. Adolescent estimates (high school students) are based on data from the Youth Risk Behavior Surveillance System (YRBSS).

\* Based on trend analyses using logistic regression models (adult models controlled for age). When significant linear and quadratic trends ($p < 0.05$) were present across years, inflection points were identified using JoinPoint software. For segments when only the linear trend was significant ($p<0.05$), the increases or decrease is noted and the percentage point change was identified using JoinPoint software.

**FIGURE 1.1.** 2008 Physical Activity Guidelines for Americans. (Adapted from Centers for Disease Control and Prevention. *U.S. Physical Activity Statistics, 2007* [Internet]. Atlanta [GA]: Centers for Disease Control and Prevention; [cited 2012 May 21]. Available from: http://www.cdc.gov/nccdphp/dnpa/physical/stats/index.htm.)

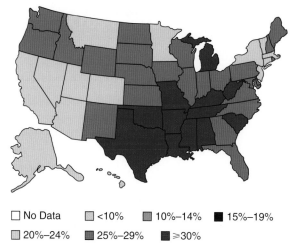

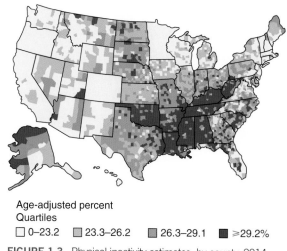

□ No Data    □ <10%    ■ 10%–14%    ■ 15%–19%

■ 20%–24%    ■ 25%–29%    ■ ≥30%

**FIGURE 1.2.** Prevalence of obesity in percentage (body mass index ≥30) and diagnosed diabetes in the U.S. adults in 2014. The data shown in these maps were collected through the CDC's Behavioral Risk Factor Surveillance System (BRFSS). Each year, state health departments use standard procedures to collect data through a series of monthly telephone interviews with the U.S. adults. Prevalence estimates generated for the maps may vary slightly from those generated for the states by the BRFSS as slightly different analytic methods are used. (From the Centers for Disease Control and Prevention. *U.S. Leisure-Time Physical Inactivity by U.S. County 2008* [Internet]. Atlanta [GA]: Centers for Disease Control and Prevention; [cited 2011 Mar 9]. Available from: http://www.cdc.gov/Features/dsPhysicalInactivity.)

Age-adjusted percent
Quartiles
□ 0–23.2    ■ 23.3–26.2    ■ 26.3–29.1    ■ ≥29.2%

**FIGURE 1.3.** Physical inactivity estimates, by county, 2014.

nationally recommended 150 minutes per week of physical education. Only 16% of states require elementary schools to provide daily recess. For middle schools/junior highs, only three states require the recommended 225 minutes per week of physical education (15).

Health care costs are rising exponentially as the medical field continues to focus more on treatment than on prevention. Food portion sizes in restaurants are increasing. According to the CDC, obesity has become a problem in every state. No state reported that less than 20% of adults were obese in 2015. The data also show that at least 30% of adults in 21 states and Guam were obese in 2015 (see Fig. 1.2). This is quite a change from 2000 when no states reached that level of obesity and in 2010 when 12 states were at that level. The data also indicate how obesity impacts some regions more than others. For example, states in the South have the highest obesity rate at 31.2%, the Midwest had an obesity rate of 30.7%, the Northeast had a rate of 26.4%, and the West had a rate of 25.2% (7,8).

> Despite the growth of the fitness industry and emerging opportunities for physical fitness, high inactivity rates among Americans have not really changed in the past 20 years.

According to the most recent National Health and Nutrition Examination Survey (NHANES), nearly 34% of adults and 17% of children aged 2–19 years in the United States are obese. When overweight is included in the statistics, an astonishing 68% of American adults, 33% of children aged 6–11 years, and nearly 34% of adolescents/teens aged 12–19 years are overweight or obese (15). For children, this is nearly triple the rate of overweight and obesity seen in the year 1963 and double the 1980 rates (8). According to the American Heart Association (5), childhood obesity is a significant health concern among the U.S. parents, even greater than the concerns of drug abuse and smoking. With so much to be done about the current health status of Americans, the time is right for highly qualified Personal Trainers (with the help of health care providers) to lead the charge toward a healthier nation. Participation in physical activity can lead to higher quality of life by decreasing risk factors associated with morbidity and mortality. Therefore, one role of the Personal Trainer is to encourage and motivate others to be more active (Box 1.1).

| Box 1.1 | Predicted Top 10 Fitness Trends from 2013 to 2017 (18) | | | |
|---|---|---|---|---|
| **2013** | **2014** | **2015** | **2016** | **2017** |
| Educated and experienced fitness professionals | High-intensity interval training | Body weight training | Wearable technology | Wearable technology |
| Strength training | Body weight training | High-intensity interval training | Body weight training | Body weight training |
| Body weight training | Educated and experienced fitness professionals | Educated and experienced fitness professionals | High-intensity interval training | High-intensity interval training |
| Children and obesity | Strength training | Strength training | Strength training | Educated and experienced fitness professionals |
| Exercise and weight loss | Exercise and weight loss | Personal training | Educated and experienced fitness professionals | Strength training |
| Fitness programs for older adults | Personal training | Exercise and weight loss | Personal training | Group training |
| Personal training | Fitness programs for older adults | Yoga | Functional fitness | Exercise is Medicine |
| Functional fitness | Functional fitness | Fitness programs for older adults | Fitness programs for older adults | Yoga |
| Core training | Group personal training | Functional fitness | Exercise and weight loss | Personal training |
| Group personal training | Yoga | Group personal training | Yoga | Exercise and weight loss |

Adapted from Thompson WR. Worldwide survey of fitness trends for 2012. *ACSM's Health Fitness J*. 2011;15(6);9–18.

## Definition of a Personal Trainer

American College of Sports Medicine's (ACSM's) job definition/scope of practice for ACSM Certified Personal Trainer is

The ACSM Certified Personal Trainer (CPT) (1) possesses a minimum of a high school diploma, and (2) works with apparently healthy individuals and those with health challenges who are able to exercise independently to enhance quality of life, improve health-related physical fitness, performance, manage health risk, and promote lasting health behavior change. The CPT conducts basic pre-participation health screening assessments, submaximal cardiovascular exercise tests, and muscular strength/endurance, flexibility, and body composition tests. The CPT facilitates motivation and adherence as well as develops and administers programs designed to enhance muscular strength/endurance, flexibility, cardiorespiratory fitness, body composition, and/or any of the motor skill related components of physical fitness (*i.e.*, balance, coordination, power, agility, speed, and reaction time).

It is crucially important to understand that a CPT's scope of practice does NOT include meal planning or diagnosing injuries or other medical conditions, nor can Personal Trainers work with individuals who cannot currently exercise independently.

As mentioned previously, the health and fitness industry is unique in that it has a wide variety of certifications available to the potential fitness professional. Organizations that offer certifications are commercial (for-profit) as well as nonprofit. Some have services and benefits that facilitate professional development, such as publications and conferences. Before committing to a specific certification, Personal Trainers should review each one for its relevance to their individual situation (see Tables 1.1 and 1.2 for more information).

Some certification organizations recognize other certifications for the purposes of continuing education. Most legitimate certifications will require their respective certified professionals to pursue educational opportunities, commonly referred to as *continuing education units* (CEUs) or *continuing education credits* (CECs). These CEUs/CECs are required in an ongoing fashion for a certified professional to maintain his or her certification status and as one way to maintain professional competence. Some certifications are complementary to others, and again, multiple certifications could make you more valuable to a potential employer. Currently, CPTs need to obtain 45 CEUs every 3 years. There is a nominal administrative fee associated with recertification.

> ACSM CPTs need to obtain 45 CEUs every 3 years. There is a nominal administrative fee associated with recertification.

## Personal Trainers' Scope of Practice

As mentioned previously, the profession of personal training is rapidly evolving, and employment opportunities are wide-ranging and will continue to increase. But what does a Personal Trainer do? Depending on the work setting, Personal Trainers have a wide range of potential activities, including, but not limited to, the following tasks:

- Screen and interview potential clients to determine their readiness for exercise and physical activity. This may involve communicating with the clients' health care team (especially for clients with special needs): physicians, nurse practitioners, registered dietitians, physical therapists, occupational therapists, and others.
- Perform fitness tests or assessments (as appropriate) on clients to determine their current level of fitness.
- Help clients set realistic goals, modify goals as needed, and provide motivation for adherence to the program.
- Develop exercise regimens and programs (often referred to as an "exercise prescription") for clients to follow and modify programs as necessary based on progression and goals.
- Demonstrate and instruct specific techniques to clients for the safe and effective performance of various exercise movements.
- Provide clients with safe and effective exercise techniques or training programs as well as educate them about exercises that may be contraindicated.
- Supervise or "spot" clients when they are performing exercise movements.
- Maintain records of clients' progress or lack thereof with respect to the exercise prescription.
- Be a knowledgeable resource to accurately answer clients' health and fitness questions.
- Educate clients about health and fitness and encourage them to become independent exercisers (provided they have medical approval to do so).

Other responsibilities not directly involving a client may be assigned or performed as needed. These usually include administrative paperwork, maintenance of equipment, and cleaning of equipment and facilities as required.

| Table 1.1 | Specialty Certifications | |
|---|---|---|
| | Scope of Practice | Minimum Requirements |
| Exercise is Medicine™ (EIM) | ■ Has three levels that range from those with low or moderate risk and cleared for independent activity to those at high risk and need to be monitored | ■ Depends on the level but ranges from current certification and bachelor's degree to current certification, hours in a clinical setting, and master's degree |
| ACSM/NCPAD Certified Inclusive Fitness Trainer℠ (CIFT) | ■ Works with people with a disability who are healthy or have medical clearance to exercise and were referred or currently under the care of a physician or health care professional<br>■ Leads and demonstrates safe, effective, and adapted methods of exercise<br>■ Writes adapted exercise recommendations, understands precautions and contraindications to exercise for people with disabilities and is aware of current ADA policy for recreation facilities and standards for accessible facility design | ■ Current ACSM certification or current NCCA-accredited, health/fitness-related certifications (e.g., ACE, NCSF, NASM, NFPT, NSCA, Cooper Institute)<br>■ Current adult CPR (with practical skills component) and AED |
| ACSM/ACS Certified Cancer Exercise Trainer℠ (CET) | ■ Trains individuals who were recently diagnosed with cancer and have not yet begun treatment, are receiving treatment or have completed treatment, and are apparently healthy or have the presence of known stable cardiovascular disease with low risk for complications with vigorous exercise and do not have any relative or absolute contraindications for exercise testing<br>■ Performs appropriate fitness assessments and makes exercise recommendations while demonstrating a basic understanding of cancer diagnoses, surgeries, treatments, symptoms, and side effects | ■ An ACSM- or NCCA-accredited exercise/fitness certification<br>■ Certification in adult CPR and AED<br>■ Choose one of the following:<br>  ■ Bachelor's degree (in any field) 500 h of experience training older adults or individuals with chronic conditions<br>  ■ 10,000 h of experience training older adults or individuals with chronic conditions[a] |
| ACSM/ NSPAPPH Physical Activity in Public Health Specialist℠ (PAPHS) | ■ Conducts needs assessments; plans, develops, and coordinates physical activity interventions provided at local, state, and federal levels<br>■ Provides leadership, develops partnerships, and advises local, state, and federal health departments on all physical activity-related initiatives | ■ A bachelor's degree in a health-related field[b] from a regionally accredited college or university<br>OR<br>■ A bachelor's degree in any subject and 1,200 h of experience in settings promoting physical activity, healthy lifestyle management or other health promotion[c] |

ACE, American Council on Exercise; NCSF, National Council on Strength & Fitness; NASM, National Academy of Sports Medicine; NFPT, National Federation of Professional Trainers; NSCA, national Strength and Conditioning Association; CPR, cardiopulmonary resuscitation; AED, automated external defibrillator.

[a]Hours of experience with older adults or individuals with chronic conditions include exercise testing, exercise prescription, group or individual training, group or individual client education, academic coursework and/or continuing education (relating to older adults or individuals with chronic conditions), internships or observational hours in an oncology setting and/or cancer rehabilitation program.

[b]Examples: exercise science; exercise physiology; kinesiology; physical education; sports management; athletic training; recreation; nutrition; health education; health promotion; public health; community health; and health care administration.

[c]Examples: education; community/public health setting; YMCA, parks and recreation, after-school programs; worksite health promotion; community health; health education or health promotion; federal, state, or local government; health care or health plan; academia or university; nonprofit organization; commercial health clubs; and corporate fitness centers.

From the Centers for Disease Control and Prevention. *U.S. Obesity Trends 1985–2010* [Internet]. Atlanta (GA): Centers for Disease Control and Prevention; [cited 2011 Apr 2]. Available from: http://www.cdc.gov/nccdphp/dnpa/obesity/trend/maps.

| Table 1.2 | ACSM Certification Requirements | | |
|---|---|---|---|
| | Education | Age | Certifications |
| **Health/Fitness Track** | | | |
| ACSM Certified Personal Trainer[SM] (CPT) | High school diploma or equivalent | 18 y of age or older | Current adult CPR certification with a practical skills component (such as the American Heart Association or the American Red Cross) |
| ACSM Certified Group Exercise Instructor[SM] (GEI) | High school diploma or equivalent | 18 y of age or older | Current adult CPR (with practical skills component) |
| ACSM Certified Exercise Physiologist[SM] (EP-C) | Bachelor's degree in kinesiology or exercise science, or other exercise-based degree | | Current adult CPR certification with a practical skills component (such as the American Heart Association or American Red Cross) |
| **Clinical Track** | | | |
| ACSM Certified Clinical Exercise Physiologist® (CEP) | Bachelor's degree in an exercise science–based field from a regionally accredited college or university (you are eligible to sit for the certification exam if you are in the last term or semester of your degree program) Examples: exercise science, kinesiology, kinesiotherapy, physiology, and exercise physiology | | ■ Current certification as a basic life support provider or CPR for the professional rescuer (available through the American Heart Association or the American Red Cross) ■ Practical experience in a clinical exercise program: ■ Minimum of 400 h from a CoAES Accredited University Curriculum Program[a] OR ■ Minimum of 500 h from a Non-CoAES Accredited University Curriculum Program[a] |
| ACSM Registered Clinical Exercise Physiologist (RCEP) | Master's degree from a college or university in exercise science, exercise physiology, or kinesiology | | ■ Current certification as a basic life support provider or CPR for the professional rescuer ■ One of the following: ■ ACSM Exercise Specialist Certification (current or expired) OR ■ 600 h of clinical experience[b] |

CPR, cardiopulmonary resuscitation.

[a]Hours of practical experience in a clinical exercise program (*e.g.*, cardiac/pulmonary rehabilitation programs, exercise testing, exercise prescription, electrocardiography, patient education and counseling, disease management of cardiac, pulmonary, and metabolic diseases, and emergency management).

[b]Recommendations for the 600 h of clinical experience:

Cardiovascular: 200 h
Pulmonary: 100 h
Metabolic: 120 h
Orthopedic/musculoskeletal: 100 h
Neuromuscular: 40 h
Immunological/hematological: 40 h

**FIGURE 1.4.** A trainer working with a client who has a physical disability.

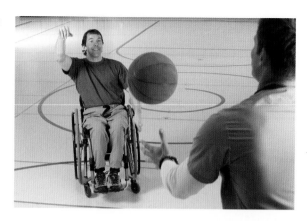

Many Personal Trainers also obtain additional instruction or specialty certifications in areas such as kickboxing, cancer, yoga, aquatic exercise, wellness coaching, studio cycling, and inclusive fitness.

Many Personal Trainers also obtain additional education or specialty certifications in areas such as kickboxing, cancer, yoga, aquatic exercise, wellness coaching, indoor cycling, and inclusive fitness (Fig. 1.4). These specialties should not be confused with "core" or primary certifications, such as ACSM CPT. Additional specialty certifications are valuable and allow Personal Trainers to have a wider variety of responsibilities, such as teaching group exercise classes.

## Becoming a Personal Trainer

Because of the large number of certification organizations, the prerequisites and eligibility requirements for becoming a Personal Trainer vary widely. Some are stand-alone certifications, whereas others, such as those offered by ACSM, are part of a progressive professional development pathway in which the scope of practice increases in both depth and scope as the prerequisites and eligibility requirements increase.

There are two tracks of ACSM certification (health/fitness and clinical) with five main certifications (not counting specialty certifications). The health/fitness certifications include (a) Group Exercise Instructor (GEI), (b) Certified Personal Trainer (CPT), and (c) Certified Exercise Physiologist (EP-C) previously Health/Fitness Specialist (HFS), whereas the clinical track certifications include (a) Certified Clinical Exercise Specialist (CES) and (b) Registered Clinical Exercise Physiologist (RCEP). Each certification level has minimum requirements (Table 1.2).

Personal Trainers should consider current career plans as well as future professional goals when determining what educational preparation and certification(s) are needed. Background and interests will combine in determining how fast and by what process a Personal Trainer can develop a career. One should ensure that the certifying agency is accredited by the National Commission for Certifying Agencies (NCCA). The NCCA is the accreditation body of the National Organization for Competency Assurance. The NCCA is a widely recognized, independent, nongovernmental agency that accredits professional certifications in a variety of professions. The NCCA comprehensively reviews the certification organization's procedures, protocols, and operations and determines if the certification properly discriminates between those who are qualified and those who are not qualified to be awarded the respective credential.

## The Backgrounds of Personal Trainers

The Committee on Accreditation for the Exercise Sciences (CoAES) was established in April 2004 under the auspices of the Commission on Accreditation of Allied Health Education Programs

The Committee on Accreditation for the Exercise Sciences (CoAES) was established in April 2004 under the auspices of the Commission on Accreditation of Allied Health Education Programs (CAAHEP).

(CAAHEP). The primary role of the CoAES is to establish standards and guidelines for academic programs that facilitate the preparation of students seeking employment in the health, fitness, and exercise industry. The secondary role of the CoAES is to establish and implement a process of self-study, review, and recommendation for all programs seeking CAAHEP accreditation.

Programmatic accreditation through the CAAHEP is specifically intended for exercise science or related departments (physical education, kinesiology, etc.), with a professional preparation tract designed for students seeking employment opportunities in the health, fitness, and exercise industry.

The CAAHEP is the largest programmatic accrediting body in the health sciences field; it reviews and accredits more than 2,000 educational programs in 28 health science occupations such as Personal Fitness Trainer. See www.coaes.org and www.caahep.org for more information or to find a CAAHEP-accredited academic institution in your state.

It is important to possess a certification from an NCCA-accredited certifying agency; because of the many different types of certifications that exist, the background of today's Personal Trainer varies significantly with respect to educational preparation and work-related experience. Some individuals commit to the profession early and pursue an appropriate course of study in college. Many of these individuals actually begin working part-time at a local health club or at the university student recreation center, gaining valuable "hands-on" practical experience to complement their studies. Other Personal Trainers enter the profession later in life as a new career, or as a second career, on a part-time basis while maintaining their primary career pursuit (Fig. 1.5). Ideally, the Personal Trainer will have a good combination of education, work-related experience, and even first-person perspective experiences as either an athlete or a former client.

## Educational Background

As the profession of personal training continues to evolve and grow, more and more educational opportunities become available. Many certification organizations offer workshops and online examination preparation opportunities. From a formal academic training perspective, there are certificate, associate's, bachelor's, master's, and doctoral degree programs available for fitness professionals. Typically, certificate programs (both in-person and online) range from 1 year to 18 months in duration. Associate degree programs range in length from 18 months to 2 years. Bachelor's degree programs are usually 4 years in duration. Master's degree programs are typically 18 months to 2 years beyond a bachelor's degree. Finally, a doctoral degree program is usually 3–4 years beyond a master's degree and involves a research project. Also internships, practicums, or student cooperative work experiences (typically unpaid opportunities to work under the direct supervision of an experienced fitness professional)

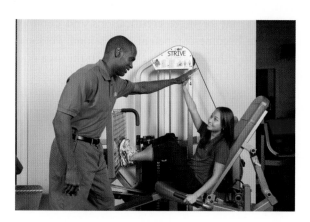

**FIGURE 1.5.** A trainer and a client have reached a goal.

The CAAHEP accredits academic programs for personal fitness trainer (certificate and associate degrees), exercise science (bachelor's degree), and clinical exercise physiology and applied exercise physiology graduate programs.

may or may not be part of these different types of programs. Common names for these academic programs include exercise science, exercise physiology, physical education, kinesiology, sport science, Personal Trainer, fitness specialist, and others. Currently, the CAAHEP accredits academic programs for personal fitness trainer (certificate and associate degrees), exercise science (bachelor's degree), and clinical exercise physiology and applied exercise physiology graduate programs.

Increasingly, more fitness programs require Personal Trainers to have college degrees. Long-term employment and management advancement often require a degree. Most fitness directors, those individuals who have management/supervisory responsibilities over the floor staff (Personal Trainers), often have master's degrees and/or experiences in training staff.

## Work-Related Background

It is possible for Personal Trainers to obtain employment without a related degree, especially if they have one or more certifications and some prior industry-related work experience. For many individuals who want a career change, pursuing a second degree or even a first degree later in life simply is not possible. Some health and fitness facilities have formal training paths and processes for their employees that may include assigning a more experienced Personal Trainer as a mentor or scheduling periodic staff training sessions, sometimes referred to as "in-services." Some health and fitness centers may even pay for continuing education opportunities for their staff as one benefit of employment. If not, look for an experienced Personal Trainer with an exemplary reputation who would consider taking on an apprentice. Many certification organizations have educational opportunities, such as workshops, which can also provide a good review of the various areas of content, especially as they relate to preparing for a certification examination. It is always advisable for all professionals working in this environment to seek a college degree whenever possible.

## Experiential Background

Some Personal Trainers pursue this field as a result of previous positive experiences. Examples would include those who were once standout high school, college, professional, elite athletes, or even former clients who had a significant positive or transformational experience. Like those who are changing careers, some may not have a related academic degree, and some may have no college degree at all. However, their passion for a particular sport or a love of exercise in general usually motivates them sufficiently to fill in any knowledge gaps they may have as they begin their personal training career. Commitment to the profession is shown by obtaining one or more certifications from reputable organizations such as ACSM as well as obtaining relevant, work-related experience under the mentorship of a proven, experienced (preferably degreed) CPT. By being proactive from a self-study perspective, obtaining one or more certifications and combining these with work-related experience, individuals can become competent professional Personal Trainers over time. Basically, if the opportunity arises to enhance your knowledge in the area of exercise science by a reputable organization or institution, do not pass it up.

Regardless of one's background, starting down the career path as a Personal Trainer does not have to be complicated. Consider current status and then professional goals for 1, 2, and 5 years in the future. Reflect on the following questions:

- Do I have an exercise science–based college degree, and is it from a CAAHEP-accredited academic institution?
- If not, is it feasible for me to go back to obtain a certificate or degree on either a part-time or full-time basis?

- Was I ever a client of a Personal Trainer, and did I have a positive experience in achieving my goals?
- Do I have experience as a high school, college, professional, or elite athlete that provides me with some first-person experiences?
- Which certifications and certifying agency are appropriate for me to pursue now and in the future? The certifying agency (such as ACSM) should be well respected, provide peer-reviewed materials, and be NCCA-accredited.
- Which certifications have study materials and/or workshops to help me accumulate a core body of knowledge?
- Where can I begin obtaining the necessary skills, either by observing a more experienced CPT or by volunteering at a local health and fitness facility?
- Which certifying organizations and, specifically, which level of certification do potential employers in my city expect to see when hiring Personal Trainers for their facilities?

# Certifications

ACSM currently offers four specialty certifications, with others in the works for the future (see Table 1.1 for details). These additional certifications can assist the Personal Trainers in their continued education as well as provide them with opportunities to add skills and increase potential client base by offering diversity.

## ACSM Exercise is Medicine™

The ACSM Exercise is Medicine™ (EIM) credential is for the fitness professional who collaborates with those in health care professions (*e.g.*, physicians, nurses, physician assistants) to provide additional assistance to clients who need fitness programming to change behavior and achieve greater fitness outcomes. There are currently three levels for this credential which depend on your current level of certification and educational background as well as the health status of the client.

## ACSM/NCPAD Certified Inclusive Fitness Trainer^SM

ACSM/National Center on Physical Activity and Disability (NCPAD) Certified Inclusive Fitness Trainer^SM (CIFT) is a fitness professional who assesses, develops, and implements an individualized exercise program for persons with a physical, sensory, or cognitive disability; who are healthy; or have medical clearance to perform independent physical activity. In addition to knowledge of exercise physiology and exercise testing and programming, a CIFT has knowledge in inclusive facility design and awareness of social inclusion for people with disabilities and the Americans with Disabilities Act (ADA).

Additionally, ACSM/NCPAD CIFT demonstrates and leads safe, effective, and adapted methods of exercise; writes adapted exercise recommendations; understands precautions and contraindications to exercise for people with disabilities; is aware of current ADA policy specific to recreation facilities (U.S. Access Board Guidelines) and standards for accessible facility design; and can utilize motivational techniques and provide appropriate instruction to individuals with disabilities to enable them to begin and continue healthy lifestyles.

## ACSM/ACS Certified Cancer Exercise Trainer^SM

ACSM/American Cancer Society (ACS) Certified Cancer Exercise Trainer^SM (CET) is a fitness professional who trains men and women who were recently diagnosed with cancer and have not yet begun treatment, are receiving treatment, have completed treatment, or are a survivor experiencing chronic or late effects from disease or treatment and are apparently healthy or have the presence of known stable cardiovascular disease with low risk for complications with vigorous exercise and do not have any relative or absolute contraindications for exercise testing. In addition, the CET performs appropriate fitness assessments and makes exercise recommendations while demonstrating a basic understanding of cancer diagnoses, surgeries, treatments, symptoms, and side effects.

### ACSM/NSPAPPH Physical Activity in Public Health Specialist^SM

ACSM/National Society of Physical Activity Practitioners in Public Health (NSPAPPH) Physical Activity in Public Health Specialist^SM (PAPHS) is a professional who promotes physical activity in public health at the national, state, and/or local level. The PAPHS engages and educates key decision makers about the impact of, and need for, legislation, policies, and programs that promote physical activity. Additionally, the PAPHS provides leadership and develops partnerships with private and public associations to catalyze the promotion of population-based physical activity.

These additional certifications can assist the Personal Trainer in continued education as well as to provide opportunities to add skills and increase potential client base by offering diversity. The kinds of fitness facilities are diverse, with the most numerous being multipurpose, commercial, for-profit clubs, followed by community, corporate, and medical fitness centers (MFCs). Although there are many core similarities between facilities, there is also great variety in size, structure, target markets, program offerings, amenities, membership fees, contracts, staffing, and equipment. This variety is necessary to attract and serve many different populations with many different interests (Fig. 1.6). With the member retention rate varying greatly across the industry, most clubs and centers must continually recruit new members. According to the IHRSA, in competitive suburban markets, in which the automobile is the primary means of commuting to a club, the majority of a club's membership base will come from within a 10- to 12-minute

**FIGURE 1.6.** A trainer spotting a squat exercise of a client who is on a BOSU ball (with light dumbbells in each hand).

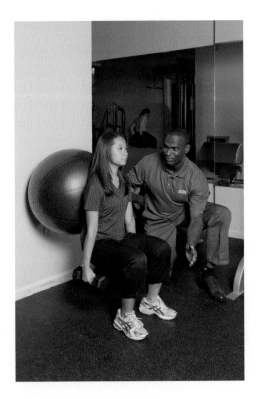

drive time from home to the club; thus, clubs that are located close to one another are typically competing for the same members (13). This means that Personal Trainers are vying for the same clients as well. However, Personal Trainers, just like clubs, can differentiate themselves from the competition in a number of ways, such as focusing on a specific clientele (*e.g.*, women, children, seniors, and athletes), developing expertise in a given area, offering small-group training in addition to individual sessions, offering a more competitive price, and using multiple locations. Many trainers make themselves more marketable by obtaining more than one primary and/or specialty certification.

# Establishing a Solid Knowledge Base

Everyone has strengths and weaknesses with respect to how much he or she knows or does not know about any given topic, including Personal Trainers. Even fitness professionals with college degrees have content areas that they are more knowledgeable. Part of the commitment to the profession is for Personal Trainers to continuously evaluate their educational foundation or knowledge base. One way to focus on an action plan for specific continuing education needs is to use the job tasks as a knowledge map.

Begin by performing a thorough review of the job tasks and corresponding knowledge, skills, and abilities for each, rating familiarity and competence against each specific job task (specific information on the job tasks for Personal Trainers can be found on ACSM Web site under Certifications [http://certification.acsm.org/get-certified]). Next, use this checklist to prioritize the job task knowledge and skill areas from weakest to strongest. Over the course of a year, seek out and participate in continuing educational opportunities that focus on weak content areas. Personal Trainers should do this on a yearly basis, at a minimum, as content areas that were once weak may become stronger over time, especially for those who devote additional study to these areas and, more importantly, develop a client base in which some content areas are relied upon more than others. By doing this consistently 1 year to the next, recertifying becomes a pleasure as opposed to a chore. Some Personal Trainers procrastinate, waiting until the last minute to accumulate the required number of CEUs/CECs. Not only does this create a great deal of stress but also it is not a very effective way to expand one's knowledge base as a Personal Trainer.

## The Exercise Sciences

The competent Personal Trainer should have a strong knowledge foundation in the exercise sciences with combined leadership and coaching training. Exercise science is a broad term that includes multiple disciplines. These disciplines often include but are not limited to anatomy and physiology; exercise physiology; motor learning/motor control; nutrition (dietetics); biomechanics/applied kinesiology; exercise prescription; fitness testing; wellness coaching; and sport, exercise, and health psychology. Good-quality educational programs (workshops or online opportunities offered by certification organizations or curriculums offered by academic institutions) may offer a course of study that includes content or courses dedicated to helping the Personal Trainer develop an understanding of these more specific disciplines.

ACSM has worked collaboratively with Fitness Education Network (FEN) to offer both 1-day and 3-day workshops to help candidates prepare for ACSM CPT certification examination. The workshops review the knowledge, skills, and abilities relevant to the content areas tested on the examination. Taking a workshop in no way guarantees passing an examination; however, many candidates find it helpful to review at the workshop what they have already learned (for more information, see www.acsm.org).

> The competent Personal Trainer should have a strong knowledge foundation in the exercise sciences.

## Developing Your Tool Kit

In addition to a strong knowledge foundation in the exercise sciences, effective Personal Trainers are constantly developing and adding skills to their "tool kit." Essential tools include the following:

- Effective communication skills (in-person, phone, and written such as e-mail)
- Ability to motivate appropriately
- Ability to influence behavior change
- Effective interviewing and screening
- Effective use of goals and objectives
- Effective and safe exercise program design
- Ability to demonstrate, instruct, spot, and supervise appropriate exercise movements
- Effective use of up-to-date technology in order to obtain continuing educational opportunities via webinars and other online resources
- Obtaining new primary or specialty certification skills
- Effective use of social networking sites, Web sites, blogs, e-mail blasts, and so on for marketing and monitoring purposes
- Using a sound business model

These are, at the minimum, the tools Personal Trainers should include in their tool kit and also master using effectively, either individually or in combination with others. Nonetheless, effective Personal Trainers continuously add tools throughout their professional career.

### Communication Skills (Motivating and Influencing Behavioral Change)

Perhaps, the most overlooked yet important skill for the Personal Trainer tool kit is that of communication. Communication is more than just verbal, as it includes nonverbal elements such as visual (what is observed) and kinesthetic (what is felt). Additionally, effective communication involves much more than information exchange. Communication also relies on the emotional state of both individuals. For example, is the client "ready" to accept information or is there temporary resistance to the new information being provided? Likewise, Personal Trainers can be effective motivators when they create an optimal emotional state for clients, so they not only are ready to take in the information provided but also are able to put it to good use. As a complex and important skill, communication is discussed throughout this book, particularly in Chapter 9.

### Screening, Assessment, and Referrals

Another set of tools required for the Personal Trainer include interviewing, screening, and recognizing when to refer a client to a medical health care provider such as a physician, physical therapist, sport psychologist, or registered dietitian. When health screening forms are used appropriately, these tools help establish a foundation of trust that facilitates the development of the trainer–client relationship. Combined with effective communication skills, these tools further improve the possibility of achieving the client's goals.

Typically, a Personal Trainer conducts an initial interview with a potential client in which basic demographic information is obtained, along with the client's health history. Two types of forms are used at a minimum: the health history form and the Physical Activity Readiness Questionnaire (PAR-Q) form. Examples of these and other forms are available in Chapter 11. In addition, it is appropriate during this initial interview to ask clients about their specific expectations for working with a Personal Trainer, what initial goals they may have, as well as any other lifestyle information they can share. Examples include the following:

- Recent and past history of physical activity (if any)
- History of previous injuries (if any)
- Level of social support from family and friends
- Potential stressors/obstacles that may impose challenges on their exercise regimen, such as excessive work hours, physically demanding work, and multiple recurring commitments within the community or with family

Finally, this initial consultation should be used to synchronize the Personal Trainer–client expectations, obtain or request any medical clearance forms (if required) as well as obtain signatures on required waivers, informed consent forms, and/or other contractual forms and agreements as required by your employer.

Assessing risk of your new client is the next step. It is important to note that Personal Trainers should not diagnose or treat disease, disorders, injuries, or other medical conditions under any circumstance. The presence of specific and/or multiple risk factors requires that the Personal Trainer refer the client to the appropriate health care professional for additional guidance and/or a medical release before designing and implementing an exercise program. Also, even if the client fails to initially disclose information that becomes known at a later time, the Personal Trainer still has a legal obligation to refer the client to a health care provider before additional training guidance can be provided. Personal Trainers who provide services outside their scope of practice place both themselves and their clients at risk. If in doubt as to whether or not a client should be referred to another health care professional before working with them, be cautious and refer them first. The old saying still holds true, "If in doubt, refer out."

Assessments are tests and measurements that Personal Trainers use with their clients to evaluate their current physical and functional status. Assessments may include the following:

- Resting and exercise heart rate
- Resting and exercise blood pressure
- Body weight and height
- Body composition estimates
- Circumference measurements of limbs, hips, and waist
- Calculation of body mass index
- Calculation of waist-to-hip ratio
- Measurements of flexibility
- Tests for muscular strength/muscular endurance
- Tests for cardiorespiratory fitness

Assessments provide a current snapshot of the functional ability of a client. When combined with the data from the PAR-Q and other health-related questionnaires, the Personal Trainer can begin developing a draft of a customized exercise regimen for the client.

## Professional Work Environments

Employment opportunities for Personal Trainers are available in more diverse settings than ever before and include (but are not limited to) the following:

- Commercial (for-profit) fitness centers
- Community (not-for-profit) fitness centers
- Corporate fitness/wellness centers

- University wellness/fitness centers
- Owner/operator (self-employed) studios, fitness centers, and in-home businesses
- MFCs
- Municipal/city recreation/public parks/family centers
- Governmental/military fitness centers
- Activity centers/retirement centers/assisted living communities for older adults
- Worksite health promotion programs
- Cruise ships, resorts, and spa fitness centers

## For Profit

Commercial (for-profit) fitness centers dominate the fitness landscape and include independently owned, chains, studios, licensed gyms, and franchises. Opportunities for gainful employment exist within the commercial club industry. Most commercial fitness centers advertise employment opportunities locally or regionally, whereas some also post them on their corporate Web sites, blogs, or social networking sites. It is wise to thoroughly investigate a company's policies concerning compensation, benefits, policies, and opportunities for advancement before accepting a position.

> Commercial (for-profit) fitness centers dominate the fitness landscape and include independents, chains, studios, licensed gyms, and franchises.

Licensed gyms and franchises are popular choices when establishing a new commercial fitness centers (Fig. 1.7). The benefits of choosing a franchise include brand recognition, access to proven operational systems, logo usage, marketing templates, in-depth training, and ongoing support. Franchisers then retain the right to dictate most aspects of the facility, including colors, layout, décor, equipment, programs, and product sales. Initial fees for fitness franchises can range from $10,000 to more than $100,000, and equipment may or may not be included in the cost. There is also a monthly franchising fee, which is either a set amount or a percentage of gross revenue (typically about 5%). Licensed gyms operate on a much simpler model. A fee is paid to use (license) the name and logo. Licensees typically have much more flexibility in how they operate the facility than do franchisees, but they also do not receive as much operational support (see Chapter 21).

## Not for Profit

Not-for-profit (or nonprofit) organizations with fitness centers make up a large proportion of the total market. Some examples of the larger nonprofit organizations in which fitness professionals

**FIGURE 1.7.** A trainer demonstrating a fly motion using a stability ball as a bench press.

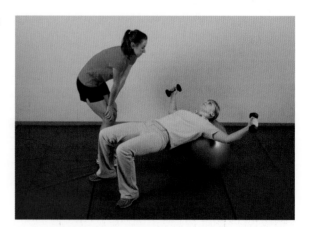

can find relevant employment include the Young Men's Christian Association (YMCA), Jewish Community Centers (JCC), hospital-based clubs, municipal and military fitness facilities, and college/university recreation centers.

Personal Trainers may find that some nonprofits may not have rates of pay comparable with those of their for-profit counterparts, but at the same time may provide better benefits. Nonprofit work (regardless of the industry) creates a strong sense of mission throughout the organization and carries a significant commitment to service with respect to their specific members or constituents. Nonprofit fitness centers fill a significant role in the fitness professional job market, and it is ultimately up to the individuals to determine the most appropriate place of employment for their personal and professional goals.

## Medical Fitness Centers

The growing relationship between the fitness industry and the health care field is evidenced by the steady growth of MFCs and the establishment of the Medical Fitness Association (MFA). The MFA is a nonprofit organization that was established to assist with medically integrated health and wellness. These types of fitness facilities tend to see older adults and focus on clients with chronic diseases and multiple risk factors. The number of MFCs has grown at an average annual rate of 4.5% since 2010. In 2014, there were approximately 1,291 medical centers compared to 950 reported in 2008. In 2014, the average number members per club reported was over 3,400 with an average member age of 49.3 years. Although these centers do provide access to hospital employees, over half of the membership is typically composed from community members.

> The growing relationship between the fitness industry and the health care field is evidenced by the steady growth of MFCs and the establishment of the MFA.

MFCs tend to be relatively large with an average size reported in 2012–2014 of just under 40,000 square feet. Growth can be seen in across the United States with the Northeast and West regions having the largest percentage increase in the number of MFCs built since 2003. However, Florida, Texas, and Illinois are the states with the highest number of MFCs. The average size of MFCs built in 2010 was 39,726 sq ft. Although they offer a number of clinical and wellness services not typically found in traditional clubs, personal training tops the list of reported nonmembership fee services, with 95% of centers offering such a program between 2012 and 2014. In addition, approximately 80% report being owned by a hospital or health system, and 69% report holding not-for-profit status (14).

A central mission of many MFCs is integration of services for both the "sick" and the "healthy." It is not uncommon for patients in cardiovascular rehabilitation or physical therapy programs to exercise next to healthy community members. Using the same space and equipment saves on overhead, space, and staffing needs. Although there currently are not any specific guidelines for hiring Personal Trainers with specific degrees or certifications in these facilities, the focus on transitional programs (*i.e.*, working with former hospital patients) may require that a Personal Trainer has higher qualifications than usual.

## Corporate

More than 50% of business profits are spent annually on employees' and dependents' health care (12). Because employers typically pay a significant portion of the nation's health care bill, about 40% in 2006, compared with 18% in 1965, businesses and industries are naturally concerned about today's rising medical costs and what they can do to decrease this liability (10). Therefore, one possible cost-containment strategy is to implement worksite health promotion programs. *Worksite health promotion* (WHP) can be defined as "a combination of educational, organizational, and environmental activities and programs designed to motivate and support healthy lifestyles among a company's employees and their families" (10). The goals of WHP programs are to

- Reduce modifiable risk factors
- Improve a person's overall health status
- Reduce demand for health care costs to the worksite

Worksite health promotion can be defined as "a combination of educational, organizational, and environmental activities and programs designed to motivate and support healthy lifestyles among a company's employees and their families" (10).

Despite the benefits of WHP programs, only about 50% of American worksites with over 750 employees provide some type of WHP program, and smaller companies are even less inclined to provide such services (10). However, the Employee Services Management (ESM) Association (formerly the National Employee Service and Recreation Association) estimates that there are more than 50,000 organizations with on-site physical fitness programs in the United States and nearly 1,000 employing full-time program directors (10).

The kinds of fitness-specific offerings vary greatly in WHP programs, ranging from steps-based walking programs to group exercise classes to fully equipped health and fitness facilities. One of the primary determinants of facility and program size is the number of employees. Companies with more than 1,000 employees working in a central location (building or campus) are much more likely to offer traditional fitness facilities because they have the financial means to do so and it makes economic sense. Smaller companies with a smaller employee base are much less likely to offer a WHP, especially one that includes fitness facilities.

Many corporate fitness programs are outsourced to companies that specialize in facility and program management. This makes it somewhat easier for the corporation because it can rely on someone else's expertise instead of having to develop it from within. Some choose to avoid development and management altogether by setting up a corporate account with an existing local fitness facility. A reduced membership fee is negotiated, and the company reimburses employees a portion or all of the fees. It is common, though, for the company to dictate that an employee must visit the facility a certain number of times per month to qualify for reimbursement.

Corporate fitness opportunities exist for Personal Trainers within both large and smaller companies. For larger companies, the typical route is to work as a traditional employee or independent contractor in the fitness center. For smaller companies, a more entrepreneurial approach is usually taken. Personal Trainers will typically need to approach the management about offering on-site services to the employees, with the employer absorbing some of the cost. Because employers are often very cost-conscious and are typically unsure about investing in preventive programs, Personal Trainers will need to educate them about the benefits of their services to the health and well-being of their employees. Reporting client's results, such as weight loss, reductions in blood pressure, and other health factors, also has a positive impact on their thinking and decision making. Because individual sessions are the most expensive option, small-group training sessions are potentially more appealing to the employer.

## Ethics and Professional Conduct

Ethics can be described as standards of conduct that guide decisions and actions based on duties derived from core values. Specifically, core values are principles used to define what is right, good, and/or just. When a professional demonstrates behavior that is consistent, or aligned, with widely accepted standards in their respective industry, that professional is said to behave "ethically." On the other hand, "unethical" behavior is behavior that is not consistent with industry-accepted standards. As a fitness professional, Personal Trainers have obligation to stay within the bounds of the defined scope of practice for a Personal Trainer as well as to abide by all industry-accepted standards of behavior at all times. Furthermore, individuals certified or registered through ACSM must be familiar with all aspects of ACSM's Code of Ethics for certified and registered professionals.

# Code of Ethics for ACSM Certified and Registered Professionals

## Purpose

This code of ethics is intended to aid all certified and registered American College of Sports Medicine Credentialed Professionals (ACSMCPs) to establish and maintain a high level of ethical conduct, as defined by standards by which ACSMCPs may determine the appropriateness of their conduct. Any existing professional, licensure, or certification affiliations that ACSMCPs have with governmental, local, state, or national agencies or organizations will take precedence relative to any disciplinary matters that pertain to practice or professional conduct.

This code applies to all ACSMCPs, regardless of ACSM membership status (to include members and nonmembers). Any cases in violation of this Code will be referred to ACSM Committee on Certification and Registry Boards (CCRB).

## Principles and Standards

### RESPONSIBILITY TO THE PUBLIC

- ACSMCPs shall be dedicated to providing competent and legally permissible services within the scope of the knowledge and skills of their respective credential/certification. These services shall be provided with integrity, competence, diligence, and compassion.
- ACSMCPs provide exercise information in a manner that is consistent with evidence-based science and medicine.
- ACSMCPs respect the rights of clients, colleagues, and health care professionals and shall safeguard client confidences within the boundaries of the law.
- Information relating to ACSMCP–client relationship is confidential and may not be communicated to a third party not involved in that client's care without the prior written consent of the client or as required by law.
- ACSMCPs are truthful about their qualifications and the limitations of their expertise and provide services consistent with their competencies.

### RESPONSIBILITY TO THE PROFESSION

- ACSMCPs maintain high professional standards. As such, an ACSMCP should never represent himself or herself, either directly or indirectly, as anything other than ACSMCP unless he or she holds other license/certification that allows him or her to do so.
- ACSMCPs practice within the scope of their job tasks. ACSMCPs will not provide services that are limited by state law to provision by another health care professional only.
- An ACSMCP must remain in good standing relative to governmental requirements as a condition of continued credentialing.
- ACSMCPs take credit, including authorship, only for work they have actually performed and give credit to the contributions of others as warranted.
- Consistent with the requirements of their certification or registration, ACSMCPs must complete approved, additional educational course work aimed at maintaining and advancing their knowledge and skills.

## Principles and Standards for Candidates of ACSM Certification Examinations

Candidates applying for a credentialing/certification examination must comply with candidacy requirements and, to the best of their abilities, accurately complete the application process. In addition, the candidate must refrain from any and all behavior that would be interpreted as "irregular" (including any behavior that undermines or threatens the integrity of the application, assessment or certification processes of ACSM CCRB) whether before, during, or after an exam.

## Public Disclosure of Affiliation

- Any ACSMCP may disclose his or her affiliation with ACSM credentialing in any context, oral or documented, provided it is currently accurate. In doing so, no ACSMCP may imply college endorsement of whatever is associated in context with the disclosure unless expressly authorized by the college. Disclosure of affiliation in connection with a commercial venture may be made, provided the disclosure is made in a professionally dignified manner; is not false, misleading, or deceptive; and does not imply licensure or the attainment of specialty or diploma status.
- ACSMCPs may disclose their credential status.
- ACSMCPs may list their affiliation with ACSM credentialing on their business cards without prior authorization.
- ACSMCPs and the institutions employing an ACSMCP may inform the public of an affiliation as a matter of public discourse or presentation.

## Discipline

Any ACSMCP may be disciplined or lose his or her certification or registry for conduct that, in the opinion of the executive council of the ACSM CCRB, goes against the principles set forth in this code. Such cases will be reviewed by the ACSM CCRB Ethics Subcommittee, which will include a liaison from the ACSM CCRB Executive Council, as appointed by the CCRB chair. The ACSM CCRB Ethics Subcommittee will make an action recommendation to the executive council of ACSM CCRB for final review and approval.

 # National Campaigns to Promote Physical Activity

Many national organizations associated with physical activity and health are actively involved promoting the benefits of physical activity. In addition, these organizations launch national campaigns, produce recommendations and guidelines, and serve as advocates for legislation related to physical activity. Discussed in the following text are examples of the ways organizations are helping to promote physical activity.

## Exercise is Medicine

In 2007, ACSM in partnership with the American Medical Association launched EIM, a program designed to encourage America's patients to incorporate physical activity and exercise into their daily routine. EIM encourages doctors to assess and review every patient's physical activity program at every visit. For those patients not already exercising, the physician is asked to prescribe exercise to their patients and to record physical activity as a vital sign during patient visits.

ACSM has developed a system to credential exercise professionals for EIM designation. The EIM Certificate contains three levels based on the health status of the patient referrals and the educational status and certifications of the candidate. Individuals who are currently certified by an NCCA accrediting organization (this would include individuals with ACSM's Personal

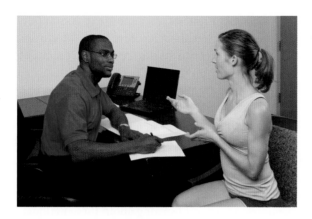

**FIGURE 1.8.** A trainer and a client doing an initial client consultation.

Trainer certification) and who successfully complete an EIM certification course and exam will meet Level 1 requirements; Level 1 includes working with individuals at low or moderate risk. For more information about the levels and the certification and educational requirements, please see http://certification.acsm.org/exercise-is-medicine-credential.

EIM has a user-friendly Web site (www.exerciseismedicine.org) providing many helpful resources for health care providers, health and fitness professionals, members of the media as well as the general public (Fig. 1.8). CPTs should become familiar with and regularly use the continually updated tools provided to them on the EIM Web site to educate themselves as well as their clients on the importance and best implementation of regular physical activity according to the most recent evidence-based research.

According to a public survey conducted by ACSM, nearly two-thirds of patients (65%) would be more interested in exercising to stay healthy if advised by their doctors and given additional resources. Patients look to their doctor first for advice on exercise and physical activity (4). Many physicians are beginning to refer patients directly to certified fitness professionals, thanks in part to the EIM initiative.

EIM has reached far beyond doctor's offices. In 2008, EIM month (May) was launched; as of 2010, 38 cities, states, and organizations have proclaimed May as EIM month in order to recognize, emphasize, and celebrate the valuable health benefits of exercise on a national scale. The "Exercise is Medicine™ on Campus" initiative was launched in 2009 as a call to action for educational institutions around the country to make a commitment supporting EIM and the benefits of physical activity. The Inaugural World Congress on EIM was held in Baltimore, Maryland, in 2010 where the U.S. Surgeon General, Vice Admiral Regina Benjamin spoke to a standing-room-only crowd on the consequences of a sedentary population and the dire need for Americans to incorporate regular physical activity into their lifestyles. Finally, EIM has a global outreach program that includes six regional centers in North America, Latin America, Africa, Australia, Europe, and Asia. The EIM initiative continues to gain momentum so Personal Trainers will benefit by keeping up on its most recent accomplishments.

## American Fitness Index

Another new public health initiative is ACSM American Fitness Index (AFI). The AFI is a program to help cities understand how the health of their residents and community assets that support active, healthy lifestyles compare to that of other cities nationwide. The overall goal of the AFI program is to improve the health, fitness, and quality of life of the nation through promoting physical activity. The AFI uses three primary means to achieve their task: (a) collection and dissemination of city health data, (b) provision of resources, and (c) community assistance to connect with health promotion partners.

The American Fitness Index is one example of a national initiative to help understand how the health of residents and community assets in a city support active, healthy lifestyles. For further information, visit www.americanfitnessindex.org (1).

The AFI reflects a composite of community indicators for preventive health behaviors, levels of chronic disease conditions, access to health care, and community support and policies for physical activity. In addition, demographic and economic diversity and levels of violent crime are shown for each metropolitan area. Cities with the highest scores are considered to have high *community* fitness, a concept akin to an individual having high *personal* fitness. In 2016, the top five cities were Washington, DC; Minneapolis, Minnesota; Denver, Colorado; Portland, Oregon; and San Francisco, California. These communities had many strengths that supported healthy living and few challenges that hindered their choices. The AFI provides ideas and goals for other cities to initiate and become healthier. Understanding and learning about these national initiatives may assist a Personal Trainer in proving support to community members concerning healthy lifestyles. Other organizations that are taking active roles in promoting healthy lifestyles include the IHRSA (www.ihrsa.org), American Council on Exercise (www.acefitness.org), and the National Strength and Conditioning Association (www.nsca-lift.org).

## Other Recent Releases of Which Personal Trainers Must Be Aware

- 2008 Physical Activity Guidelines for Americans is the first such report put forward by the U.S. government. The 2008 guidelines state that adults aged 18–64 years should do 2 hours and 30 minutes per week of moderate-intensity or 1 hour and 15 minutes per week of vigorous-intensity aerobic physical activity. Children and adolescents aged 6–17 years should do 1 hour or more of physical activity every day. All of these groups are encouraged to do muscle-strengthening activities weekly, and older adults aged 65 years and older should do the same as adults with the addition of exercises to maintain or improve balance if they're at risk for falling (20).
- 2015 Dietary Guidelines for Americans has five overarching themes: (a) Follow a healthy eating pattern across the lifespan; (b) focus on variety, nutrient density, and amount; (c) limit calories from added sugars and saturated fats and reduce sodium intake; (d) shift to healthier food and beverage choices; and (e) support healthy eating patterns for all. Decreasing consumption of some foods such as those with added sugars, saturated fats and sodium are recommended (19). More information on dietary choices is found in Chapter 6 and at http://www.choosemyplate.gov.
- *The Surgeon General's Vision for a Healthy and Fit Nation 2010* has several recommendations on how to decrease obesity and increase physical activity in our country. Recommendations include creating healthy home environments by having healthy food choices on hand, increasing physical activity, decreasing television and computer use, as well as creating healthy child care settings, schools, and worksites. The report emphasizes mobilization of the medical community, recommending EIM concepts, and collaborative ways to improve communities (22).
- Healthy People 2020 was released by the U.S. Department of Health and Human Services at the end of 2010 (see http://www.healthypeople.gov/2020/default.aspx). The report includes the nation's new 10-year goals and objectives for health promotion and disease prevention. The Healthy People initiative is grounded in the principle that setting national objectives and monitoring progress can motivate action, and indeed, in just the last decade, preliminary analyses indicate that the country has either progressed toward or met 71% of its Healthy People targets (21).

## ACSM's Role and the Educational Continuum

ACSM is a professional member association headquartered in Indianapolis, Indiana, and composed of a multidisciplinary mix of more than 50,000 exercise science researchers, educators, and medical practitioners in more than 90 countries. More specifically, member categories include exercise physiologists, physicians, nurses, athletic trainers, dietitians, and physical therapists, as well as many other allied health care professionals with an interest in sports medicine and the exercise sciences. The mission statement for ACSM is

> ACSM promotes and integrates scientific research, education and practical applications of sports medicine and exercise science to maintain and enhance physical performance, fitness, health, and quality of life.

ACSM was founded in 1954, was the first professional organization to begin offering health and fitness certifications (in 1975), and continues to deliver the most respected NCCA-accredited certifications within the health and fitness industry. Because of the multidisciplinary nature and diversity of its members, ACSM has evolved into the unique position of an industry leader for creating evidence-based best practices through the original research of its members as well as disseminating this information through its periodicals, meetings and conferences, position stands and consensus statements, and certification workshops. ACSM's respect has earned them numerous health-initiative partnerships and collaborative efforts with groups such as the American Heart Association (AHA), American Medical Association, NSF International, ACS, CDC, IHRSA, National Intramural-Recreational Sports Association, National Academy of Sports Medicine, the CAAHEP, the NCCA, the National Collegiate Athletic Association, the NCPAD, and many others.

> ACSM was founded in 1954, was the first professional organization to begin offering health and fitness certifications (in 1975), and continues to deliver the most respected, NCCA-accredited certifications within the health and fitness industry.

## Identification of a Core Body of Knowledge

Shortly after ACSM began offering certifications, the first edition of *ACSM's Guidelines for Exercise Testing and Prescription* (2) was published along with its companion publication *ACSM's Resource Manual for Guidelines for Exercise Testing and Prescription* (3). These publications included, for the first time anywhere, the consensus of subject matter experts (SMEs) and so defined the core body of knowledge with respect to standards and guidelines for assessing fitness and prescribing exercise. Generally, all professions, regardless of the industry, have a core body of knowledge that provides guidance and clarity and also helps establish a specific profession's scope of practice. This initial publication proved so effective for practitioners that periodic review and revision of this book now takes place every 4 years. The year 2017 marks the publication of the 10th edition of *ACSM's Guidelines for Exercise Testing and Prescription*, as well as the 5th edition of the *ACSM's Certification Review Book*.

## Continuous Revision of Knowledge and Skills

In the past, included in the appendices of every edition of *ACSM's Guidelines for Exercise Testing and Prescription* was a comprehensive list of knowledge, skills, and abilities (KSAs) relative to each ACSM certification. These categories are now called Performance Domains for each ACSM Certification Level and can be found on ACSM Web site (www.acsm.org/get-certified). Each domain has a percentage attached to it that expresses the relative importance or weighting of that particular domain in the workplace and on the certification exam as well (see Table 1.3 for the current domains).

ACSM CPT certification domains contain several job tasks, each requiring knowledge and skills statements (KSs). These job tasks represent the specific attributes necessary for success as a practitioner (practicing personal trainer). The general process for the ongoing revision and/or addition to the job tasks follows industry-accepted best-practice models for ongoing quality assurance. Box 1.2 describes the development of the knowledge and skills required of the Personal Trainer.

| Table 1.3 | ACSM Certified Personal Trainer Performance Domains | |
|---|---|---|
| Domain | Content Areas | Percentage |
| I | Initial client consultation and assessment | 26 |
| II | Exercise programming and implementation | 27 |
| III | Exercise leadership and client education | 27 |
| IV | Legal, professional, business, and marketing | 20 |

All certification examination candidates are encouraged to visit the American College of Sports Medicine Web site (www.acsm.org). Follow the links through certification to view the latest certification examination blueprint and job tasks.

| Box 1.2 | Description of the Development of the Personal Trainer Skills |
|---|---|

1. A group of subject matter experts, including practitioners, academicians, and potential employers, review the current set of job tasks for a particular occupation (*i.e.*, personal training).
2. Updated job tasks from the review are evaluated through a "job task analysis," in which a large sample of randomly selected practitioners and employers further comment on the importance, frequency, and relevance of each specific job task compared with the typical job demands and requirements in the real-world setting.
3. Subject matter experts then revise the job tasks as needed, based on the results and comments from the job task analysis.
4. The job tasks are assigned to their appropriate performance domain, the necessary knowledge and skills to accomplish each job task are determined, and each performance domain is weighted, representing the combined work of the content experts and the results of the job task analysis.
5. The weighted domains serve as the certification exam blueprint for the creation of legally defensible exam questions. The exam has multiple-choice questions delivered in a computer-based testing format.

## SUMMARY

The rapidly expanding fitness industry offers Personal Trainers many potential work environments in which they gain experience and develop a career, including commercial (for-profit) fitness center, not-for-profit fitness centers, university recreation centers, corporate fitness centers, MFCs, and more. Although compensation varies greatly for trainers, they are overall very satisfied with their career choice and see opportunities for advancement and growth. With a nation on the verge of a health care crisis due primarily to the prevalence of lifestyle-related conditions, highly qualified and motivated Personal Trainers are needed now more than ever to lead individuals down the road to good health and well-being. As the fitness industry grows and the demographics/characteristics of the population continue to change, it is likely that the role of Personal Trainers will change too. This changing role will likely be an expansion of Personal Trainers' scope of practice so that Personal Trainers may soon be seen as allied health care professionals. Personal Trainers are beginning to be more commonplace in areas where they were seldom seen in the past, such as medical clinics, with a role of helping low-risk individuals capable of independent exercise to become more active, as the medical profession turns to the prevention of disease and not just the treatment of it. As an emerging professional in this rapidly growing field, Personal Trainers can contribute to this expanding sphere of influence by being the utmost professional at all times for clients and for the best interests of the profession.

# REFERENCES

1. American College of Sports Medicine. *ACSM's American Fitness Index: Actively Moving U.S. Cities to Better Health — The 2016 Report* [Internet]. Indianapolis (IN): American College of Sports Medicine; [cited 2017 Jan 25]. Available from: http://www.americanfitnessindex.org

2. American College of Sports Medicine. *ACSM's Guidelines for Exercise Testing and Prescription*. 10th ed. Philadelphia (PA): Wolters Kluwer; 2018.

3. American College of Sports Medicine. *ACSM's Resource Manual for Guidelines for Exercise Testing and Prescription*. 6th ed. Baltimore (MD): Wolters Kluwer Health/Lippincott Williams & Wilkins; 2009. 896 p.

4. American College of Sports Medicine. *Exercise Is Medicine®: A Global Health Initiative* [Internet]. Indianapolis (IN): American College of Sports Medicine; [cited 2017 Jan 25]. Available from: http://www.exerciseismedicine.org/

5. American Heart Association. *Overweight in Children* [Internet]. Dallas (TX): American Heart Association; [cited 2011 Mar 29]. Available from: http://www.heart.org/HEARTORG/Getting Healthy/Overweight-in-Children_UCM_304054_Article.jsp

6. Bureau of Labor Statistics. *Occupational Outlook Handbook, 2016-17 Edition* [Internet]. Washington (DC): U.S. Bureau of Labor Statistics; [cited 2016 Jul 13]. Available from: https://www.bls.gov/ooh/personal-care-and-service/fitness-trainers-and-instructors.htm

7. Centers for Disease Control and Prevention. *Nutrition, Physical Activity and Obesity: Data, Trends and Maps* [Internet]. Atlanta (GA): U.S. Department of Health and Human Services; [cited 2017 Jan 25]. Available from: https://nccd.cdc.gov/NPAO_DTM/IndicatorSummary.aspx?category=71&indicator=36

8. Centers for Disease Control and Prevention. *U.S. Obesity Trends 1985–2010* [Internet]. Atlanta (GA): U.S. Department of Health and Human Services; [cited 2017 Jan 23]. Available from: https://www.cdc.gov/obesity/data/prevalence-maps.html

9. Central Intelligence Agency. Life expectancy. In: *The CIA World Factbook 2010*. [Internet]. New York (NY): Skyhorse Publishing; [cited 2016 Jul 13]. Available from: https://www.cia.gov/library/publications/the-world-factbook/geos/us.html

10. Chenoweth D. *Worksite Health Promotion*. 2nd ed. Champaign (IL): Human Kinetics; 2007. 192 p.

11. Ekblom-Bak E, Hellenius M, Ekblom B. Are we facing a new paradigm of inactivity physiology? *Br J Sports Med*. 2010;44:834–5.

12. Ethics Resource Center [Internet]. Arlington (VA): Ethics Resource Center; [cited 2008 Aug 21]. Available from: http://www.ethics.org

13. International Health, Racquet and Sportsclub Association. *Industry Statistics. IHRSA 2016 Global Report: The State of the Health Club Industry*. Boston (MA): International Health, Racquet and Sportsclub Association; 2016. 128 p.

14. Medical Fitness Association. *Medical Fitness Centers Benchmarks for Success 2015*. 9th ed. Richmond (VA): Medical Fitness Association; 2015. 97 p.

15. Ogden CL, Carroll MD, Kit BK, Flegal KM. *Prevalence of Obesity in the United States, 2009–2010* (NCHS Data Brief No. 82). Hyattsville (MD): National Center for Health Statistics; 2012. 8 p.

16. Pennington B. Baby boomers stay active, and so do their doctors. *The New York Times* [Internet]. [cited 2006 Apr 16]. Available from: http://www.nytimes.com/2006/04/16/sports/16boomers.html

17. Tharrett SJ, Peterson JA. *Fitness Management: A Comprehensive Resource for Developing, Leading, Managing, and Operating a Successful Health/Fitness Club*. Monterey (CA): Healthy Learning; 2006. 511 p.

18. Thompson, WR. Worldwide survey of fitness trends for 2017. *ACSM's Health Fitness J*. 2016;20(6):8–17.

19. U.S. Department of Agriculture, Center for Nutrition Policy and Promotion. *Dietary Guidelines for Americans: 2015-2020* [Internet]. Washington (DC): U.S. Department of Agriculture; [cited 2017 Jan 23]. Available from: https://health.gov/dietary guidelines/2015/guidelines/executive-summary/

20. U.S. Department of Health and Human Services. *At-A-Glance: A Fact Sheet for Professionals* [Internet]. Washington (DC): U.S. Department of Health and Human Services; [cited 2008 Oct 7]. Available from: http://www.health.gov/Paguidelines/factsheetprof.aspx

21. U.S. Department of Health and Human Services. *Healthy People 2020* [Internet]. Washington (DC): U.S. Department of Health and Human Services; [cited 2010 Dec 2]. Available from: http://www.healthypeople.gov/2020/about/new2020.aspx

22. U.S. Department of Health and Human Services. *The Surgeon General's Vision for a Healthy and Fit Nation*. Rockville, MD: U.S. Department of Health and Human Services, Office of the Surgeon General, January 2010 [Internet]. Washington (DC): U.S. Department of Health and Human Services; [cited 2010 Jan]. Available from: https://www.surgeongeneral.gov/priorities/healthy-fit-nation/obesityvision2010

# 2

# Career Track for Personal Trainers

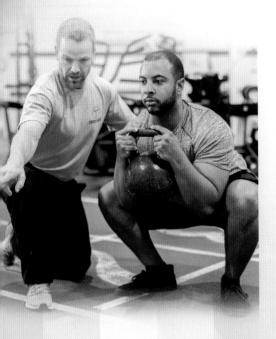

## OBJECTIVES

**Personal Trainers should be able to:**

- Discuss common client expectations of a Personal Trainer.
- Examine potential career starting points and career paths.
- Highlight options for continuing education and career development.
- Examine expectations of a career as a Personal Trainer.

## INTRODUCTION

The iconic Jack LaLanne was undoubtedly one of the first professional Personal Trainers to bring personal training to the masses through television. He created the identifiable persona as an expert and motivated millions of people to exercise through the power of television. He then parlayed that success into a 74-year career that spanned from health clubs to jump ropes and juicers.

Although popularized in the late 1970s with the advent of celebrity Personal Trainers for stars of movie screens and tennis courts, personal training gained notoriety as a stand-alone business through the work of pioneers in New York City and Hollywood, California. These pioneers founded personal training studios that provided personal training in 30- or 60-minute bouts of strength and endurance training. They catered to the elite, including movie stars, tennis pros, television news anchors, business leaders, and ballerinas. The personal approach to fitness was so successful that professional athletic teams employed strength coaches (leading to the formation of the National Strength and Conditioning Association [NSCA] in 1978). Movie stars hired Personal Trainers to work with them on location. Financial firms brought trainers in-house to push their corporate athletes.

At the same time, in health clubs, training facilities, gymnasiums, and sporting arenas around the world, people were seeing and feeling the benefits of having an educated and dedicated fitness professional (1). Personal training evolved into a career that was waiting to happen. A career that allowed exercise experts, cajoling coaches, tenacious teachers, and master motivators to make a living by guiding their clients to a specific set of goals and objectives that would eventually lead to a better body but more importantly, better health.

## Client Expectations of a Personal Trainer

Most evaluations of service professionals utilize the concept of how the individual performs in relation to expectations. If Personal Trainers do not know what clients expect from them, it is virtually impossible to meet, no less exceed, those expectations. The following are categories and examples of reasonable client expectations. The scope and scale of the service-level agreement with the client should clearly describe goals and an acceptable "range of results." Chapters throughout this book provide background and information on how to assist clients to achieve great results (Fig. 2.1).

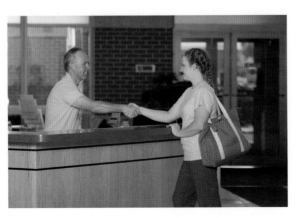

**FIGURE 2.1.** A Personal Trainer and client meeting for the first time.

## Know the Goal

As defined by James Prochaska's transtheoretical model of behavior change (5), personal-training clients typically arrive in the "action" stage (see Chapter 7 for more information on the stages of change, processes of change, and decisional balance). They have decided that they will take their physical activity behaviors to a new level, and they are employing the Personal Trainer as the expert to guide them to their vision of success. This is an important assignment and a very difficult one. Implementing lasting behavior change is difficult even under the best circumstances.

> Goals can be discussed as part of the intake process and serve as a foundation for the development of objectives.

Goals can be discussed as part of the intake process and serve as a foundation for the development of objectives. The contractual business agreement Personal Trainers make with their clients reflects these objectives regarding the following:

- Number of sessions
- Cost per session
- Length of session
- Unsupervised training requirements outside of each session
- Length of agreement
- Cancellation policies
- Refund policies
- Performance guarantees

For example, if the Personal Trainer is training a client to compete in a marathon, a schedule should be created in reverse from the day of the race to the start of the training. One-to-one sessions may be more frequent in the beginning, at critical mileage differentiators, at low points in the client's motivational cycle, or at other junctures in the training when both parties agree are appropriate. Training for a 20-lb weight reduction might require a very different, regimented schedule that includes nutritional check-ups, weigh-ins, and disciplined combinations of supervised high-intensity training with partially supervised aerobic exercise bouts. Each situation is determined by the goal. After maintaining the safety and well-being of the client, attainment of goals is the next top priority.

Many clients have a goal or set of goals in mind when they hire a Personal Trainer. Some come to a Personal Trainer with an unrealistic and unfounded expectation for what they can reasonably achieve in a defined period of time. The Personal Trainer must manage these expectations in a way that encourages the path to success and does not further distort already unhealthy images of what can be achieved, especially in the area of body image and weight loss. For a much broader and in-depth description of goal setting and the achievement of goals, please see Chapter 7.

By making goals measurable (clearly quantifiable), the Personal Trainer demonstrates having listened to the reason the clients have sought the assistance of a Personal Trainer. The clients' goals must be translated by the Personal Trainer into achievable objectives and outcomes. The outcomes are a way to measure success. It is important to acknowledge that goal setting and behavior change in general are dynamic processes that vary from client to client and even from day to day within each individual client. Setbacks should be anticipated, and Personal Trainers should work with clients to reevaluate training and take the opportunity to improve the client's program rather than to simply view a setback as a failure.

> By making goals measurable (clearly quantifiable), the Personal Trainer demonstrates having listened to the reason the clients have sought the assistance of a Personal Trainer. The clients' goals must be translated by the Personal Trainer into achievable objectives and outcomes.

Another long-term objective related to the client's training goals is to enable clients to exercise independently. The underlying, unspoken question "When will you be able to maintain your goals without me?" is often not addressed. The long-term objective of Personal Trainers is to prepare their clients for the day when they can successfully become their own "expert." Good teachers teach their students to succeed without supervision. Good coaches teach players to perform successfully with little or no supervision as the player becomes his or her own coach. In many ways, Personal Trainers combine the characteristics of a good teacher and a good coach. Specifically, a Personal Trainer can bolster a client's self-efficacy and provide them with a high level of mastery of skills regarding their exercise habits. For more information regarding self-efficacy and behavior change see Chapter 7.

## Be Knowledgeable and Experienced

In 2002, commercial health club's largest trade organization, The International Health, Racquet and Sportsclub Association (IHRSA) persuaded the industry into rethinking how Personal Trainers would be certified for the betterment of their careers and the safety of their clients. Faced with literally hundreds of certification options, Personal Trainers and their clients were unsure which certification processes were well-designed, unbiased, valid, and reliable. IHRSA, in concert with most of the certifying organizations, crafted a position statement in 2004. This statement recommended that by January 2006, member clubs hire only the Personal Trainers who hold certification from an organization that was in the process of obtaining third-party accreditation of its certification procedures and policies from an independent and nationally recognized accrediting body. The goal was to ensure that the certificate held by Personal Trainers accurately and appropriately measured their competence and provided the industry with a means toward improving the growing business of personal training. With the new standard of accredited certification taking hold, certifying agencies felt comfortable establishing the high school diploma (or its equivalent) and cardiopulmonary resuscitation (CPR)/automated external defibrillator (AED) training as the prerequisite for their entry-level personal training certificate (1) (Box 2.1).

> Experience is meaningful if the Personal Trainer is successful in documenting the outcomes, acquiring references from employers and clients alike, and building a resume to a stated career objective.

Experience requires time that is well-spent. The process of discovering a specialty, obtaining a degree, completing internship hours for certification, performing volunteer work, and actual employment will provide the Personal Trainer with many professional opportunities. Experience is meaningful if the Personal Trainer is successful in documenting the outcomes, acquiring references from employers and clients alike, and building a resume to a stated career objective. Sometimes, these experience-based opportunities require the Personal Trainer to work for little or no compensation and seek situations that may be outside of the typical comfort zone. For example, a Personal Trainer may lack experience working with an older population. However, the demographic trends point toward a larger number of clients who are older and who may possess orthopedic and metabolic conditions as a result of their age. Therefore, the Personal Trainer may search out opportunities to work in retirement homes or assisted living facilities as most offer exercise therapy for their residents. Many of these facilities feature well-equipped fitness centers with robust programming, giving the Personal Trainer an opportunity to gain valuable experience with this market segment.

## Box 2.1    For More Information

For the most up-to-date list of accredited personal training certification programs, go to the Institute of Credentialing Excellence (ICE; http://www.credentialingexcellence.org) (3). Note that ICE was formerly the National Organization for Competency Assurance (NOCA).

## Present a Clear and Concise Plan

Football coach Vince Lombardi once said, "Plan your work and work your plan." A simple-sounding strategy but it conveys one of the most important qualities for success in the art and science of personal training. The pretraining assessment, screening, and goal discovery phase with a client provides the foundation for the exercise prescription.

Once the mode, frequency, duration, intensity, and general components (*e.g.*, warm-up, flexibility, balance, agility, strength, endurance, aerobic power, specific skills, and cool-down) of the exercise prescription are determined, a written plan is presented to the client. The plan includes the exercise session date(s), primary goal(s) for each session, exercise mode, the order of exercises, the name of the exercises, duration (in repetitions, sets, exercise time), and intensities (target heart rate, rating of perceived exertion, amount of resistance).

The last line of each completed exercise prescription plan should be the Personal Trainer's signature. It is a sign that the Personal Trainer has developed the plan and has incorporated any pertinent observations, notes, adjustments, and comments from the client and the session for future reference. This can also be helpful in case another Personal Trainer works with that client in the future. More importantly, the signature reflects the work put forth by the Personal Trainer, similar to an artist signing a painting.

A good time to review the overall strategy and individual session plan with clients is during the warm-up phase, while they are walking on a treadmill or riding the bike. This is also an opportunity to get their general level of readiness for the day's exercises; check nutritional and hydration status; ask about any recent injuries, aches, or pains that may impact the plan; and set the stage for a great workout.

In addition to the exercise prescription, the Personal Trainer should include a communication plan; establish policies for late, cancelled, or abbreviated sessions; share health history data; communicate nutrition and hydration habits; and in general establish the ground rules for how the Personal Trainer and client will work together. Information on referring when needed is covered in Chapters 11 and 22.

## Be Innovative, Creative, and Resourceful

Effective Personal Trainers demonstrate both innovation and creativity (1). An innovator is defined as one who continually introduces new methods and techniques. The personal training experience provides many opportunities for such innovation in ways that are simple to execute. Yet, it is imperative the Personal Trainer ensure the safety of any new methods and techniques before the use with clients. Safety of the client should be the most important aspect for any exercise prescribed.

Creativity is another behavioral trait of effective Personal Trainers. The opportunity for the Personal Trainer to be creative frequently comes when a piece of equipment or area of the

---

### Box 2.2    Manual Resistance

One technique that seems to demonstrate creativity is when a Personal Trainer substitutes his or her strength to provide resistance to the client's exercise movement. This technique is called "manual resistance." The client can push against a trainer, but a trainer should avoid pushing against a client. Another innovation is to manipulate speed of movement. Speed of contraction is as relevant a variable as reps, sets, and weight in the completion of a strength training exercise, so manipulating the speed of the pushing or pulling (or both) phases of a movement is an effective way to change the stimulus for the muscle complex and surprise the client in regard to his or her expectations of what action is coming next at the same time.

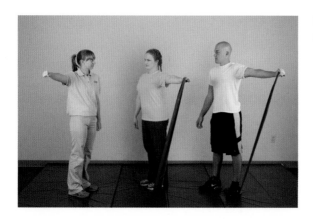

**FIGURE 2.2.** A Personal Trainer demonstrates the use of resistance bands.

facility is unexpectedly out of service. A creative Personal Trainer will always have a back-up exercise ready to accomplish a particular exercise objective. This is usually a substitution of a free-weight movement for a machine-based exercise or the same with a manual resistance exercise option (Box 2.2).

A competent Personal Trainer is also resourceful. Discovering new, cutting-edge equipment and adapting an ordinary device such as resistance bands to accommodate clients with orthopedic limitations convey to clients that the Personal Trainer is thinking about their goals well in advance (Fig. 2.2). Clients will see that the Personal Trainer is current with the profession and is always looking for the latest developments. Offering variety provides a level of stimulation that keeps the client engaged and less likely to be bored with the repetitive routine that exercise training can follow.

## Educate

Good health is a lifelong journey. An important goal for any Personal Trainer is to teach clients the basic tenants of safe and effective physical activity so they can apply these principles for themselves and eventually teach others these same concepts. These concepts include the components of a complete workout, including warm-up and cool-down, flexibility/stretching, balance, agility, strength, endurance, and aerobic power. For example, when learning the progression of a properly designed program for developing muscular fitness, the client should learn progression from large muscle groups to small muscle groups. They should be familiar with the differences between pushing and pulling movements, proper breathing, effective stretching techniques, determination of exercise intensity (training heart rate, rating of perceived exertion or amount of resistance), various modes of exercise, and proper program progression (intensity, duration, and frequency of workouts) in accordance with established exercise goals. An appropriate and safe exercise mode is of importance to the effectiveness of a training session.

A working knowledge of human anatomy, kinesiology, and physiology is essential for a Personal Trainer to describe what is happening inside the body through the bout of exercise.

A working knowledge of human anatomy, kinesiology, and physiology is essential for a Personal Trainer to describe what is happening inside the body through the bout of exercise. The ability to translate the science of exercise into terminology that the layman will understand is an important skill for Personal Trainers as they will work with a range of clients with varying backgrounds.

Effective Personal Trainers are patient, are prepared, know the knowledge level of their clients, provide handouts and background reading/research notes, and use questions to elicit thoughtful answers. These teaching techniques, when used effectively by the Personal Trainer, apply to facts, theories, and concepts (cognitive learning) and acquisitions of exercise movements (motor learning).

| Box 2.3 | For More Information |
|---------|---------------------|

Simon Sinek describes in his video "Start with Why — How Great Leaders Inspire Action" (6) that although most people can deftly describe what they do and how they do it, the thorough conviction, the passion, and a "dream" of WHY a person became a Personal Trainer are what will really stand out to a potential client.

## Inspire

For many people, exercising regularly at a level that will yield visible results is difficult. One of the reasons why personal training has been so popular is because of the customized, concentrated, safe, and effective elements that the person in the Personal Trainer role provides to the client.

Personal Trainers who have taken up the profession because of their personal, positive experience as a personal training client have a built-in story for inspiration. If they have overcome a physical challenge themselves, the empathy they can convey to clients who are in similar situations is also a very powerful source of inspiration for prospective clients and clients in training especially when the compassion is delivered at just the right moment of need (Box 2.3). This oftentimes happens when a client is stuck at a certain training level or cannot easily attain the goals they seek.

Each and every training client is motivated to succeed for very different reasons. Personal Trainers can take their time to discover what the driving force is for each client on an individual level and then customize the appropriate levers to accelerate this success. For example, some clients like the competitive challenge and respond to the desire to excel over and above others. The Personal Trainer could assemble a group of clients, categorized by sex, weight, and training experience and provide each member of the team with unique identifiers to protect each client's privacy (often referred to in experimental settings as blind coding). The Personal Trainer ranks the clients by a select category of performance, for example, a personal record (PR) on a bench press one repetition maximum (1-RM). At periodic intervals or when the client needs a "competitive" push, the Personal Trainer posts the team rankings and thus uses the client's internal competitive spirit as a motivator to work harder to achieve a new PR (Fig. 2.3). If the Personal Trainer knows that a client is motivated by competition, using a competitive game to leverage that knowledge and help that client succeed is an example of how a trainer becomes personal. Individual enjoyment is especially employed in training programs that are long in term and duration. Mixing in specialty classes, team sports, individual sports, or partner sports can provide a welcome relief and a quick dose of motivation to endure and eventually succeed in the long-term training objective such as a triathlon, half marathon, or marathon. More about motivation and adherence is discussed later in Chapter 8.

> Each and every training client is motivated to succeed for very different reasons. Personal Trainers can take their time to discover what the driving force is for each client on an individual level and then customize the appropriate levers to accelerate this success.

**FIGURE 2.3.** A Personal Trainer using a team ranking chart to show the client her latest position after the last posting of their personal record.

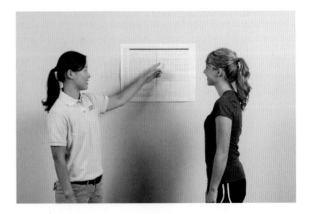

## Focus

When it comes to personal training, one of the most important features of this service is individual attention. Undivided, undistracted, unencumbered, and eye-to-eye focus on their form, speed, posture, grip, stance, breathing, and even facial expressions may help differentiate an easy exercise from one that is pushing the client to the highest levels of exercise intensity.

Preparation is the first step in creating an environment, which indicates to the client that the Personal Trainer is focused. If the session is well-planned and the Personal Trainer has reviewed the elements and sequences, then there is no worry what will be done next, so the concentration can center on the client's performance. "Now and how" is a great mantra to replay as preparations are made mentally to launch each set of exercises for the client.

The Personal Trainer should set the ground rules for clients on distractions during the session. Alert clients that the Personal Trainer will not answer their questions while training another client. Personal Trainers should give clients their contact information (*e.g.*, e-mail, phone number) so clients can easily contact them if they have questions. The client being trained should also be restricted from taking phone calls, texting, and checking e-mail, especially during key sets/reps in the training session.

The Personal Trainer should have charts, stop watches, small exercise equipment, towels, and water set up in advance so that stocking the training area during a workout is not necessary. This is part of the overall session preparation.

Clients want Personal Trainers to have a proactive awareness and be able to anticipate a client's needs. Hospitality will become a part of the unique selling proposition, the feature that makes individuals different from the competition and that provides added value (Box 2.4). In addition to hospitality, Personal Trainers can make their services distinctive by specializing in one or several niche markets (*e.g.*, Personal Trainer who specializes in working with female triathletes). Creating unique markets within an overall business model can help to set on Personal Trainer apart from others.

## Track and Recognize Progress

A Personal Trainer determines all the appropriate metrics of success for each and every individual client in the intake process. As described in the SMART goal concept (see Chapter 7 for more details), while establishing key success metrics, the Personal Trainer sets critical benchmarks used to evaluate whether or not the training programs are effective. These metrics are also used to motivate the client to forge ahead toward these very important goals. Clients are often after "big-impact" results (*e.g.*, lose 20 lb [9 kg], reduce body fat by 7%, serve a tennis ball at 75 mph [121 kph], or hit a golf drive 275 yards [251.5 m]). The Personal Trainer's challenge is to lead clients toward their long-term goals through attainment of several smaller ones. The Personal Trainer's job is to make clients aware of the small advances they are achieving and how they all contribute toward their desired endpoint.

Simple charts and graphs are very effective in demonstrating client progress toward a desired goal. The simplest example of how this works is usually seen when working with clients who have a weight loss goal. Clients set weight loss goals that are too high and too fast. Safe and effective

| Box 2.4 | For More Information |
| --- | --- |

To become an expert in hospitality, study service organizations that are best in delivering customer service. Hotels and internet retailers are two examples of organizations that thrive as a result of the highest standards when it comes to servicing their customers. Successful examples of organizations that have achieved legendary levels of customer service are well-documented in *The New Gold Standard* (4) and *Delivering Happiness: A Path to Profits, Passion and Purpose* (2).

| Box 2.5 | Client Spotlight |
|---------|------------------|

Have a small budget for incentive rewards to use with your clients. Free training sessions, 30-minute massage gift certificates, training gear, a motivational or instructional book, and training diaries are all effective rewards. Regardless, your recognition of their accomplishments is the most effective strategy.

weight loss strategies typically recommend 1–2 lb (0.5–1 kg) of weight loss per week, although this can vary depending on the initial body weight of the client. If a client wants to lose 20 lb (9 kg), this may take up to 20 weeks and that does not account for any muscle weight gain that may occur as a result of the training regimen. Twenty weeks equals 5 months. Because clients read advertisements on the Internet and listen to late night television that claims weight loss of 20 lb (9 kg) in 1 month without exercise, getting clients to acknowledge a 5-month wait for a weight-loss goal is a challenge. Educate clients on the safety of slow weight loss and chart their weight weekly or every other week on the same day to display slow and steady progress and keep the client focused and motivated that the long-range goal is in sight, one small step at a time.

Recognition and positive reinforcement is also part of the Personal Trainer's responsibilities and expectations. The Personal Trainer has to respond and react to clients when they do their job as well. Keep them motivated by pointing out their successes and accomplishments, whether small or large, that they may overlook in order to bolster self-efficacy. Establish a pattern of noting PRs for critical exercises. Set rituals for recording and then celebrating the big accomplishments such as losing not only the first 10 lb (4.5 kg) but the second 2 lb (1 kg) as well (Box 2.5).

# Where Do I Start My Career?

## Background

The prerequisites for employment will depend on the employer, job description, and types of clients' serviced while performing the scope of work. Many employers in commercial health clubs expect a personal training certificate from an accredited organization. *ACSM's Health/Fitness Facility Standards and Guidelines* indicates that facilities should hire trainers with demonstrable competence as evidenced by, among others, holding certification from a recognized organization. Facilities (*e.g.*, medical wellness centers and rehabilitation clinics) that serve clients with multiple risk factors and orthopedic limitations typically require both a degree (graduate or undergraduate) in a health- or fitness-related field *and* a certificate that is related to their scope of responsibilities.

## First Find Your "Why"

Most trainers start their careers as a result of personal experience, direct or related. Trainers with direct experience include the athlete who has been positively affected by a coach, Personal Trainer, teacher, or even a highly regimented and effective self-imposed routine. They can be sport athletes on any level, cosmetic athletes who are performing a total body makeover, or corporate athletes who are sold on the concept that their bodies are as important as their minds for success in their business pursuits. The success and even the disappointing failure of those experiences serve as a catalyst for the future as a Personal Trainer. Someone who works in the health, fitness, or medical field as an allied professional (*e.g.*, registered dietitian, physical therapist, clinical exercise physiologist, athletic trainer, licensed massage therapist, occupational therapist, and physical therapy aide) or a support person (*e.g.*, receptionist, maintenance person, membership sales person, or administrator, such as operations manager, office assistant, bookkeeper, accountant, or human resources administrator) can also use their proximity to and familiarity with the personal training profession as a springboard to their entrance as a career Personal Trainer.

Personal Trainers face a challenging profession, including long hours, starting early in the morning and extending into the evening; focusing attention on individual clients and their needs for 45 minutes at a time and more than 8–10 clients per day; hours of reading, researching, and attending webinars and conferences; and keeping in a healthy physical condition required to meet the demands of training and to serve as a positive role model for current and prospective clients. Understanding why this career is appealing is the first step. After uncovering the compelling "WHY" for entering a personal training career, the next strategy is to get ready for the first experiences in the field training clients. The most effective strategy is multidimensional, and although occurring at the same time, the degree of emphasis depends on the personal life stage, budget, and time constraints of the Personal Trainer.

## Next: Start Your "How"

The next steps include certification as well as finding a mentor.

### Certification

Start by identifying two to three accredited certification programs and do some background research on each.

1. Do you meet their eligibility requirements?
2. Are their fees within your budget?
3. Are the logistics required to obtain their certification reasonable for you to achieve (*e.g.*, travel, Internet access, time, internship requirements)?
4. Does the certification match with your prospective field of training specialty or is it a general Personal Trainer certificate?

> Whether working for a national health and fitness chain, a specialty franchise, a small privately held studio, or opening up a private practice, attaining certification is the most important first step to be accomplished.

Whether working for a national health and fitness chain, a specialty franchise, a small privately held studio, or opening up a private practice, attaining certification is the most important first step to be accomplished. When applying for a personal training position, it is important to ask if the employer requires a particular certification. The requirements may have been established based on the certifications held by the employer or those recommended to him or her by others in the industry.

What if you are already certified? Make sure that the certification is current as most require some level of documented continuing education. Next, make sure that the certification matches the requirements of the job openings. Many certifying agencies are offering multiple levels of certification with subspecialties in weight management, wellness coaching, health coaching, and behavior change. Great Personal Trainers are lifelong learners. They adapt to the need of the clients in the markets they serve, and they make sure to be current with the techniques required to serve those clients safely and effectively. Lastly, remember that most personal training facilities require a CPR/AED certification in order to train clients.

### Find a Mentor

A mentor invests time, energy, and personal experience into another's career development. Find a mentor that most closely matches the background and experiences needed. It is in the best interest of an effective Personal Trainer to have a mentor who has been in the business of personal training.

The mentor can provide a Personal Trainer with the guidance necessary to avoid both training and business mistakes. Make sure that expectations from a mentor are clearly defined, including the estimated time required, right from the beginning. Find a mentor who is working with the types of clients in your preferred Personal Trainer practice specialty, although a signed nonsolicitation agreement with them, if their business is within your catchment area, may be required. One hour every 2 weeks is a reasonable amount of time to ask from a mentor and make sure that questions are written in advance and that plenty of time to respond to the inquiries is provided. In today's electronic communication environment, mentorships can be accomplished effectively via text and e-mail. This capability greatly expands the universe of prospective mentors.

## What Are Some Examples of Rewarding Career Paths?

There so are many types of clients, working venues, schedules, and unique opportunities in the personal training field today that a Personal Trainer can extend a career over many years and even more geographies. The next logical step in a career path, especially if working in an environment that employs many other personal training professionals, is personal training management. This path generally can consist of two distinct elements: administration and clinical. Administration requires a Personal Trainer to hire staff, manage and evaluate performance, set schedules and policies, interface with clients, and oversee the sales and financial performance of a personal training department. On the clinical path, Personal Trainers with specialty expertise (*e.g.*, yoga, Pilates, sports-specific training) are often responsible for the education, certification, and programming in specific areas. In these situations, a Personal Trainer may be required to evaluate staff's clinical capabilities and even deliver (or at a minimum coordinate) the continuing education curriculum for the team. Depending on the size of the organization, these roles may be combined proportionally to individual expertise.

> There so are many types of clients, working venues, schedules, and unique opportunities in the personal training field today that a Personal Trainer can extend a career over many years and even more geographies.

Although Personal Trainers work as commissioned employees in some commercial health and fitness centers, they may also serve as independent contractors. As a result, Personal Trainers may seek the career path of an entrepreneur. Being your own boss is rewarding and has many advantages, but it also has challenges and responsibilities. Of course, the easiest way to this path is to train clients privately in public facilities, in their own homes, or even your own home gym.

To minimize some of the risks of entrepreneurship, Personal Trainers can explore the option to become franchisees. Entering into a contract with a franchise has many branding, marketing, and operating advantages, but they come with a cost and commitment to the franchise. Good legal advice is always recommended when considering this career path.

The boldest entrepreneur opens up his or her own personal training business. Finding, renting, and renovating or, alternatively, buying the land and then building the physical location are obviously the most expensive journeys on this career path. Searching the newspaper or on the Internet for an existing business to buy and place under management is also an option worth exploring and may even come with a built-in client base.

Personal Trainers can also seek to set up a business inside another service facility such as a commercial health and fitness center, spa, medical office, hospital wellness center, salon, nutritional consultation practice, or physical therapy practice. They most likely have clients in need of a Personal Trainer's service, locker/shower rooms, equipment, and a comfortable operating environment so the Personal Trainer can focus on building a business.

In every case, the Personal Trainer who is going to create a new business needs a very capable team of real estate agents, lawyers, construction professionals, accountants, information technology professionals, and sales and marketing consultants and a high tolerance for risk. Risk decreases and reward increases in proportion to every celebrity or professional athlete that a Personal Trainer has on a client list. It also helps to have approximately 30% more startup cash on hand than the most conservative estimate (1).

Career paths for Personal Trainers can also take very successful detours down the related professional paths requiring higher levels of education. Personal Trainers who have an interest in clinical work and who are academically inclined enter the allied health professions. The careers most closely aligned with personal training are physical therapy assistants, health promotion professionals, nutritional counselors, and health/wellness coaches. Other potential allied health professional paths include physician assistants, nurses, occupational therapists, clinical exercise physiologists, and physical therapists. Most allied health careers require an advanced degree, additional certifications, a state license, and/or extensive internship hours.

# What Are My Best Options for Continuing Education and Career Development?

The best way to a long, successful, and fulfilling career is to establish a disciplined strategy for reading, research, clinics, conferences, conventions, and course work right from the beginning.

## Reading and Research

The Personal Trainer must consistently read professional journals to stay current on the research in the field. The American College of Sports Medicine (ACSM) has several publications that will provide a wide range of information, from the more practical in their *Health & Fitness Journal* to the newly launched *Translational Journal of the American College of Sports Medicine* and the latest peer-reviewed research published in *Medicine & Science in Sports & Exercise*. The *American Journal of Health Promotion* publishes an excellent peer-reviewed research journal every 2 months that is focused on health and wellness. The Institute for Health and Productivity Management publishes a quarterly journal that explores the effect of health on all aspects of employee productivity. Most professional organizations (*e.g.*, International Dance and Exercise Association [IDEA], the American Council on Exercise [ACE], IHRSA, the National Academy of Sports Medicine [NASM], ACSM, the National Business Group on Health [NBGH], NSCA) offer frequently updated electronic publications including newsletters, articles, blogs, and national professional organization position papers (Box 2.6). Access to information varies for members and nonmembers. Many very reputable publications and organizations will provide quick and easy access to their latest articles via Twitter. The Harvard Business Review and the Centers for Disease Control and Prevention are two examples of organizations that will deliver information to a smart phone.

| **Box 2.6** | **For More Information** |
| --- | --- |

Learn how to use the U.S. National Library of Medicine's PubMed at http://www.ncbi.nlm.nih.gov/pubmed/. This free resource comprises more than 20 million citations for biomedical literature from MEDLINE, life science journals, and online books. Citations may include links to full-text content from PubMed Central and publisher Web sites. The resource also provides updates of the latest research by keyword to e-mail accounts.

## Clinics, Conferences, and Conventions

There are many opportunities on the local, regional, national, and international level to attend (in person and virtually) educational sessions held over a one-to-several-day format, sponsored by professional membership organizations, certifying agencies, suppliers, customers, government agencies, and academic institutions. Membership in a relevant professional organization such as ACSM or a trade association such as IHRSA allows you to stay informed about these opportunities. Annual conferences or conventions typically provide a broad curriculum, including keynote speakers, poster presentations of research studies, topical lectures and demonstrations, and supplier trade shows to showcase products/services/software and networking/recruiting opportunities. Regional clinics are shorter in duration (from 1 h to 1 d) and are typically focused on a specific issue or topic. Many are available via teleconference, using WebEx and Skype platforms.

## Coursework

The first place to look for continuing education opportunities is the employer. Today, almost every organization has an internal training department that offers formal and informal courses that assist in performing day-to-day responsibilities and also to prepare for advancement within the company. In conjunction with maintaining a professional certification, certifying agencies require continuing educational credits (CECs). To achieve the required CECs, the agencies, either directly or through affiliated suppliers, offer courses that upon completion award CECs. Identifying, planning, and scheduling the courses needed to receive the number of CECs required to maintain (or attain) a certification is the most efficient path to follow for coursework.

Specialty courses are also available from schools and organizations that specialize in continuing education like IDEA, ACE, and the Cooper Clinic, and even some suppliers like Nike, Adidas, and Cybex (exercise equipment). For subject matter outside of the health and fitness disciplines, continuing education courses can be found at local colleges and universities, commercial organizations that offer education.

# What Can I Expect from a Career as a Personal Trainer?

The evolution of personal training as a career has been very rapid and dynamic. With less than 30 years of existence in the modern day, the profession experienced a major change for the better with the requirement of accredited certification. This requirement has drastically changed what a professional must expect as a result of pursuing personal training career. The increased requirements of certification have promoted a "better" (more qualified) Personal Trainer who can provide a safe and improved experience for clients. Although national certification has helped, there are only a few states that have attempted to mandate certification or licensing requirements. This can often be frustrating for the certified trainer if competing for positions with others without certifications.

## The Satisfaction of Seeing Healthy Results

Working with a Personal Trainer has always provided clients with quicker and more effective results (1). The most satisfying part of this career is that the Personal Trainer gets to see and be an integral part of positively affecting the clients' health. Client responses vary depending on initial fitness and individual goals; structuring a regular exercise routine can promote higher energy levels, increased levels of aerobic capacity, flexibility, and muscular fitness.

## Exceeding Client Expectations

The opening chapter objective delineated in detail what clients expect from a Personal Trainer. Realize these are the baseline expectations. Clients will want the Personal Trainer, and the trainer should aspire, to exceed these expectations.

If a Personal Trainer is successful in knowing the clients' goals, the likelihood of success for the client increases. Fine-tuning the program in relation to the actual results will have the most significant impact on the real reason for using a Personal Trainer in the first place—efficient, effective, and relevant attainment of individual goals. The more a Personal Trainer works with a particular client and understands the client's readiness to change and ability levels, the greater will be the potential to inspire and motivate the client.

Planning exercise sessions and documenting workouts are minimum expectations. Charting and graphing results and using them as motivational and educational presentations to clients are a plus. Expect to work long hours at either ends of the day (morning and evening). Most clients train either before the start of their work day or after. Weekends are popular as well. Some markets can be contained to a normal daily schedule but will always mirror the peak usage times for a health and fitness facility, fitness center, or other training facility.

## Entering the World of Lifelong Learning

As a certified Personal Trainer, a higher level of education is now expected. This will require that the Personal Trainer devote much more time and effort into reading, research, and continuing education. The Personal Trainer will be expected to put this time in on a regular basis. As summarized earlier in this chapter, reading and research can take considerable time. The Personal Trainer should plan on attending at least one major conference every year or every other year at a minimum. This is a 2- to 4-day commitment away from clients, and travel, hotel, meals, and registration expenses need to be included in the annual budget. Local conferences are an option minimizing travel and eliminating some other related expenses. The Personal Trainer will have to maintain a certification, and this will require a minimum amount of course work to obtain the necessary CECs.

## SUMMARY

Personal training is now well established as a viable professional career option for those interested in helping clients experience healthy results efficiently and effectively. The Personal Trainer's job description is based on a foundation of expertise that is relevant to the client's goals and on the ability to exceed the client's service expectations. Successful Personal Trainers combine the qualities of a good teacher with those of a good coach. Gaining certification and eliciting the assistance of a mentor are two important first steps. These steps are best achieved concurrently. Fortunately, the most rewarding aspect of embarking on a personal training career is the act of personal training itself. The personal satisfaction that comes with empowering clients to achieve their health goals is well worth the effort and hours required to stay up on the latest research and plan the most effective exercise prescriptions. A personal training career requires a strategy of lifelong learning combined with the rigors of facilitating individual behavior change.

# REFERENCES

1. Baechle T, Earle R. editors. *NSCA's Essentials of Personal Training. National Strength and Conditioning Association.* Champaign (IL): Human Kinetics; 2004. 688 p.
2. Hsieh T. *Delivering Happiness: A Path to Profits, Passion and Purpose.* New York (NY): Hachette Book Group; 2010. 272 p.
3. Institute for Credentialing Excellence. *Accredited Certification Programs* [Internet]. Washington (DC): Institute for Credentialing Excellence; [cited 2011 Oct 25]. Available from: http://www.credentialingexcellence.org/
4. Michelli JA. *The New Gold Standard: 5 Leadership Principles for Creating a Legendary Customer Experience Courtesy of the Ritz Carlton Hotel Company.* New York (NY): McGraw Hill; 2008. 304 p.
5. Prochaska JO, Norcross J, DiClemente C. *Changing for Good: A Revolutionary Six-Stage Program for Overcoming Bad Habits and Moving Your Life Positively Forward.* New York (NY): Avon Books; 1994. 304 p.
6. Sinek S. Start with why — how great leaders inspire action [Internet]. Puget Sound (WA): TEDx Talks; [cited 2011 Oct 25]. Available from: http://www.youtube.com/watch?v=u4ZoJKF_VuA

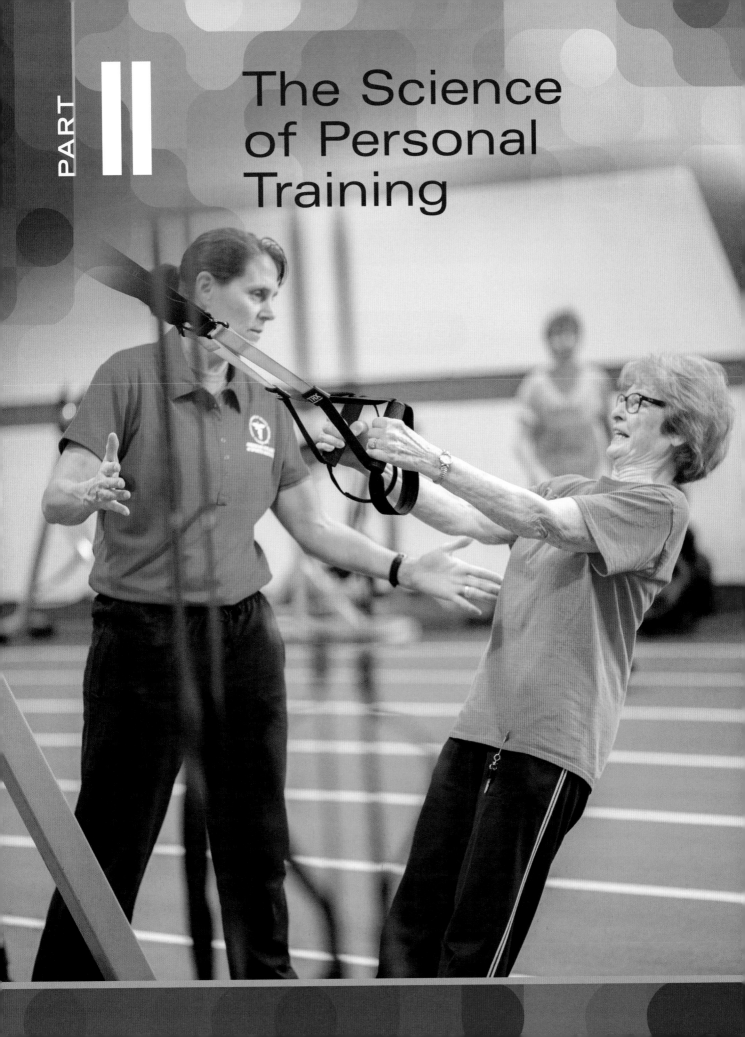

# PART II

# The Science of Personal Training

# 3

# Anatomy and Kinesiology

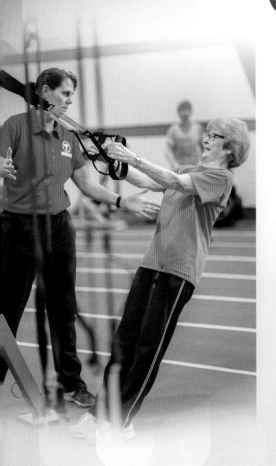

## OBJECTIVES

**Personal Trainers should be able to:**

- Provide an overview of anatomical structures of the musculoskeletal system.

- Explain the underlying biomechanical and kinesiological principles of musculoskeletal movement.

- Identify the key terms used to describe body position and movement.

- Describe the specific structures, movement patterns, range of motion, muscles, and common injuries for each major joint of the body.

## INTRODUCTION

A major goal of exercise training is to improve cardiovascular and musculoskeletal fitness. The physiological adaptation of muscle to exercise training is evidenced by improvements in muscle strength, endurance, flexibility, and resistance to injury (12). The objective of this chapter is to gain an understanding of musculoskeletal functional anatomy of the major joint structures during exercise movements, with emphasis on body alignment and kinesiological principles. A thorough understanding of these principles is essential for the Personal Trainer to design safe, effective, and efficient exercise training programs to improve musculoskeletal fitness.

Kinesiology is the study of the mechanics of human movement and specifically evaluates muscles, joints, and skeletal structures and their involvement in movement (38).

The disciplines primarily involved in describing and understanding human movement are biomechanics and kinesiology. Personal Trainers teach clients how to perform exercise movements and how to use exercise or rehabilitation equipment. Kinesiology is the study of the mechanics of human movement and specifically evaluates muscles, joints, and skeletal structures and their involvement in movement (38). Kinesiology is primarily based on three fields of science — biomechanics, musculoskeletal anatomy, and neuromuscular physiology. Kinesiology includes the study of gait, posture and body alignment, ergonomics, sports and exercise movements, and activities of daily living and work. Biomechanics is the study of the motion and causes of motion of living things, using a branch of physics known as mechanics (31). The study of biomechanics is essential for Personal Trainers because it forms the basis for documenting human motion (kinematics) and understanding the causes of that motion (kinetics). Chapter 4 covers this information in more detail. A variety of health care practitioners, including Personal Trainers, exercise physiologists, athletic trainers, physicians, physical educators, occupational therapists, physical therapists, chiropractors, and ergonomists, use biomechanical and kinesiological principles (4).

 ## Describing Body Position and Joint Movement

### Anatomical Position

Anatomical position is the universally accepted reference position used to describe regions and spatial relationships of the human body and to refer to body positions (*e.g.*, joint motions) (18). In the anatomical position, the body is erect with feet together and the upper limbs positioned at the sides, palms of the hands facing forward, thumbs facing away from the body, and fingers extended (Fig. 3.1). Other common terms to describe anatomical spatial relationships and positions are shown in Table 3.1 (4).

### Planes of Motion and Axes of Rotation

There are three basic imaginary planes that pass through the body (Fig. 3.2). The sagittal plane divides the body or structure into the right and left sides. The frontal plane (also called the coronal plane) divides the body or structure into anterior and posterior portions. The transverse plane (also called the cross-sectional, axial, or horizontal plane) divides the body or structure into superior and inferior portions (18). Activities of daily living, exercise, and sports usually involve movement

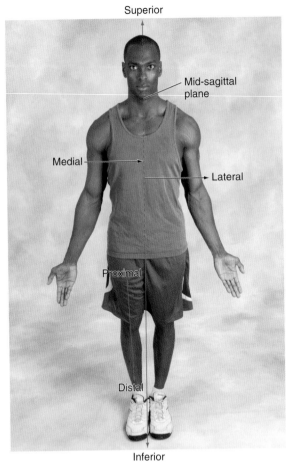

FIGURE 3.1. Anatomical position. Body is erect with the feet together, upper limbs hanging at the sides, palms of the hands facing anteriorly, thumbs facing laterally, and fingers extended. Typically, all anatomical references to the body are relative to this position.

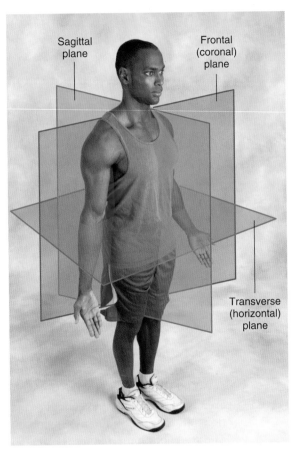

FIGURE 3.2. Anatomical planes of the body.

in more than one plane at a given joint structure. If movement occurs in a plane, it must rotate about an axis that has a 90° relationship to that plane. Thus, movement in the sagittal plane rotates about an axis with a frontal arrangement, movement in the frontal plane rotates about an axis with a sagittal arrangement, and movement in the transverse plane rotates about an axis with a vertical arrangement (38).

## Center of Gravity, Line of Gravity, and Postural Alignment

An object's center of gravity is a theoretical point where the weight force of the object can be considered to act. Center of gravity changes with movement and depends on body position. When a person is standing in a neutral position, the body's center of gravity is approximately at the second sacral segment (31). The kinematics (variation in height and horizontal distance) of the center of gravity relative to the base of support (31) is often studied to examine balance exhibited by the performer. In a sit-to-stand movement, for example, the center of gravity is shifted over the base of support when there is a transition from primarily horizontal motion to a vertical or lifting motion (Fig. 3.3).

| Table 3.1 | Definitions of Anatomical Locations and Positions |
|-----------|---------------------------------------------------|
| **Term** | **Definition** |
| Anterior | The front of the body; ventral |
| Posterior | The back of the body; dorsal |
| Superficial | Located close to or on the body surface |
| Deep | Below the surface |
| Proximal | Closer to any reference point |
| Distal | Farther from any reference point |
| Superior | Toward the head; higher (cephalic) |
| Inferior | Away from the head; lower (caudal) |
| Medial | Toward the midline of the body |
| Lateral | Away from the midline of the body; to the side |
| Ipsilateral | On the same side |
| Contralateral | On the opposite side |
| Unilateral | One side |
| Bilateral | Both sides |
| Prone | Lying face down |
| Supine | Lying face up |
| Valgus | Distal segment of a joint deviates laterally |
| Varus | Distal segment of a joint deviates medially |
| Arm | The region from the shoulder to elbow |
| Forearm | The region from the elbow to the wrist |
| Thigh | The region from the hip to the knee |
| Leg | The region from the knee to the ankle |

The line of gravity of the body is an imaginary vertical line passing through the center of gravity and is typically assessed while the subject is standing (18). The line of gravity helps define proper body alignment and posture, using various superficial landmarks from the head, upper extremity, trunk, and lower extremity regions as guides. From the lateral view, the line of gravity should be slightly posterior to the apex of the coronal suture, through the mastoid process, through the midcervical vertebral bodies, through the shoulder joint, through the midlumbar vertebral bodies, slightly posterior to the axis of the hip joint, slightly anterior to the axis of the knee joint, and slightly anterior to the lateral malleolus. From the posterior view, the line of gravity should pass through the midline of the body, and bilateral structures such as the mastoid, shoulder, iliac crest, knee, and ankles should be in the same horizontal plane (18) (Fig. 3.4). Personal Trainers should consider the ideal line of gravity when describing postural abnormalities.

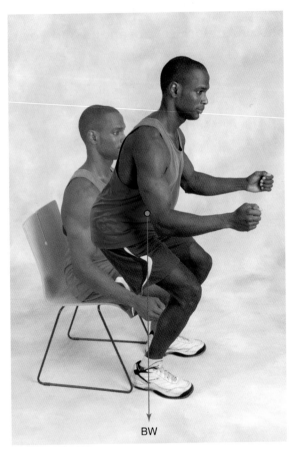

**FIGURE 3.3.** The initial phase of the sit-to-stand movement involves trunk lean and horizontal weight shift to position the center of gravity over the new base of support (feet). The movement of the center of gravity in several directions is often used to study balance. BW, body weight.

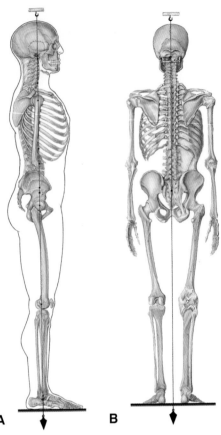

**FIGURE 3.4.** Line of gravity of the skeletal system. **A.** Lateral view. **B.** Posterior view. (Reprinted with permission from Anatomical Chart Company. *ACC's Skeletal System Chart*. Baltimore [MD]: Lippincott Williams & Wilkins; 2000.)

## Joint Movement

Joint movement is often described by its spatial movement pattern in relation to the body, typically in terms of anatomical position. Terms used to describe joint movement are listed in Table 3.2 (18) and discussed in detail for the major joints in the next section.

 ## Musculoskeletal Anatomy

The three primary anatomical structures of the musculoskeletal system that are of interest to the Personal Trainer are bones, joints, and muscles. Mechanically, the interaction of the bones, joints, and muscles determines the range of motion (ROM) of a joint, the specific movement allowed, and the force produced. This section provides an overview of these structures. For in-depth study, the reader is referred to a variety of excellent sources (1,16,28,29,33).

## Skeletal System

The skeletal system consists of cartilage, periosteum, and bone (osseous) tissue. The bones of the skeletal system support soft tissue, protect internal organs, act as important sources of nutrients

| Table 3.2 | Joint Movement |
|---|---|
| **Term** | **Description** |
| Flexion | Movement resulting in a decrease of the joint angle, usually moving anteriorly in the sagittal plane |
| Extension | Movement resulting in an increase of the joint angle, usually moving posteriorly in the sagittal plane |
| Abduction | Movement away from the midline of the body, usually in the frontal plane |
| Adduction | Movement toward the midline of the body, usually in the frontal plane |
| Horizontal abduction | Movement away from the midline of the body in the transverse plane, usually used to describe horizontal humerus movement when the shoulder is flexed at 90° |
| Horizontal adduction | Movement toward the midline of the body in the transverse plane, usually used to describe horizontal humerus movement when the shoulder is flexed at 90° |
| Internal (medial) rotation | Rotation in the transverse plane toward the midline of the body |
| External (lateral) rotation | Rotation in the transverse plane away from the midline of the body |
| Lateral flexion (right or left) | Movement away from the midline of the body in the frontal plane, usually used to describe neck and trunk movement |
| Rotation (right or left) | Right or left rotation in the transverse plane, usually used to describe neck and trunk movement |
| Elevation | Movement of the scapula superiorly in the frontal plane |
| Depression | Movement of the scapula inferiorly in the frontal plane |
| Retraction | Movement of the scapula toward the spine in the frontal plane |
| Protraction | Movement of the scapula away from the spine in the frontal plane |
| Upward rotation | Superior and lateral movement of the inferior angle of the scapula in the frontal plane |
| Downward rotation | Inferior and medial movement of the inferior angle of the scapula in the frontal plane |
| Circumduction | A compound circular movement involving flexion, extension, abduction, and adduction, circumscribing a cone shape |
| Radial deviation | Abduction of the wrist in the frontal plane |
| Ulnar deviation | Adduction of the wrist in the frontal plane |
| Opposition | Diagonal movement of thumb across the palmar surface of the hand to make contact with the fifth digit |
| Eversion | Abducting the ankle |
| Inversion | Adducting the ankle |
| Dorsiflexion | Flexing the ankle so that the foot moves anteriorly in the sagittal plane |
| Plantarflexion | Extending the ankle so that the foot moves posteriorly in the sagittal plane |
| Pronation (foot/ankle) | Combined movements of abduction and eversion resulting in lowering of the medial margin of the foot |
| Supination (foot/ankle) | Combined movements of adduction and inversion resulting in raising of the medial margin of the foot |

and blood constituents and serve as rigid levers for movement. There are 206 bones in the human body, 177 of which engage in voluntary movement. The skull, hyoid, vertebral column, sternum, and ribs are considered the axial skeleton; the remaining bones, in particular those of the upper and lower limbs and their respective girdles, are considered the appendicular skeleton (36). The major bones of the body are illustrated in Figure 3.5.

The structure of a bone can be explained using a typical long bone such as the femur (the long bone of the thigh). The main portion of a long bone or shaft is called the "diaphysis" (Fig. 3.6). The ends of the bone are called the "epiphyses" (singular is "epiphysis"). The epiphyses are covered by articular cartilage. Cartilage is a resilient, semi-rigid form of connective tissue that reduces the friction and absorbs some of the shock in synovial joints. The region of mature bone where the diaphysis joins each epiphysis is called the "metaphysis." In an immature bone, this region includes the epiphyseal plate, also called the "growth plate." The medullary cavity, or marrow cavity, is the space inside the diaphysis. Lining the marrow cavity is the endosteum, which contains cells necessary for bone development. The periosteum is a membrane covering the surface of bones, except at the articular surfaces. The periosteum is composed of two layers: an outer fibrous layer and an inner highly vascular layer that contains cells for the creation of a new bone. The periosteum serves as a point of attachment for ligaments and tendons and is critical for bone growth, repair, and nutrition (31).

There are two types of bones (2): cortical (compact) and trabecular (spongy). The main differences between the two types are the architecture and amount of matter and space they contain. Compact bone is architecturally arranged in "osteons" that contain few spaces. It forms the external layer of all bones of the body and a large portion of the diaphysis of the long bones, where it provides support for bearing weight. In contrast, spongy bone is characterized as being much

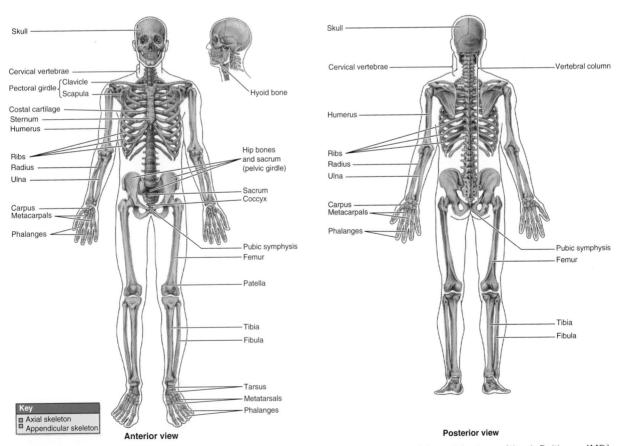

**FIGURE 3.5.**  Divisions of the skeletal system. (From Moore KL, Dalley AF II. *Clinically Oriented Anatomy.* 4th ed. Baltimore [MD]: Lippincott Williams & Wilkins; 1999, with permission.)

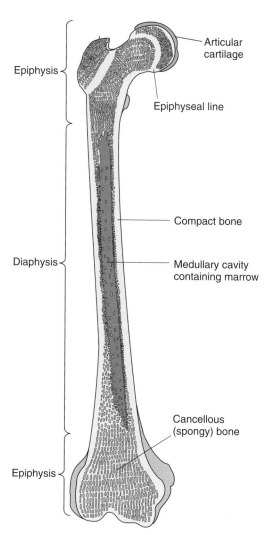

Epiphysis

Articular
cartilage

Epiphyseal line

Compact bone

Diaphysis

Medullary cavity
containing marrow

Cancellous
(spongy) bone

Epiphysis

**FIGURE 3.6.** Bone anatomy. (From Willis MC. *Medical Terminology: A Programmed Learning Approach to the Language of Health Care.* 2nd ed. Baltimore [MD]: Lippincott Williams & Wilkins; 2011, with permission.)

less dense. It consists of a three-dimensional lattice composed of beams or struts of bone called "trabeculae." Open spaces are present between the trabeculae, unlike in compact bone. The trabeculae are oriented to provide strength against the stresses normally encountered by the bone. In some bones, the space within these trabeculae is filled with red bone marrow, which produces blood (31).

Bones are also classified according to their shape. Long bones contain a diaphysis with a medullary canal (*e.g.*, femur, tibia, humerus, ulna, and radius). Short bones are relatively small and thick (*e.g.*, carpals and tarsals). Flat bones are plate-like (*e.g.*, sternum, scapulae, ribs, and pelvis). Irregular bones are oddly shaped (*e.g.*, vertebrae, sacrum, and coccyx). Finally, sesamoid bones are found within tendons and joint capsules and are shaped like sesame seeds (*e.g.*, patella) (38).

## Articular System

Joints are the articulations between bones, and along with bones and ligaments, they constitute the articular system. Ligaments are tough, fibrous connective tissues anchoring bone to bone. Joints are classified as synarthrodial, amphiarthrodial, or diarthrodial (synovial) (31). Synarthrodial joints (*e.g.*, sutures of the skull) do not move appreciably. Amphiarthrodial joints move slightly and are held together by ligaments (syndesmosis; *e.g.*, inferior tibiofibular joint) or fibrocartilage (synchondrosis; *e.g.*, pubic symphysis). Synarthrodial and amphiarthrodial joints do not contain an articular cavity, synovial membrane, or synovial fluid (31).

## Synovial Joints

The most common type of joint in the human body is the synovial joint. Synovial joints contain a fibrous articular capsule and an inner synovial membrane that encloses the joint cavity. Figure 3.7 illustrates a synovial joint's unique capsular arrangement. There are five distinct features of a synovial joint (31):

1. It is enclosed by a fibrous joint capsule.
2. The joint capsule encloses the joint cavity.
3. The joint cavity is lined with synovial membrane.
4. Synovial fluid occupies the joint cavity.
5. The articulating surfaces of the bones are covered with hyaline cartilage, which helps absorb shock and reduces friction.

The synovial membrane produces synovial fluid, which provides constant lubrication during movement to minimize the wearing effects of friction on the cartilaginous covering of the articulating bones (31). Ligaments sometimes reinforce synovial joints. These ligaments are either separate structures (extrinsic) or a thickening of the outer layer of the joint capsule (intrinsic). The collagen fibers of ligaments are typically arranged to counteract multidimensional stresses. Some synovial joints have other structures such as articular discs (*e.g.*, meniscus of the knee), bursae, or fat pads. There are seven major types of synovial joints classified by the shape of the articulating surfaces or types of movement allowed. Table 3.3 summarizes the joint classifications and examples in the human body. Table 3.4 summarizes the motions of the major joints and the planes in which they occur.

Synovial joints are typically perfused by numerous arterial branches and are innervated by branches of the nerves supplying the adjacent muscle and overlying skin. Proprioceptive feedback is a

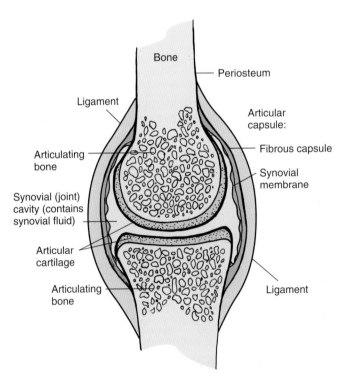

**FIGURE 3.7.** Synovial joint. (From Oatis CA. *Kinesiology: The Mechanics and Pathomechanics of Human Movement*. 3rd ed. Baltimore [MD]: Lippincott Williams & Wilkins; 2016, with permission.)

| Table 3.3 | Classification of Joints in the Human Body |
|---|---|
| **Joint Classification** | **Features and Examples** |
| **Fibrous** | |
| Suture | Tight union unique to the skull |
| Syndesmosis | Interosseous membrane between bones (*e.g.*, the union along the shafts of the radius and ulna, tibia and fibula, and distal tibiofibular joint) |
| Gomphosis | Unique joint at the tooth socket |
| **Cartilaginous** | |
| Primary (synchondroses; hyaline cartilaginous) | Usually temporary to permit bone growth and typically fuse (*e.g.*, epiphyseal plates); some do not (*e.g.*, at the sternum and rib [costal cartilage]) |
| Secondary (symphyses; fibrocartilaginous) | Strong, slightly movable joints (*e.g.*, intervertebral discs, pubic symphysis) |
| **Synovial** | |
| Plane (arthrodial) | Gliding and sliding movements (*e.g.*, acromioclavicular joint) |
| Hinge (ginglymus) | Uniaxial movements (*e.g.*, elbow extension and flexion) |
| Ellipsoidal (condyloid) | Biaxial joint (*e.g.*, radiocarpal extension, flexion at the wrist) |
| Saddle (sellar) | Unique joint that permits movements in all planes, including opposition (*e.g.*, the carpometacarpal joint of the thumb) |
| Ball-and-socket (enarthrodial) | Multiaxial joints that permit movements in all directions (*e.g.*, hip and shoulder joints) |
| Pivot (trochoidal) | Uniaxial joints that permit rotation (*e.g.*, proximal radioulnar and atlantoaxial joints) |
| Bicondylar | Allow movement primarily around one axis with some limited rotation in a second axis (*e.g.*, knee flexion and extension with limited internal and external rotation) |

significant joint sensation, as is pain, because of the high density of sensory fibers in the joint capsule. This feedback has obvious importance in regulating human movement and preventing injury (31).

## Joint Movements and Range of Motion

Joint movement is a combination of rolling, sliding, and spinning of the joint surfaces (4). "Open chain" movements occur when the distal segment of a joint moves in space. An example of an open chain movement for the knee joint is leg extension exercise on a machine. "Closed chain" movements occur when the distal segment of the joint is fixed in space. An example of a closed chain movement for the knee joint is standing barbell squats. A joint is in a "closed pack" position when there is both maximal congruency of the joint surfaces and maximal tautness of the joint capsule and ligaments (4). A joint is in an "open pack" (loose) position when there is the least joint congruency and the joint capsule and ligaments are most loose. Movement at one joint may influence the

| Table 3.4 | Major Joint Motions and Planes of Motion | | |
|-----------|-------------------------------------------|---|---|
| **Major Joints** | **Type of Joints** | **Joint Movements** | **Planes** |
| Scapulothoracic | Not a true joint ("physiological" or "functional" joint) | Elevation–depression<br>Upward–downward rotation<br>Protraction–retraction<br>Medial–lateral rotation<br>Anterior–posterior tilting | Frontal<br>Frontal<br>Frontal<br>Transitional<br>Sagittal |
| Glenohumeral | Synovial: ball-and-socket | Flexion–extension<br>Abduction–adduction<br>Internal–external rotation<br>Horizontal abduction–adduction<br>Circumduction | Sagittal<br>Frontal<br>Transverse<br>Transverse<br>Multiple |
| Elbow | Synovial: hinge | Flexion–extension | Sagittal |
| Proximal radioulnar | Synovial: pivot | Pronation–supination | Transverse |
| Wrist | Synovial: ellipsoidal | Flexion–extension<br>Abduction–adduction | Sagittal<br>Frontal |
| Metacarpophalangeal | Synovial: ellipsoidal | Flexion–extension<br>Abduction–adduction | Sagittal<br>Frontal |
| Proximal and distal interphalangeal | Synovial: hinge | Flexion–extension | Sagittal |
| Intervertebral | Cartilaginous | Flexion–extension<br>Lateral flexion<br>Rotation | Sagittal<br>Frontal<br>Transverse |
| Hip | Synovial: ball-and-socket | Flexion–extension<br>Abduction–adduction<br>Internal–external rotation<br>Circumduction | Sagittal<br>Frontal<br>Transverse<br>Multiple |
| Knee | Synovial: bicondylar | Flexion–extension<br>Internal–external rotation | Sagittal<br>Transverse |
| Ankle: talocrural | Synovial: hinge | Dorsiflexion–plantarflexion | Sagittal |
| Ankle: subtalar | Synovial: gliding | Inversion–eversion | Frontal |

extent of movement at adjacent joints because a number of muscles and other soft tissue structures cross multiple joints. For example, finger flexion decreases in the presence of wrist flexion because muscles that flex both the wrist and fingers cross multiple joints (4).

"Open chain" movements occur when the distal segment of a joint moves in space. "Closed chain" movements occur when the distal segment of the joint is fixed in space. The degree of movement within a joint is called the ROM. It can be active (the range that can be reached by voluntary movement from contraction of skeletal muscle) or passive (the ROM that can be achieved by external means). Joints with excessive ROM are called "hypermobile," and joints with restricted ROM are called "hypomobile" (4). Joint ROM is quantified using goniometers or inclinometers, and each joint has normal ROM values for reference purposes (18). ROM measures at baseline help guide the exercise prescription, and ROM measures at follow-up help document progress.

## Joint Stability

The stability of a joint is its resistance to displacement. All joints do not have the same degree of stability, and in general, ROM is gained at the expense of stability. Five factors account for joint stability (4):

1. Ligaments facilitate normal movement and resist excessive movement.
2. Muscles and tendons that span a joint also enhance stability, particularly when the bony structure alone contributes little stability (*e.g.*, shoulder).
3. Fascia contributes to joint stability (*e.g.*, iliotibial band of the tensor fasciae latae).
4. Atmospheric pressure creates greater force outside of the joint than internal pressure exerts within the joint cavity (the suction created by this pressure is an important factor in aiding joint stability).
5. The bony structure of a joint is an important contributor to joint stability (*e.g.*, limitation of elbow extension by the olecranon process of the ulna) (4).

# Muscular System

Bones provide support and leverage to the body, but without muscles, movement would not be possible. There are three types of muscle tissue: skeletal, cardiac, and smooth muscle. Skeletal muscle is primarily attached to bones and is under voluntary control. Skeletal muscle is responsible for moving the skeletal system and stabilizing the body (*e.g.*, maintaining posture). There are more than 600 skeletal muscles in the human body (38), approximately 100 of which are primary movement muscles with which Personal Trainers should be familiar (4). The superficial muscles of the body are shown in Figures 3.8 and 3.9.

Skeletal muscles are generally anchored to the skeleton by tendons. Tendons are dense cords of connective tissue that attach a muscle to the periosteum of the bone. The collagen fibers of tendons are in parallel arrangement, which makes the tendon suitable for unidirectional stress. When the tendon is flat and broad, it is called an "aponeurosis." Tendons and aponeuroses provide the mechanical link between skeletal muscle and bone. Bursae are often positioned between tendons and bony prominences to allow the tendons to slide easily across the bones (31).

## Classification of Skeletal Muscles

Skeletal muscles can be classified according to their muscle fiber architecture (*i.e.*, the arrangement of muscle fiber relative to the line of pull of the muscle) (Fig. 3.10). Muscles typically have either a parallel arrangement or a pennate arrangement. In parallel muscle, the muscle fibers run in line with the pull of the muscle. Fusiform muscles have a parallel arrangement and are spindle shaped, tapering at each end (*e.g.*, biceps brachii). Longitudinal muscles are strap-like, with parallel fibers (*e.g.*, sartorius). Quadrate muscles are four-sided, are usually flat, and consist of parallel fibers (*e.g.*, rhomboids). Fan-shaped or triangular muscles contain fibers that radiate from a narrow attachment at one end to a broad attachment at the other (*e.g.*, pectoralis major) (38).

In pennate muscle, the fibers run obliquely or at an angle to the line of pull. Pennate muscles can be classified as unipennate (fibers only on one side of the tendon; *e.g.*, flexor pollicis longus), bipennate (fibers on both sides of a centrally positioned tendon; *e.g.*, rectus femoris), or multipennate (two or more fasciculi attaching obliquely and combined into one muscle; *e.g.*, subscapularis) (38).

Muscles can also be described on the basis of the number of joints upon which they act. For example, a muscle that causes movement at one joint is uniarticular (*e.g.*, brachialis). Muscles that cross more than one joint are referred to as biarticular (having actions at two joints, *e.g.*, hamstring

There are more than 600 skeletal muscles in the human body (38), approximately 100 of which are primary movement muscles with which Personal Trainers should be familiar (4).

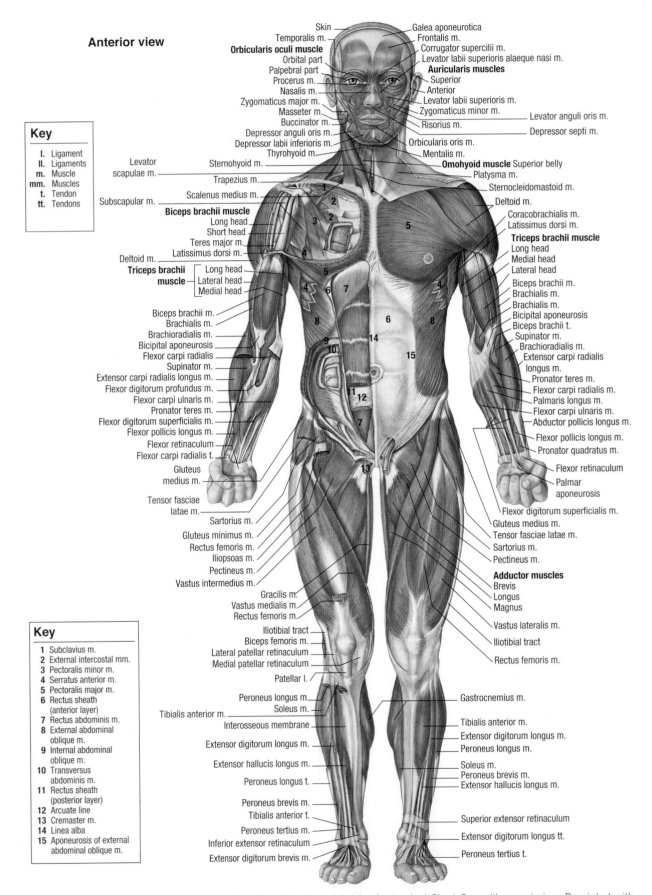

**Anterior view**

**Key**

| | |
|---|---|
| **l.** | Ligament |
| **ll.** | Ligaments |
| **m.** | Muscle |
| **mm.** | Muscles |
| **t.** | Tendon |
| **tt.** | Tendons |

**Key**

1 Subclavius m.
2 External intercostal mm.
3 Pectoralis minor m.
4 Serratus anterior m.
5 Pectoralis major m.
6 Rectus sheath (anterior layer)
7 Rectus abdominis m.
8 External abdominal oblique m.
9 Internal abdominal oblique m.
10 Transversus abdominis m.
11 Rectus sheath (posterior layer)
12 Arcuate line
13 Cremaster m.
14 Linea alba
15 Aponeurosis of external abdominal oblique m.

**FIGURE 3.8.** Superficial muscles — anterior view. (Asset provided by Anatomical Chart Co., with permission. Reprinted with permission from Anatomical Chart Company. *ACC's Muscular System Chart.* Baltimore [MD]: Lippincott Williams & Wilkins; 2002.)

**Posterior view**

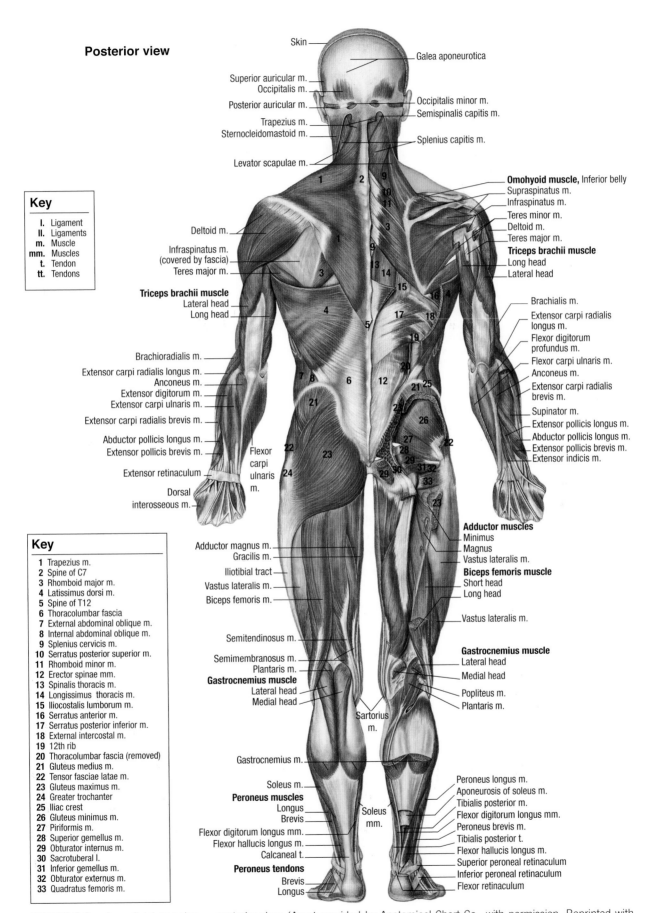

Skin
Galea aponeurotica
Superior auricular m.
Occipitalis m.
Posterior auricular m.
Occipitalis minor m.
Semispinalis capitis m.
Trapezius m.
Sternocleidomastoid m.
Splenius capitis m.
Levator scapulae m.

**Omohyoid muscle,** Inferior belly
Supraspinatus m.
Infraspinatus m.
Teres minor m.
Deltoid m.
Teres major m.
**Triceps brachii muscle**
Long head
Lateral head

Deltoid m.
Infraspinatus m.
(covered by fascia)
Teres major m.

**Triceps brachii muscle**
Lateral head
Long head

Brachialis m.
Extensor carpi radialis
longus m.
Flexor digitorum
profundus m.
Flexor carpi ulnaris m.
Anconeus m.
Extensor carpi radialis
brevis m.
Supinator m.
Extensor pollicis longus m.
Abductor pollicis longus m.
Extensor pollicis brevis m.
Extensor indicis m.

Brachioradialis m.
Extensor carpi radialis longus m.
Anconeus m.
Extensor digitorum m.
Extensor carpi ulnaris m.
Extensor carpi radialis brevis m.
Abductor pollicis longus m.
Extensor pollicis brevis m.
Extensor retinaculum
Flexor
carpi
ulnaris
m.
Dorsal
interosseous m.

**Adductor muscles**
Minimus
Magnus
Vastus lateralis m.
**Biceps femoris muscle**
Short head
Long head
Vastus lateralis m.

Adductor magnus m.
Gracilis m.
Iliotibial tract
Vastus lateralis m.
Biceps femoris m.

**Gastrocnemius muscle**
Lateral head
Medial head
Popliteus m.
Plantaris m.

Semitendinosus m.
Semimembranosus m.
Plantaris m.
**Gastrocnemius muscle**
Lateral head
Medial head
Sartorius
m.

Gastrocnemius m.
Soleus m.
**Peroneus muscles**
Longus
Brevis
Flexor digitorum longus mm.
Flexor hallucis longus m.
Calcaneal t.
**Peroneus tendons**
Brevis
Longus
Soleus
mm.

Peroneus longus m.
Aponeurosis of soleus m.
Tibialis posterior m.
Flexor digitorum longus mm.
Peroneus brevis m.
Tibialis posterior t.
Flexor hallucis longus m.
Superior peroneal retinaculum
Inferior peroneal retinaculum
Flexor retinaculum

**Key**

I. Ligament
II. Ligaments
m. Muscle
mm. Muscles
t. Tendon
tt. Tendons

**Key**

1 Trapezius m.
2 Spine of C7
3 Rhomboid major m.
4 Latissimus dorsi m.
5 Spine of T12
6 Thoracolumbar fascia
7 External abdominal oblique m.
8 Internal abdominal oblique m.
9 Splenius cervicis m.
10 Serratus posterior superior m.
11 Rhomboid minor m.
12 Erector spinae mm.
13 Spinalis thoracis m.
14 Longissimus thoracis m.
15 Iliocostalis lumborum m.
16 Serratus anterior m.
17 Serratus posterior inferior m.
18 External intercostal m.
19 12th rib
20 Thoracolumbar fascia (removed)
21 Gluteus medius m.
22 Tensor fasciae latae m.
23 Gluteus maximus m.
24 Greater trochanter
25 Iliac crest
26 Gluteus minimus m.
27 Piriformis m.
28 Superior gemellus m.
29 Obturator internus m.
30 Sacrotuberal l.
31 Inferior gemellus m.
32 Obturator externus m.
33 Quadratus femoris m.

**FIGURE 3.9.** Superficial muscles — posterior view. (Asset provided by Anatomical Chart Co., with permission. Reprinted with permission from Anatomical Chart Company. *ACC's Muscular System Chart*. Baltimore [MD]: Lippincott Williams & Wilkins; 2002.)

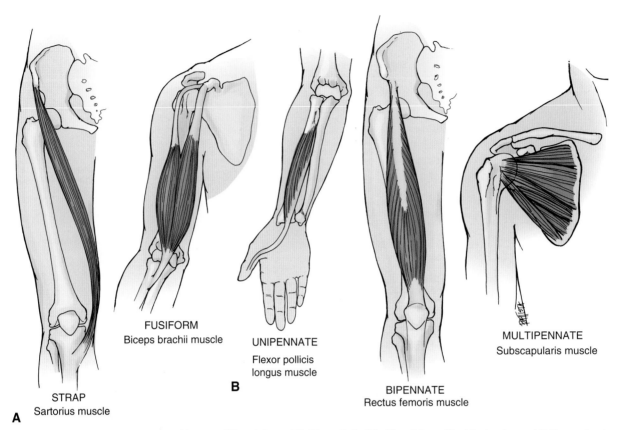

FUSIFORM
Biceps brachii muscle

UNIPENNATE

Flexor pollicis
longus muscle

**B**

MULTIPENNATE
Subscapularis muscle

BIPENNATE
Rectus femoris muscle

STRAP
Sartorius muscle

**A**

**FIGURE 3.10.** Skeletal muscle architecture **(A)** and shape **(B)**. (From Oatis CA. *Kinesiology: The Mechanics and Pathomechanics of Human Movement.* 3rd ed. Baltimore [MD]: Lippincott Williams & Wilkins; 2016, with permission.)

muscles and biceps brachii) or multiarticular (*e.g.,* erector spinae). The main advantage of bi- and multiarticular muscles is that only one muscle is needed to generate tension in two or more joints. This is more efficient and conserves energy. In many instances, the length of the muscle stays within 100% to 130% of the resting length. As one side of the muscle shortens, the other side lengthens, maintaining a near constant overall length. This property of bi- and multiarticular muscles enhances tension production (4).

## How Muscles Produce Movement

Skeletal muscles produce force that is transferred to the tendons, which in turn pull on the bones and other structures, such as the skin. Most muscles cross a joint, so when a muscle contracts, it pulls one of the articulating bones toward the other. Usually, both articulating bones do not move equally; one of the articulating bones remains relatively stationary. The attachment that is usually more stationary and proximal (especially in the extremities) is called the "origin." The muscle attachment located on the bone that moves more and is usually located more distally is called the "insertion" (4).

## Muscle Roles

Movements of the human body generally require several muscles working together rather than a single muscle doing all the work. Keep in mind that muscles cannot push, they can only pull;

therefore, most skeletal muscles are arranged in opposing pairs such as flexor–extensor, internal–external rotator, and abductor–adductor. Muscles can be classified according to their roles during movement (38). When a muscle or a group of muscles is responsible for the action or movement, it is called a "prime mover" or "agonist." For example, during a biceps curl, the prime movers are the elbow flexors, which include the biceps brachii, brachialis, and brachioradialis muscles. The opposing group of muscles is called the antagonist (*e.g.*, the triceps brachii and anconeus muscles in biceps curl). Antagonists relax to permit the primary movement and contract to act as a brake at the completion of the movement. In addition, most movements also involve other muscles called "synergists." The role of synergists is to prevent unwanted movement, which helps the prime movers perform more efficiently. Synergists can also act as fixators or stabilizers. In this role, the muscles stabilize a portion of the body against a force (38). For example, the scapular muscles (*e.g.*, rhomboids, serratus anterior, and trapezius) must provide a stable base of support for the upper extremity muscles during the throwing motion. Co-contraction is the simultaneous contraction of the agonist and antagonist. Co-contraction of the abdominal and lumbar muscles, for example, helps stabilize the lower trunk during trunk movements (25).

##  Specific Joint Anatomy and Considerations

Muscle actions produce force that causes joint movement during exercise. Personal Trainers need a solid working knowledge of the functional anatomy and kinesiology of major joint structures. Tables 3.5 and 3.6 summarize the major joint movements, muscles that produce those movements, normal ROM values, and examples of resistance exercises for the muscles. This knowledge is the basis for the development of exercise programs to be used in training (8). In this section, we describe the structure and function of each of the major joints of the body in four steps:

1. Structure: What are the initial considerations of the joint's structure (*e.g.*, bones, muscles, tendons, ligaments, cartilage, bursae) and ability to move?
2. Movements: What movements occur at the joint? What are the normal ROMs for each movement?
3. Muscles: What specific muscles are being used to create the movements? How are the muscles being used (*e.g.*, agonist, synergist, stabilizer)?
4. Injuries: What common injuries occur to the joint structure?

### Upper Extremity

The shoulder complex is a multijoint structure that provides the link between the thoracic cage and upper extremity. The shoulder has a high degree of mobility; as a result, the shoulder region is very unstable.

#### *Shoulder*

The shoulder complex is a multijoint structure that provides the link between the thoracic cage and upper extremity. The shoulder is a ball-and-socket joint. It has a high degree of mobility and, as a result, is very unstable. Because the bony structures of the shoulder provide relatively little support, much of the responsibility for stabilizing this region falls on the soft tissues — the muscles, ligaments, and joint capsules. Thus, the shoulder is more likely to be injured than the hip (3).

| Table 3.5 | **Major Upper Extremity Joints: Movements, Range of Motion, Muscles, and Example Resistance Exercises** | | | |
|---|---|---|---|---|
| Joint | Movement | Range of Motion (°) | Major Agonist Muscles | Examples of Resistance Exercises |
| Scapulothoracic | Fixation | | Serratus anterior, pectoralis minor, trapezius, levator scapulae, rhomboids | Push-up, parallel bar dip, upright row, shoulder shrug, seated row |
| | Upward rotation | | Trapezius | |
| | Downward rotation | | Rhomboids, pectoralis minor, levator scapulae | |
| | Elevation | | Rhomboids, levator scapulae, trapezius | Shoulder shrug |
| | Depression | | Pectoralis minor, trapezius | |
| | Protraction | | Serratus anterior, pectoralis minor | Supine dumbbell serratus press, push-up |
| | Retraction | | Rhomboids, trapezius | Seated row |
| Glenohumeral (shoulder) | Flexion | 90–100 | Anterior deltoid, pectoralis major (clavicular head), biceps brachii (long head) | Dumbbell front raise, incline bench press |
| | Extension | 40–60 | Latissimus dorsi, teres major, pectoralis major (sternocostal head), posterior deltoid and triceps brachii (long head) | Dumbbell pullover, chin-up |
| | Abduction | 90–95 | Middle deltoid, supraspinatus | Dumbbell lateral raise, dumbbell press |
| | Adduction | 0 | Latissimus dorsi, teres major, pectoralis major | Lat pull-down, seated row, cable crossover, flat bench dumbbell fly |
| | Horizontal abduction | 45 | Posterior deltoid, teres major, latissimus dorsi | Prone reverse dumbbell fly, reverse cable fly |
| | Horizontal adduction | 135 | Pectoralis major, anterior deltoid | Flat bench chest fly, pec dec, cable crossover |
| | Internal rotation | 70–90 | Latissimus dorsi, teres major, subscapularis, pectoralis major, anterior deltoid | Lat pull-down, bent over row, dumbbell row, rotator cuff exercises, dumbbell press, parallel bar dip, front raises |
| | External rotation | 70–90 | Infraspinatus, teres minor, posterior deltoid | External rotator cuff exercises — dumbbell side-lying, cable in; rotator cuff exercises — dumbbell side-lying, cable |

| Table 3.5 | Major Upper Extremity Joints: Movements, Range of Motion, Muscles, and Example Resistance Exercises *(continued)* | | | |
|---|---|---|---|---|
| Joint | Movement | Range of Motion (°) | Major Agonist Muscles | Examples of Resistance Exercises |
| Elbow | Flexion | 145–150 | Biceps brachii, brachialis, brachioradialis | Dumbbell curl, preacher curl, hammer curl |
| | Extension | 0 | Triceps brachii, anconeus | Dip, pulley triceps extension, close grip bench press, push-downs, dumbbell kickback |
| Radioulnar | Supination | 80–90 | Biceps brachii, supinator | Dumbbell curl (with supination) |
| | Pronation | 70–90 | Pronator quadratus, pronator teres | Dumbbell pronation |
| Wrist | Flexion | 70–90 | Flexor carpi radialis and ulnaris, palmaris longus, flexor digitorum superficialis | Dumbbell wrist curl |
| | Extension | 65–85 | Extensor carpi radialis longus, brevis, and ulnaris, extensor digitorum | Dumbbell reverse wrist curl |
| | Adduction | 25–40 | Flexor and extensor carpi ulnaris | Wrist curl, reverse wrist curl |
| | Abduction | 15–25 | Extensor carpi radialis longus and brevis, flexor carpi radialis | Wrist curl, reverse wrist curl |

## STRUCTURE

### Bones

The bones of the shoulder region include humerus, scapula, and clavicle (Fig. 3.11). The humerus is a long bone and is the major bone of the arm. The humeral head is rounded and articulates with the glenoid fossa of the scapula. The greater and lesser tubercles of the humerus are attachment sites for many of the muscles that act on the shoulder. The scapula is a large triangular bone that rests on the posterior thoracic cage between the second rib and the seventh rib in the normal position. The scapula lies in the scaption plane, that is, obliquely at 30° to the frontal plane. The glenoid fossa of the scapula faces anterolaterally. The acromion process is located at the superior aspect of the scapula and articulates with the clavicle. The clavicle runs obliquely at 60° to the scapula and provides the link between the upper extremity and the axial skeleton. The clavicle provides protection for the neural bundle called the "brachial plexus" and the vascular system supplying the upper extremity, supports the weight of the humerus, and helps maintain the position of the scapula and the humerus (36).

### Ligaments and Bursae

The ligaments and bursae of the shoulder region are shown in Figure 3.12, and some of these structures are discussed in this section. The coracohumeral ligament spans the bicipital groove of the humerus and provides anteroinferior stability to the glenohumeral joint. The glenohumeral ligament (anterior, middle, and anteroinferior bands) reinforces the anterior capsule and provides stability to the shoulder joint in most planes of movement. The coracoacromial ligament, located

| Table 3.6 | | Major Spine and Lower Extremity Joints: Movements, Range of Motion, Muscles, and Example Resistance Exercises | | |
|---|---|---|---|---|
| **Joint** | **Movement** | **Range of Motion (°)** | **Major Agonist Muscles** | **Examples of Resistance Exercises** |
| Cervical spine | Flexion | 50 | Sternocleidomastoid, anterior scalene, longus capitis/colli | Machine neck flexion |
| | Extension | 60 | Suboccipitals, splenius capitis/cervicis, erector spinae | Machine neck extension |
| | Lateral flexion | 45 | Unilateral contraction of flexor–extensor muscles above | Machine neck lateral flexion |
| | Rotation | 80 | Unilateral contraction of flexor–extensor muscles above | Machine neck rotation |
| Lumbar spine | Flexion | 60 | Rectus abdominis, internal–external oblique abdominis | Crunch, leg raise, machine crunch, high pulley crunch |
| | Extension | 25 | Erector spinae, multifidus | Roman chair, machine trunk extension, dead lift, squat, good morning |
| | Lateral flexion | 25 | Quadratus lumborum, internal–external oblique abdominals, unilateral erector spinae | Roman chair side bend, dumbbell side bend, hanging leg raise |
| | Rotation | | Internal–external oblique abdominals, intrinsic spinal rotators, multifidus | Broomstick twist, machine trunk rotation |
| Hip | Flexion | 130 | Iliopsoas, rectus femoris, sartorius, pectineus, tensor fasciae latae | Leg raise, sit-up, machine crunch |
| | Extension | 30 | Gluteus maximus, hamstrings | Squat, leg press, lunge, machine leg extension |
| | Abduction | 35 | Tensor fasciae latae, sartorius, gluteus medius and minimus | Cable or machine hip abduction |
| | Adduction | 30 | Adductor longus, brevis, and magnus, gracilis, and pectineus | Power squats, cable or machine hip adduction, lunge |
| | Internal rotation | 45 | Semitendinosus, semimembranosus, gluteus medius and minimus, tensor fasciae latae | |
| | External rotation | 50 | Biceps femoris, sartorius, gluteus maximus, deep rotators (piriformis, superior and inferior gemelli, internal and external obturators, quadratus femoris) | |

| Table 3.6 | **Major Spine and Lower Extremity Joints: Movements, Range of Motion, Muscles, and Example Resistance Exercises** (continued) | | | |
|---|---|---|---|---|
| **Joint** | **Movement** | **Range of Motion (°)** | **Major Agonist Muscles** | **Examples of Resistance Exercises** |
| Knee | Flexion | 140 | Hamstrings, gracilis, sartorius, popliteus, gastrocnemius | Leg curl (standing, seated, prone) |
| | Extension | 0–10 | Quadriceps femoris | Lunge, squats, machine leg extension |
| | Internal rotation | 30 | Gracilis, semimembranosus, semitendinosus | |
| | External rotation | 45 | Biceps femoris | |
| Ankle: talocrural | Dorsiflexion | 15–20 | Tibialis anterior, extensor digitorum longus, extensor hallucis longus, peroneus (fibularis) tertius | Ankle dorsiflexion resistance band |
| | Plantarflexion | 50 | Gastrocnemius, soleus, tibialis posterior, flexor digitorum longus, flexor hallucis longus | Standing/seated calf raise, donkey calf raise |
| Ankle: subtalar | Eversion | 5–15 | Peroneus (fibularis) longus and brevis | Elastic band eversion |
| | Inversion | 20–30 | Tibialis anterior and posterior | Elastic band inversion |

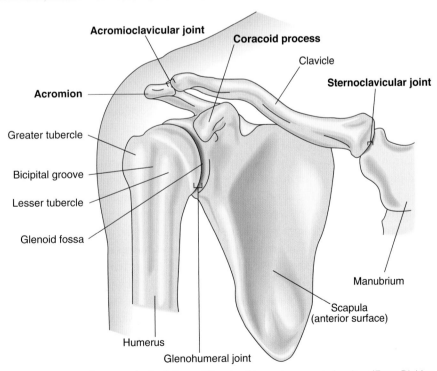

**FIGURE 3.11.**  Bones and articulations of the shoulder region — anterior view. (From Bickley LS, Szilagyi P. *Bates' Guide to Physical Examination and History Taking.* 8th ed. Philadelphia [PA]: Lippincott Williams & Wilkins; 2003, with permission.)

**FIGURE 3.12.** Ligaments and bursae of the shoulder region — anterior view. (From Hendrickson T. *Massage for Orthopedic Conditions.* Baltimore [MD]: Lippincott Williams & Wilkins; 2003, with permission.)

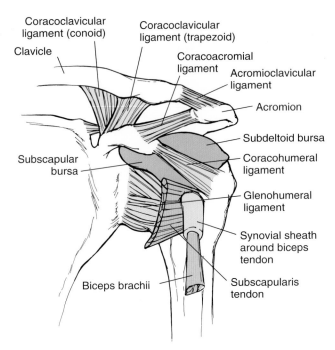

superior to the glenohumeral joint, protects the muscles, tendons, nerves, and blood supply of the region and prevents superior dislocation of the humeral head. The acromioclavicular ligament is the major ligament that provides stability to the acromioclavicular joint. The coracoclavicular ligament (trapezoid and conoid bands) prevents superior dislocation of the acromioclavicular joint. The sternoclavicular ligaments (anterior and posterior) help strengthen the capsule of the sternoclavicular joint. The costoclavicular ligament connects the first rib and clavicle, and the interclavicular ligament connects the two clavicles and manubrium. The subacromial (subdeltoid) bursa, which lies between the supraspinatus and deltoid tendons and the acromion, allows gliding and cushioning of these structures, especially upon shoulder abduction (4).

## Joints

The shoulder region is a complex of four joints: the glenohumeral (shoulder), acromioclavicular, sternoclavicular, and scapulothoracic joints (see Fig. 3.12). The glenohumeral joint is a ball-and-socket joint and is the most freely moveable joint in the body. It consists of the articulation of the spherical head of the humerus with the small, shallow, and somewhat pear-shaped glenoid fossa of the scapula. The glenoid labrum (which is composed of fibrocartilage) of the scapula deepens the fossa and cushions against impact of the humeral head in forceful movements (4) (Fig. 3.13).

The acromioclavicular joint is a plane synovial joint of the articulation of the acromion and the distal end of the clavicle. The acromioclavicular joint moves in three planes simultaneously with scapulothoracic motion. The sternoclavicular joint, the articulation of the proximal clavicle with the sternum and cartilage of the first rib, is a saddle synovial joint. The sternoclavicular joint moves in synchronization with the other three joints of the shoulder region and, importantly, provides the only bony connection between the humerus and the axial skeleton (38).

The scapulothoracic joint is not a true joint but a physiological (functional) joint. It is formed by the articulation of the scapula with the thoracic cage. In the kinematic chain, any movement of the scapulothoracic joint results in movement of the acromioclavicular, sternoclavicular, and glenohumeral joints. The scapulothoracic joint provides mobility and stability for the orientation of the glenoid fossa and the humeral head for arm movements in all planes (31).

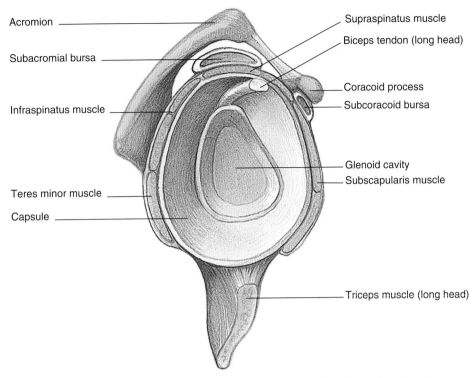

Acromion

Subacromial bursa

Infraspinatus muscle

Teres minor muscle

Capsule

Supraspinatus muscle

Biceps tendon (long head)

Coracoid process

Subcoracoid bursa

Glenoid cavity

Subscapularis muscle

Triceps muscle (long head)

**FIGURE 3.13.** Shoulder joint socket. (Reprinted with permission from Anatomical Chart Company. *ACC's Shoulder and Elbow Anatomical Chart.* Baltimore [MD]: Lippincott Williams & Wilkins; 2003.)

## MOVEMENTS

Because the glenohumeral joint is a ball-and-socket joint, it is capable of motion in three planes: abduction–adduction in the frontal plane, flexion–extension in the sagittal plane, and internal–external rotation and horizontal abduction–adduction in the transverse plane. Furthermore, the multiplanar movement of circumduction is possible at the glenohumeral joint (38). Glenohumeral movements are demonstrated in Figure 3.14, and normal ROM values are listed in Table 3.5.

The center of rotation of the glenohumeral joint occurs at the humeral head within the glenoid fossa. At 0°–50° of abduction, the lower portion of the humeral head is in contact with the glenoid fossa, whereas at 50°–90° of abduction, the upper portion of the humeral head is in contact with the glenoid fossa. Because shear force creates friction across surfaces, the rolling of the humeral head within the glenoid reduces stress on the joint (4).

The scapulothoracic joint is also capable of motion in three planes. These motions include upward–downward rotation, retraction–protraction, elevation–depression, anterior–posterior tilting, and medial–lateral rotation (4). Scapulothoracic joint movements are shown in Figure 3.15.

### Scapulohumeral Rhythm

Full abduction of the arm requires simultaneous movement of the glenohumeral and scapulotho-racic joints. This dual movement is called "scapulohumeral rhythm" (Fig. 3.16). Scapulohumeral rhythm allows a greater abduction ROM, maintains optimal length–tension relationships of the glenohumeral muscles, and prevents impingement between the greater tubercle of the humerus and the acromion. After 100°–120° of abduction, upward rotation of the scapula in the frontal plane causes the glenoid fossa of the scapula to face upward, making further elevation of the arm above the head possible (32). Overall, in every 3° elevation of the arm, 2° occurs at the glenohumeral joint and 1° occurs at the scapulothoracic joint (37).

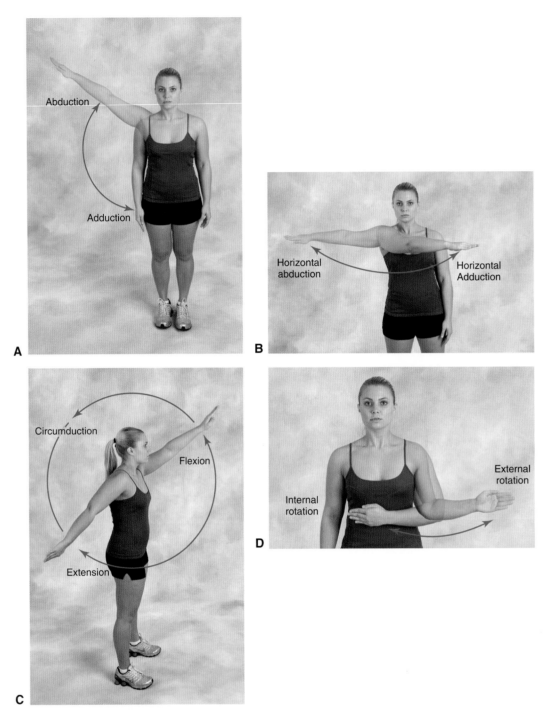

**FIGURE 3.14.** Movements of the shoulder. **A.** Abduction–adduction. **B.** Horizontal abduction–adduction. **C.** Flexion–extension and circumduction. **D.** Internal–external rotation.

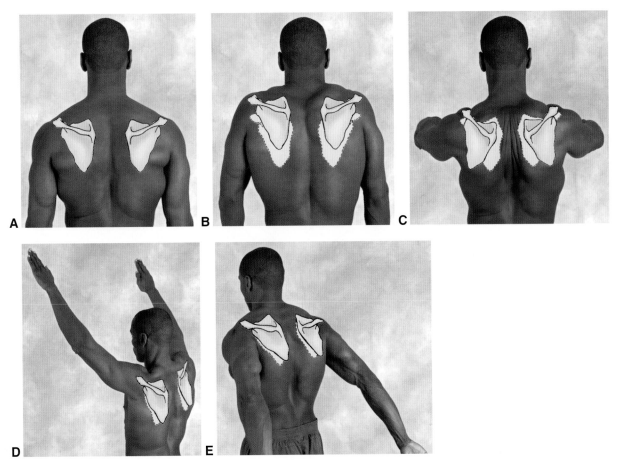

**FIGURE 3.15.** Movements of the scapulothoracic joint. **A.** Starting position. **B.** Elevation–depression. **C.** Protraction–retraction. **D.** Internal–external rotation. **E.** Anterior–posterior tilt.

### MUSCLES

The numerous muscles of the shoulder region are typically characterized as either shoulder joint muscles or shoulder girdle muscles. The shoulder joint and shoulder girdle muscles work together to contribute to upper extremity movements. The shoulder joint muscles directly move the arm, whereas the shoulder girdle muscles mainly stabilize the scapula on the thoracic cage and are particularly important in maintaining proper posture (38). The muscles of the shoulder region are shown in Figures 3.17 and 3.18.

### Anterior

The anterior muscles of the shoulder joint are the pectoralis major, subscapularis, coracobrachialis, and biceps brachii. The posterior muscles of the shoulder joint are the infraspinatus and teres minor. The superior muscles are the deltoid and supraspinatus, and the inferior muscles include the latissimus dorsi, teres major, and long head of the triceps brachii. The pectoralis major is a large and powerful muscle that is a prime mover in adduction, horizontal adduction, and internal rotation of the humerus. The pectoralis major is triangular, originating along the medial clavicle and sternum and attaching to the intertubercular groove of the humerus. The clavicular portion of the muscle primarily flexes the humerus, whereas the sternocostal portion extends the humerus from a flexed position (4). The coracobrachialis, a small muscle, assists with shoulder flexion and adduction. The biceps brachii is a two-joint, two-head muscle that crosses the shoulder and elbow. At the shoulder, the coracobrachialis assists with horizontal adduction, flexion,

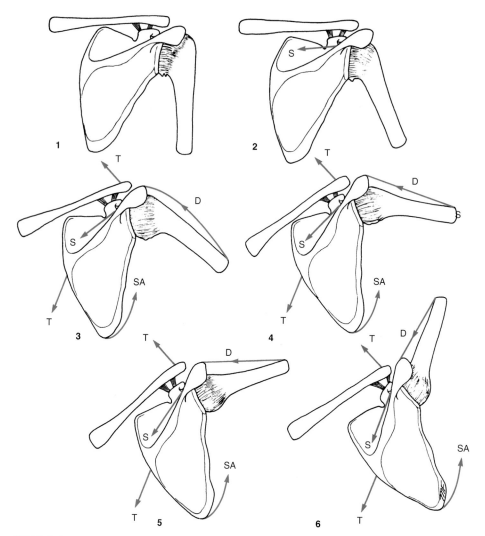

**FIGURE 3.16.**   Scapulohumeral rhythm: movements of shoulder abduction and scapular upward rotation and the muscles that produce these movements at various stages of abduction. For every 3° elevation of the arm, 2° occurs at the glenohumeral joint and 1° occurs at the scapula. S, supraspinatus; T, trapezius; D, deltoid; SA, serratus anterior. (From Snell RS. *Clinical Anatomy.* 7th ed. Baltimore [MD]: Lippincott Williams & Wilkins; 2003, with permission.)

and internal rotation (4). Its primary functions and anatomical considerations are discussed in the section "Elbow" in this chapter.

## Superior

The deltoid muscle has three heads: anterior, middle, and posterior. All heads insert at the deltoid tuberosity on the lateral humerus. The anterior deltoid originates from the anterolateral aspect of the clavicle. It is chiefly responsible for shoulder flexion, horizontal adduction, and internal rotation of the glenohumeral joint. The middle deltoid originates from the lateral aspect of the acromion and is a powerful abductor of the glenohumeral joint. The posterior deltoid originates from the inferior aspect of the scapular spine, and its actions of glenohumeral extension, horizontal abduction, and external rotation oppose those of the anterior deltoid (18). The anterior and posterior deltoids should be approximately the same size. However, in most individuals, the anterior deltoid is much more developed than the posterior deltoid. This imbalance can cause postural abnormalities (shoulder forward and internally rotated) and may be related to shoulder problems such as impingement syndrome (4).

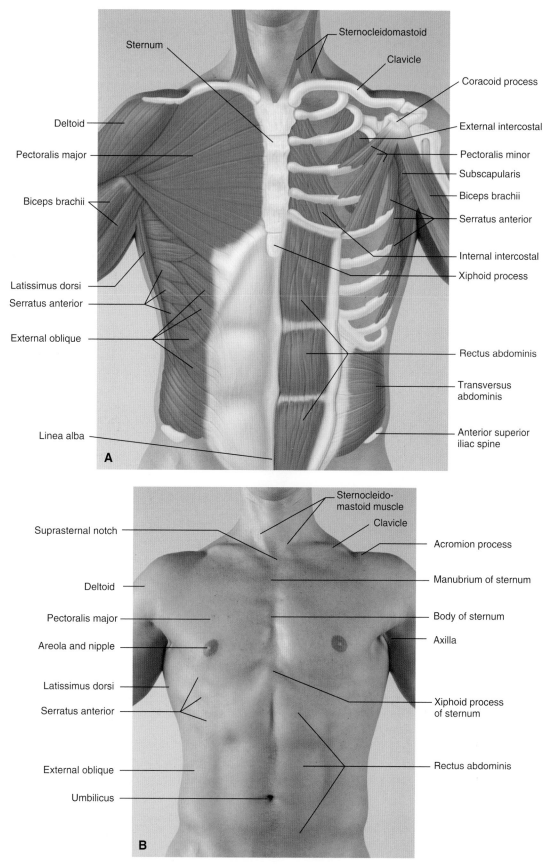

**FIGURE 3.17.** Muscles of the neck, shoulder, and trunk — anterior view. **A.** Superficial *(right)* and deep *(left)* muscles. **B.** Surface landmarks. (From Premkumar K. *The Massage Connection: Anatomy and Physiology*. 3rd ed. Baltimore [MD]: Lippincott Williams & Wilkins; 2011, with permission.)

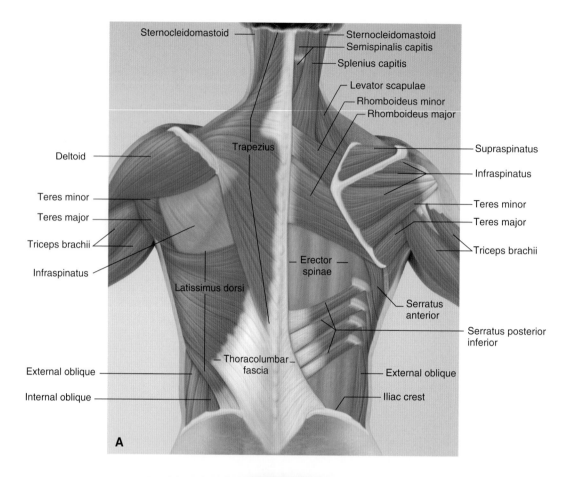

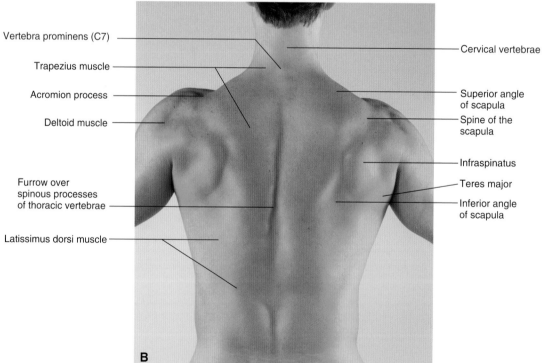

**FIGURE 3.18.** Muscles of the neck, shoulder, and trunk — posterior view. **A.** Superficial *(right)* and deep *(left)* muscles. **B.** Surface landmarks. (From Premkumar K. *The Massage Connection: Anatomy and Physiology*. 3rd ed. Baltimore [MD]: Lippincott Williams & Wilkins; 2011, with permission.)

## Rotator Cuff

The rotator cuff muscles include the supraspinatus, infraspinatus, teres minor, and subscapularis, often remembered by the acronym "SITS," which describes their insertions on the greater and lesser tubercles of the humerus (Fig. 3.19). The rotator cuff muscles originate from the scapula and insert at the greater or lesser tubercle of the humerus (6). The supraspinatus primarily initiates abduction at the glenohumeral joint, the infraspinatus and teres minor externally rotate the glenohumeral joint, and the subscapularis internally rotates the glenohumeral joint.

The rotator cuff muscles are important stabilizers of the glenohumeral joint and aid in glenohumeral positional control (6). These muscles act like a strong ligament, holding the humeral head tightly in the glenoid fossa during arm movements initiated by the larger shoulder muscles. The rotator cuff stabilizes the shoulder through four mechanisms: (a) passive muscle tension, (b) contraction of the muscles causing compression of the articular surface, (c) joint motion that result in secondary tightening of the ligamentous restraints, and (d) the barrier effect of contracted muscle (2).

> The rotator cuff muscles include the supraspinatus, infraspinatus, teres minor, and subscapularis, often remembered by the acronym "SITS."

## Posterior

The latissimus dorsi is a large fan-shaped muscle that originates from the iliac crest and the posterior sacrum (via thoracolumbar fascia), lower six thoracic vertebrae, and lower three ribs. It inserts at the intertubercular groove of the humerus. The latissimus dorsi is a strong extensor, internal rotator, and adductor of the glenohumeral joint. The angle of pull of the latissimus dorsi increases when the arm is abducted to 30°–90°. The teres major muscle has actions similar to those of the latissimus dorsi. The triceps brachii is typically known as an elbow muscle, but its long head acts to extend the shoulder as well (18).

## Scapular

The muscles of the anterior shoulder girdle include the pectoralis minor, serratus anterior, and subclavius. The pectoralis minor originates from the anterior aspects of the third to fifth ribs and inserts at the coracoid process of the scapula. Contraction of the pectoralis minor causes protraction,

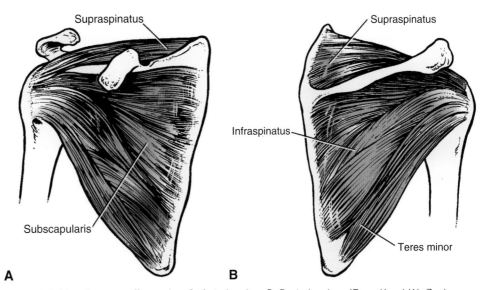

**FIGURE 3.19.** Rotator cuff muscles. **A.** Anterior view. **B.** Posterior view. (From Koval KJ, Zuckerman JD. *Atlas of Orthopaedic Surgery: A Multimedia Reference.* Philadelphia [PA]: Lippincott Williams & Wilkins; 2004, with permission.)

downward rotation, and depression of the scapula. The pectoralis minor has a lifting effect on the ribs during forceful inspiration and postural control. The serratus anterior contains several bands that originate from the upper nine ribs laterally and insert on the anterior aspect of the medial border of the scapula. The serratus anterior protracts the scapula and is active in reaching and pushing. Winging of the scapula results from serratus anterior dysfunction, which is possibly related to long thoracic nerve dysfunction. The subclavius is a small muscle that protects and stabilizes the sternoclavicular joint (18).

The posterior shoulder girdle muscles are the levator scapulae, rhomboids (major and minor), and trapezius. The levator scapulae originate from the transverse processes of the upper four cervical vertebrae, run obliquely, and insert at the medial border superior to the scapular spine. The levator scapulae produce elevation and downward rotation of scapula and also act on the neck. The rhomboids originate from the spinous processes of the last cervical and upper five thoracic vertebrae and insert on the medial border of the scapula from the spine to the inferior angle. Rhomboid action results in scapular retraction, downward rotation, and slight elevation. Along with the trapezius, proper rhomboid activity is necessary for good posture (*i.e.*, squeezing shoulder blades together) (4).

The trapezius muscle is a large triangular muscle and one of the largest muscles of the shoulder region. It contains three distinct regions: the upper, middle, and lower fibers. The origin of the trapezius covers a broad area from the base of the occiput to the spinous process of the twelfth thoracic vertebra, and its insertion runs from the lateral clavicle, medial border of the acromion, and scapular spine. Contraction of the upper trapezius causes scapular elevation, of the middle trapezius causes scapular retraction, and of the lower trapezius causes scapular depression (18). Together, the upper and lower fibers cause upward rotation of the scapula.

## INJURIES

Impingement syndrome is probably the most common nontraumatic cause of shoulder pain (17). Impingement syndrome results from approximation of the acromion and greater tubercle of humerus, which causes entrapment of the rotator cuff tendons (6). Shoulder impingement may also be associated with subacromial bursitis, biceps tendonitis, and degenerative tears of the rotator cuff tendons (3). A primary factor of impingement syndrome is muscular imbalance at the shoulder exacerbated by external rotator cuff muscle weakness and highly trained internal rotator muscles (particularly the prime movers) (17). This imbalance can lead to postural abnormalities, such as anterior shoulder carriage with excessive internal rotation (shoulder rounded forward), adaptive shortening and fibrosis of the internal rotators, and inflamed rotator cuff tendons. The progressive loss of external rotation, because of fibrosis or adaptive shortening of the internal rotators, is the most common factor in chronic rotator cuff disorders. Some of the predisposing factors for impingement syndrome include biomechanically unsound exercises, sports activities (*e.g.*, swimming), lifting weights with poor form, and training the same area of the body too often (overtraining anterior deltoids, pectoralis major, and latissimus dorsi) (17). Treatment of impingement syndrome is heavily focused on retraining proper exercise and posture. This includes strengthening and improving the function of the external rotators, stretching the internal rotators, and eliminating the training errors that started the dysfunction in the first place (17). All too often, however, a person who suffers from impingement syndrome is noncompliant with appropriate rehabilitation, and the condition becomes chronic, leading to permanent degenerative changes and dysfunction. A primary factor of impingement syndrome is muscular imbalance at the shoulder exacerbated by external rotator cuff muscle weakness and highly trained internal rotator muscles (particularly the prime movers) (17).

Thoracic outlet syndrome is another condition of the shoulder that can be related to faulty biomechanics, poor posture, and shoulder muscle imbalance (7). Thoracic outlet syndrome is compression of the neurovascular bundle (brachial plexus and axillary artery/vein) in the axillary (arm pit) region and results in symptoms such as pain, numbness, and tingling in the upper extremity, usually in the fourth and fifth digits of the hand. The three sites of compression in thoracic outlet syndrome occur between the first rib and anterior scalene muscle, pectoralis minor muscle or clavicle (7). Treatment of thoracic outlet syndrome includes correcting faulty biomechanics, strengthening the rotator cuff, and stretching the shoulder internal rotators and scalenes. As with impingement syndrome, complete recovery may take several months or longer.

The shoulder is also susceptible to traumatic injuries such as joint separation or dislocation and tearing of tendons, ligaments, or joint capsules. Glenohumeral joint dislocation usually occurs anteriorly because of capsular tears (4). The mechanism of glenohumeral joint dislocation is typically excessive abduction, external rotation, and extension of the shoulder. Stabilizing the shoulder after suspected glenohumeral joint dislocation is important to prevent any further damage, particularly to the neurological structures. Acromioclavicular joint separation is classically because of a direct blow to the shoulder or fall on an outstretched arm (3). Signs and symptoms of acromioclavicular joint separation include elevation of the distal clavicle and sharp pain in the joint. Rotator cuff tendon tears (particularly of the supraspinatus muscle) can be caused by forceful throwing (*e.g.*, baseball) and improper weightlifting techniques (3).

## Elbow

The elbow is an important joint involved in lifting, carrying, throwing, swinging, and most upper extremity exercise movements. The elbow is commonly injured and is the second most injured joint from overuse or repetitive motion (15,23).

### STRUCTURE

### Bones

The bones of the elbow joint include the humerus, radius, and ulna. The humeroulnar joint is the articulation of the distal humerus with the proximal ulna, the humeroradial joint is the articulation of the distal humerus with the proximal radius, and the proximal radioulnar joint is the articulation of the proximal radius with the proximal ulna (38) (Fig. 3.20).

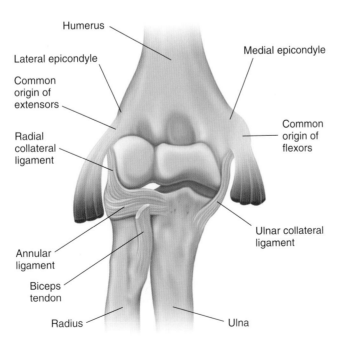

**FIGURE 3.20.** Bones and ligaments of the elbow joint — anterior view. (From Premkumar K. *The Massage Connection: Anatomy and Physiology*. 3rd ed. Baltimore [MD]: Lippincott Williams & Wilkins; 2011, with permission.)

The elbow is an important joint involved in lifting, carrying, throwing, swinging, and most upper extremity exercise movements. The elbow is commonly injured and is the second most injured joint from overuse or repetitive motion (15,23).

With the arms held at the side of the body and the palms of the hand facing anteriorly, the forearm and hands are usually held slightly away from the body. This is because of the carrying angle of the elbow, which is normally 5°–15° in males and 20°–25° in females. Carrying angle allows the forearm to swing free of the side of the hips during walking and provides a mechanical advantage when carrying objects (4).

## Ligaments

Three major ligaments stabilize the elbow: the ulnar (medial) collateral ligament, which connects the humerus with the ulna; the radial (lateral) collateral ligament, which connects the humerus with the radius; and the annular ligament, which connects the radius with the ulna. The collateral ligaments provide support for stresses in the frontal plane, the medial collateral for valgus forces, and the lateral collateral for varus forces. The annular ligament provides stability for the radius, securing it to the ulna (38) (see Fig. 3.20).

## Joints

The elbow joint complex is a compound synovial joint that consists of two articulations: humeroulnar and humeroradial. It is continuous with the proximal radioulnar joint, responsible for allowing the radial head to rotate during pronation and supination of the forearm. The distal humerus articulates with both the proximal ulna and proximal radius, and the two articulations are enclosed by one capsule and share a single synovial cavity. On the lateral side of the elbow, the capitulum of the humerus articulates with the head of the radius to form the humeroradial joint; medially, the trochlea of the humerus articulates with the trochlear notch of the ulna to form the humeroulnar joint. The proximal radioulnar joint, whose joint capsule is continuous with that of the humeroulnar and humeroradial joints, is the articulation of the radial head with the radial notch of the ulna (38) (see Fig. 3.20).

### MOVEMENTS

Both the humeroulnar and humeroradial are hinge joints that flex and extend the elbow in the sagittal plane (Fig. 3.21). The normal ROM for flexion–extension is 145°–150°, with the fully flexed position (elbow bent) represented by 145°–150° and the fully extended position (arm straight with forearm) represented by 0°. During sagittal movement of the elbow, the trochlear notch of the humerus slides into the trochlear groove of the ulna. Upon full flexion, the coronoid process of the ulna approximates the coronoid fossa of the humerus. At full extension, the olecranon process of the ulna hits the olecranon fossa of the humerus, which enhances stability of the elbow in full extension. The proximal radioulnar joint is a pivot joint, which permits axial rotation of the radial head during supination and pronation of the forearm. Normal ROM for supination (forearm rotated laterally — palms facing anteriorly) is 80°–90°; normal ROM for pronation (forearm rotated medially — palms facing posteriorly) is 80°–90° (38).

### MUSCLES

### Anterior

The anterior muscles of the arm mainly flex the elbow joint (5) and include the biceps brachii, brachialis, and brachioradialis (Fig. 3.22). The biceps brachii is a two-head, two-joint muscle that acts on both the shoulder and elbow. Its long head originates from the supraglenoid tubercle of the scapula, and the short head originates from the coracoid process of the scapula, with both heads inserting at the tuberosity of the radius. The biceps brachii is a strong supinator and flexes the elbow most effectively when the forearm is in supination. The long head of the biceps brachii also assists in shoulder flexion. To optimally train the biceps brachii, exercise movements should

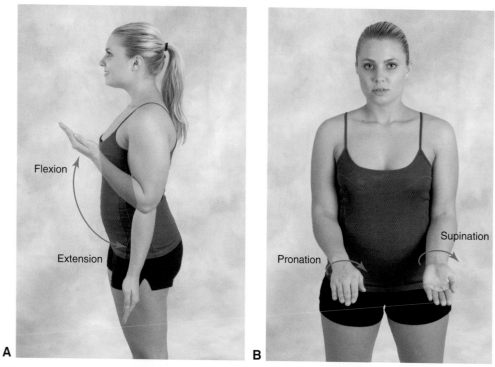

**FIGURE 3.21.** Movements of the elbow. **A.** Flexion–extension. **B.** Pronation–supination.

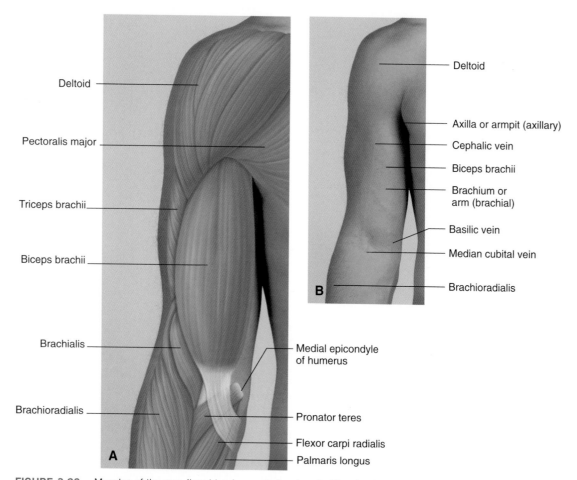

**FIGURE 3.22.** Muscles of the arm (brachium) — anterior view. **A.** Muscles. **B.** Surface landmarks. (From Premkumar K. *The Massage Connection: Anatomy and Physiology.* 3rd ed. Baltimore [MD]: Lippincott Williams & Wilkins; 2011, with permission.)

include both elbow flexion and forearm supination (*e.g.*, dumbbell biceps curl). The brachialis is considered the elbow flexor workhorse (4). Hammer curls, with the forearms maintained in a neutral position, are ideal to develop the brachialis and brachioradialis. In the forearm, the pronator quadratus and pronator teres, as their names suggest, cause pronation. The pronator quadratus is the stronger of the two.

## Posterior

The posterior muscles of the elbow primarily extend the elbow joint and include the triceps brachii and anconeus (Fig. 3.23). The triceps brachii is a three-head, two-joint (long head) muscle that acts on the elbow and shoulder. Its long head originates from the infraglenoid tubercle of the scapula, whereas the medial and lateral heads originate from the upper humerus. All three heads insert on the olecranon of the ulna. The triceps brachii is the main elbow extensor, getting minor assistance from the anconeus. The anconeus, a small muscle, also adds stability to the posterior elbow joint (18).

### INJURIES

Because of its use in most upper extremity daily living activities, exercise, and sport activities, the elbow is frequently injured from chronic overuse or repetitive motion (3). Tendonitis is evident in a variety of muscular insertion points at the elbow. "Tennis elbow" (lateral epicondylitis), which

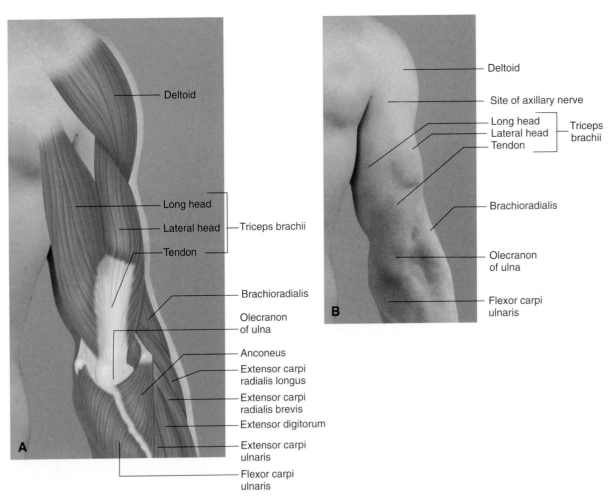

**FIGURE 3.23.**    Muscles of the arm (brachium) — posterior view. **A.** Muscles. **B.** Surface landmarks. (From Premkumar K. *The Massage Connection: Anatomy and Physiology.* 3rd ed. Baltimore [MD]: Lippincott Williams & Wilkins; 2011, with permission.)

creates lateral elbow pain, is the most widespread overuse injury of the adult elbow (15,23). It is usually caused by eccentric overload of the forearm extensor muscles (*e.g.*, gripping a racquet too tightly, wrong grip size, faulty backhand technique, excessive racquet weight) (11). "Golfer's elbow" (medial epicondylitis), which produces medial elbow pain, is often caused by repeated valgus stresses placed on the arm during swinging of racquets or clubs. Triceps tendonitis, which produces pain over the olecranon, is caused by repetitive posterior stresses during elbow extension. Resistance and flexibility exercises for elbow flexion, extension, pronation, and supination are often incorporated to prevent and treat these injuries. Medial collateral ligament sprain often results from repetitive microtrauma and excessive valgus force (3).

The elbow is also the site for traumatic injuries. Olecranon bursitis, which typically produces a large red swelling over the posterior elbow, usually results from a fall directly on the elbow. Ulnar dislocation typically results from violent hyperextension or varus or valgus forces. Ulnar dislocation, which is most common in individuals younger than 20 years, results in obvious elbow deformity and may present with neurological symptoms into the hand (fifth digit) because of entrapment of the ulnar nerve at the elbow (3).

## Wrist, Hand, and Fingers

The wrist, hand, and fingers are required for most daily living, work, and sports activities, including tasks such as gripping, lifting, writing, typing, eating, and throwing. Because adequate wrist and hand function is necessary for these activities, injuries to the wrist and hand are often disabling. This section focuses mainly on the functional anatomy of the wrist. The reader is referred to other sources (1,16,28,29,33) for the functional anatomy of the intrinsic hand and fingers.

### STRUCTURE

### Bones

The wrist, hand, and fingers consist of 29 bones: a distal ulna, a distal radius, 8 carpals, 5 metacarpals, and 14 phalanges (36) (Fig. 3.24). The carpals are small oddly shaped bones arranged in two rows. The proximal row from lateral to medial includes scaphoid (navicular), lunate, triquetrum, and pisiform. The distal row from lateral to medial includes trapezium, trapezoid, capitate, and hamate. There is one metacarpal per digit, which connects the carpals to the phalanges. Each digit has three phalanges, except the thumb, which has two (36).

### Ligament

The volar radiocarpal, dorsal radiocarpal, radial collateral, and ulnar collateral ligaments support the radioulnar joint. The radiocarpal ligaments provide stability in the sagittal plane, whereas the collateral ligaments provide stability in the frontal plane (36). There are numerous other ligaments that stabilize the wrist, hand, and fingers, many of which have clinical implications for health care professionals other than Personal Trainers.

### Joints

The primary wrist joint (radiocarpal joint) is a condyloid (ellipsoidal) joint consisting of the articulation of the distal radius with three proximal carpal bones: scaphoid, lunate, and triquetrum. The joint surface of the radius is concave, allowing the convex carpals to approximate it. The proximal and distal rows of carpal bones form the complex midcarpal joint. The distal radioulnar joint, a pivot joint, is situated medial to the radiocarpal joint and allows forearm supination and pronation (36).

### Movement

The wrist allows approximately 70°–90° of flexion and 65°–85° of extension in the sagittal plane and 15°–25° of abduction (radial deviation) and 25°–40° of adduction (ulnar deviation)

**FIGURE 3.24.** Bones of the wrist and hand — anterior view. (From Anderson M, Hall SJ. *Sports Injury Management.* 2nd ed. Baltimore [MD]: Lippincott Williams & Wilkins; 2000, with permission.)

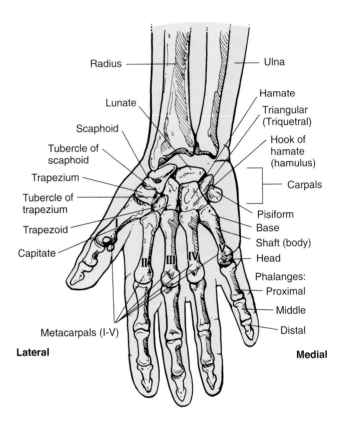

in the frontal plane (Fig. 3.25). Flexion–extension and abduction–adduction movements occur mainly at the radiocarpal joint. However, gliding motions at the midcarpal joint, which are facilitated by ligaments, allow full ROM in both planes. Circumduction of the wrist is also possible through the compound action of the radioulnar and midcarpal joints. The closed pack position of the wrist joint is full extension, whereas the open pack position is 0° of extension with slight adduction (4).

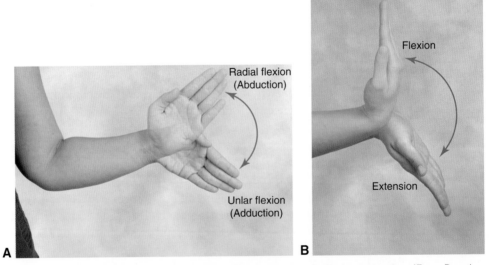

**FIGURE 3.25.** Movements of the wrist. **A.** Abduction–adduction. **B.** Flexion–extension. (From Premkumar K. *The Massage Connection: Anatomy and Physiology.* 3rd ed. Baltimore [MD]: Lippincott Williams & Wilkins; 2011, with permission.)

### MUSCLES

#### Anterior

The wrist flexor muscles, which are located on the anteromedial aspect of the wrist and generally originate from the medial epicondyle of the humerus, include the flexor carpi radialis, flexor carpi ulnaris, flexor digitorum superficialis, and palmaris longus (Fig. 3.26). In addition to the flexor activity, the flexor carpi radialis abducts the wrist, the flexor carpi ulnaris adducts the wrist, and the flexor digitorum superficialis flexes the phalanges as well (18).

#### Posterior

The wrist extensor muscles, which are located on the posterolateral aspect of the wrist and generally originate at or near the lateral epicondyle of the humerus, include the extensor carpi radialis longus and brevis, extensor digitorum, extensor digiti minimi, and the extensor carpi ulnaris (Fig. 3.27).

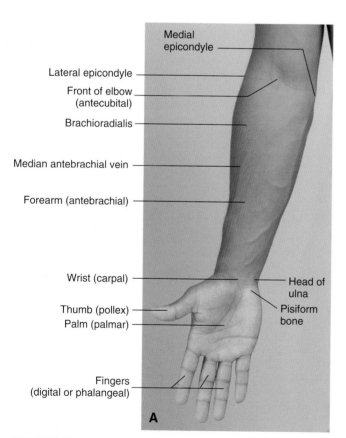
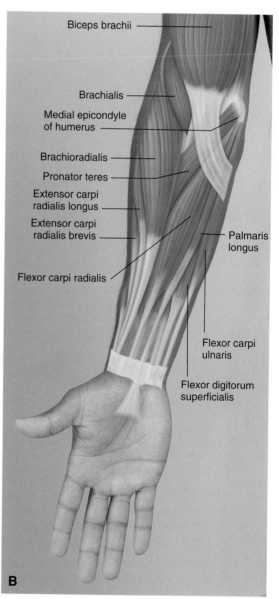

**FIGURE 3.26.**   Muscles of the forearm (antebrachium) — anterior view. **A.** Muscles. **B.** Surface landmarks. (From Premkumar K. *The Massage Connection: Anatomy and Physiology*. 3rd ed. Baltimore [MD]: Lippincott Williams & Wilkins; 2011, with permission.)

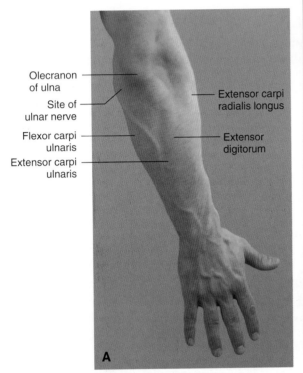
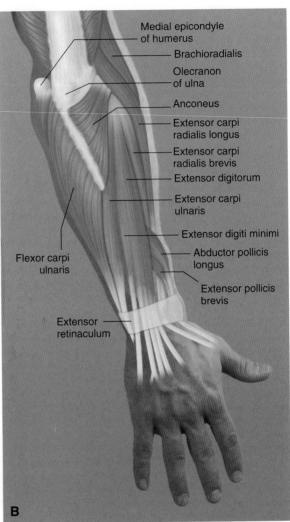

**FIGURE 3.27.** Muscles of the forearm (antebrachium) — posterior view. **A.** Muscles. **B.** Surface landmarks. (From Premkumar K. *The Massage Connection: Anatomy and Physiology.* 3rd ed. Baltimore [MD]: Lippincott Williams & Wilkins; 2011, with permission.)

In addition to their extensor activity, the extensor carpi radialis longus abducts the wrist and the extensor carpi ulnaris adducts the wrist, and extensor digitorum, extensor digiti minimi extend the phalanges as well (18).

### INJURIES

Dislocations, fractures, and sprains are common at the wrist after falls. Falling on an outstretched arm with the wrist extended may cause lunate bone dislocation (usually anteriorly) or scaphoid bone fracture. Colles and Smith fractures are serious fractures affecting both the distal ulna and radius, which many times require fixation with rigid screws and plates to restore function (14). Wrist ligament sprains are frequently caused by axial loading of the palm during a fall on an outstretched arm (3).

Carpal tunnel syndrome is a widespread cumulative trauma disorder that is caused by median nerve entrapment at the anterior wrist (7). It usually results from repeated microtrauma to the carpal tunnel and flexor retinaculum due to prolonged

Carpal tunnel syndrome usually results from repeated microtrauma to the carpal tunnel and flexor retinaculum because of prolonged manual work with the wrist in a flexed position (*e.g.,* in individuals who work with computer keyboards, assembly line workers, cyclists).

manual work with the wrist in a flexed position (*e.g.*, in individuals who work with computer keyboards, assembly line workers, cyclists). Its symptoms include pain, numbness, tingling, and weakness in thumb, index, and middle finger (median nerve distribution). Carpal tunnel syndrome usually requires physical rehabilitation, surgery, or ergonomic correction to restore function.

## Lower Extremity

### Pelvis and Hip

The pelvic girdle is the link between axial skeleton (trunk) and lower extremities. This region assists with motion, stability, and shock absorption and helps distribute body weight evenly to the lower extremities (4). The pelvic girdle is the link between the axial skeleton (trunk) and lower extremities.

#### BONES

The bones of the pelvic girdle (pelvis) are the sacrum and innominate (os coxae). The innominate bone includes the fused ilium (largest pelvic bone), ischium, and pubis on each side (which typically fuse by the end of puberty). The two sides of the pelvis join anteriorly at the pubic symphysis and posteriorly at the sacroiliac joints, where the sacrum and coccyx serve as the inferior foundation for the lumbosacral spine. The pelvis of females is usually wider than that of males, which contributes to the increased "Q angle" of the knee in females (4). The anterior superior iliac spine (ASIS) of the ilium is a bony protuberance that provides an attachment point for several muscles of the anterior thigh. The sacrum articulates with the pelvis on each side, forming the sacroiliac joints. The pelvis articulates with each femur at the acetabulum, forming the hip joints (36) (Fig. 3.28).

**Anterior view**

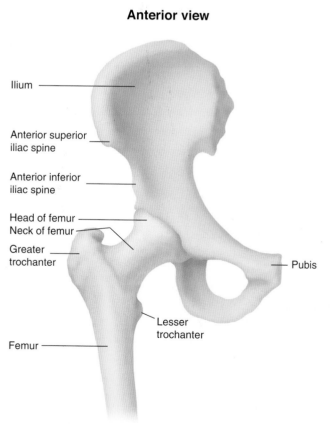

Ilium

Anterior superior
iliac spine

Anterior inferior
iliac spine

Head of femur
Neck of femur

Greater
trochanter

Pubis

Lesser
trochanter

Femur

**FIGURE 3.28.** Bones of the pelvis and hip region — anterior view. (Reprinted with permission from Anatomical Chart Company. *ACC's Joints of the Lower Extremities Anatomical Chart.* Baltimore [MD]: Lippincott Williams & Wilkins; 2003.)

## LIGAMENTS

The anterior, posterior, and interosseous ligaments bind the sacroiliac joint. The highly mobile hip joint is stabilized by several intrinsic ligaments, forming a strong, dense joint capsule (38). They include iliofemoral, pubofemoral, and ischiofemoral ligaments. The iliofemoral ligament ("Y" ligament) is an extraordinarily strong band that checks hip extension and rotation. The pubofemoral ligament prevents excessive abduction. The ischiofemoral ligament is triangular and limits hip rotation and adduction in the flexed position (38) (Fig. 3.29). The transverse acetabular ligament is a sturdy band that bridges the acetabular notch and completes the acetabular ring of the hip joint. The ligamentum teres ligament (ligament of the femoral head) ties the head of the femur to the acetabulum, providing reinforcement from within the joint (Fig. 3.30).

## JOINTS

The pubic symphysis connects each side of the pelvic girdle anteriorly and is an amphiarthrodial joint. The sacroiliac joint connects the sacrum to the ilium on each side and is sometimes described as a gliding joint. These joints are capable of relatively little movement (38).

The hip joint is a ball-and-socket (enarthrodial) joint and is one of the most mobile joints in the body. The hip joint is formed by the articulation of the proximal femur (femoral head) with the acetabulum of the pelvis. The femoral head is covered with hyaline cartilage, except at the fovea capitis, and the acetabulum is lined with hyaline cartilage as well. The acetabular labrum is a fibrocartilaginous "lip" that adds depth to the acetabulum and serves as a cushion for the femoral head (4) (see Fig. 3.30).

## MOVEMENTS

The pelvic girdle allows movement in three planes. These movements are shown in Figure 3.31. Movement at the pelvis during normal activities usually involves simultaneous motion of the hip and lumbar spine (38). In the sagittal plane, the pelvis is capable of anterior–posterior tilt.

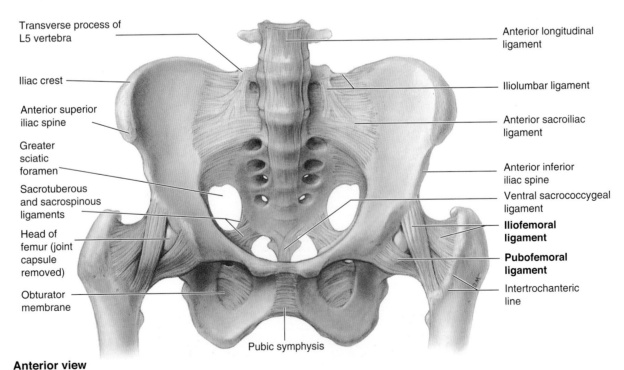

**Anterior view**

**FIGURE 3.29.**  Ligaments of the pelvis and hip regions — anterior view. (From Moore KL, Dalley AF II. *Clinically Oriented Anatomy.* 4th ed. Baltimore [MD]: Lippincott Williams & Wilkins; 1999, with permission.)

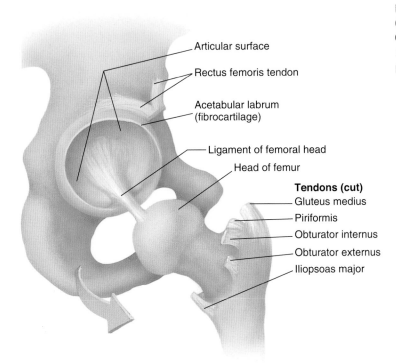

**FIGURE 3.30.** Acetabulum of the hip joint. (Reprinted with permission from Anatomical Chart Company. *ACC's Joints of the Lower Extremities Anatomical Chart*. Baltimore [MD]: Lippincott Williams & Wilkins; 2003.)

With anterior pelvic tilt, the pubic symphysis moves inferiorly, the lumbar spine extends, and the hips flex, resulting in an increased lumbosacral angle. With posterior pelvic tilt, the pubic symphysis moves superiorly, the lumbar spine flexes, and the hips extend, resulting in a decreased lumbosacral angle. Lateral tilt of the pelvis occurs in the frontal plane, and rotation of the pelvis occurs in the axial plane. Locomotion (walking or running) typically involves small oscillations of the pelvis in all three planes (38).

The highly mobile hip joint allows movement in three planes: flexion–extension in the sagittal plane, abduction–adduction in the frontal plane, internal–external rotation in the axial plane, and the combined plane movement of circumduction (38). Hip movements are shown in Figure 3.32.

### MUSCLES

#### Pelvis

The muscles of the pelvis include the muscles that act on the lumbar spine, lower trunk, and hip, which are discussed elsewhere in this chapter. In general, anterior pelvic tilt results from contraction of the hip flexors and lumbar extensors. Posterior pelvic tilt results from contraction of the hip extensors and lumbar flexors. Lateral tilt results from contraction of the lateral lumbar muscles (*e.g.*, quadratus lumborum) and hip abductor–adductor muscles, and axial rotation occurs through the action of the hip and spinal rotator muscles (4).

#### Hip

The muscles that act on the hip are shown in Figures 3.33 through 3.36.

#### Anterior

The anterior muscles of the hip region include the iliopsoas, pectineus, rectus femoris (a component of the quadriceps femoris), sartorius, and tensor fasciae latae. The iliopsoas muscle group, which consists of the psoas major and iliacus muscles, is a strong hip flexor. The pectineus is a small muscle that attaches the anterior pubis to the posteromedial side of the proximal femur. It assists

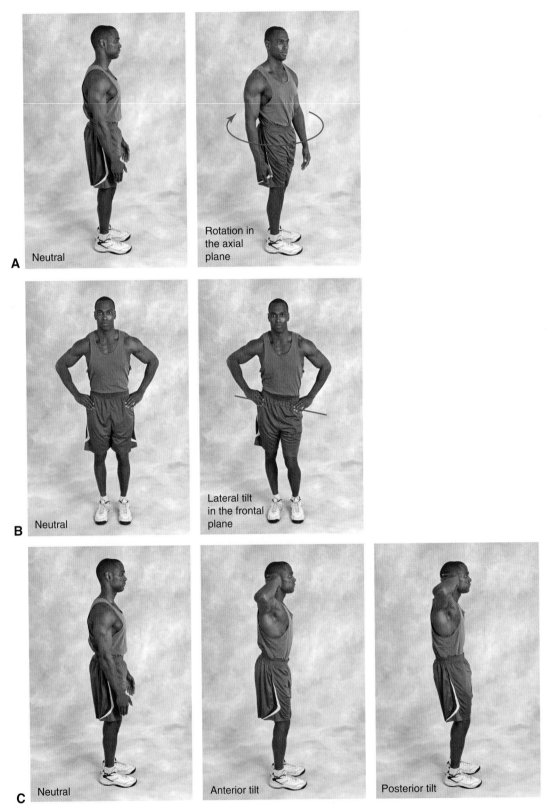

**FIGURE 3.31.** Movements of the pelvis. **A.** Rotation in the axial plane. **B.** Lateral tilt in the frontal plane. **C.** Anterior and posterior tilt in the sagittal plane.

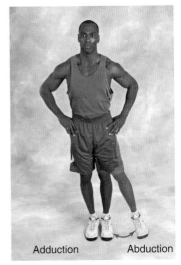

A      Adduction      Abduction

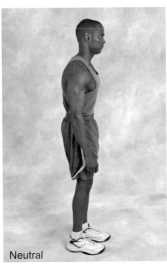
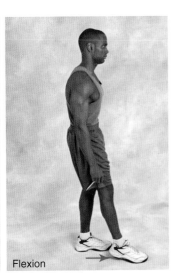

B      Extension      Neutral      Flexion

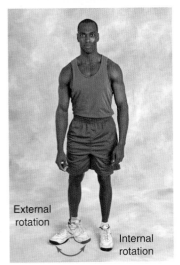

External rotation      Internal rotation

C

**FIGURE 3.32.** Movements of the hip joint. **A.** Abduction–adduction. **B.** Flexion–extension. **C.** Internal–external rotation.

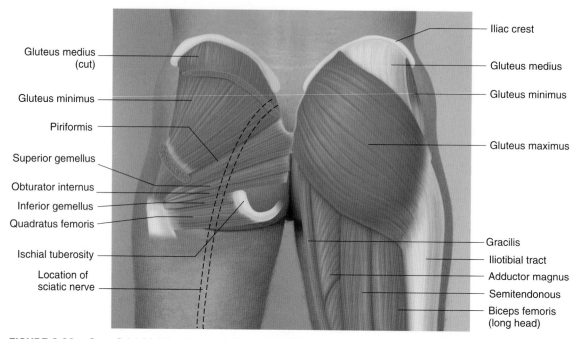

**FIGURE 3.33.** Superficial *(right)* and deep *(left)* muscles of the hip and pelvis — posterior view. (From Premkumar K. *The Massage Connection: Anatomy and Physiology.* 3rd ed. Baltimore [MD]: Lippincott Williams & Wilkins; 2011, with permission.)

in hip flexion, adduction, and internal rotation. The rectus femoris is a large two-joint muscle that flexes the hip and extends the knee. The rectus femoris originates from the anterior inferior iliac spine (AIIS) and inserts at the tibial tuberosity via the patellar ligament. The sartorius, a two-joint muscle, is the longest muscle in the body, originating from the ASIS and inserting at the medial tibial surface (pes anserinus). The sartorius flexes, abducts, and externally rotates the hip (it also assists with knee flexion). The tensor fasciae latae, a two-joint muscle, originates from the anterior iliac crest of the ilium and inserts at the anterolateral tibial condyle via a long band of fascia — the iliotibial band. The tensor fasciae latae abducts and flexes the hip and stabilizes the hip against external rotation when the hip is flexed (18) and also assists with extension and stabilization of the knee.

## Medial

Medial muscles of the hip include gracilis and the adductors longus, brevis, and magnus. These muscles primarily adduct the hip. Variably, they may participate in hip flexion (adductor longus and brevis, upper fibers of adductor magnus) or extension (lower fibers of adductor magnus) and medial rotation (adductors longus, brevis, and magnus). Pectineus, a muscle previously considered with the anterior hip muscles, also participates in hip adduction. These muscles originate generally from the pubis and insert on the linea aspera of the femur. Gracilis, which is a two-joint muscle inserting on tibia (pes anserine), may also assist with knee flexion.

## Posterior

The posterior muscles of the hip include gluteus maximus, medius, and minimus; six deep lateral rotators (piriformis, gemellus superior and inferior, obturators internus and externus, and quadratus femoris); and hamstrings (biceps femoris, semimembranosus, and semitendinosus). Gluteus maximus, which forms the bulk of the buttock regions, has an extensive origin from ilium, sacrum, and coccyx and inserts on the gluteal tuberosity, located on the lateral aspect of femur. In addition to being a powerful extensor of the hip, it also participates in lateral rotation and abduction and lower fibers may participate in adduction. Gluteus medius and minimus lie deep to gluteus maximus and are abductors and medial rotators of the hip. Additionally, these muscles are important postural muscles

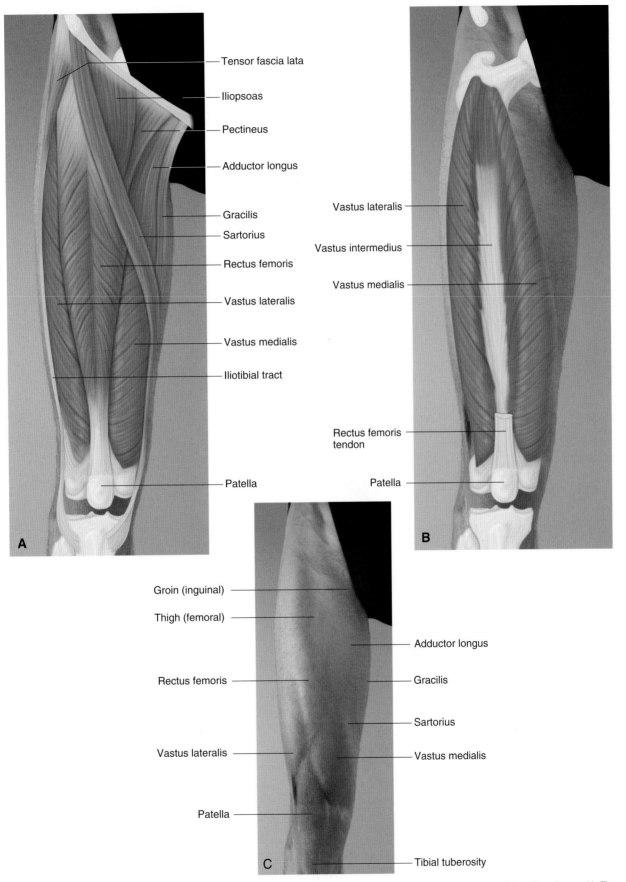

**FIGURE 3.34.** Muscles of the thigh — anterior view. **A.** Muscles. **B.** Quadriceps femoris. **C.** Surface landmarks. (From Premkumar K. *The Massage Connection: Anatomy and Physiology.* 3rd ed. Baltimore [MD]: Lippincott Williams & Wilkins; 2011, with permission.)

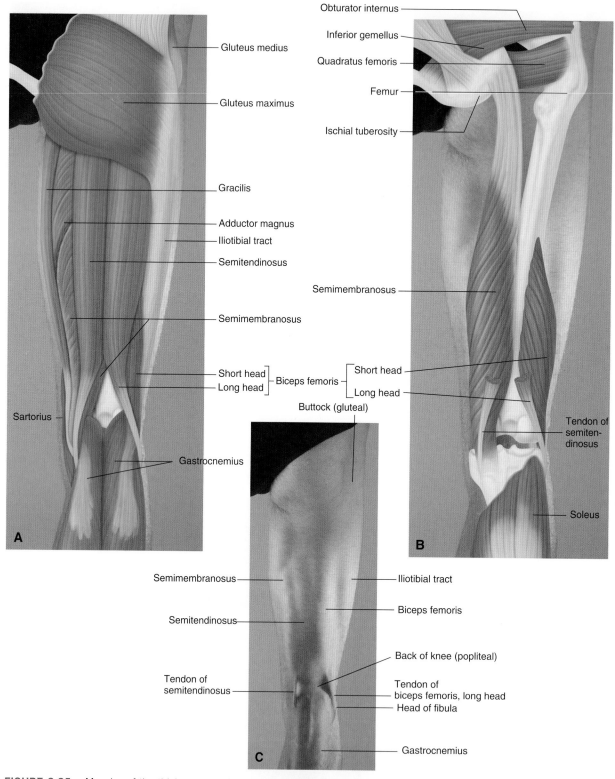

**FIGURE 3.35.** Muscles of the thigh — posterior view. **A.** Superficial muscles. **B.** Deep muscles. **C.** Surface landmarks. (From Premkumar K. *The Massage Connection: Anatomy and Physiology*. 3rd ed. Baltimore [MD]: Lippincott Williams & Wilkins; 2011, with permission.)

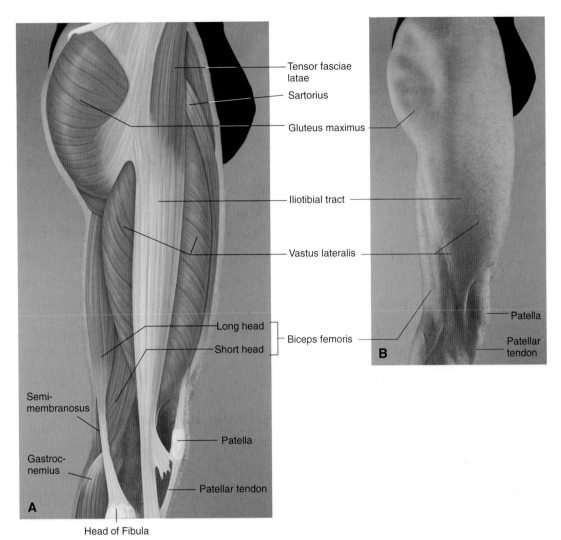

Tensor fasciae latae

Sartorius

Gluteus maximus

Iliotibial tract

Vastus lateralis

Long head

Short head

Biceps femoris

Semi-membranosus

Gastroc-nemius

Patella

Patellar tendon

**A**

Head of Fibula

Patella

Patellar tendon

**B**

**FIGURE 3.36.** Muscles of the thigh — lateral view. **A.** Muscles. **B.** Surface landmarks. (From Premkumar K. *The Massage Connection: Anatomy and Physiology*. 3rd ed. Baltimore [MD]: Lippincott Williams & Wilkins; 2011, with permission.)

Hip and pelvis have a strong structural anatomy, so traumatic sports injuries at these locations are relatively infrequent compared with injuries to other joints (3). However, the soft tissues of the thigh are often injured in sports (3), and the hip and pelvis are sites of several chronic overuse disorders.

to keep the pelvis level during locomotion. They arise from the external surface of ilium and insert on the greater trochanter of femur with most of the deep lateral rotators. Hamstrings (semimembranosus, semitendinosus, and biceps femoris) are two-joint muscles, which extend the hip (except the short head of biceps femoris) and flex the knee. Biceps femoris originates from the ischial tuberosity (long head) and proximal femur (short head) and inserts on the lateral tibial condyle and fibular head. The long head extends the hip, flexes the knee, and causes lateral rotation at both joints, whereas the short head acts only on the knee. Semimembranosus and semitendinosus are also two-joint muscles that extend the hip, flex the knee, and internally rotate both joints. They originate on the ischial tuberosity and insert on the medial aspect of the tibia.

### INJURIES

Hip and pelvis have a strong structural anatomy, so traumatic sports injuries at these locations are relatively infrequent compared with injuries to other joints (3). However, the soft tissues of the thigh are often injured in sports (3), and the hip and pelvis are sites of several chronic overuse disorders.

Traumatic injuries of the pelvis and hip include dislocation, fracture, contusion, and muscle strain. Hip dislocation results from falls, violent twisting of the hip, or jamming the knee into the dashboard of a car. Some 85% of hip dislocations are posterior. Hip fractures (fractures of the femoral neck) are common in older adults with osteoporosis and can cause permanent disability. Contusions (crush injuries of muscle against bone) are common in the region. Iliac crest contusion ("hip pointer") is caused by a direct blow to the pelvis region. Quadriceps contusion ("charley horse") and tearing can result in permanent muscle abnormality called "myositis ossificans," in which bone tissue is deposited within the muscle (3). Hamstring muscle strains and tears are often caused by sudden changes in direction and speed, with underlying factors of muscular imbalance, fatigue, and a deconditioned athlete (3). Hamstring injuries are frequent in preseason or early season activities.

Chronic and overuse injuries to the hip and pelvis include arthritis, bursitis, and tendonitis. Degenerative arthritis of the hip results from abnormal articular cartilage wear from either too much or too little resistance. Avascular necrosis of the hip is caused by the lack of proper blood flow to the femoral head and typically results in severe hip degeneration. Trochanteric bursitis involves irritation of the bursa between the iliotibial band and greater trochanter of the femur. Chronic bursitis in this region can lead to "snapping hip syndrome" (3). Iliotibial band friction syndrome is a chronic overuse injury that causes pain along the lateral aspect of the thigh. Piriformis syndrome is a myofascial disorder that can be caused by overuse and faulty lower extremity biomechanics. The hypertonic piriformis muscle may compress the sciatic nerve because the nerve may course through the muscle. This results in pain and neurological symptoms of the posterior aspect of the lower extremity (sciatica) (7).

### Knee

The knee joint is the largest joint in the body. Because the knee joint bears the load of the upper body and trunk and is crucial for locomotion, it is frequently subject to overuse and traumatic injuries (38).

#### STRUCTURE

##### Bones

The knee joint consists of the distal femur, proximal tibia, and patella (Fig. 3.37). The tibia is the major weight-bearing bone of the leg. The fibula is not considered part of the knee joint (38). The patella (kneecap) is a triangular sesamoid bone that is located within the patellar tendon of the quadriceps muscle group. The patella protects the anterior knee (3) and creates an improved angle of pull for the quadriceps muscles, which results in a mechanical advantage during knee extension (38).

##### Ligaments

There are two major pairs of ligaments in the knee: the cruciate and collateral ligaments (see Fig. 3.37). The cruciate ligaments cross within the joint cavity between the femur and tibia and are important in maintaining anterior–posterior and rotational stability at the knee. The anterior cruciate ligament is slightly longer and thinner than the posterior ligament (4).

The collateral ligaments connect the femur with the leg bones — the medial collateral with the tibia and the lateral collateral with the fibula. The collateral ligaments aid in stability of the knee, counteracting valgus (lateral deviation) and varus (medial deviation) forces. The medial collateral ligament attaches to the medial meniscus of the knee, but the lateral collateral ligament does not attach to the lateral meniscus (4).

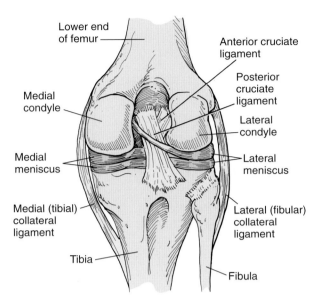

Lower end
of femur

Anterior cruciate
ligament

Posterior
cruciate
ligament

Medial
condyle

Lateral
condyle

Medial
meniscus

Lateral
meniscus

Medial (tibial)
collateral
ligament

Lateral (fibular)
collateral
ligament

Tibia

Fibula

**FIGURE 3.37.** Bones, ligaments, and menisci of the knee region — posterior view — with the knee extended. (From Cipriano J. *Photographic Manual of Regional Orthopaedic and Neurological Tests*. 5th ed. Baltimore [MD]: Lippincott Williams & Wilkins; 2014, with permission.)

## Joints

The knee consists of the tibiofemoral and patellofemoral joints (see Fig. 3.37). The proximal tibiofibular joint, although an important attachment site for knee structures, is typically not considered a compartment of the knee joint (38). The tibiofemoral joint is the primary joint of the knee and primarily a hinge joint allowing flexion and extension; however, with its rotational components about the vertical axis, it is better considered bicondylar. The tibiofemoral joint is formed by the articulation of the medial and lateral femoral condyles with the medial and lateral tibial plateaus. The knee is equipped with fibrocartilage discs (menisci) that are attached to the tibial plateaus and knee joint capsule (4) (see Fig. 3.37). The menisci improve congruency of the joint surfaces (allowing better distribution of joint pressure), add stability, aid in shock absorption, provide joint lubrication, aid in load bearing, add anterior–posterior stability, and protect articular cartilage. The medial meniscus is larger, thinner, and more "C"-shaped than the lateral meniscus (4). The medial femoral condyle typically extends more distally than the lateral condyle, giving the knee a slight valgus arrangement (38).

The patellofemoral joint is an arthrodial joint formed by the posterior aspect of the patella and patellofemoral groove between the condyles of the femur. "Q angle" is the angle formed from the line connecting ASIS to the center of the patella and the line connecting the center of the patella to the tibial tuberosity (4) (Fig. 3.38). It determines the line of pull of the patella at the patellofemoral joint. A normal Q angle is 18° in females and 13° in males. A Q angle that is below normal (negative) results in a genu varum position of the knee (bow-legged), whereas a Q angle that is above normal results in a genu valgum position (knock-kneed) (4).

### MOVEMENTS

The major movements at the tibiofemoral joint are flexion and extension in the sagittal plane (Fig. 3.39). The knee has a normal ROM of 140° in the sagittal plane, with 0° representing full extension (knee straight) and 140° representing full flexion (knee bent). When the knee is flexed, the tibiofemoral joint is also capable of internal and external rotation in the transverse plane. Approximately 30° of internal rotation and 45° of external rotation can be achieved at the knee (4). During the final few degrees of extension, the tibia externally rotates on the femur, which brings the knee into a close-packed, or locked, position. This phenomenon is known as the "screwing home" mechanism (3).

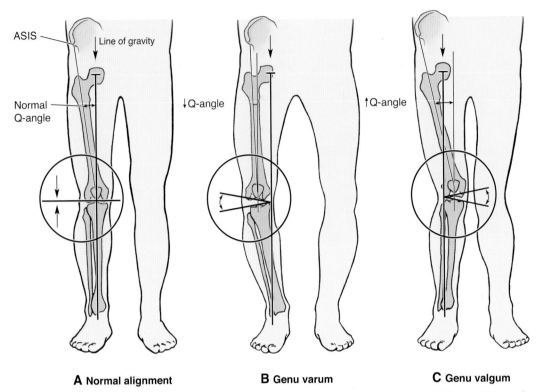

**A Normal alignment**    **B Genu varum**    **C Genu valgum**

**FIGURE 3.38.**    Q angle of the knee: normal alignment, genu varum, and genu valgum. ASIS, anterior superior iliac spine. (From Moore KL, Dalley AF II. *Clinically Oriented Anatomy*. 5th ed. Baltimore [MD]: Lippincott Williams & Wilkins; 2006, with permission.)

**FIGURE 3.39.**    Movements of the knee joint (flexion–extension).

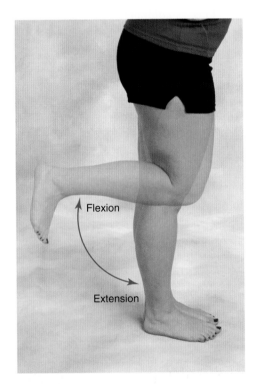

## MUSCLES

### Anterior

Large and powerful thigh muscles cross the knee joint, several of which are two-joint muscles acting on the hip joint as well. The quadriceps muscles (*i.e.*, rectus femoris, vastus lateralis, vastus intermedius, and vastus medialis) are anterior knee muscles and act to extend the knee joint (see Fig. 3.34). The quadriceps muscles insert into the superior aspect of the patella and ultimately to the tibial tuberosity by the patellar ligament. The rectus femoris is a large, two-joint muscle that originates from the AIIS. The rectus femoris flexes the hip in addition to extending the knee. The three vasti muscles originate from the proximal femur. The vastus lateralis and vastus medialis are pennate muscles that pull on the patella at oblique angles (20).

### Posterior

The muscles of the posterior knee joint are the hamstrings (biceps femoris, semitendinosus, and semimembranosus), sartorius, gracilis, popliteus, and gastrocnemius (see Fig. 3.35). The biceps femoris (lateral hamstrings) muscle contains a long head (which originates from the ischial tuberosity and is a two-joint muscle) and a short head (which originates from the mid-femur). The biceps femoris inserts into the lateral condyle of the tibia and head of the fibula. It acts to flex and externally rotate the knee and extend and externally rotate the hip. The semimembranosus and semitendinosus (medial hamstrings) are two-joint muscles that act to flex and internally rotate the knee and extend and internally rotate the hip. The sartorius muscle, which originates from the ASIS, acts on both the knee and hip joints. The tendons of the sartorius, gracilis, and semimembranosus join together to form the pes anserinus, which inserts to the anteromedial aspect of the proximal tibia, just inferior to the tibial tuberosity. The gastrocnemius muscle is a two-head and two-joint muscle that acts to flex the knee and plantarflex the ankle (18). The gastrocnemius is discussed in detail in the "Ankle and Foot" section of this chapter. The popliteus is a weak flexor of the knee but, more importantly, "unlocks" the extended knee by laterally rotating the femur on the fixed tibia.

## INJURIES

As mentioned earlier, the knee is a frequently injured joint, with its ligaments, menisci, and patellofemoral joint vulnerable to acute and repetitive use damage. Most knee injuries require exercise training for rehabilitation, and some require surgery as well. Predisposing factors to knee injury include the following (3,7,36):

- Lower extremity malalignment (*e.g.*, Q angle abnormalities, flat feet)
- Limb length discrepancy
- Muscular imbalance and weakness
- Inflexibility
- Previous injury
- Inadequate proprioception
- Joint instability
- Playing surface and equipment problems
- Slight predominance in females (particularly for patellofemoral problems)

Ligamentous sprains and tears are common in the knee, particularly in athletes. Because of its structure and insertion points, the anterior cruciate ligament is more frequently injured compared with the posterior cruciate ligament. Classically, the anterior cruciate ligament is injured when external rotation of the tibia is coupled with a valgus force on the knee (*e.g.*, direct force from the lateral side of the knee, planting the foot and twisting the knee) (3). Ligamentous sprains and tears are common in the knee, particularly in athletes.

The menisci are also frequently injured, particularly in athletes. The medial meniscus is more frequently torn than the lateral meniscus due in part to its attachment to the medial collateral ligament. The menisci are poorly innervated and relatively avascular; thus, they are not very pain sensitive and are slow to heal following injury. The "terrible triad" is a traumatic sports injury in which the anterior cruciate ligament, medial collateral ligament, and medial meniscus are damaged simultaneously (4).

Patellofemoral pain syndrome is a common disorder in young athletes (particularly females) that produces anterior knee pain. Often, patellofemoral pain syndrome is caused by an off-center line of pull of the patella, which irritates the joint surfaces and retinaculum of the knee (40). An off-center pull of the patella can result from insufficiency muscular imbalance during knee extension (24) and from excessive varus and valgus stresses from Q angles outside of the normal range of 13°–18°.

### Ankle and Foot

Ankles and feet are responsible for weight bearing and ambulation. Proper function and mechanics of ankles and feet are essential for most sports activities and performance of activities of daily living. Slight abnormalities in the feet and ankles (*e.g.*, muscular imbalance, proprioceptive dysfunction, and structural changes) are transmitted via the kinetic chain to most joints superior to them in the body (4). Thus, knee, hip, low back, neck, shoulder, and body alignment and postural problems can at times be traced to dysfunctional ankles and feet. This section focuses on ankle functional anatomy. For the functional anatomy of the intrinsic foot, the reader is referred to other sources (1,16,28,29,31). Proper function and mechanics of ankles and feet are essential for most sports activities and performance of activities of daily living.

### STRUCTURE

### Bones

The foot has 26 articulating bones contained in three functional units: the anterior (forefoot), middle (midfoot), and posterior (hindfoot) (Fig. 3.40). The forefoot contains the five metatarsals

**FIGURE 3.40.** Bones of the ankle and foot regions. **A.** Lateral view. **B.** Medial view. (From Moore KL, Dalley AF II. *Clinically Oriented Anatomy*. 4th ed. Baltimore [MD]: Lippincott Williams & Wilkins; 1999, with permission.)

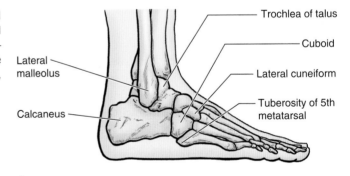

**A Lateral foot**

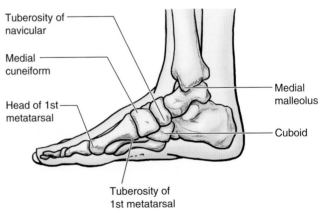

**B Medial foot**

(one for each digit) and 14 phalanges (toes), three each for digits 2–5 and two for the great toe. The midfoot contains the five tarsal bones: a navicular, a cuboid, and three cuneiforms. The hindfoot contains the talus and calcaneus bones. The dome of the talus articulates with the distal tibia and fibula and provides the link between the leg and foot at the talocrural joint. The ankle is formed by the fibrous union of the distal tibia, the medial malleolus of the tibia, and the lateral malleolus of the fibula (7). The location of the talus is superior to the calcaneus, between the malleoli of the tibia and fibula. Most of the calcaneus represents the posterior projection of the heel. The calcaneus provides important attachment sites for the ankle plantarflexor muscles.

## Ligaments

There are approximately 100 ligaments in the ankle and foot region (Fig. 3.41). On the lateral side of the ankle, the major ligaments include the anterior and posterior talofibular and the calcaneofibular ligaments. The deltoid ligament complex is on the medial ankle and includes the tibiocalcaneal, anterior and posterior tibiotalar, and tibionavicular ligaments. The plantar calcaneonavicular ligament (spring ligament) of the foot helps support the talus and maintains the longitudinal arch (36).

There are two arches on the plantar aspect of the foot that give the foot its shape and distribute body weight from the talus to the foot during various load-bearing conditions (3). The various ligaments and bones primarily support the arches, with muscles providing secondary support. The longitudinal arch extends from the calcaneal tuberosity to the five metatarsals, whereas the transverse arch extends crosswise from medial to lateral in the midtarsal region. The plantar fascia, or plantar aponeurosis, is a strong fibrous connective tissue that provides support for the longitudinal arch. The plantar fascia acts as an extension of the calcaneal (Achilles) tendon of the plantarflexor muscles. During weight-bearing phase of gait, the plantar fascia acts like a spring to store mechanical energy that is then released during foot push-off (38).

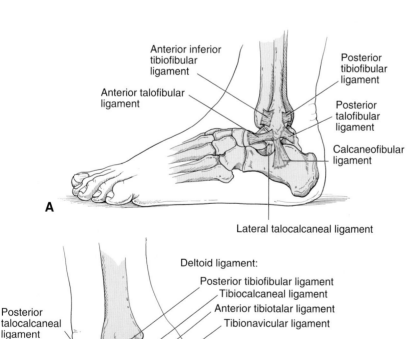

**FIGURE 3.41.** Ligaments of the ankle and foot regions. **A.** Lateral view. **B.** Medial view. (From Cipriano J. *Photographic Manual of Regional Orthopaedic and Neurological Tests.* 5th ed. Baltimore [MD]: Lippincott Williams & Wilkins; 2014, with permission.)

## Joints

The ankle joint is a synovial, hinge-type joint between the distal tibia and fibula and the dome of talus. A tight fibrous syndesmosis between tibia and fibula unites the distal ends of the bones and forms a "malleolar mortise" into which the trochlea or "dome" of talus fits. The subtalar joint is a plane synovial joint between talus and calcaneus. There are many other joints between the other tarsal bones that allow varying degrees and types of movements. Additionally, there are tarsometatarsal, intermetatarsal, metatarsophalangeal, and interphalangeal joints (36).

### MOVEMENTS

The talocrural joint allows approximately 15°–20° of dorsiflexion and 50° of plantarflexion in the sagittal plane. The subtalar joint allows approximately 20°–30° of inversion and 5°–15° of eversion in the frontal plane. The midtarsal and tarsometatarsal joints permit gliding motion. The metatarsophalangeal and interphalangeal joints primarily allow flexion and extension of the digits in the sagittal plane. Pronation and supination are combination movements at the ankle and foot that allow the foot to maintain contact with the ground in a variety of stances or on uneven ground. Pronation is a combination of talocrural dorsiflexion, subtalar eversion, and forefoot abduction. Supination is a combination of talocrural plantarflexion, subtalar inversion, and forefoot adduction (38) (Fig. 3.42).

### MUSCLES

The major muscles that act on the ankle and foot are located in the leg, and these muscles are typically grouped by their compartmental location — anterior, lateral, superficial posterior, and deep posterior (38).

### Anterior and Lateral

The anterior muscles, tibialis anterior, peroneus (fibularis) tertius, extensor digitorum longus, and extensor hallucis longus, are ankle dorsiflexors (Fig. 3.43). The tibialis anterior also inverts the foot, whereas the peroneus tertius everts the foot. The extensor hallucis longus acts to extend the big toe, and extensor digitorum longus extend digits 2–5. The lateral muscles, peroneus longus and brevis, evert the foot and assist with plantarflexion as well (18) (Fig. 3.44).

### Superficial and Deep Posterior

The superficial posterior muscles, gastrocnemius, soleus, and plantaris, are ankle plantarflexors (Fig. 3.45). The gastrocnemius is a two-head and two-joint muscle and is a powerful plantarflexor of the ankle as well as a flexor of the knee. The gastrocnemius has relatively faster twitch fibers than the soleus. Thus, the gastrocnemius is used more during dynamic, higher force activities, and the soleus is more active during postural and static contractions (4). Because the gastrocnemius

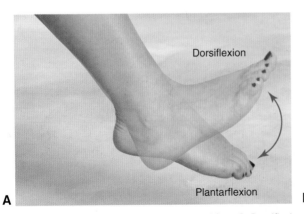

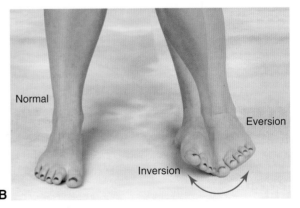

**FIGURE 3.42.**    Movements of the ankle and foot. **A.** Dorsiflexion–plantarflexion. **B.** Normal, inversion, and eversion.

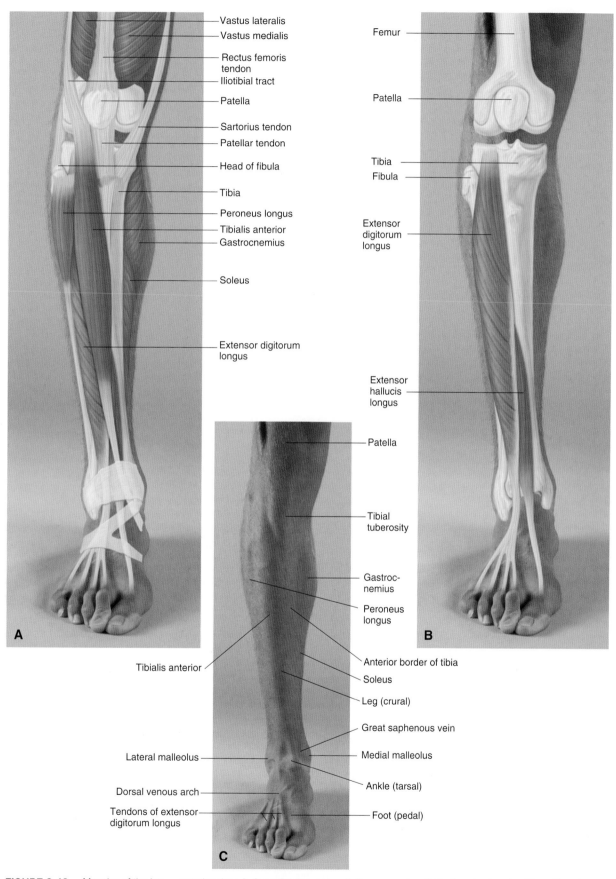

**FIGURE 3.43.** Muscles of the leg — anterior view. **A.** Superficial muscles. **B.** Deep muscles. **C.** Surface landmarks. (From Premkumar K. *The Massage Connection: Anatomy and Physiology.* 3rd ed. Baltimore [MD]: Lippincott Williams & Wilkins; 2011, with permission.)

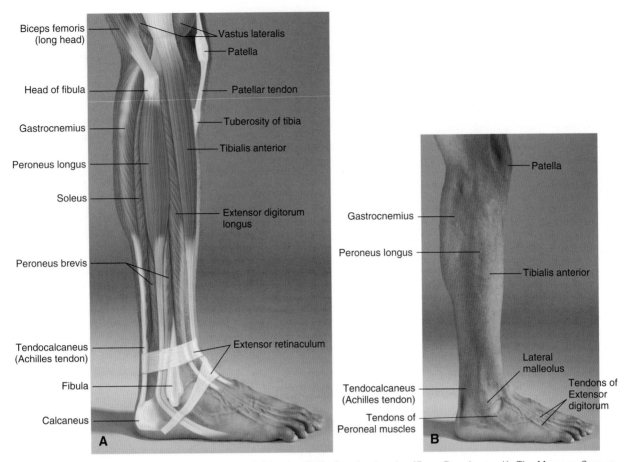

**FIGURE 3.44.**   Muscles of the leg — lateral view. **A.** Muscles. **B.** Surface landmarks. (From Premkumar K. *The Massage Connection: Anatomy and Physiology*. 3rd ed. Baltimore [MD]: Lippincott Williams & Wilkins; 2011, with permission.)

crosses the knee and ankle, the position of the knee during plantarflexion resistance exercise affects the activity of the gastrocnemius. At 90° of knee flexion, the gastrocnemius experiences passive insufficiency and thus is less active than when the knee is straight (0° of flexion). In other words, during calf raise exercise, keep the knees straight to emphasize the gastrocnemius and bend the knees to emphasize the soleus. The deep posterior muscles are flexor digitorum longus, flexor hallucis longus, tibialis posterior, and popliteus. All except for popliteus are ankle plantarflexors and inverters. Additionally, the tibialis posterior inverts the foot. The flexor digitorum and hallucis longus flex their respective digits.

### INJURIES

Because of the burden placed on the ankle and foot during activities such as walking, running, jumping, and lifting, traumatic and overuse injuries frequently occur to these structures (3). Numerous acute muscular strains and cramps occur in the leg and foot, and many ligament sprains occur in this region as well. Ankle sprains are more common on the lateral side than on the medial side because there is less bony stability and ligamentous strength on the lateral side. The mechanism of injury for lateral ankle sprains is excessive inversion (rolling out of the ankle), as occurs when landing on someone's foot after jumping in basketball. The anterior talofibular ligament is the most frequently sprained ligament in inversion injuries (3).

Because of the burden placed on the ankle and foot during activities such as walking, running, jumping, and lifting, traumatic and overuse injuries frequently occur to these structures (3).

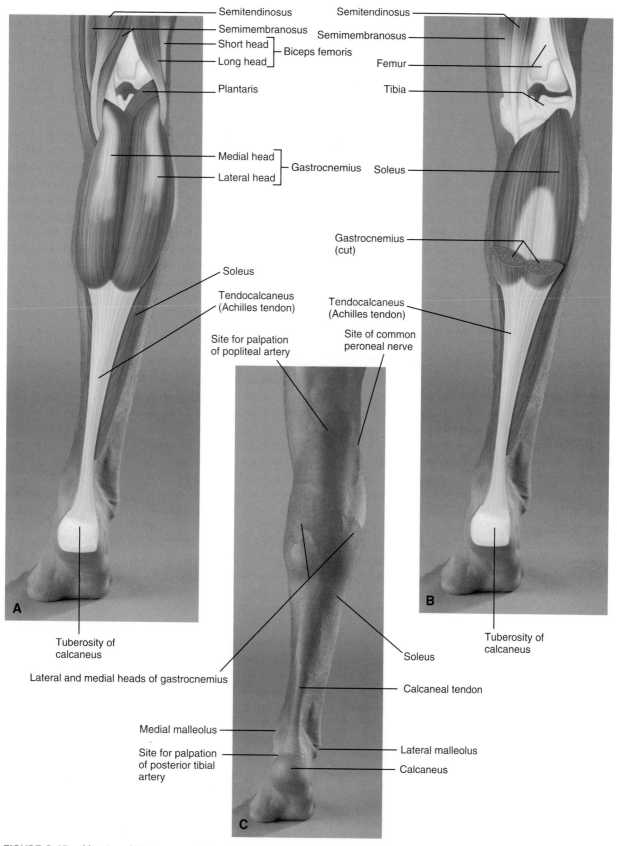

**FIGURE 3.45.** Muscles of the leg — posterior view. **A.** Superficial muscles. **B.** Soleus. **C.** Surface landmarks. (From Premkumar K. *The Massage Connection: Anatomy and Physiology.* 3rd ed. Baltimore [MD]: Lippincott Williams & Wilkins; 2011, with permission.)

Achilles tendon rupture is possibly the most serious acute injury of the leg (3). Nearly 75% of Achilles tendon ruptures are seen in male athletes between 30 and 40 years of age. The typical mechanism is forceful plantarflexion while the knee is extended. These injuries almost always require surgical repair and extensive long-term rehabilitation. Achilles tendon rupture is often a career-ending injury for athletes, especially if it occurs in the later stages of their careers (3).

Plantar fasciitis is a chronic inflammatory condition that typically results in pain at the calcaneal insertion of the plantar fascia (3). Plantar fasciitis is usually caused by chronic pulling on the plantar fascia, tight Achilles tendon, hyperpronation (flat feet or pes planus), or other factors that overload the fascia (*e.g.*, obesity). Treatment of plantar fasciitis includes stretching and strengthening exercises for the posterior calf muscles, orthoses to correct hyperpronation, and physiotherapy modalities and medication to reduce inflammation. Sometimes, surgery is required to release the plantar fascia. Plantar fasciitis is often associated with calcaneal heel spurs (3).

Other chronic conditions of the foot and ankle include bunions, neuromas, Achilles tendonitis, and calcaneal bursitis. These conditions are frequently related to structural problems of the foot and ankle, such as hyperpronation or hypersupination (high arch or pes cavus). Unilateral hyperpronation or hypersupination may cause instability and proprioceptive difficulties at the ankle and postural imbalances and mechanical problems to proximal joint structures in the kinetic chain.

## Spine

The spine is an intricate multijoint structure that plays a crucial role in functional mechanics. The spine provides the link between the upper and lower extremities, protects the spinal cord, and enables trunk motion in three planes (3). Moreover, the rib cage of the thoracic spinal region protects the internal organs of the chest. Because of its intricacies, the spine is susceptible to injuries that may severely impair physical function.

### STRUCTURE

### Bones

The spinal column contains a complex of irregular bones called "vertebrae" that are stacked on one another (Fig. 3.46). There are 24 individual vertebrae: 7 cervical (neck), 12 thoracic (mid-back), and 5 lumbar (low back) (36). The most superior cervical vertebra (C1) articulates with the occipital bone of the skull, whereas the most inferior lumbar vertebra (L5) articulates with the sacrum. The size of the vertebrae increases from the cervical to the lumbar region because of an increase in load-bearing responsibilities. Each vertebra contains anterior and posterior elements. The anterior element, called the "vertebral body," is oval with flat superior and inferior surfaces for articulation with the adjacent vertebral bodies. The posterior element, or posterior arch, consists of pedicles and laminae, which join anteriorly at the body and posteriorly at the spinous process to form the vertebral foramen (canal). The vertebral foramen provides a space through which the spinal cord passes. The posterior arch also contains facets on each side and top and bottom for articulation with adjacent vertebra. The spinous and transverse processes are bony protuberances that provide attachment points for the spinal musculature (36).

Ribs attach to each of the 12 thoracic vertebrae bilaterally and form the thoracic cage (Fig. 3.47). The seven most superior pairs of ribs are considered true ribs and attach directly to the sternum. The five lower pairs of ribs are considered false ribs. Three pairs of false ribs attach indirectly to the sternum by the costal cartilages. Two most inferior pairs of false ribs do not attach to the sternum and are considered floating ribs (38).

The spinal column also contains a sacrum and coccyx, which are situated at the lower spine, immediately inferior to the fifth lumbar vertebra. The sacrum is a large triangular bone that acts as the transition point between the spine and pelvis. The coccyx is a bone formed of three to five fused vertebrae located at the distal sacrum (36).

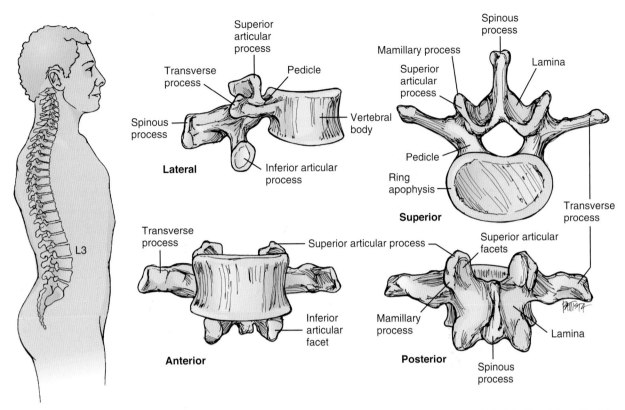

**FIGURE 3.46.** A typical lumbar vertebra (L3) in four views identifying the relevant landmarks. (From Oatis CA. *Kinesiology: The Mechanics and Pathomechanics of Human Movement*. 3rd ed. Baltimore [MD]: Lippincott Williams & Wilkins; 2016, with permission.)

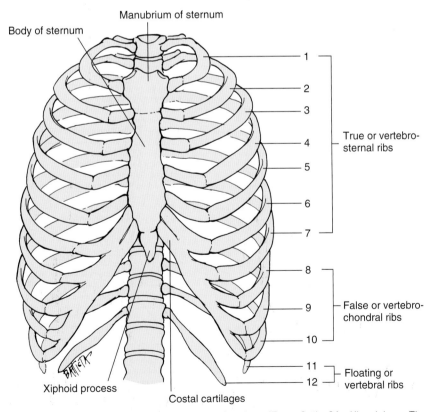

**FIGURE 3.47.** The thoracic cage — anterior view. (From Oatis CA. *Kinesiology: The Mechanics and Pathomechanics of Human Movement*. 3rd ed. Baltimore [MD]: Lippincott Williams & Wilkins; 2016, with permission.)

In the sagittal plane, the spinal column normally demonstrates four curves instead of a straight line (Fig. 3.48). These curves give the spine mechanical advantage and improved load-bearing capabilities. When the convexity of the curve is posterior, the curve is known as kyphosis, and when the convexity of the curve is anterior, the curve is known as lordosis. The cervical and lumbar regions have lordosis, and the thoracic and sacral regions have kyphosis. Deviations in the sagittal plane are referred to as "hyperlordosis" or "hyperkyphosis." In the frontal plane, the spinal column should normally be positioned in the midline. Lateral deviation is referred to as "scoliosis" (Fig. 3.49) (4).

## Ligaments

The main supporting ligaments of the spinal column are the anterior and posterior longitudinal ligaments and the ligamentum flavum, which span from the upper cervical to lower lumbar region (Fig. 3.50). The anterior and posterior longitudinal ligaments attach to the vertebral bodies, and the ligamentum flavum connects the posterior arches and forms the posterior border of the vertebral canal. The interspinous and supraspinous ligaments attach to adjacent posterior arch structures (4).

## Intervertebral Discs

The intervertebral discs are important structures that provide load bearing, shock absorption, and stability to the vertebral column. The discs are located between the vertebral bodies and constitute

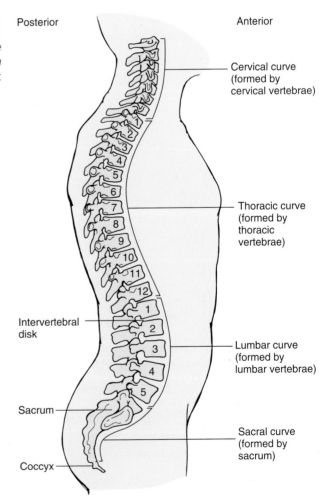

**FIGURE 3.48.** Vertebral column — lateral view showing the four normal curves and regions. (From Oatis CA. *Kinesiology: The Mechanics and Pathomechanics of Human Movement.* 3rd ed. Baltimore [MD]: Lippincott Williams & Wilkins; 2016, with permission.)

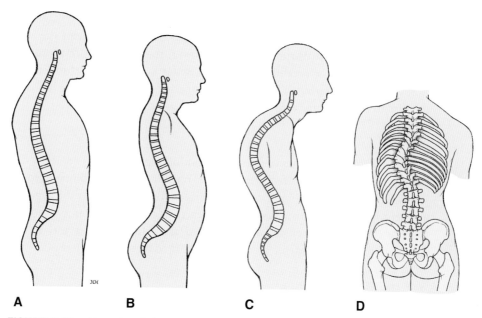

**FIGURE 3.49.** Normal and abnormal curves of the vertebral column. **A.** Normal. **B.** Hyperlordosis. **C.** Hyperkyphosis. **D.** Scoliosis. (Courtesy of Neil O. Hardy, Westport, CT).

about 20%–33% of the height of the vertebral column (31) (see Fig. 3.50). Each intervertebral motion segment contains a disc, except for the articulation between the first and second cervical vertebrae (the atlas and axis, respectively). The intervertebral disc consists of the nucleus pulposus, annulus fibrosis, and endplates. These structures are composed of various concentrations of water, collagen, and proteoglycans. The nucleus pulposus, located in the center of the disc, is gel-like and more liquid than the annulus fibrosis. The nucleus pulposus dehydrates with age, which is one of the reasons why overall body height reduces with age (31). The annulus fibrosis, located at the

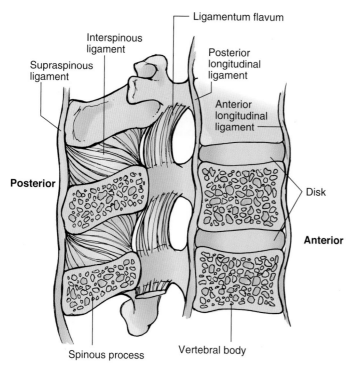

Ligamentum flavum
Interspinous ligament
Supraspinous ligament
Posterior longitudinal ligament
Anterior longitudinal ligament
Posterior
Disk
Anterior
Spinous process
Vertebral body

**FIGURE 3.50.** Ligaments and discs of the lumbar spine — mid-sagittal view. (From Oatis CA. *Kinesiology: The Mechanics and Pathomechanics of Human Movement.* 3rd ed. Baltimore [MD]: Lippincott Williams & Wilkins; 2016, with permission.)

periphery of the disc, is a more rigid structure and contains more collagen fibers than the nucleus. The oblique arrangement of the collagen fibers of the annulus helps the annulus resist tensile and compressive forces in various planes. However, the annulus is most susceptible to tearing with movements involving rotation and flexion under load. The vertebral endplates are thin layers of fibrocartilage that cover the inferior and superior aspects of the vertebral body and help anchor the disc to the vertebrae (25).

### Joints

The spinal column consists of numerous motion segments (two adjacent vertebrae). Each motion segment of spine contains five articulations: one intervertebral joint and four zygapophysial (facet) joints. The intervertebral joint connects adjacent bodies, whereas the zygapophysial joints connect adjacent facets (superior and inferior on each side). The lumbar zygapophysial joints are angled to allow flexion and extension and restrict axial rotation. The cervical and thoracic zygapophysial joints, on the other hand, are angled to accommodate axial rotation (4).

### MOVEMENTS

The spine is capable of motion in all planes, and the extent of motion varies with region. In the cervical spine, the atlantooccipital joint allows flexion and extension and slight lateral flexion. The atlantoaxial joint allows primarily rotation. The remaining cervical joints allow flexion and extension, lateral flexion, and rotation. The thoracic joints allow moderate flexion, slight extension, moderate lateral flexion, and rotation. The lumbar joints allow flexion and extension, lateral flexion, and slight rotation (4) (Fig. 3.51). Refer to Table 3.6 for normal cervical and lumbar ROM values.

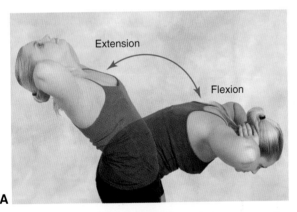

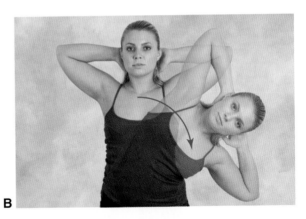

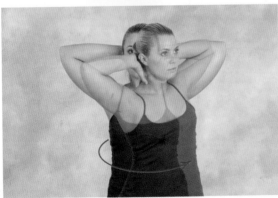

**FIGURE 3.51.**    Movements of the lower trunk. **A.** Flexion–extension. **B.** Lateral flexion. **C.** Rotation.

## Compound Trunk Extension

Trunk motion in the sagittal plane during normal activities, such as lifting and bending, requires the compound movement of the lumbar spine, pelvis, and hip joints (22). This action is called "compound trunk extension" or "lumbopelvic rhythm." From a position of full trunk flexion, the lumbar extensors (erector spinae and multifidus) and hip extensors (gluteals and hamstrings) work together to actively rotate the trunk through approximately 180° in the sagittal plane (7) (Fig. 3.52). Lumbar movement accounts for approximately 72° of this motion, whereas hip and pelvis movement accounts for the remaining 108° (34). The relative contribution of individual muscle groups to force production during compound trunk extension is unknown, but it is assumed that the larger hip extensors generate most of the force (7). Because the pelvis remains free to move during activities of daily living such as lifting and bending, it is assumed that the small lumbar muscles play only a minor role in trunk extension torque production. Thus, they are considered to be the weak link in trunk extension movements (13). The rationale behind isolating the lumbar spine through pelvic stabilization mechanisms during exercise training is to force the lumbar muscles to be the primary trunk extensors, thereby providing the overload stimulus for strength gains (13). Dynamic progressive resistance exercise protocols on devices that stabilize the pelvis have produced unusually large gains (greater than 100%) in lumbar extension strength, even with training frequencies as low as one time per week (13). Clinically, patients with low back pain have displayed significant improvements in symptoms, disability, and psychosocial function following intensive exercise training with pelvic stabilization (19,26).

### MUSCLES

The spine and trunk muscles exist in pairs, one on each side of the body. In general, bilateral contraction results in movement in the sagittal plane. The anterior muscles flex the spine, whereas the posterior muscles extend the spine. Unilateral contraction results in lateral bend or axial rotation.

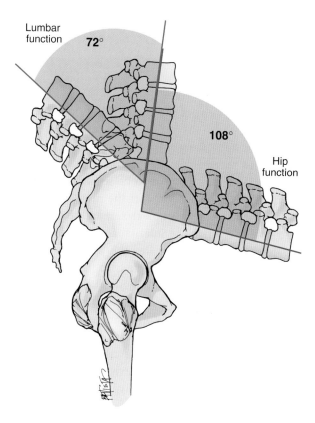

Lumbar function 72°

108°

Hip function

**FIGURE 3.52.** Compound trunk extension (lumbopelvic rhythm). Compound trunk extension involves the simultaneous movement of the lumbar spine (72°) and pelvis/hips (108°).

### CERVICAL

#### Anterior

The major anterior muscles of the cervical region include the sternocleidomastoid, scalenes (anterior, middle, and posterior), longus capitis, and longus colli muscles. On unilateral contraction, these muscles laterally flex and rotate the neck and head. On bilateral contraction, the anterior scalene, longus capitis and colli, and sternocleidomastoid muscles flex the neck and head. The scalenes attach proximally to the upper cervical transverse processes and distally to the upper two ribs. The sternocleidomastoid attaches proximally to the mastoid process of the occiput and distally to the sternum (medial head) and clavicle (lateral head) (see Fig. 3.17). The longus muscles run from the transverse processes of the upper cervical vertebrae to the anterior aspect of the superior cervical vertebrae (longus colli) or the base of the occiput (longus capitis) (18).

#### Posterior

The suboccipital muscles, which attach the upper cervical vertebrae to the occiput, extend the head when they contract bilaterally and laterally bend and rotate the neck when they contract unilaterally. Similarly, the splenius (capitis and cervicis) and erector spinae (spinalis, longissimus, and iliocostalis) muscles extend the neck when they contract bilaterally and laterally bend and rotate the neck when they contract unilaterally (18) (see Fig. 3.18).

#### Lateral

The lateral muscles of the neck and head include the levator scapulae and upper trapezius muscles, both of which laterally bend and rotate the neck on unilateral contraction. The upper trapezius extends the neck as well on bilateral contraction. The levator scapulae attaches superiorly to the transverse processes of the upper four cervical vertebrae and inferiorly to the vertebral border of the scapula above the spine. The upper trapezius attaches proximally to the occiput and spinous processes of the cervical vertebrae and distally to the clavicle and acromion of the scapula (18). The levator scapulae and upper trapezius muscles also cause movement of the scapulothoracic joint, as discussed in the section "Shoulder" in this chapter.

### LUMBAR

#### Anterior

The anterior muscles of the lumbar region consist of the abdominal group: the rectus abdominis, internal and external abdominal oblique, and transversus abdominis (see Fig. 3.17). The rectus abdominis originates from the pubic bone and inserts at the fifth through seventh ribs and xiphoid process. The rectus abdominis exists as two vertical muscles separated by a connective tissue band, the linea alba. Horizontally, the rectus abdominis appears to be separated by three distinct lines. These lines represent areas of connective tissue that support the muscle in place of attachment to bones (38). The rectus abdominis is the primary trunk flexor, and through its attachment to the pubic bone, it also tilts the pelvis posteriorly. The internal and external obliquus abdominis muscles rotate the trunk on unilateral contraction and flex the trunk on bilateral contraction. The transversus abdominis runs horizontally, attaching medially to the linea alba via the abdominal aponeurosis and laterally to the thoracolumbar fascia, inguinal ligament, iliac crest, and the lower six ribs. Contraction of the transversus abdominis stabilizes the lumbar spine and increases intra-abdominal pressure, and aberrant firing patterns of the transversus abdominis appear to be related to low back pain (35).

To isolate the abdominal muscles during trunk flexion exercise, it is advisable to shorten the psoas and other hip flexor muscles (active insufficiency) by flexing the hips and knees (38). Thus, crunches with the hips and knees flexed may be more effective in conditioning the abdominals than straight knee sit-ups (18).

## Posterior

The posterior musculature of the lumbar spine consists of three muscle groups, namely, the erector spinae, multifidus muscles, and intrinsic rotators (Fig. 3.53). Additionally, the latissimus dorsi, which is usually considered a muscle that acts on the shoulder, extends and stabilizes the lumbar spine through its attachment to the thoracolumbar fascia (25). The erector spinae group, which lies lateral and superficial to the multifidus, is divided into the iliocostalis lumborum and longissimus thoracis muscles (5). These muscles are separated from each other by the lumbar intramuscular aponeurosis, with the longissimus lying medially. The longissimus and iliocostalis are composed

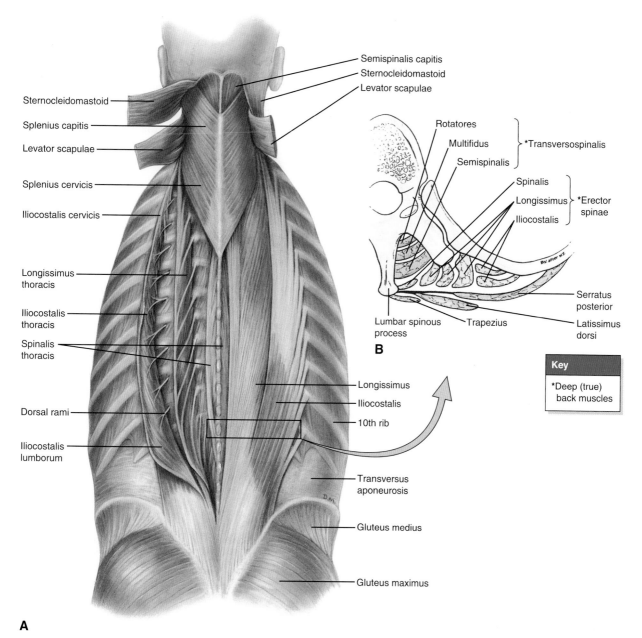

**FIGURE 3.53.** Deep muscles of the back. **A.** Right, the three columns of the erector spinae. Left, the spinalis is displayed by reflecting the longissimus and iliocostalis. **B.** Transverse section of the back showing arrangement of the erector spinae, multifidus, and rotator muscles. (From Moore KL, Dalley AF II. *Clinically Oriented Anatomy*. 4th ed. Baltimore [MD]: Lippincott Williams & Wilkins; 1999, with permission.)

of several multisegmental fascicles, which allow for extension and posterior translation when the muscles are contracted bilaterally. The fascicular arrangement of the multifidus muscle suggests that the multifidus acts primarily as a sagittal rotator (extension without posterior translation) (21). Lateral flexion and axial rotation are possible for both the multifidus and erector spinae musculature during unilateral contraction. The iliocostalis may be better suited to exert axial rotation on the lumbar vertebral motion segment than either the longissimus or multifidus muscles (5). Because of their anatomical and biomechanical properties, the posterior lumbar muscles are particularly adapted to maintain posture and stabilize the spine and trunk (5). The intrinsic rotators, rotators, and intertransversarii muscles, are primarily length transducers and position sensors for the vertebral segment (30).

### Lateral

The lateral muscles of the lumbar spine include the quadratus lumborum and psoas (major and minor). The quadratus lumborum originates from the iliac crest and inserts at the 12th rib and transverse process of the lower four lumbar vertebrae. The quadratus lumborum produces lateral bending of the lumbar spine with unilateral contraction and stabilizes the trunk with bilateral contraction. The psoas major muscle originates from the anterior surfaces of the transverse processes of all the lumbar vertebrae and inserts at the lesser trochanter of the femur. The psoas major flexes the trunk and the hip (18).

### INJURIES

### Cervical

The cervical region is the most mobile region of the spine, and relatively small cervical muscles are responsible for supporting the head. These factors make the cervical region vulnerable to instability and injury (3). The most dangerous injuries to the cervical region are traumatic fractures and dislocations that result in instability of the column. The combination of axial compression and hyperflexion is a common mechanism for severe cervical injuries such as these (39). Examples of activities with these mechanisms include diving into a shallow pool or a football player making a head-on tackle. The direct consequence of upper cervical dislocation or fracture is neural damage to the upper spinal cord, which may result in paralysis or death (3). Thus, any traumatic neck injury should be treated as a medical emergency (41).

Sprains and strains of the neck muscles and ligaments are frequently the result of violent hyperextension–hyperflexion from sudden acceleration–deceleration, such as a head-on car collision. This condition, commonly called "whiplash," can cause tears of the anterior and posterior structures of the cervical region, including the muscles (*e.g.*, sternocleidomastoid, upper trapezius, and cervical paraspinals) and ligaments (7). After ruling out fracture, dislocation, instability, and disc herniation, treatment of whiplash usually includes passive modalities, stretches, and strengthening exercises for the neck.

### Lumbar

Low back pain is one of the leading causes of disability and consistently ranks as one of the top reasons for visits to physicians. Low back pain affects 60%–80% of the general population at some point during their lifetime, and 20%–30% suffer from this disorder at any given time (9,10). Attaching a specific diagnosis to low back pain is difficult and elusive because there often is no identifiable source of the pain or injury (27). It should not be assumed that all low back pain is musculoskeletal in nature. Back pain can be experienced secondary to a wide variety of other medical conditions that are not musculoskeletal in nature (*e.g.*, abdominal aneurysm, kidney infection, cancer). These should be ruled out by the appropriate medical professionals.

Some of the causes of low back pain include intervertebral disc herniation, facet joint inflammation, muscular strains, and ligamentous sprains. Injury to these structures can be traumatic, caused by events such as inappropriately lifting or falling, or degenerative, caused by a deconditioned lumbar spine, poor posture, prolonged mechanical loading, or poor body mechanics during work, home, or sports activities (3,7). A common cause of lumbar disc herniation is forceful flexion and rotation of the lumbar spine. A protruded lumbar disc that encroaches on the lumbar nerve roots may result in lower extremity sensory and motor problems such as pain, numbness, and muscular weakness and atrophy. Bowel and bladder dysfunction are serious conditions that can result from herniated lumbar discs and require immediate medical treatment (3).

Restorative exercise designed to improve the structural integrity of the lower trunk is commonly used for the treatment of low back pain, and generally, the efficacy of this approach has been supported (20). Many types of exercises, including aerobic, flexibility, muscular strength and endurance, and core stability, are used. The Personal Trainer should be particularly well versed in low back exercise techniques, incorporating those needed when appropriate.

## SUMMARY

This chapter provides an overview of musculoskeletal functional anatomy of the major joint structures of the human body. These principles play a major role in nearly all aspects of the Personal Trainer's practice, including exercise testing, exercise prescription, and analysis of exercise movements. Thus, the Personal Trainer is urged to master these principles so that safe, effective, and efficient exercise training programs can be designed to improve musculoskeletal fitness.

## REFERENCES

1. Agur A, Lee M, Anderson J. *Grant's Atlas of Anatomy.* 9th ed. Baltimore (MD): Williams & Wilkins; 1991. 650 p.
2. An K, Morrey B. Biomechanics of the shoulder. In: Matsen F, editor. *The Shoulder.* Philadelphia (PA): WB Saunders; 1990. p. 213–65.
3. Anderson M, Hall S. *Fundamentals of Sports Injury Management.* Baltimore (MD): Williams & Wilkins; 1997. 689 p.
4. Baldwin K. *Kinesiology for Personal Fitness Trainers.* New York (NY): McGraw-Hill; 2003.
5. Bogduk N, Twomey LT. *Clinical Anatomy of the Lumbar Spine.* New York (NY): Churchill Livingstone; 1990. 197 p.
6. Burkhead W. *Rotator Cuff Disorders.* Baltimore (MD): Williams & Wilkins; 1996. 422 p.
7. Cailliet R. *Soft Tissue Pain and Disability.* 3rd ed. Philadelphia (PA): FA Davis; 1996. 545 p.
8. DeLavier F. *Strength Training Anatomy.* Champaign (IL): Human Kinetics; 2001. 124 p.
9. Deyo R, Tsui-Wu Y. Descriptive epidemiology of low-back pain and its related medical care in the United States. *Spine (Phila Pa 1976).* 1987;12:264–8.
10. Frymoyer J, Cats-Baril WL. An overview of the incidences and cost of low back pain. *Orthop Clin North Am.* 1991;22:263–71.
11. Garrick J, Webb D. *Sports Injuries: Diagnosis and Management.* Philadelphia (PA): WB Saunders; 1990. 347 p.
12. Graves J, Franklin B. Introduction. In: Graves J, Franklin B, editors. *Resistance Training for Health and Rehabilitation.* Champaign (IL): Human Kinetics; 2001. p. 1–12.
13. Graves JE, Webb DC, Pollock ML, et al. Pelvic stabilization during resistance training: its effect on the development of lumbar extension strength. *Arch Phys Med Rehabil.* 1994;75(2):210–15.
14. Griggs S, Weiss A. Bony injuries of the wrist, forearm, and elbow. In: Plancher KD, editor. *Clin Sports Med.* 1996;15(2):373–400.
15. Halikis M, Taleisnik J. Soft-tissue injuries of the wrist. In: Plancher KD, editor. *Clin Sports Med.* 1996;15(2):235–259.
16. Hall-Craggs E. *Anatomy as the Basis for Clinical Medicine.* 3rd ed. Baltimore (MD): Williams & Wilkins; 1995. 587 p.
17. Horrigan J, Robinson J. *The 7-Minute Rotator Cuff Solution.* Los Angeles (CA): Health for Life; 1990. 64 p.
18. Kendall F, McCreary E, Provance P. *Muscles: Testing and Function.* 4th ed. Philadelphia (PA): Lippincott Williams & Wilkins; 1993. 448 p.
19. Leggett S, Mooney V, Matheson L, et al. Restorative exercise for clinical low back pain: a prospective two-center study with 1-year follow-up. *Spine (Phila Pa).* 1999;24(9):889–98.
20. Liemohn W, editor. *Exercise Prescription and the Back.* New York (NY): McGraw-Hill; 2001. 254 p.
21. MacIntosh J, Bogduk N. The attachments of the lumbar erector spinae. *Spine (Phila Pa).* 1991;16(7):783–92.
22. Mayer L, Greenberg B. Measurement of the strength of trunk muscles. *J Bone Joint Surg.* 1942;4:842–56.
23. McCue F, Hussamy O, Gieck J. Hand and wrist injuries. In: Zachazewski J, Magee D, Quillen W, editors. *Athletic Injuries and Rehabilitation.* Philadelphia (PA): WB Saunders; 1996. p. 585–98.

24. McGee D. *Orthopedic Physical Assessment*. Philadelphia (PA): WB Saunders; 1987.

25. McGill S. *Low Back Disorders: Evidence-Based Prevention and Rehabilitation*. Champaign (IL): Human Kinetics; 2002. 295 p.

26. Mooney V. Functional evaluation of the spine. *Curr Opin Orthop*. 1994;5(2):54–7.

27. Mooney V, Kron M, Rummerfield P, Holmes B. The effect of workplace based strengthening on low back injury rates: a case study in the strip mining industry. *J Occup Rehabil*. 1995;5:157–67.

28. Moore K, Agur A. *Essentials of Clinical Anatomy*. 2nd ed. Baltimore (MD): Williams & Wilkins; 2002. 691 p.

29. Moore K, Dalley AF. *Clinically Oriented Anatomy*. 4th ed. Baltimore (MD): Williams & Wilkins; 2004. 1164 p.

30. Nitz A, Peck D. Comparison of muscle spindle concentrations in large and small human epaxial muscles acting in parallel combinations. *Am Surg*. 1986;52:273–7.

31. Norkin C, Levangie P. *Joint Structure & Function*. 2nd ed. Philadelphia (PA): FA Davis; 1992. 512 p.

32. Oatis C. *Kinesiology: The Mechanics and Pathomechanics of Human Movement*. Baltimore (MD): Lippincott Williams & Wilkins; 2004. 899 p.

33. Olson T, Pawlina W. *A.D.A.M. Student Atlas of Anatomy*. Baltimore (MD): Williams & Wilkins; 1996. 492 p.

34. Pollock ML, Leggett SH, Graves JE, et al. Effect of resistance training on lumbar extension strength. *Am J Sports Med*. 1989;17(5):624–9.

35. Richardson C, Jull G, Hodges P, Hides J. *Therapeutic Exercise for Spinal Segmental Stabilization in Low Back Pain*. Edinburgh, Scotland: Churchill Livingstone; 1999. 191 p.

36. Rosse C, Clawson D. *The Musculoskeletal System in Health and Disease*. Hagerstown (MD): Harper & Row; 1980. 462 p.

37. Snell R. *Clinical Anatomy*. 7th ed. Baltimore (MD): Lippincott Williams & Wilkins; 2003. 1012 p.

38. Thompson C, Floyd R, editors. *Manual of Structural Kinesiology*. 14th ed. New York (NY): McGraw-Hill; 2001. 288 p.

39. Torg J, Vegso J, O'Neill MJ, Sennett B. The epidemiologic, pathologic, biomechanical, and cinematographic analysis of football-induced cervical spine trauma. *Am J Sports Med*. 1990;18(1):50–7.

40. Westfall D, Worrell T. Anterior knee pain syndrome: role of the vastus medialis oblique. *J Sports Rehabil*. 1992;1(4):317–25.

41. Wiesenfarth J, Briner W. Neck injuries: urgent decisions and actions. *Phys Sports Med*. 1996;24(1):35–41.

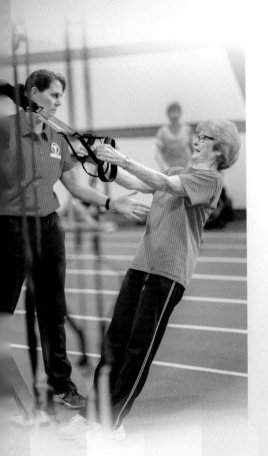

# Biomechanical Principles of Training

## OBJECTIVES

**Personal Trainers should be able to:**

- Introduce the field of biomechanics as an important tool for Personal Trainers to assess, teach, and correct exercise technique.
- Describe the relationship between proper biomechanics and the application of the overload principle of physical training.
- Describe the use of mechanical levers as a visual aid and description of the human musculoskeletal system.
- Introduce the three laws of motion as a method of understanding the mechanical nature of the human musculoskeletal system.
- Describe scalar and vector quantities and their relationship to mechanical variables that determine physical responses to exercise and activity.
- Describe the concept of a rotational moment or torque to measure the effects of muscles as they create angular movements of the body's articulations.
- Describe mechanical work and its use in quantifying training volume of physical activity.
- Describe the use of mechanical work in rotational (angular) movements and its relation to positive and negative work.
- Describe mechanical power and its importance in training rate.
- Describe the use of mechanical power for rotational (angular) movements.
- Explain the importance of an understanding of muscular anatomy in training and utilizing all sources of muscular force.

# INTRODUCTION

Biomechanics is the branch of science that applies the principles of mechanics (the study of forces) to living (Greek: βίος "bios") organisms (8). When considering physical activity, the human body is often compared to a machine. A machine needs fuel for energy to power the engine. Similarly, the human body requires the proper fuel to power muscles that enables the skeleton to move. The body may also be compared to a machine in terms of the physical laws that govern its performance. Operating an engine beyond its limits is readily observable by the red line displayed on the tachometer of most cars. Similarly, the human body may be loaded beyond the limits of the skeletal system and muscles that act on the moving human frame. Unfortunately, most people are not aware of the mechanical risks of physical activity until an injury has resulted. Biomechanics views the human body as a mechanical system of movable parts put in motion by the application of forces. The educated professional understands the consequences of physical exercise related to potential injury due to improperly imposed forces.

> Biomechanics views the human body as a mechanical system of movable parts put in motion by the application of forces.

An understanding of biomechanics provides a great advantage to the Personal Trainer, beyond the ability to predict possible injuries. Biomechanics can be used to maximize the benefits of physical performance in sports, work, and activities of daily living as well as for increases in physical strength or muscle size (hypertrophy) (3). This link between an understanding of biomechanical concepts and maximal training effect can be seen with the overload principle of physical training. The overload principle states that in order for a training adaptation to take place (an increase in muscular strength or muscle size), a greater-than-normal stress (force or load) must be applied to produce this adaptation. This may seem to imply that one simply needs to use progressively heavier weights to produce increasing strength gains; however, a better understanding of biomechanical principles will reveal that the amount of weight used to exercise is only one of many factors that results in the stress placed on the muscles. A lack of understanding of these biomechanical principles can often lead to inferior results and to acute or chronic injury resulting in significant lost training time.

## ◖● Training Illustration 1

In the illustration given in Figure 4.1, a woman is performing a common barbell curl to strengthen the elbow flexors (biceps brachii, brachialis, and brachioradialis). During the execution of the exercise, she observes that there are positions in the range of motion (ROM) of the elbows that appear more difficult than other positions — often referred to as a "sticking point." She asks her Personal Trainer, what causes the sticking point?

How should the Personal Trainer answer this training question? The answer is based on a proper understanding of the biomechanics of the human body. The explanation will be developed throughout this chapter, revisiting the question as each new biomechanical concept is introduced.

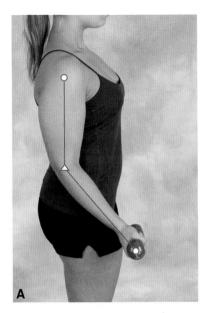
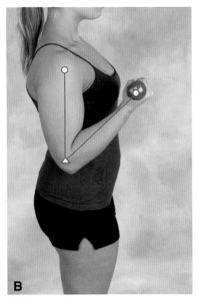
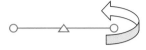

**A**    **B**    **C**

**FIGURE 4.1.** Barbell biceps curl. The musculoskeletal system of the arm is visualized as a lever system rotating around a fulcrum (Δ), moving from the starting position **(A)** to the finish position **(B)**. Note that each lever consists of one of more rigid bars representing the skeletal system (*e.g.,* humerus) rotating around a fulcrum as in a teeter-totter **(C)**.

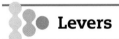

## Levers

The exercise scenario in Case Study 4.1 presents a training question in which the solution will require the Personal Trainer to view the anatomy of the elbow complex — upper and lower arm as a *lever system*. Figure 4.1 illustrates the elbow complex, including the humerus, elbow joint, and ulna-radius, as a mechanical or lever system. A lever is a simple machine consisting of a rigid bar used about a point of rotation or *fulcrum* to multiply the effect of a mechanical force (make it greater), or increase the distance across which the force is applied (*lever arm*). In effect, the lever is used to increase the amount of resistance that can be overcome by the application of a force.

Levers are commonly classified according to the arrangement of the two forces acting on them (effort and resistance) and the point of rotation or fulcrum (3). Figure 4.2 illustrates these three classes of levers. The rotational joints of the human body all fall into one of these three classes of levers. A full understanding of their effects will be presented later in the chapter. First, the concept of a force as it is used in the application of a lever system or created by the contraction of a muscle will be discussed.

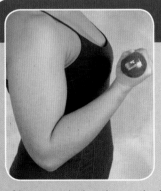

## Case Study 4.1

### What Causes the "Sticking Point" during a Lift?

A woman is performing a common biceps curl with a barbell as shown in Figure 4.1. After several repetitions of the exercise, she notices that the barbell seems to be heavier, and the exercise more difficult at the 90° elbow angle position than at any other position in the ROM. She has heard the term "sticking point" to describe the hardest point of the lift. She asks her Personal Trainer what causes this sticking point — is it simple fatigue, a mental block, or something else related to the position of her arm during the motion? How should the Personal Trainer respond?

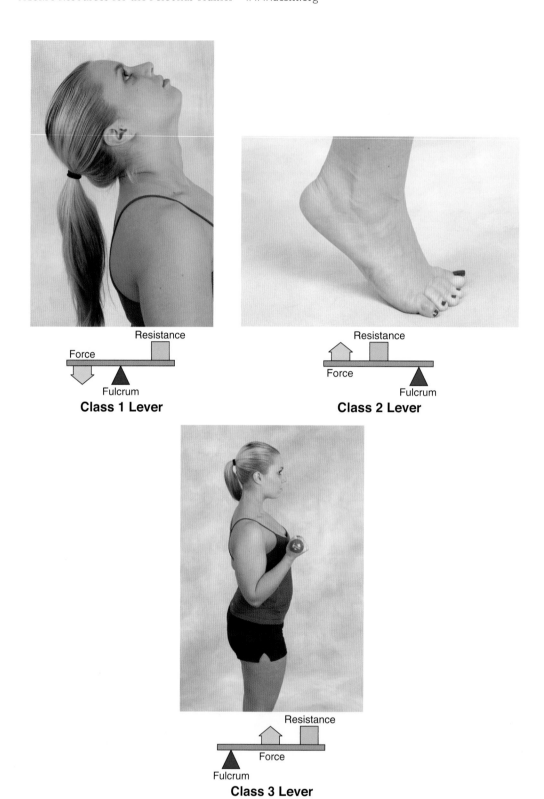

**Class 1 Lever**

**Class 2 Lever**

**Class 3 Lever**

**FIGURE 4.2.** The three classes of lever systems. Class 1: fulcrum in the middle; class 2: load or resistance in the middle; and class 3: effort force in the middle.

# Mechanical Laws of Motion

In Case Study 4.1, a woman created a contraction force using the elbow flexors to forcefully flex her elbows against the load of a barbell (see Fig. 4.1). Understanding the mechanical effects of these movements depends on knowing the concept of force. A definition of force as well as its mathematical expression was first given by Isaac Newton (1643–1727) in a historic text titled, *Philosophiæ Naturalis Principia Mathematica*, or in more common usage, *The Principia* (6). The Latin translation of the book's title is *Mathematical Principles of Natural Philosophy*, the term for what is known as physics today. In this text, Isaac Newton built on earlier work of other scientists such as Galileo Galilei (1564–1642) to provide the mathematical laws that allow for the calculation of the physical laws of motion caused by forces. These laws are summarized for both straight line (linear) and rotational (angular) movement in Table 4.1. These mechanical terms are explained throughout this chapter. A brief explanation of the nature of each of these laws and their importance in physical activity is provided here.

**Force**

Standard International Unit: Newtons (N) = $1 \, kg \cdot 1 \, m \cdot s^{-2}$

English: pound (lb)

Conversion: 1 lb ≈ 4.45 N

**Law of Inertia (First Law):** explains the physical nature of a force. Inertia is defined as a resistance an object has, to change its state of motion (velocity). To overcome an object's inertia, a force must be applied. An object's linear (straight line) inertia is proportional to its mass.

**Law of Acceleration (Second Law):** provides the mathematical equation to calculate the size of magnitude of a force. A force is proportional to the product of an object's mass multiplied by its acceleration ($F = ma$). Force is measured in Newtons: $1 \, kg \cdot 1 \, m \cdot s^{-2}$.

$$F = m \cdot a$$

(Eq. 4.1)

**Law of Reaction (Third Law):** explains that a force cannot act alone on an object. Any force acting on an object is always accompanied by another (reaction) force. This reaction force is equal in magnitude (size) and opposite in direction to the force.

| Table 4.1 | Newton's Three Laws of Linear Motion | |
|---|---|---|
| **Law** | **Linear Movement** | **Angular Movement** |
| 1. Law of Inertia | An object at rest stays at rest and an object in motion stays in motion with the same speed and in the same direction (velocity) unless acted on by an external *force*. | An object will maintain a constant angular velocity unless acted on by an external torque (moment). |
| 2. Law of Acceleration | The linear acceleration of an object is produced by a force directly proportional to that force and inversely proportional to the object's mass. Equation: $F = m \cdot a$ | The angular acceleration of an object is produced by a torque (moment) directly proportional to that torque and inversely proportional to the object's moment of inertia. Equation: $M = I \cdot \alpha$ |
| 3. Law of Reaction | For every force, there is a reaction force equal in magnitude and opposite in direction. | For every torque (moment), there is a reaction torque (moment) equal in magnitude and opposite in direction. |

## Vector Quantities

Equation 4.1 defined force as the product of a body's mass times its acceleration:

$$F = m \cdot a$$

Mathematically, this provides a method for calculating the numerical value of a force. However, it is often just as important to understand the physical significance of a force as it is to calculate its magnitude. For example, in Figure 4.3, the force of muscular contraction of the biceps brachii of the elbow flexor muscles created to complete a barbell curl first introduced in Case Study 4.1 is broken into component parts directed parallel and perpendicular to the forearm. This division of the muscular contraction force reveals an important feature of force — it is a *vector* quantity (4).

A vector quantity is one that requires both a *magnitude* (size) and *direction* to define. This is in contrast to *scalar* quantities that are completely determined by their magnitude. Examples of scalar quantities include number of students in a class, the speed a car is traveling, and the volume of water in a jar. Each of these scalar quantities are completely represented by a single number (*e.g.,* 25 students in a class).

Vector quantities also have a magnitude or size, but in addition, they also require a direction. For example, consider the man attempting to lift the barbell in an angled Smith machine from a squatting position in Figure 4.4. The desired direction of the barbell is at an angle relative to vertical. However, as the man rises to a standing position, the force he produces is likely directed vertically. A portion (component) of this force will be directed along the slide path of the bar in the Smith machine. Another component of the force will be directed perpendicular to this slide path, not contributing to the lifting of the bar. The direction of each vector in Figure 4.4 is essential in understanding its physical effect in performing the Smith machine squat. The process whereby the force created by the individual performing the Smith machine squat was broken into component vectors is known as *vector resolution*. Vectors are commonly designated in bold (*e.g.,* **F**) to distinguish them from scalar quantities.

Vectors are commonly designated in bold (*e.g.,* **F**) to distinguish them from scalar quantities.

**FIGURE 4.3.** Illustration of the muscle contraction force (**F**) created by the biceps brachii while performing a barbell curl. The forces directed perpendicular (**F**$_\perp$) and parallel (**F**$_\parallel$) to the forearm are explained in the text.

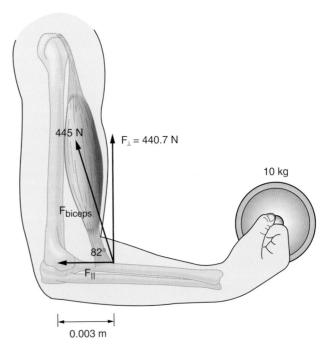

445 N

$F_\perp = 440.7$ N

10 kg

F$_{biceps}$

82°

F$_\parallel$

0.003 m

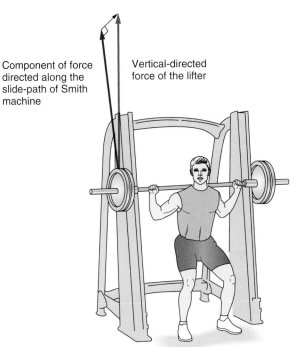

Component of force directed along the slide-path of Smith machine

Vertical-directed force of the lifter

**FIGURE 4.4.** Vector resolution of forces showing wasted muscular force in raising a bar in an angled Smith machine when pushing directly upward (vertical).

In Figure 4.3 the force of contraction of the biceps brachii ($\mathbf{F}_{biceps}$) was resolved into two components: $\mathbf{F}_{\parallel}$, applied parallel to the forearm, and $\mathbf{F}_{\perp}$, applied perpendicular to the forearm. In vector language, $\mathbf{F}_{biceps} = \mathbf{F}_{\parallel} + \mathbf{F}_{\perp}$. Thus, the contraction force of the biceps brachii produces both the force directed perpendicular to the elbow ($\mathbf{F}_{\perp}$) and the force directed parallel to the forearm ($\mathbf{F}_{\parallel}$) simultaneously. Physically, $\mathbf{F}_{\perp}$ rotates (flexes) the forearm, whereas $\mathbf{F}_{\parallel}$ compresses (stabilizes) the elbow. The Personal Trainer's ability to understand the vector nature of muscular force greatly enhances understanding of the physical effects of muscles as they contract.

> The Personal Trainer's ability to understand the vector nature of muscular force greatly enhances understanding of the physical effects of muscles as they contract.

## The Rotational Effect of a Force: Moments

The training activity examples applied so far have all illustrated an important feature of the human musculoskeletal system: Many articulations rotate. The kinesiology terms for the various movements of body joints introduced in Chapter 3 demonstrate this point. Flexion, extension, abduction, adduction, dorsiflexion, and plantarflexion all have one common feature — they are all rotations. Earlier in the chapter, force as a linear concept was introduced. Forces measure the physical effects in a straight line such as the guide path of the bar in the Smith machine example. Rotational movements are measured using the *moment of force* or *torque*.

**Moment or Torque**
Standard International Units: N · m
English: lb–foot (ft) (lb · ft)
Conversion: 1 N · m ≈ 0.738 lb · ft

The moment of force (torque) is a measure of the rotational effect of a force. Mathematically, it is the product of the magnitude of a force and the perpendicular distance from that force to the fulcrum.

$$M = F \cdot \mathrm{d}_{\perp} \tag{Eq. 4.2}$$

Returning to the barbell curl example first presented in Case Study 4.1, the total rotational effect (moment) of the elbow flexion created by the contraction of the biceps brachii (see Fig. 4.3) can be calculated. For this example, assume the biceps brachii is contracting with a force of 445 N (100 lb). The distance from the attachment of the biceps brachii on the forearm (insertion) to the center of rotation of the elbow (fulcrum) is 0.003 m. The angle the biceps brachii forms with the forearm is 82°. Using the equation for the calculation of the moment of force,

$$M = F \cdot d_\perp$$

The distance from point A (elbow) to point B (insertion), or moment arm is not perpendicular to the force ($\mathbf{F}_{biceps}$) as required by Equation 4.1. Therefore, $\mathbf{F}_{biceps}$ can be divided, or *resolved*, into components perpendicular ($\mathbf{F}_\perp$) and parallel ($\mathbf{F}_\parallel$) to the forearm which may be calculated as the magnitude of the moment.

$$\mathbf{M}_{biceps} = \mathbf{F}_\perp \cdot 0.003 \text{ m}$$

$$\mathbf{M}_{biceps} = 440.7 \text{ N} \cdot 0.003 \text{ m}$$

$$\mathbf{M}_{biceps} = 1.32 \text{ N} \cdot \text{m}$$

Return now to the training question posed in Case Study 4.1 related to the cause of the sticking point. The answer lies in an understanding of the rotational moment. The biceps brachii creates a contraction force that when multiplied by its moment arm produces a moment during the performance of a barbell curl. Assume a contraction force of 100 lb, as in the previous example for the biceps brachii. To increase or decrease this moment and thus the amount of effort used to perform the exercise, it may seem that this contraction force must either increase or decrease. However, recall that elbow flexion is a rotational movement. Therefore, to measure the effort that must be produced to lift the barbell, use a moment to measure the effort rather than the force.

Figure 4.5 provides a picture of the force of contraction of the biceps brachii being applied to the forearm, similar to Figure 4.3. However, in addition to the 90° elbow angle shown earlier, the moment about the elbow is illustrated at 45° and 135°. At each of these elbow angles, assume the same 100-lb contraction force used in the earlier example. Recall that the magnitude of the perpendicular component of the biceps brachii force ($\mathbf{F}_\perp$) for the 90° elbow angle was 440.7 N or 99.1 lb. However, Figure 4.5 shows that the perpendicular component of the biceps brachii force for the 45° and 135° elbow angles would be 79.9 lb. The amount of the muscular

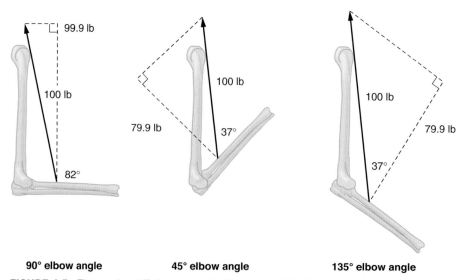

| 90° elbow angle | 45° elbow angle | 135° elbow angle |

**FIGURE 4.5.** The rotational ($\mathbf{F}_\perp$) component of force of a 100-lb biceps brachii contraction force at elbow angles of 90°, 45°, and 135°.

contraction force that is creating the rotation (elbow flexion) has decreased as a result of a changing elbow angle. This demonstrates that muscle geometry, which changes throughout the ROM of body joints, affects the effort that must be exerted during an exercise as much as the amount of resistance used in that exercise (4). This concept is essential to a proper understanding of training, including prescription and injury prevention. An example of how this changing muscle force due to body position can be used to positively affect training is given in the next training illustration.

## Training Illustration 2

Consider a resistance machine which uses a "cam" (Fig. 4.6). A cam is an oblique-shaped pulley. To understand its function, contrast it with a conventional round-shaped pulley. Figure 4.6 illustrates the contrast in the moment arms created by a round pulley and a cam. Notice that a round pulley, due to its shape, has the same length moment arm at any place in its circumference. The cam, however, has a moment arm that changes depending on which point on its circumference the cable is contacting. When the moment arm is longer, the moment created by the resistance weight will be greater even though the weight has not increased. Because this will increase the moment the lifter must overcome, the lifter will have to increase the amount of muscular effort to produce the same result. This is similar to the changes that occur in the rotational moment produced by muscular contraction when a joint angle changes. Resistance machines using a cam system have been designed for just this purpose. The idea is to use the changes in the resistance moment produced by the cam's changing moment arm to mimic the changes the moment created by muscular contraction to keep the effort the same through the ROM (8).

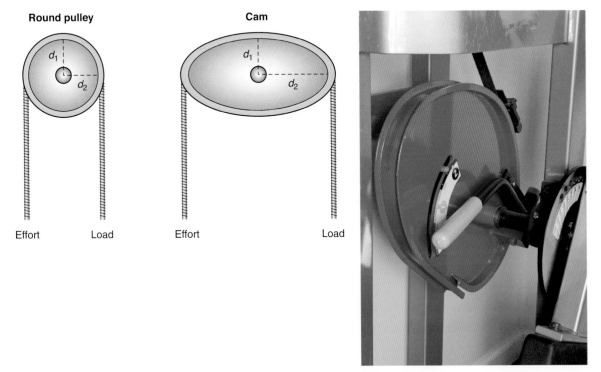

**FIGURE 4.6.** The moment arm ($d$) distance of a round pulley and a cam. Note that the moment arm remains constant for a round pulley ($d_1 = d_2$) versus changing constantly ($d_1 < d_2$) for a cam. The changing moment arm length creates a changing moment as the cam is rotated.

## Quantifying Training Effects

One challenge the Personal Trainer faces is maximizing each training session for each client. Today's busy schedules often leave limited time for extended workouts. Training prescription will require an understanding of each client's goals, physical fitness, limitations, and, importantly, the physical demands of training exercises. These demands are often described in terms of metabolic effort using measures such as calories or metabolic equivalents (METs) (5). However, one of the features of many of today's sophisticated training machines is the calculation of biomechanical measures of total effort. Perhaps, the simplest example can be found on many stair climbing machines that provide a display of the total number of "floors" ascended during an exercise bout. This number can often be equated with caloric expenditure to provide both a mechanical and metabolic measure of total exercise quantity. Mechanical measures quantify the effort in terms of forces created during the training bout, whereas metabolic measures are related to the amount of nutritional energy required to complete the exercise. Although each is valuable for the Personal Trainer for maximizing training results and motivating clients, the mechanical measures are equally valuable when the goals of training are muscle strength and/or size gains as such results are dependent on mechanically loading the musculoskeletal system beyond its normal use, and these same mechanical measures are often motivating factors (*e.g.*, amount of weight) to the user (8). Also, consider the importance of mechanical factors in activities of daily living as well as work and athletic performance.

## Training Illustration 3

The training scenario in Case Study 4.2 presents two training options. The first option, higher weight (load) and lower repetitions, is called the *strength training routine*. The second option, lower weight (load) and higher repetitions, is called the *endurance training routine*. The question the Personal Trainer must answer for the client is "Which training routine produces the most total volume of training?" To answer this question, two new mechanical terms, work and power, must be understood.

---

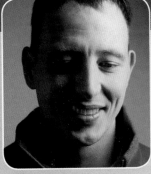

### Case Study 4.2

### Comparison of Training Routines

A new client found two strength training routines in a popular training magazine and asks which he should implement. He states that his goal is to find the routine that provides the greatest *total training volume* in his designated training time. The two training routines he presents are a *strength training routine*, which includes the use of higher weights (loads) with lower numbers of repetitions, and an *endurance training routine*, which includes the use of lower weights (loads) and higher numbers of repetitions.

The specifics of the two routines applied to this man's one repetition maximum (1-RM) are the following:

| Strength Training Routine | Endurance Training Routine |
|---|---|
| 3 sets | 3 sets |
| 10 reps | 15 reps |
| 200 lb | 150 lb |

Based on this information, which training routine has the greatest total training volume?

## Mechanical Work

The term *work* in everyday usage usually refers to some metabolic measure of the volume of activity a person has completed (*e.g.*, the total caloric expenditure). Although such a definition may be common, mechanically, it is inaccurate. Mechanical work is defined as the product of the magnitude of a force that creates a change in position, and the linear displacement (straight-line distance) defines the change in position (4).

$$\text{Mechanical work } (W) = \mathbf{F} \cdot \mathbf{d} \tag{Eq. 4.3}$$

For example, if in Figure 4.7 a wagon is pulled with a force of 100 lb to produce a linear change in position (displacement) of 20 ft, the resulting mechanical work would be,

$$W = \mathbf{F} \cdot \mathbf{d},$$

$$W = 100 \text{ lb} \cdot 20 \text{ ft}$$

$$W = 2,000 \text{ ft} \cdot \text{lb}$$

In this example, notice the force in Figure 4.7 was applied in the same direction as the resulting change in position (displacement). What would happen if the wagon in Figure 4.7 was pulled with the handle in another position?

**Mechanical Work**

Standard International Unit: N · m or Joule (J)
English: ft · lb
Conversion: 1 N · m (J) = 0.738 ft · lb

In Figure 4.8, the force is pulling the wagon with the handle at a 45° angle relative to horizontal. If it is assumed that force is pulling the wagon with the same 100-lb force, force can be divided (resolved) into horizontal and vertical components. Notice that each of these components would have a magnitude of 70.7 lb. This illustrates that scalars and vectors do not add together in the same way because 70.7 lb + 70.7 lb ≠ 100 lb. To complete the same amount of work as in Figure 4.7 (2,000 ft · lb), the wagon would have to cover a distance of 28.3 ft because a smaller amount of force (70.7 lb) is being applied in the direction the wagon is moving.

## Training Volume

Training illustration 3 (Case Study 4.2) asked the question, "Which training routine produces the most total volume of training?" To answer this question, calculate the amount of *work* done using each training regimen.

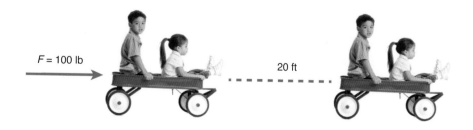

$F = 100$ lb          20 ft

(W)ork = $F$ x $d$

$W = 100$ lb x 20 ft

$W = 2,000$ lb · ft

**FIGURE 4.7.** The mechanical work created by a 100-lb (45.5-kg) force applied to a wagon to produce a displacement (straight-line distance) of 20 ft (6.1 m) is 2,000 lb · ft (278 kg · m).

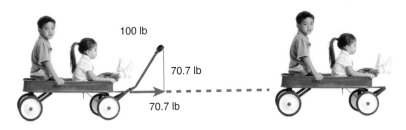

Total (W)ork = 2,000 lb · ft

2,000 lb · ft = 70.7 lb x *d*

*d* = 28.3 ft

**FIGURE 4.8.** Resolution of a 100-lb pulling force on a wagon into components parallel and perpendicular to the direction of the wagon; to complete the same 2,000 lb · ft of work (278 kg · m) as in Figure 4.7, the wagon would have to have a displacement of 28.3 ft (8.6 m) due to the smaller pulling force of 70.7 lb (32.1 kg) created by the direction of the handle.

Work is the product of force (**F**) and displacement (**d**),

$$W = \mathbf{F} \cdot \mathbf{d}$$

However, the strength routine includes 10 repetitions and the endurance routine includes 15 repetitions, while each routine includes three sets. Table 4.2 shows the calculation of mechanical work for each resistance training regimen. The strength routine would produce 18,000 ft · lb of mechanical work and the endurance routine would produce 20,250 ft · lb of mechanical work. Mechanical work, then, answers the question of which resistance training routine produces the greatest total training volume. For more information on matching training volume with client goals, see Chapter 15.

 **Mechanical Work for Rotational (Angular) Movements**

Mechanical work was defined as the product of the magnitude of a force that creates a change in position, and the *linear* displacement that defines that change in position.

$$\text{Mechanical work} = \mathbf{F} \cdot \mathbf{d} \qquad\qquad \text{(Eq. 4.3)}$$

Note in this definition the use of the word "linear." Equation 4.3 calculates the linear work as the displacement measures a change in position in a straight line. However, as discussed in the

| Table 4.2 | Calculation of Total Mechanical Work for Two Resistance Training Routines | |
|---|---|---|
| | **Strength Routine** | **Endurance Routine** |
| **S**ets | 3 | 3 |
| **R**epetitions | 10 | 15 |
| **F**orce–Load | 200 lb | 150 lb |
| **D**isplacement | 3 ft | 3 ft |
| Total Work: (F × D) × R × S | (200 × 3) × 10 × 3 = 18,000 lb · ft | (150 × 3) × 15 × 3 = 20,250 lb · ft |

section on rotational moments, most movements of the human body are *rotational* (*e.g.,* flexion, abduction). To measure rotational or *angular* work, the appropriate terms can be replaced in the equation for linear work.

$$W = \mathbf{F} \text{ (linear force)} \cdot \mathbf{d} \text{ (linear displacement)}$$

Replacing with angular terms,

$$\text{Angular work} = \mathbf{M} \text{ (angular moment)} \cdot \Delta\theta \text{ (angular displacement)} \qquad \text{(Eq. 4.4)}$$

The application of angular work can be illustrated by considering the barbell curl described in Case Study 4.1. The rotational moment flexing the elbow was calculated to be 1.0 lb · ft. If it is assumed that the woman's ROM for elbow flexion to be equal to the average for a female −150° (5), the angular work performed during the barbell curl can be calculated as,

$$\text{Mechanical work} = \mathbf{M} \cdot \Delta\theta$$

$$= 1.0 \text{ ft} \cdot \text{lb} \cdot 150°$$

$$= 150 \text{ ft} \cdot \text{lb}$$

Interestingly, note that if the same woman were to lower the barbell (elbow extension) back to the starting position (Fig. 4.9), the angular displacement would be the same (150°), but the biceps brachii would not be required to create the same rotational moment (1.0 ft · lb) because it does not have to overcome the resistance load (moment) but only control the rate at which it is lowered (extended).

Figure 4.9 demonstrates that muscles can only *actively* contract. Thus, the direction of the force they create will be the same relative to a body segment regardless of the movement. In Figure 4.9A, the biceps brachii *creates* elbow flexion by producing a rotational moment *greater* than the resistance moment created by the barbell. Notice the direction of the muscular force and movement (flexion) are the *same*. This is an example of *positive work* — performed when the motive force and movement direction are the *same*. In Figure 4.9B, the biceps brachii *resists* elbow extension by producing a rotational moment *less* than the resistance moment created by the barbell. Notice the direction of the muscular force and movement (extension) are *opposite*. This is an example of *negative work* — performed when the motive force and movement direction are *opposite*.

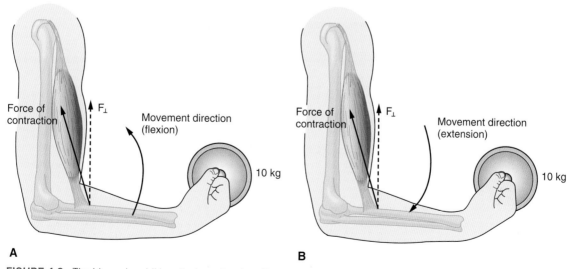

**FIGURE 4.9.** The biceps brachii is actively contracting. The perpendicular component of the muscular force ($\mathbf{F}_\perp$) is directed upward, with the direction of movement of the forearm in the same direction in **(A)** creating elbow flexion and *positive work*; and the direction of movement of the forearm in the opposite direction in **(B)** creating elbow extension and *negative work*.

The term "negative" has a common usage in resistance training. A simple definition might be a resistance movement in which the weight is lowered (8). Physiologically, this is an example of an *eccentric* contraction. Eccentric contractions occur when an active muscle (contracting) is lengthened by an external force or moment. A common training use of lengthening a muscle against resistance is to load the muscle beyond its 1-RM and lower the weight in a controlled manner. The common term for this type of movement *negative* is derived from the fact that this is defined as negative work.

## Training Illustration 4

The training scenario in Case Study 4.3 presents a typical athlete's questions. The question the Personal Trainer must answer is "What do the three physical tests have in common?" The answer to this question will allow the Personal Trainer to optimize training time. Analyzing the three physical tests, mechanical variables in common include the following:

- Force (jumping force, sprinting force, lifting force)
- Displacement (height jumped, distance ran)
- Time (length of time to complete sprint distance, time to complete squats)

The first two variables were used to calculate mechanical work ($W = \mathbf{F} \cdot \mathbf{d}$). In addition to these two variables, the physical tests also include time ($t$) as a variable. Time suggests that these physical tests are measuring the rate at which the work is being performed ($W \div t$). In equation form, the rate at which work is performed is power,

$$P = W \div t \qquad \text{(Eq. 4.5)}$$

Inserting the definition of work earlier,

$$P = \mathbf{F} \cdot \mathbf{d} \div t$$

Using the equation for velocity ($v = d/t$), power can be written as,

$$P = \mathbf{F} \cdot \mathbf{v} \qquad \text{(Eq. 4.6)}$$

or the rate ($\mathbf{v}$) at which force ($\mathbf{F}$) can be produced.

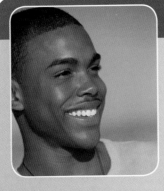

## Case Study 4.3

### Using Testing Data

A client interested in training to make a varsity football team approaches a Personal Trainer to design a proper preseason training program to optimize his chances to become a starting running back. As part of the initial interview, the potential client shares a list of physical tests used by the football coaches to assess the players' talent, including the following:

- A jump-and-reach for vertical height test
- A roll from a lying position upward to sprint through an obstacle course for time test
- The number of complete squats that can be performed with a certain weight in 2 minutes.

The potential client wants a training routine that will maximize both his chances of earning the starting running back position as well as increasing his performance on these tests. What advice could be offered based on this information?

Designing a training routine that maximizes the power requirement based on the client's abilities is an essential skill for an effective Personal Trainer.

**Mechanical Power**
Standard International Units: J/s or Watt (W)
English: horsepower
Conversion: 1 horsepower ≈ 746 W

The common factor, then, in each of these three physical tests is power. To optimize the training time for this client, the training regimen should focus on exercises that increase power, or the ability to create muscular force quickly.

A simple example of the calculation of power can be taken from Case Study 4.2 (answers in Table 4.2). The total work volumes for the two training regimens were found to be the following:

Strength routine = 18,000 ft · lb
Endurance routine = 20,250 ft · lb

Because the endurance routine included 15 repetitions versus 10 repetitions for the strength routine, assume it takes longer to complete the endurance routine. For this example, assume the endurance routine takes 30 minutes versus 25 minutes for the strength routine to complete. Power can now be calculated for each training routine.

Strength routine     $P = 18{,}000 \text{ ft} \cdot \text{lb}/25 \text{ min } (1{,}500 \text{ s})$

$P = 12.0 \text{ ft} \cdot \text{lb/s}$

Endurance routine     $P = 20{,}250 \text{ ft} \cdot \text{lb}/30 \text{ min } (1{,}800 \text{ s})$

$P = 11.25 \text{ ft} \cdot \text{lb/s}$

The strength routine does require more power (12.0 ft · lb/s) than the endurance routine (11.25 ft · lb/s). Designing a training routine that maximizes the power requirement based on the client's abilities is an essential skill for an effective Personal Trainer.

## Power for Rotational (Angular) Movements

Linear power was defined as the rate of linear work,

$$P = W / t$$

(Eq. 4.5)

or the product of force and linear velocity.

$$P = \mathbf{F} \cdot \mathbf{v}$$

(Eq. 4.6)

Linear power then is defined using linear velocity. To define the rotational equivalent of power, use either the rotational expression of work.

$$\text{Angular power} = \text{angular work} / \text{time}$$

(Eq. 4.7)

Or replace the linear variables force and velocity with angular equivalents:

$$P = \mathbf{F} \text{ (linear force)} \cdot \mathbf{v} \text{ (linear velocity)}$$

Replacing with angular terms,

$$\text{Angular power} = \mathbf{M} \text{ (angular moment)} \cdot \omega \text{ (angular velocity)}$$

(Eq. 4.8)

An interesting example of the use of rotational power can be seen in training individuals in wheelchair propulsion. Many sports popular with wheelchair athletes require training aimed at producing the maximal torque to the wheelchair rim to create maximal velocity. Training for this activity creates a unique muscular activity pattern commonly leading to overuse injuries in the shoulder region (2). The reason for this overuse pattern is unequal agonist/antagonist muscle use

**FIGURE 4.10.** Calculation of rotational power for wheelchair propulsion. The product of the tangent force (**F**) and the wheel radius ($d_\perp$) gives the rotational moment (**M**). The product of the rotational moment (**M**) and the angular velocity (ω) gives the rotational power.

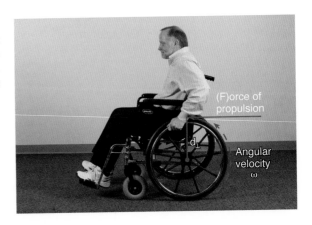

specific to wheelchair propulsion. Biomechanically, producing forward movement of a wheelchair requires a powerful internal rotation at the shoulder. The recovery phase involves a far less powerful external rotation. Repeated forceful propulsion of the wheelchair would train the internal rotation muscles of the shoulder to a much greater degree than the external rotators.

An investigation of the isokinetic strength of the shoulder rotator muscles in wheelchair athletes documented the mean *rotational power* of these muscles at three angular velocities (1). Figure 4.10 illustrates how the power would be calculated for wheelchair propulsion. The muscular force (**F**) applied tangent to the wheel rim is multiplied by the radius of the wheel ($d_\perp$) to give the rotational moment (torque) applied to the wheel. The product of this moment and the resulting angular velocity (ω) gives the rotational power (10). Table 4.3 presents the means and standard deviations of the isokinetic rotational power for the wheelchair athletes at three angular velocities.

At each angular velocity in Table 4.3, the rotational power of the internal rotator muscles was greater than the external rotators. This is shown in the ratio (*R*) of the internal/external rotator's rotational power. Clearly, the challenge to the Personal Trainer for the wheelchair athlete is to develop a more well-balanced training regimen that attempts to develop the agonist/antagonist muscles used for propulsion equally.

 ## Muscular Anatomy and Force

The previous sections presented definitions and examples of several biomechanical measures of muscular force. Choosing the appropriate measure will depend on the training factors to be considered such as strength, power, and volume. These biomechanical measures are also dependent on

| Table 4.3 | Rotational Isokinetic Power Values of the Dominant Side for Wheelchair Athletes to Create Propulsion at Three Angular Velocities (1) | | |
|---|---|---|---|
| Angular Velocity (°/sec) | Internal Rotation (Watts)[a] | External Rotation (Watts)[a] | R[b] |
| 60 | 45.99 (13.48) | 28.4 (7.51) | 1.67 |
| 180 | 101.1 (39.2) | 58.89 (19.86) | 1.71 |
| 300 | 118.5 (44.1) | 67.3 (20.99) | 1.75 |

[a]Values provided as mean (standard deviation).
[b]Ratio of internal/external isokinetic shoulder rotation mean power.

the anatomical nature of human muscle. Muscle has an architecture that determines the amount of contraction force that can be created (10). This architecture is directly related to the two types of muscular force: active and passive.

## Active Muscle Force

Active force (tension) refers to the muscular contraction force created through the so-called sliding filament theory (see Chapter 5). In active muscular tension, a stimulus from the neural system initiates a muscular contraction. The amount of this contraction force is under the control of the individual as it is proportional to the strength of the neural signal used to generate the contraction. The active component of muscle force is readily understandable as a greater amount of force to lift a heavier object. Creating greater muscle force requires only a stronger neural signal which is under the direct control of the brain. Of course, there is a limit to the ability to generate greater contraction force which is the reason for resistance training.

## Passive Muscle Force

It is important for the Personal Trainer to know there is another way to generate muscle force. In addition to the active tension generated by the neuromuscular system, muscles can also create passive force. Passive refers to the fact that this force is generated not by the muscle itself, but by the application of an outside force to prestretch the muscle. In simpler terms, by placing a muscle in a stretched position, it creates passive muscle force that can be utilized when the muscle is shortened. This works much like a rubber band that when stretched can be released to produce an elastic force. Muscle also has an elastic force that when used properly can add to the active force defined earlier to produce additional muscle force that may be used to lift greater weight, run faster, or jump higher (10).

## The Length–Tension Relationship of Muscle

The length–tension relationship of muscle is a physiological consequence of a muscle's ability to produce both active and passive force (tension). The elastic component will begin creating muscle force as a muscle is stretched from its resting length. This force will increase as long as the muscle is further stretched as shown in Figure 4.11. The active component of muscle force can be generated throughout the ROM of a muscle, but is maximal at the resting length (not shortened or lengthened) of a muscle, and becomes less as the muscle is either shortened or lengthened.

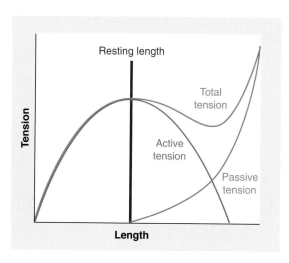

**FIGURE 4.11.** The length–tension relationship of human muscle. Note that the active and passive components of muscle force (tension) are additive, reaching their peak in a slightly elongated position.

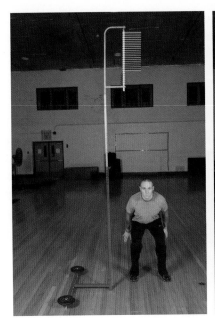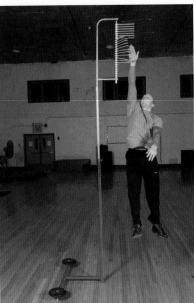

**FIGURE 4.12.** An individual performing a jump-and-reach test for vertical height. Note the prestretch of the jumping muscles by assuming a partial squat position prior to the jump. (From Ratamess N. *ACSM's Foundations of Strength Training and Conditioning.* Philadelphia [PA]: Lippincott Williams & Wilkins; 2012. p. 474.)

This is due to the loss of cross-bridges between the anatomical structures (myofilaments) that connect to generate muscle force. The total tension, or muscle force actually used in the performance of physical movement, is the arithmetic sum of the active and passive forces. Important for the Personal Trainer, this total muscle force is maximal at a slightly elongated position of a muscle or muscle group. This means that in order to produce the greatest amount of muscle force possible, the muscle or muscles that will be utilized should be placed in a slightly stretched position prior to the movement (4).

An example of using the length–tension relationship of muscle to maximize performance can be found in the jump-and-reach test in which an individual jumps against a tape measure to record the maximum vertical jumping height (Fig. 4.12). Before executing the jump, the jumper first lowers the body down in a partial squat position. This lowering of the body prestretches the muscles used for jumping (*e.g.,* hamstrings, quadriceps, gastrocnemius) in order to use the elastic or passive muscle force of these muscles as they forcefully jump upward. It is important to understand that each muscle and muscle group will have an optimal prestretch length as will each individual. Prestretching beyond this level will not only hurt performance but also may result in a potential injury. The role of the Personal Trainer is to help the client understand the proper use of a prestretch to maximize performance safely.

## Biomechanics of Selected Physical Activities

The application of the biomechanical principles presented in this chapter present an ongoing challenge for the Personal Trainer. To illustrate how these principles can be used to analyze and correct the training techniques used for physical activities and exercises commonly encountered as a Personal Trainer, consider the following physical activity examples, evaluated for correct technique.

The magnitude of a load being lifted is not equal to the load placed on the body.

## Lifting and Carrying Objects

Common advice for individuals lifting objects from a standing position includes "keep the back straight" and "lift with the legs." As a Personal Trainer, what if a client was to ask for an explanation of this advice? Is this advice correct from a biomechanical perspective?

Figure 4.13A shows an incorrect method of lifting an object from a standing position. For this example, consider the most often injured area of the human body during lifting: the lower back. The load (weight) being lifted does not change due to improper lifting technique. So, if the force (load) applied to the body does not increase with improper lifting technique, how does the risk of injury increase? The answer is that the magnitude of a load being lifted is not equal to the load placed on the body. Remember that if a load (force) is applied at a distance relative to a point of rotation (fulcrum), measure the effect using a moment, not a force. In the example illustrated in Figure 4.13A, the load (100 lb) is transmitted through the lifter's arms to the upper body. The perpendicular distance from the arms to the fulcrum point (the lower back) is given as 2 ft for this example. The flexion moment at the low back would be,

$$\mathbf{M}_{\text{flexion}} = 100 \text{ lb} \cdot 2 \text{ ft}$$

$$\mathbf{M}_{\text{flexion}} = 200 \text{ ft} \cdot \text{lb}$$

To counter the flexion moment, the extensor muscles of the lower back would have to produce an equal and opposite (Newton's third law) moment = 200 ft · lb of extension, significantly larger than the 100-lb load being lifted. Figure 4.13A shows that the longer the anatomical moment arm due to improper lifting technique becomes, the larger the moment imposed on the muscles and structures of the low back.

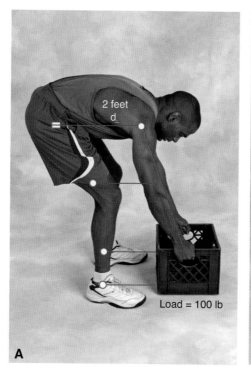 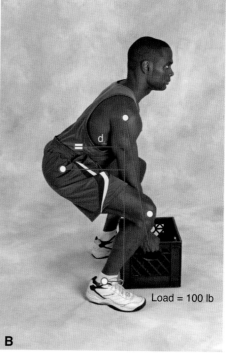

**FIGURE 4.13.** Improper **(A)** and proper **(B)** biomechanical lifting technique for lifting an object from a standing position. Improper technique **(A)** produces a large rotational moment at the low back due to the large moment arm ($d_{\perp}$) from the low back to the loading point at the arms. Proper technique **(B)** aligns the hips, knees, and ankles as close to the line of force as possible to minimize any rotational moment on the low back.

Proper biomechanical lifting technique from the standing position is illustrated in Figure 4.13B. The weight of the load to be lifted, which acts vertically due to the force of gravity, intersects the articulations of the low back, hip, knee, and ankle as close as possible in order to minimize the length of any moment arm. If the moment arm of any joint of the body is equal to zero while performing the lift, the moment would also be equal to zero. This means that only a linear force would be applied to that joint, specifically, a *compressive* force. The anatomical design of the articulations of the spine is well suited for compressive forces, whereas rotational moments create potentially harmful stresses to these same structures (11).

## Standing Calf Raises

The standing calf raise is a common resistance exercise for strengthening the plantarflexors that act at the ankle joint (*i.e.*, gastrocnemius, soleus). Improper form while performing this exercise, often produced by leaning forward and keeping the knees extended, produces two important biomechanical problems. First, the vertical line of force extending from the point of contact of the shoulders with the machine creates a moment arm with the low back similar to the previous example. This flexion moment on the low back will again have to be countered by the extensor muscles of the low back.

The second biomechanical consequence of this poor exercise technique is a hyperextension moment at the knee joints. The line of force passes anterior to the knees creating a backward (posterior)–directed hyperextension moment at the knees. The human knee reaches the limit of its ROM at 1.0° of hyperextension for men and 1.6° of hyperextension for women (7). The "locked" knee in this position which is subjected to a large hyperextension moment will counter this moment primarily with soft tissues such as ligaments that if stretched can potentially result in injury.

Correct biomechanical technique for the standing calf raise includes placing the hips, knees, and ankles in line with the line of force and keeping a slightly flexed position of the knees throughout the exercise.

## Walking Gait

Normal walking gait includes both a stance and swing phase (Fig 4.14). In stance, there is initial contact, which is frequently heel contact in most people. Initial contact is also the initiation of the "braking" subphase of the gait cycle. Initial contact is preceded by the eccentric action of the

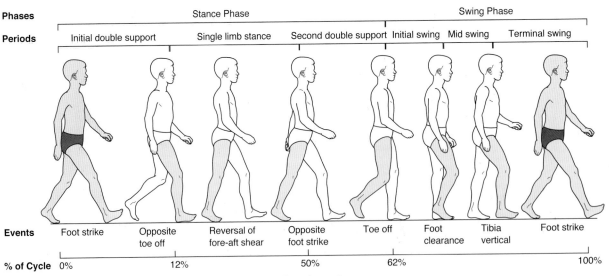

**FIGURE 4.14.** Normal walking gait. (Taken from biometrics.derawi.com.)

| Table 4.4 | **Common Gait Abnormalities and Associated Biomechanical Responses** | |
|---|---|---|
| **Gait Abnormality** | **Description** | **Biomechanical Response** |
| Antalgic (painful) gait | A self-protective result of injury to the pelvis, hip, knee, ankle, or foot | Stance phases of two limbs are not equal in time (swing phase of the unaffected limb is shorter). |
| Arthrogenic (stiff hip or knee) gait | Results from stiffness, laxity, or deformity | Unequal step lengths of the two limbs Circumduction of the affected limb |
| Equinus gait | Inadequate dorsiflexion range | Weight bearing on lateral edge of the foot Decreased stance time on affected side Pelvis and femur may be laterally rotated |
| Short leg gait | Leg length difference | Pelvic obliquity (rotation to one side) Exaggerated flexion of knee and hip of unaffected limb Hip "hiking" during swing phase for foot clearance Transverse plane movement of arm on one side |

hamstrings to slow extension of the knee on the support side so appropriate foot placement can occur. Braking is halted around the time of midsupport. Following initial contact, there is a loading response when lower extremity muscle activation is high to provide support for stabilization of the pelvis. At initial contact the foot generally rolls to the medial side followed by some magnitude of supination. The loading response is followed by midstance, terminal stance, and toe off. Midstance is the time when the body begins to become propelled forward. Midstance ends at toe-off. On the swing side, there is initial swing, midswing, and then a slowing of the foot prior to initial contact before initiating the stance phase again. Although a common daily activity, many gait abnormalities may be observed (9). Some common gait abnormalities, along with the biomechanical response, are briefly summarized in Table 4.4.

## SUMMARY

Biomechanics is the branch of science that applies the principles of mechanics to living organisms. An understanding of biomechanics provides a great advantage to the Personal Trainer, as this understanding provides the framework for viewing the human body in terms of a lever system acted on by forces internally by the muscles and externally by interaction with the environment. Because levers rotate around an axis, forces imposed on the human body create torque, or moments, when forces are magnified by the length of these levers. This chapter defines the mechanical terminology associated with the biomechanics of human movement and provides several training scenarios designed to show the application of these principles to personal training.

# REFERENCES

1. Bernard PL, Codine P, Minier J. Isokinetic shoulder rotator muscles in wheelchair athletes. *Spinal Cord.* 2004; 42(4):222–9.
2. Burnham RS, May L, Nelson E, Steadward R, Reid DC. Shoulder pain in wheelchair athletes: the role of muscle imbalance. *Am J Sports Med.* 1993;21(2):238–42.
3. Hall S. *Basic Biomechanics.* 6th ed. Boston (MA): McGraw-Hill; 2011. 560 p.
4. Hamill J, Knutzen KM. *Biomechanical Basis of Human Movement.* 3rd ed. Philadelphia (PA): Lippincott Williams & Wilkins; 2008. 491 p.
5. McArdle WD, Katch FI, Katch VL. *Exercise Physiology: Energy, Nutrition, and Human Performance.* 6th ed. Philadelphia (PA): Lippincott Williams & Wilkins; 2007. 1068 p.
6. Newton I. *Philosophiæ Naturalis Principia Mathematica.* London (United Kingdom); 1687. 991 p.
7. Soucie JM, Wang C, Forsyth A, et al. Range of motion measurements: reference values and a database for comparison studies. *Haemophilia.* 2011;17(3):500–7.
8. Wilson DJ. *The Kinesiology Activity Book.* Boston (MA): McGraw-Hill, 2011.
9. Wilson DJ. Principles of gait rehabilitation and the efficacy of partial body-weight supported training. *Crit Rev Phys Rehabilitative Med.* 2007;19(3):169–94.
10. Winter DA. *Biomechanics and Motor Control of Human Movement.* 4th ed. New York (NY): Wiley; 2009. 384 p.
11. Wisleder D, Smith MB, Mosher TJ, Zatsiorsky V. Lumbar spine mechanical response to axial compression load in vivo. *Spine.* 2001;26(18):E403–9.

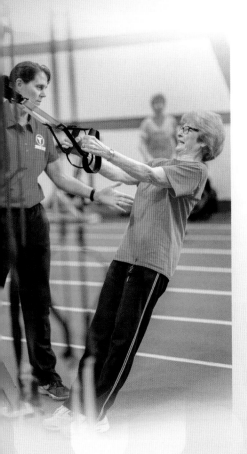

# 5

# Exercise Physiology

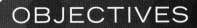

## OBJECTIVES

**Personal Trainers should be able to:**

- Provide fundamental background about the biological function of the human body.

- Introduce the physiological mechanism of various systems of the body and how they relate to exercise training.

- Identify key elements of how the body reacts and adapts to exercise stimulus so that effective exercise training can be prescribed.

# INTRODUCTION

Understanding the basic principles of how the body systems behave during the stress of exercising is paramount for the safe development of an effective exercise prescription for any client and will assist in explaining to clients how to improve their personal fitness levels. Understanding the physiological changes, and how these changes occur, allows a Personal Trainer to better understand how each exercise and movement prescribed for a client can be effective and safe for any type of individuals, regardless of their goals. This chapter will introduce essential concepts of exercise physiology and how different biological systems (*e.g.*, cardiovascular, respiratory, metabolic, muscular and skeletal, and neurological) play intricate roles during exercise performance and physical activity.

## Overview

Exercise physiology is the study of how the body systems react to the "stress" of exercise. Exercise physiology takes into account the effects of exercise on various systems of the body, including the cardiovascular, respiratory, muscular, skeletal, and nervous systems.

Consider what happens at the start of exercise (*i.e.*, heart rate rises, blood volume and respiration increase). Multiple systems work interactively to respond to an exercise stimulus so that an efficient and effective outcome is produced. Similarly, when prescribing an exercise to improve muscular strength, knowing the structure of the muscle and how muscular contraction works, a Personal Trainer is able to provide appropriate exercises for that muscle group. Knowledge of energy metabolism and how muscles adapt allows the Personal Trainer to determine the appropriate frequency, intensity, and duration of the exercise training bout and prescribe an appropriate training plan.

Another example involves the use of exercise for a weight loss program. Armed with an understanding of energy metabolism, a Personal Trainer determines the appropriate type of exercise that will maximize weight loss and decrease body fat. As explained later in this chapter, understanding the concept of energy metabolism allows the Personal Trainer to select the appropriate intensity of the work to maximize the number of calories burned.

With rapid advances in technology and research, the depth and breadth of the field of exercise physiology is growing rapidly. Traditional beliefs may be challenged as new ideas and concepts are generated. Thus, it is important for personal trainers not only to master the basic concepts of exercise physiology but also to stay abreast of new developments that will challenge what is known today.

## Definition of Exercise Physiology

Exercise physiology is a branch of physiology that deals with the study of how the body responds and adapts to the stress of exercise. Exercise physiologists are interested not only in the immediate effects of exercise (acute) but also in the long-term (chronic) effects on the body. Not one system in the body works independently from another, instead they all work together to allow the body to be as effective and efficient as possible during a bout of exercise.

## Cardiovascular System

Cardiovascular exercise physiology, a subdiscipline of exercise physiology, examines how oxygen and nutrients are transported through the cardiovascular system and into the working muscle during exercise. The cardiovascular system consists of the heart and the blood vessels. It is estimated that if stretched, an average-sized adult has enough blood vessels to encircle the Earth about two times (32). The primary purpose of the cardiovascular system is to deliver nutrients to and remove metabolic waste products from the tissues. The cardiovascular system performs the following specific functions (31):

1. Transportation of deoxygenated (depleted in oxygen) blood from heart to lungs and oxygenated (full of oxygen) blood from the lungs to the heart
2. Transportation of oxygenated blood from the heart to tissues and deoxygenated blood from the tissues to the heart
3. Distribution of nutrients (*e.g.,* glucose, free fatty acids, amino acids) to cells
4. Removal of metabolic wastes (*e.g.,* carbon dioxide, urea, lactate) from the working cells for elimination or reuse
5. Regulation of pH to control acid–base balance
6. Transportation of hormones and enzymes to regulate physiological function
7. Maintenance of fluid balance to prevent dehydration
8. Maintenance of body temperature by absorbing heat and redistributing to the surface of the body

## The Heart

Figure 5.1 shows the anatomy of the heart. The heart sits in the chest cavity at an angle, with the larger left ventricle (LV) pointed toward the left foot. It is surrounded by the thoracic vertebral column in the back, the lungs on both sides, and the chest wall (sternum/ribs) in the front.

The heart has four chambers that serve as reservoirs and pumps. The upper two chambers are called the atria, and the lower two are the ventricles (29). The chambers of the heart are separated

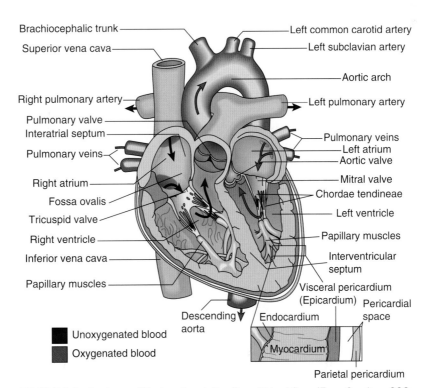

**FIGURE 5.1.** Anatomy of the heart and direction of blood flow. (From Smeltzer SCO, Bare BG. *Brunner and Suddarth's Textbook of Medical–Surgical Nursing.* 9th ed. Philadelphia [PA]: Lippincott Williams & Wilkins; 2002, with permission.)

by the coronary sulcus, and the interventricular sulcus separates right ventricle (RV) and LV. The sulci also contain the major arteries and veins that provide circulation to the heart (29).

The base of the heart consists of the structures on the top portion of the heart, such as the left atrium (LA), the right atrium (RA), and parts of the large veins that enter the heart from behind. The base is located above and close to the right sternal border at the level of the second and third ribs. The apex of the heart is located at the level of the fifth intercostal space (29). On average, the heart weighs about 11 oz and 9 oz for males and females, respectively, pumps 2.4 oz (70 mL) in each beat (32) and is about the size of a closed fist.

## Tissue Coverings and Layers of the Heart

The heart is covered by a double-walled, loose-fitting membranous sac called the pericardium. The outer wall of the pericardium has both a fibrous (tough) layer and a serous (smooth) layer. The pericardium helps anchor the heart within the chest, maintaining its positioning (29). The thickest layer of the cardiac muscle is known as the myocardium. The blood vessels and nerves that supply the heart are embedded in this layer. In addition, within the myocardium, there is a network of connective tissue fibers, a fibrous skeleton that separate the atria from the ventricles. This skeleton provides support for the myocardium and the valves of the heart.

## Chambers, Valves, and Blood Flow

In simple terms, the heart is composed of two pumps (right and left), with two chambers or cavities in each pump. The right side of the heart is composed of the RA and RV. The right side is responsible for collecting blood coming from the body (deoxygenated) and pumping the blood through the lungs (pulmonary circulation). On the other side, the left side of the heart, LA and LV collects blood from the lungs and pumps it to all parts of the body (through the arteries) (32).

In addition to the right- and left-side chambers, the heart has four valves, whose function is to maintain blood flow in a single direction. The atrioventricular (AV) valves separate the atria from the ventricles, whereas the semilunar valves separate the ventricles from the aorta and pulmonary artery. The right AV valve is called the tricuspid valve and controls the flow of blood from the RA to the RV. The left AV valve is called the mitral (or bicuspid) valve and controls blood flow between the LA and LV. The papillary muscles and the string-like chordae tendineae help the AV valves stay closed, preventing them from swinging back into the atria, which would result in reversed blood flow when the ventricles contract (29).

Two additional valves in the heart prevent backflow of blood to the ventricles. The pulmonic and aortic valves lie between the RV and the pulmonary artery and the LV and the aorta, respectively. Blood flow through the heart, depicted by the arrows in Figure 5.1, begins with the return of systemic blood from the body to the RA:

1. Deoxygenated blood flows into the RA through the superior and inferior vena cava, the coronary sinus, and the anterior cardiac veins.
2. The RA contracts and blood moves through the tricuspid valve into the RV.
3. The RV contracts, the tricuspid valve closes, and blood flows through the pulmonic valve into the pulmonary arteries and the branches of the pulmonary system.
4. Blood enters the alveolar capillaries from the pulmonary arteries, where gas exchange occurs. Oxygen is absorbed and carbon dioxide is removed.
5. Blood flows back to the LA through the pulmonary veins.
6. The LA contracts and blood flows through the mitral valve and into the LV.
7. The LV contracts, the mitral valve closes, and blood flows through the aortic valve into the aorta and its branches, where it is distributed to the heart (coronary circulation) and the rest of the body (systemic circulation) (39).

Unlike skeletal muscle, cardiac muscle has unique properties that allow it to contract without an external nervous system impulse. The heart's conduction system includes specialized cells that initiate the heart beat and electrically coordinate contractions of the heart chamber (29). The sinoatrial (SA) node is considered the intrinsic pacemaker because this is where most normal electrical impulses originate. The AV node is responsible for delaying the electrical impulses for approximately 0.12 second between the atria and the ventricles. This allows the atria to contract and fill the ventricles with blood. After a brief pause, the electrical impulse moves rapidly to the apex of the heart through the Bundle of His, the right and left bundle branches, and through the Purkinje fibers in the myocardium of both ventricles. This rapid conduction allows the two ventricles to contract at approximately the same time.

## The Blood Vessels

Once the blood exits the heart, it enters the vascular system, which is composed of numerous blood vessels. The blood vessels deliver blood to the tissues; help promote the delivery of nutrients and oxygen as well as the exchange of metabolic wastes, hormones, and other substances with cells; and return blood to the heart. Arteries carry blood away from the heart, with large arteries (aorta) branching into smaller arteries and eventually to smaller arterioles. Arterioles branch into capillaries, and it is here where the exchange of blood and other nutrients happens with various tissues (*e.g.*, digestive system, liver, kidneys, and muscles). Unlike the arterial side, the venous side of the circulation starts with the capillaries converging into small venules, which join to form larger vessels called veins. The larger veins (venae cavae) return blood to the heart.

Arterioles, or smaller arteries, are made up of smooth muscle and play a major role in regulating blood flow and pressure to the capillaries because of their ability to constrict or dilate, controlling the amount of blood entering the capillaries at one time. Capillaries have extremely thin walls and are the site of exchange of nutrients between blood and the interstitial fluid. Veins receive blood from the venules and, in general, they are thinner and more compliant than arteries; they act as blood reservoirs. The walls of some veins, such as those in the legs, contain one-way valves that help maintain venous return to the heart by preventing backward blood flow even under relatively low pressures (32).

## Cardiac Function

### Heart Rate

Heart rate (HR) is the number of times the heart beats per minute, and it is measured in beats per minute (bpm). The average normal resting HR is approximately 60–80 bpm, and at rest, the average heart pumps 1,900 gallons of blood daily or over 50 million gallons over a lifetime of 75 years (32). However, differences exist between men and women and between adults and children. The resting HR of women is typically 10 bpm higher than that of men. Children have higher HRs than adults do. One of the primary adaptations to exercise training can be seen with HR when comparing fit with unfit individuals. When comparing individuals of the same age and sex, fit individuals have a lower resting HR due to a larger stroke volume (SV; the volume of blood ejected from the heart per beat); therefore, the heart of a fit person does not have to beat as many times to maintain the same output of blood from the heart (cardiac output) (27). HR can be measured by counting the number of pulses over a given time period.

### Blood Pressure

Blood pressure (BP) is the product of the amount of blood pumped from the heart (cardiac output) and the resistance of flow encountered in the vessel (total peripheral resistance). When the heart beats, blood is propelled from the LV into the systemic circulation. As the ventricle contracts, the force exerted by the blood against the arteries is the BP. BP is measured in millimeters of mercury (mm Hg). Systolic blood pressure (SBP) is the pressure exerted on the arterial wall during the ventricles' contraction phase, and diastolic blood pressure (DBP) is the pressure exerted on the arteries during the relaxation phase of the ventricles (2). Average value for SBP and DBP is >120/80 mm Hg. A condition known as hypertension may be present when SBP and DBP measures exceed 140/90 mm Hg at rest (28).

### Stroke Volume

The amount of blood ejected from the LV in a single contraction is the SV. The SV is equal to the difference between the amount of blood in the ventricle before contraction (end-diastolic volume [EDV]) and the amount of blood left in the ventricle at the end of contraction (end-systolic volume [ESV]). In an upright posture, SV is lower in untrained individuals than in trained individuals. The SV of men is usually greater than that of women because of their larger heart size. SV is also sensitive to body position. In the supine or prone postures, SV increases.

### Cardiac Output

Cardiac output ($\dot{Q}$) is the volume of blood pumped by the heart per minute in liters ($L \cdot min^{-1}$). It is calculated by multiplying the HR by the SV ($\dot{Q} = HR \times SV$). The typical $\dot{Q}$ for adults is $4$–$5\ L \cdot min^{-1}$. However, when measuring maximal values, $\dot{Q}$ is higher in aerobically fit individuals than in untrained individuals.

## Acute Response to Cardiovascular Exercise

Many mechanisms function collectively to support the increased oxygen demands required to perform such activities. Oxygen delivery to the working muscle during activity is accomplished by changes in HR, SV, $\dot{Q}$, blood flow, BP, arteriovenous oxygen (a-$\bar{v}O_2$) difference, and pulmonary function. As exercise intensity increases, oxygen consumption and carbon dioxide production by working muscles increase. The cardiorespiratory system is tasked with the delivery of oxygen and removal of carbon dioxide to and from these tissues in an attempt to maintain cellular homeostasis. This exchange occurs in the gas-exchanging surfaces of the alveoli in the lungs. The central nervous system (CNS) plays an important role in this process, increasing neural ventilatory and cardiac drive, which causes an increase in cardiac and respiratory muscle activity, resulting in an increased blood and air flow.

## Heart Rate

The normal HR response during an acute bout of dynamic exercise is a linear increase with increasing exercise intensity and oxygen uptake. The magnitude of the HR response is related to age, body position, fitness, type of activity, presence of heart disease, medications, blood volume, and environmental factors such as temperature and humidity (32). Maximum attainable HR ($HR_{max}$) usually decreases with age. In the field, the most common equation used to estimate $HR_{max}$ in men and women is the equation $220 -$ age in years. Although this equation has been used extensively over the years, it has a great deal of variability ($\geq 12$ bpm) (3). Another equation ($HR_{max} = 207 - [0.7 \times age]$) has been suggested for both men and women, with a broad range of age and fitness (22).

## Stroke Volume

During dynamic exercise, SV increases curvilinearly with intensity until reaching near-maximal levels approximately at 40%–50% of maximum aerobic capacity, increasing only slightly thereafter (34). Once SV reaches its maximum levels, the increase in oxygen demand is met by increasing the HR.

At very high HR, SV may actually decrease because of the disproportionate shortening of diastolic filling time in the heart (14).

## Cardiac Output

In healthy adults, $\dot{Q}$ increases linearly with an increase in exercise intensity. Maximum levels, however, are dependent on many factors including age, posture, body size, presence of cardiovascular disease or other chronic diseases and conditions, and the level of physical conditioning. At the lower intensities (<50% of maximum), $\dot{Q}$ is controlled by increases in HR and SV (34). Thereafter, increases in $\dot{Q}$ results primarily from the continued rise in HR.

## Arteriovenous Oxygen Difference

a-$\bar{v}$O$_2$ difference represents the amount of oxygen extracted by the tissues and reflects the difference between the oxygen content of arterial blood and the oxygen content of venous blood. At rest, a-$\bar{v}$O$_2$ difference is usually about 5 mL O$_2 \cdot$ dL$^{-1}$ (5 mL of oxygen per 100 mL of blood) and represents about 25% of the oxygen content in arterial blood (total content is about 20 mL O$_2 \cdot$ dL$^{-1}$). During exercise to exhaustion, arterial oxygen content does not change significantly; however, the venous oxygen content typically decreases to about 5 mL O$_2 \cdot$ dL$^{-1}$ of blood, thus widening the a-$\bar{v}$O$_2$ difference from 5 to 15 mL O$_2 \cdot$ dL$^{-1}$ of blood, corresponding to a use coefficient of 75% (34). In other words, during vigorous exercise, the active muscle extracts greater amounts of oxygen from the arterial blood and reduces the oxygen content in the venous blood (32).

## Blood Flow

At rest, 15%–20% of the $\dot{Q}$ is distributed to the skeletal muscles; the remainder goes to the visceral organs, the heart, and the brain. However, during exercise, as much as 85%–90% of the $\dot{Q}$ is selectively delivered to working muscles and shunted away from the skin and the internal organs. Blood flow to the heart may increase 4–5 times with exercise, whereas blood supply to the brain is maintained at resting levels.

## Blood Pressure

Similar to HR, SBP increases in a linear fashion with exercise intensity (3). Maximal SBP values typically reach 190–220 mm Hg (36); however, maximal SBP should not exceed 250 mm Hg (3). An SBP that fails to rise or that falls (>10 mm Hg) with increasing workloads may signal a plateau or decrease in $\dot{Q}$ (10). Exercise testing should be terminated in persons demonstrating a decrease in SBP during further exercise (exertional hypotension). Unlike SBP, DBP may decrease slightly or remain unchanged during exercise (3) because of the decrease in peripheral resistance caused by the enlargement of arterioles in the active muscles during exercise (18). DBP should not exceed 115 mm Hg (3).

## Maximal Oxygen Consumption

Maximal oxygen consumption, or $\dot{V}$O$_{2max}$, is the most widely recognized measure of cardiorespiratory endurance. $\dot{V}$O$_{2max}$ is defined physiologically as the highest rate of oxygen transport and use that can be achieved at maximal physical exertion. Oxygen consumption ($\dot{V}$O$_2$) may be expressed mathematically by a rearrangement of the Fick equation (32):

$$\dot{V}O_2 \ (mL \cdot kg^{-1} \cdot min^{-1}) = HR \ (bpm) \times SV \ (mL \cdot beat^{-1}) \times (\text{a-}\bar{v}O_2 \ \text{difference})$$

Thus, it is apparent that both central (*i.e.*, $\dot{Q}$) and peripheral (*i.e.*, a-$\bar{v}$O$_2$ difference) regulatory mechanisms affect the magnitude of $\dot{V}$O$_{2max}$.

## Box 5.1  Absolute versus Relative $\dot{V}O_{2max}$

To illustrate the difference between absolute and relative expressions of $\dot{V}O_{2max}$, consider two individuals with the same absolute $\dot{V}O_{2max}$ but who have different body weights.

**Jim**
45 years old, 200 lb (90.9 kg)
Absolute $\dot{V}O_{2max}$: 3.5 L $\cdot$ min$^{-1}$
Relative $\dot{V}O_{2max}$: 38.5 mL $\cdot$ kg$^{-1}$ $\cdot$ min$^{-1}$

$$3.5 \text{ L} \cdot \text{min}^{-1} \times 1{,}000 \text{ mL/1 L} = 3{,}500 \text{ mL} \cdot \text{min}^{-1}/90.9 \text{ kg} = 38.5 \text{ mL} \cdot \text{kg}^{-1} \cdot \text{min}^{-1}$$

$$38.5 \text{ mL} \cdot \text{kg}^{-1} \cdot \text{min}^{-1}/3.5 \text{ mL} \cdot \text{kg}^{-1} \cdot \text{min}^{-1} = 11 \text{ METs}$$

**Amber**
45 years old, 120 lb (54.5 kg)
Absolute $\dot{V}O_{2max}$: 3.5 L $\cdot$ min$^{-1}$
Relative $\dot{V}O_{2max}$: 64.2 mL $\cdot$ kg$^{-1}$ $\cdot$ min$^{-1}$

$$3.5 \text{ L} \cdot \text{min}^{-1} \times 1{,}000 \text{ mL/1 L} = 3{,}500 \text{ mL} \cdot \text{min}^{-1}/54.4 \text{ kg} = 64.2 \text{ mL} \cdot \text{kg}^{-1} \cdot \text{min}^{-1}$$

$$64.2 \text{ mL} \cdot \text{kg}^{-1} \cdot \text{min}^{-1}/3.5 \text{ mL} \cdot \text{kg}^{-1} \cdot \text{min}^{-1} = 18 \text{ METs}$$

Even though Jim and Amber both have the same absolute $\dot{V}O_{2max}$, Amber has a greater oxygen capacity in relation to her body mass.

$\dot{V}O_{2max}$ may be expressed either on an absolute or a relative basis (see example in Box 5.1). Absolute $\dot{V}O_{2max}$ reflects the total body energy output and energy expenditure (*i.e.*, 1 L O$_2$ consumption $\approx$ 5 kcal) and uses the units of (L $\cdot$ min$^{-1}$) without taking in consideration body weight. Relative $\dot{V}O_{2max}$ reflects the individual's oxygen consumption based on the body weight, dividing the absolute $\dot{V}O_{2max}$ value by body weight in kilograms (mL $\cdot$ kg$^{-1}$ $\cdot$ min$^{-1}$). Because large persons usually consume larger absolute amounts of oxygen by virtue of a larger muscle mass, expressing $\dot{V}O_{2max}$ values as "relative" is appropriate for comparisons between individuals of different body masses (*i.e.*, men and women). This measure is widely considered the single best index of physical work capacity or cardiorespiratory fitness (18). In terms of cardiorespiratory endurance, the higher the $\dot{V}O_{2max}$, the better.

Another term commonly used to express exercise intensity is the metabolic equivalent (MET). MET is a simple way to estimate the energy cost of an activity and is equivalent to 3.5 mL $\cdot$ kg$^{-1}$ $\cdot$ min$^{-1}$, which equals resting metabolism.

## Respiratory System

The respiratory system is responsible for filtering the air that enters the body and allow gas exchange within the alveoli, which are microscopic air sacs in the lungs. The primary structures of the respiratory system are depicted in Figure 5.2. The lungs provide the surface for gas exchange and are situated inside the chest cavity above the diaphragm and protected by the ribs and pectoral muscles. The lungs of an average sized adult weigh approximately 1 kg and have a volume between 4 and 6 L, which is similar to the air in a basketball (32). Breathing is an involuntary action controlled by movements of the respiratory muscles, diaphragm, and changes in pressure. At rest and during inspiration, the pressure inside the lungs is less than the atmospheric pressure. Therefore, when one takes a breath, an active process, the lower pressure inside the lungs allows them to inflate and prevents the collapse of the fragile air sacs within the lung. These pressure differences reverse during exhalation, a passive process, where the lungs deflate and push air out.

## Control of Breathing

Respiratory muscles lack the ability to regulate their own contractions, and thus, the control of breathing results from the interaction of brainstem and respiratory pathways (18). Autonomic control structures are located in the brainstem, and voluntary control structures are located in the cerebral cortex of the brain.

## Distribution of Ventilation

Ventilation of the pulmonary system is accomplished in two major divisions, the upper and lower respiratory tracts, illustrated in Figure 5.2.

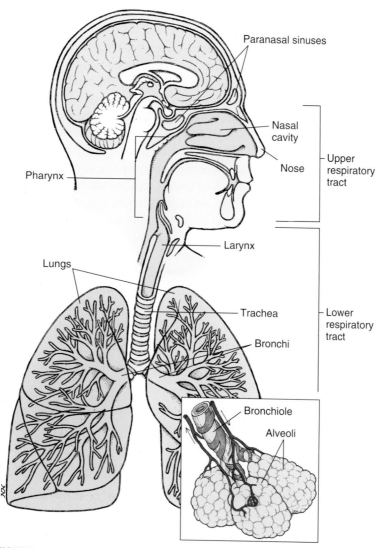

**FIGURE 5.2.** The structures of the respiratory system (anterior view). (From Thomas LS. *Stedman's Medical Dictionary*. 27th ed. Baltimore [MD]: Lippincott Williams & Wilkins; 2000, with permission.)

### Upper Respiratory Tract

The upper respiratory tract acts as a pathway for air to move into the lower respiratory tract. The upper respiratory tract is composed of the nose, sinuses, pharynx, and larynx, and its sole function is to purify, warm, and humidify the air before it reaches the gas exchange units (*i.e.*, alveoli). During normal, quiet breathing, inspired air passing through the nose is heated to body temperature, and the relative humidity is increased to more than 90%.

The pharynx is divided by the soft palate into the nasopharynx and the oropharynx. The epiglottis, located at the base of the tongue, protects the laryngeal opening during swallowing. The larynx contains the vocal cords, which contribute to speech and participate in coughing.

### Lower Respiratory Tract

The lower respiratory tract begins in the trachea just below the larynx and includes the bronchi, bronchioles, and alveoli (see Fig. 5.2). There are approximately 23 divisions of airways: The first 16 are conducting airways, and the last 7 are respiratory airways, ending in approximately 300 million alveoli, which form the gas exchange surface. The structural components of the airways coincide with their functional properties. For example, the volume of the conducting zone is approximately 1 mL of air per pound of body weight and does not contribute to gas exchange, whereas gas exchange areas occupy a proportionately greater volume in the lungs. The trachea is anterior to the esophagus and begins at the base of the neck, extending approximately 4–4.5 in (10–12 cm) before it divides into the right and left main bronchi. The trachea consists of a series of anterior horseshoe-shaped cartilaginous rings and a posterior longitudinal muscle bundle.

The major bronchi contain cartilage that keeps the airway open, as well as large numbers of mucous glands that produce secretions in response to irritation, infection, and/or inflammation. In the large airway, irritant receptors initiate the cough reflex when stimulated. The right main bronchus divides into three lobar bronchi: upper, middle, and lower. The left main bronchus divides into upper and lower lobar bronchi. Fissures separate the two lobes with two layers of visceral pleura. The lobar bronchi divide into segmental bronchi and segments, 10 on the right and 10 on the left.

Columnar cells lining the epithelium (inner lining) of the bronchi consist predominantly of ciliated cells containing motile cilia, which move or beat in a coordinated manner to move the mucous layer toward the mouth ("mucociliary escalator"). The columnar epithelium is an important barrier for lung defense. Goblet cells interspersed among the ciliated cells secrete mucus. Segmental bronchi divide further into the terminal bronchioles, which have a diameter of about 1 mm. Beyond the terminal bronchioles are respiratory bronchioles, alveolar ducts, and the alveoli. Air flows through the conducting airways and at the level of the alveolar ducts and alveoli. Movement of air or gas from the lungs into the bloodstream occurs by diffusion.

## Ventilatory Pump

The ventilatory pump provides the mechanisms for breathing and consists of the chest wall, the respiratory muscles, and the pleural space.

### Chest Wall

The chest wall includes the muscles of ventilation (primarily intercostal muscles) and bones (spine, ribs, and sternum). The ribs are hinged on the spine by ligaments and cartilage so that the ribs move upward and outward during inspiration and downward and inward during expiration. The hinging movement results in a change in thoracic volume and pressures. At rest and at the end of a normal expiration, the elastic properties of the chest wall exert an outward (expansion) force, whereas the elastic properties of the lung structures exert an inward (recoil) force. Inspiration (airflow into the lungs) occurs by activation of the respiratory muscles, particularly the diaphragm, which creates a more negative pressure in the pleural space and the lungs than that in the atmosphere. Air enters the lungs until the intrapulmonary gas pressure equals atmospheric pressure. During expiration, when the ventilatory muscles relax, air flows from the lungs into the atmosphere because of the positive pressure generated by the elastic recoil of the lungs.

## Ventilatory Muscles

The muscles of respiration are the only skeletal muscles essential to life. The diaphragm, the major muscle of inspiration, is innervated by the phrenic nerve, which originates from the third to fifth cervical spinal segments. A spinal cord injury, at or above this level, compromises respiratory muscle function and, consequently, ventilation. Figure 5.3 depicts the role of the diaphragm in ventilation. The diaphragm functions as a piston, with contraction and relaxation of the vertical muscle fibers. With contraction, the muscle fibers move downward and displace the abdominal contents so that the abdomen moves outward, as does the chest wall. Expiration is normally passive under quiet breathing because of elastic recoil of the lung; it requires no work and is therefore passive. However, during active breathing, when ventilatory requirements are increased (*e.g.*, during exercise), the internal intercostals and the abdominal muscles (rectus abdominis, external and internal oblique, and transverse abdominis) are recruited to actively pull down on the ribs. In clients with airflow obstruction (*e.g.*, asthma or emphysema), hyperinflation of the lungs stretches the lung tissue and leads to additional elastic recoil, thus impairing the diaphragm's ability to contract.

## Distribution of Blood Flow

The lungs receive blood from the pulmonary arteries, which contain systemic venous blood from the RV and bronchial arteries. The pulmonary artery emerges from the RV and divides into the right and left main pulmonary arteries. The pulmonary arteries divide into branches corresponding

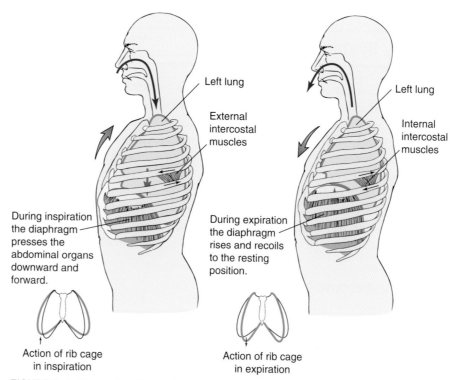

**FIGURE 5.3.** Mechanics of normal — not deep, not shallow — inspiration *(left)* and expiration *(right)*. (From Weber J, Kelley J. *Health Assessment in Nursing*. 2nd ed. Philadelphia [PA]: Lippincott Williams & Wilkins; 2003, with permission.)

to the divisions of the bronchial tree and supply the pulmonary arterioles. The pulmonary circulation is a low-pressure system with a normal mean pressure of approximately 15 mm Hg at rest (compared to systolic pressure that is about 120 mm Hg). Most blood flow to the alveoli is derived from the pulmonary circulation, whereas the bronchial arteries supply the walls of the bronchi and bronchioles to the level of the alveoli. Pulmonary arterioles divide into pulmonary capillaries that form networks in the walls of the alveoli, where gas exchange occurs. The pulmonary veins carry oxygenated blood from the pulmonary capillaries and converge into the main pulmonary veins, which empty into the LA.

### Pulmonary Ventilation

Pulmonary ventilation ($\dot{V}_E$) is the volume of air exchanged in 1 minute. For an average, sedentary adult male, the volume of air exchanged at rest is approximately 6 L $\cdot$ min$^{-1}$. However, at maximal exercise, $\dot{V}_E$ often increases 15- to 25-fold over resting values. Even though oxygen delivery is vital, $\dot{V}_E$ may be more regulated by the requirement for carbon dioxide removal than by oxygen consumption.

### Ventilatory Changes

Several ventilatory adaptations result from physical conditioning regimens. Aerobically trained persons demonstrate larger lung volumes and diffusion capacity at rest and during exercise than their sedentary counterparts. However, ventilation is either unaffected or only modestly affected by cardiorespiratory training. Maximal ventilatory capacity may be increased by exercise training, but it is unclear that this provides any advantage other than increased buffering capacity for lactate. Submaximal ventilation is probably not affected at all, but it may be decreased in some circumstances because a decrease in the production of lactate coincides with a decrease in the need to buffer lactate, which results in decreased ventilation.

 **Energy Systems**

Energy is essential to produce mechanical work, maintain body temperature, and fulfill all biological and chemical activities inside the body. To release energy, foodstuff that is consumed (*i.e.*, protein, carbohydrate, and fat) must be metabolized to yield a high-energy compound called adenosine triphosphate (ATP). In the human body, all mechanical work produced by physical activity relies on the continuous supply of ATP. The manufactured ATP is stored inside muscles so that it is immediately available to produce movement when a stimulus is given to the muscles. However, the storage of ATP in the muscles is limited. If the ATP in the muscle was the only energy available, physical activity would only last for a few seconds. Therefore, for movement that lasts longer than a few seconds, ATP must be further manufactured through other means outlined in this section. The relationship between exercise duration and energy sources is illustrated in Figure 5.4.

## Aerobic and Anaerobic Metabolism

In the transition from rest to maximal exertion, the energy requirements of the exercising muscle increase substantially; therefore, ATP must be constantly resynthesized to maintain the energy requirements of the movement. Hence, the exercising muscle must possess a large capacity of energy to produce sufficient ATP so that increased activity can continue. Energy production relies heavily on the respiratory and cardiovascular systems for the delivery of oxygen and nutrients and for the removal of waste products to maintain the internal equilibrium of cells.

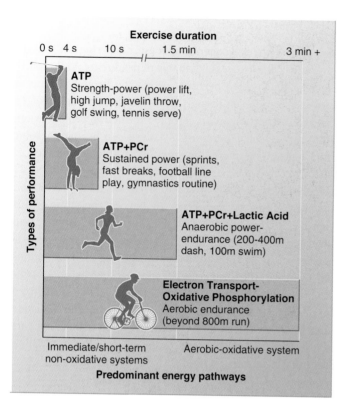

**Predominant energy pathways**

**FIGURE 5.4.** Comparison of activity with the energy pathways used (ATP = adenosine triphosphate, PCr = creatine phosphate, ATP + PCr + lactic acid = anaerobic glycolysis, electron transport-oxidative phosphorylation = aerobic oxidation). (From Premkumar K. *The Massage Connection: Anatomy and Physiology.* 3rd ed. Baltimore [MD]: Lippincott Williams & Wilkins; 2011, with permission.)

## Anaerobic Metabolism

### Adenosine Triphosphate

ATP serves as the ideal energy-transfer agent that powers all of the cell's energy needs (32). The energy released through hydrolysis of the high-energy compound ATP to form adenosine diphosphate (ADP) and inorganic phosphate (Pi) powers skeletal muscle contractions. This reaction is catalyzed by the enzyme ATPase:

$$ATP \xrightarrow{\text{ATPase}} ADP + Pi + energy$$

The amount of ATP directly available in muscle at any time is small, so it must be resynthesized continuously if exercise lasts for more than a few seconds. Muscle fibers contain the metabolic machinery to produce ATP by three pathways: creatine phosphate (CP), anaerobic glycolysis, and aerobic oxidation of nutrients to carbon dioxide and water.

### Creatine Phosphate

The CP system transfers high-energy phosphate from CP to rephosphorylate ATP from ADP (using the enzyme creatine kinase) as follows:

$$ADP + CP \xrightarrow{\text{Creatine kinase}} ATP + C$$

This system is rapid because it involves only one enzymatic step (*i.e.,* one chemical reaction). However, CP exists in finite quantities in cells as well, so the total amount of ATP that can be produced is limited, enough for only 5–10 seconds of strenuous exercise. Oxygen is not involved in the rephosphorylation of ADP to ATP, so the CP system is considered anaerobic (without oxygen).

### Anaerobic Glycolysis

The rapid breakdown of carbohydrate molecules, either glycogen or glucose, occurring without the presence of oxygen, is called anaerobic glycolysis. This process is capable of producing ATP rapidly. The degradation of carbohydrate (glycogen or glucose) to pyruvate or lactate through glycolysis involves a series of enzymatically catalyzed steps, and even though glycolysis does not use oxygen and is considered anaerobic, pyruvate can readily participate in aerobic production of ATP when oxygen is available in the sufficient quantity in the cell. Therefore, glycolysis can be an anaerobic pathway capable of producing ATP without oxygen, or the first step in the aerobic degradation of carbohydrate (18,32) (Fig. 5.5).

Lactate, a byproduct of anaerobic glycolysis, can also be resynthesized for ATP production during exercise (23). Although the details of how this process occurs are beyond the scope of this chapter, it is important to understand that lactate is produced with the initiation of exercise and accumulates in the muscle during intense exercise. During rest or moderate exercise, lactate is oxidized in muscles with high oxidizing capacity (*i.e.*, heart and ventilatory muscles) (30). In strenuous exercise, when energy demand is high and ventilation is at its peak, lactate accumulates contributing to fatigue (26). During recovery, when enough oxygen becomes available, lactate is oxidized and used for ATP production in the muscle or in the liver (24,41). Unlike popular belief, lactate accumulation does not cause soreness after intense exercise. This soreness, which usually appears after an intense bout of exercise and can last various days, is most commonly due to muscle fiber damage and is referred to as delayed onset muscle soreness (DOMS) (37).

## Aerobic Oxidation

The final metabolic pathway for ATP production combines two complex metabolic processes: the Krebs cycle and the electron transport chain (ETC) residing inside the mitochondria as illustrated in Figure 5.5. Unlike glycolysis, aerobic metabolism can use fat, protein, and carbohydrate as substrates to produce ATP. Conceptually, the Krebs cycle can be considered a primer for oxidative phosphorylation. The primary function of the Krebs cycle is to remove hydrogen from four of the reactants involved in the cycle. The electrons from these hydrogens follow a chain of cytochromes (ETC) in the mitochondria, and the energy released from this process is used to rephosphorylate ADP to form ATP. Oxygen is the final acceptor of hydrogen to form water, and this reaction is catalyzed by cytochrome oxidase (18). Although not all ATP is formed aerobically, the amount of ATP yielded by anaerobic glycolysis is extremely small (32). Nevertheless, anaerobic mechanisms provide a rapid source of ATP, which is particularly important at the beginning of any exercise bout and during high-intensity activity that can be sustained only for a brief period. As the duration of exercise increases, the relative contribution of anaerobic energy sources decreases (18).

The aerobic system requires adequate delivery and use of oxygen and uses carbohydrate, fats, and proteins as energy substrates, sustaining high rates of ATP production for muscular energy over long periods of time. The relative contributions of anaerobic and aerobic metabolism depend on oxygen exchange (ventilation), delivery (cardiovascular), and use (muscular extraction) at rates commensurate with the energy demands of activity. *Steady state* is the term used to depict a balance between the energy required by the muscle to perform work and the production of ATP via aerobic metabolism. Steady state corresponds to the flattening or plateau seen in the oxygen consumption curve during submaximal exercise. Although proteins can be used as a fuel for aerobic exercise, carbohydrates and fats are the primary energy substrates during exercise in a healthy, well-fed individual. In general, carbohydrates are used as the primary fuel at the onset of exercise and during high-intensity work (18). However, during prolonged exercise of low to moderate intensity (longer than 30 minutes), a gradual shift occurs from carbohydrate toward an increasing reliance on fat as a substrate.

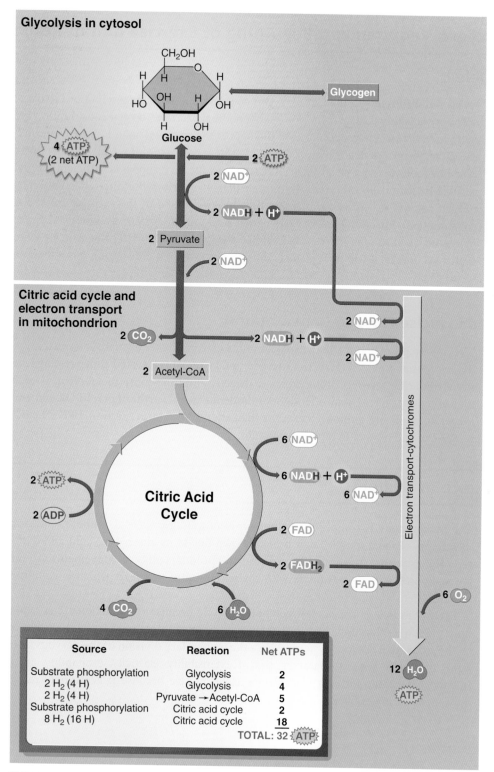

**FIGURE 5.5.** A net yield of 32 ATPs from energy transfer during the complete oxidation of one glucose molecule in glycolysis, the citric acid cycle, and electronic transport. (From Katch VL, McArdle WD, Katch FI. *Essentials of Exercise Physiology*. 4th ed. Baltimore [MD]: Lippincott Williams & Wilkins; 2011, with permission.)

# Oxygen Requirement: Beginning of Exercise and in Recovery

## Oxygen Deficit

Oxygen deficit refers to the lag in oxygen consumption at the beginning of exercise. At the initial stage or transitional stage from rest to submaximal exercise, oxygen consumption builds up gradually until it reaches an optimal level to support the energy demand of the exercise (steady state); therefore, oxygen deficit is incurred. During this stage, part of the ATP supply relies on the anaerobic metabolism. Once steady state is reached, all the ATP supply is sufficiently provided through aerobic oxidation. In other words, oxygen deficit describes the difference between the required oxygen amount necessary for meeting the energy demand of the exercise and the actual oxygen consumption. An additional oxygen deficit accumulates whenever energy demand is abruptly increased, as in sudden increase in exercise pace or intensity. After the exercise stops, the oxygen deficit accumulated will be replenished during recovery by consuming more than usual amounts of oxygen.

## Excess Postexercise Oxygen Consumption

The consumption of more than usual amounts of oxygen after exercise is termed *excess postexercise oxygen consumption* (EPOC) (18). Oxygen uptake remains elevated above resting levels for several minutes during recovery from exercise. In general, postexercise metabolism is higher following high-intensity exercise than after light or moderate work. Furthermore, EPOC remains elevated for longer duration after prolonged exercise than after shorter term exertion. EPOC helps to restore CP in muscles and oxygen in blood and tissues.

# Muscular System

The human body is composed of three types of muscles: skeletal, smooth, and cardiac. Skeletal muscle, or "striated muscle" as it is also known due to its alternating light and dark fibers, is the type of muscle that attaches to the skeleton and produces physical movements. All internal organs are composed of smooth muscle with the exception of the heart which is composed of cardiac muscle.

Skeletal muscle is considered voluntary muscle because the individual can control it, for the most part. Smooth muscle and cardiac muscle are involuntary muscles because they are controlled by the autonomic nervous system (ANS), the involuntary division of the nervous system. All three kinds of muscle possess characteristics of extensibility, elasticity, excitability, and contractility. In this chapter, the focus is placed on skeletal muscle because it is strongly related to human movement during exercise.

## Skeletal Muscles

The structure of skeletal muscle is shown in Figure 5.6. Individual skeletal muscles are composed of a varying number of muscle bundles referred to as "fasciculi" (an individual bundle is a fasciculus). Fasciculi are likewise covered and thus separated by the perimysium. Individual muscle fibers are enveloped by the endomysium. Immediately beneath the endomysium is the thin, membranous sarcolemma, the cell membrane that encloses the cellular contents of the muscle fiber, nuclei, local stores of fat and carbohydrate (stored glucose is referred to as glycogen), enzymes, contractile proteins, and other specialized structures such as the mitochondria.

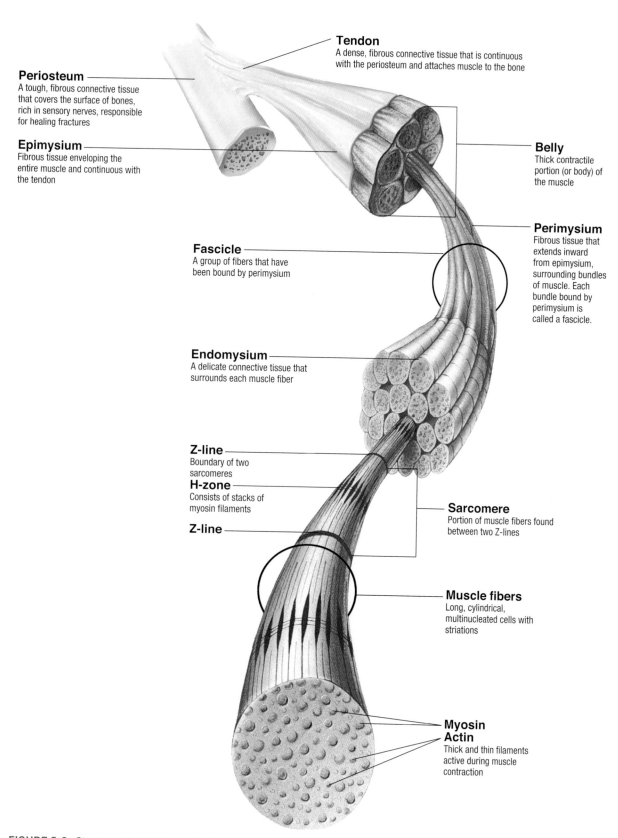

**Tendon**
A dense, fibrous connective tissue that is continuous with the periosteum and attaches muscle to the bone

**Periosteum**
A tough, fibrous connective tissue that covers the surface of bones, rich in sensory nerves, responsible for healing fractures

**Epimysium**
Fibrous tissue enveloping the entire muscle and continuous with the tendon

**Belly**
Thick contractile portion (or body) of the muscle

**Fascicle**
A group of fibers that have been bound by perimysium

**Perimysium**
Fibrous tissue that extends inward from epimysium, surrounding bundles of muscle. Each bundle bound by perimysium is called a fascicle.

**Endomysium**
A delicate connective tissue that surrounds each muscle fiber

**Z-line**
Boundary of two sarcomeres

**H-zone**
Consists of stacks of myosin filaments

**Z-line**

**Sarcomere**
Portion of muscle fibers found between two Z-lines

**Muscle fibers**
Long, cylindrical, multinucleated cells with striations

**Myosin**
**Actin**
Thick and thin filaments active during muscle contraction

**FIGURE 5.6.** Structure of skeletal muscle. (Reprinted with permission from Anatomical Chart Company. *ACC's Illustrated Pocket Anatomy: The Muscular & Skeletal Systems Study Guide*. Baltimore [MD]: Lippincott Williams & Wilkins; 2007.)

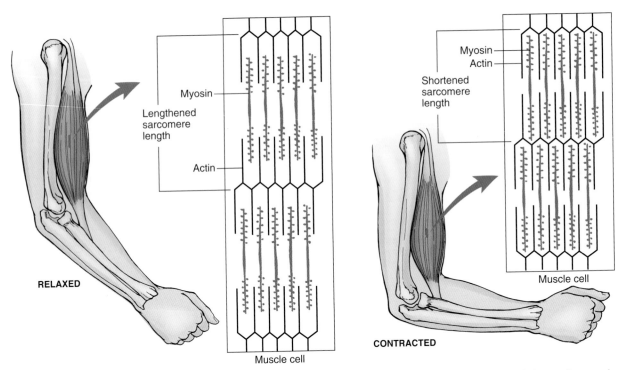

**FIGURE 5.7.** The sliding-filament model (contraction of skeletal muscle results from the sliding of the actin chains on the myosin chains). (From Oatis CA. *Kinesiology: The Mechanics and Pathomechanics of Human Movement.* 3rd ed. Baltimore [MD]: Lippincott Williams & Wilkins; 2016, with permission.)

## Muscle Contraction

The smallest contractile unit of a muscle cell is the sarcomere. A sarcomere is composed of two types of muscle protein: actin (the thin filament) and myosin (the thick filament). Actin contains two other components: troponin and tropomyosin. Myosin contains many cross-bridges where the actin attaches. Figure 5.7 illustrates the relationship between muscle contraction and microscopic action within the sarcomere. Two major principles describe the mechanism of muscle contraction: the sliding-filament theory and the all-or-none principle.

The sliding-filament theory describes the events that occur between the actin and myosin filaments during muscle contraction and relaxation. When a nerve impulse is received, the cross-bridges of the myosin pull the actin filaments toward the center of the sarcomere and tension is created. The sliding motion between the actin and myosin causes the shortening of a sarcomere and subsequently the entire muscle fiber. Moreover, the nerve impulse that applies to the muscle cell, regardless of its "strength," causes the sarcomere to contract maximally or not all. This is called the all-or-none principle. The length of a muscle fiber during a contraction is determined by the number of muscle fibers (cells) being recruited for the contraction. The more the sarcomeres are recruited for contraction, the shorter the contracted muscle length. The amount of force that is produced from a muscle contraction is determined by the number of motor units (one motor nerve together with all the muscle fibers that it innervated) that are recruited and the number of fibers contained in each motor unit (18).

## Muscle Contraction and Training

During static (isometric) contractions, the muscle or muscle group maintains a constant length as resistance is applied, and no change in the joint position occurs. Research has demonstrated that static training produces significant improvements in muscular strength. The strength gains, however, are limited to the specific joint angles at which the static contractions are performed (18). As a result, static training may have limited value in enhancing functional strength. "Functional strength" is defined as work performed against a resistance in such a way that the strength gained directly benefits the execution of activities of daily life and/or movements associated with sports. Static training has also been associated with short-term elevations in BP, perhaps because of increased intra-thoracic pressure during static contractions. Despite the limitations, static training appears to play a positive role in physical rehabilitation. For example, static training is effective in maintaining muscular strength and preventing atrophy associated with the immobilization of a limb (*e.g.*, application of a cast, splint, or brace) (15,18).

Dynamic (isotonic) resistance training is another common method of muscular training. The term *dynamic* is used because movement occurs at the joint of action. If force is sufficient to overcome the external resistance (*e.g.*, dumbbell) and the muscle shortens (*e.g.*, the lifting phase of a biceps curl), the muscle action is called concentric. When the resistance is greater than force applied by the muscle and the muscle lengthens, it is known as eccentric muscle action (*e.g.*, the lowering phase of the biceps curl). Most dynamic resistance training includes both concentric and eccentric actions. Significantly heavier loads can be moved eccentrically; in fact, in nonfatigued muscle, the ratio of eccentric to concentric strength can be as high as 1.4:1 (15,18). For example, maximal eccentric weight is 1.4 times the maximal concentric weight in the same muscle group/movement. The greater force production occurring during the eccentric action compared with the concentric action probably results from the greater recruitment of motor units and a slow movement velocity. Individuals who are eccentrically trained are often subjected to DOMS (18). Eccentric training can, however, play an important role in preventing or rehabilitating certain musculoskeletal injuries. For example, eccentric training has been demonstrated to be effective for treating hamstring strains, tennis elbow, and patellofemoral pain syndrome (40).

Isokinetic exercise is the other major type of resistance training and entails a muscular contraction at a constant speed against accommodating resistance. The speed of movement is controlled, and the amount of resistance is proportional to the amount of force produced throughout the full range of motion. The theoretical advantage of isokinetic exercise is the potential for development of maximal muscle tension throughout the range of motion. Research documents the effectiveness of isokinetic training (18). Strength gains achieved during high-speed training (*i.e.*, contraction velocities of $180° \cdot s^{-1}$ or faster) appear to carry over to all speeds below that specific speed (13). Improvement in strength at slow speeds of movement, however, has not been shown to carry over to faster speeds.

## Muscle Fiber Types

The human body has the ability to perform a wide range of physical tasks, combining varying composites of speed, power, and endurance. No single type of muscle fiber possesses the characteristics that would allow optimal performance across this continuum of physical challenges. Rather, muscle fibers possess certain characteristics that result in relative specialization. For example, certain muscle fibers are selectively recruited by the body for tasks of short duration that require speed and power, whereas others are recruited for endurance tasks of long duration and relatively low intensity. When the challenge requires elements of speed or power but also has an endurance component, yet another type of muscle fiber is recruited. These different fiber types should not be thought of as mutually exclusive. In fact, intricate recruitment and switching occurs within the muscle over the performance of many tasks, and fibers designed to be optimal for one type of task can contribute to the performance of another. The net result is a functioning muscle that can respond to a wide variety of tasks, and although the composition of the muscle may lend itself to performing best in endurance activities, it still can accomplish speed and power tasks to a lesser degree (42).

Although there is a fair amount of controversy about the classification of muscle fiber types, there is general agreement that two distinct fiber types exist; type I or slow twitch and type II or fast twitch, with their proposed subdivisions. These fibers have been identified and classified by contractile and metabolic characteristics such as the chemical breakdown of carbohydrate, fat, and protein for energy within the muscle cell (8).

### Slow-Twitch Muscle Fibers

The characteristics of slow-twitch muscle fibers are consistent with those of muscle fibers that resist fatigue. Thus, type I fibers are selected for activities of low intensity and long duration. In addition to their inherent resistance to fatigue, endurance is prolonged by the constant switching that occurs to ensure freshly charged muscle fibers are activated as the exercise stimulus continues. The average person has approximately 50% slow-twitch fibers, and this distribution is generally equal throughout the major muscle groups of the body (32). Individuals most successful at endurance activities generally have a higher proportion of slow-twitch fibers, and this is most likely due to genetic factors supplemented through appropriate exercise training. From a metabolic perspective, slow-twitch fibers are those frequently called "aerobic" because the generation of energy for continued muscle contraction is met through the ongoing oxidation (chemical breakdown using oxygen) of available energy substrates. Thus, with minimal accumulation of anaerobically (chemical breakdown without oxygen) produced metabolites; continued submaximal muscle contraction is favored in slow-twitch fibers.

### Fast-Twitch Muscle Fibers

At the opposite end of the continuum, those who achieve the greatest success in power and high-intensity speed tasks usually have a greater proportion of fast-twitch muscle fibers distributed through the major muscle groups. Because force generation is so important, fast-twitch fibers shorten and develop tension considerably faster than type I fibers (44). These fibers are typically thought of as type IIx fibers (9). Metabolically, these fibers have minimal aerobic capacity due to a small amount of mitochondria. When an endurance component is introduced, such as in events lasting upward of several minutes (*e.g.*, 800- to 1,500-m races), a second type of fast-twitch fiber, type IIa, is recruited. The type IIa fibers represent a transition of sorts between the needs met by the type I and type IIb fibers. Metabolically, although type IIa fibers have the ability to generate a moderately large amount of force, they also have some aerobic capacity. In addition, type IIa fibers are adaptable with training. For example, with significant endurance training, it is possible for type IIa fibers to increase their aerobic capacity such that these type IIa fibers behave much more like type I fibers (38). This is a logical and necessary bridge between the types of muscle fibers and the ability to meet the variety of physical tasks imposed.

## Neuromuscular Activation

Physical activity involves purposeful, voluntary movement. The stimulus for this voluntary muscle activation comes from the brain, where the signal is relayed through the brainstem, through the spinal cord and transformed into a specific motor unit activation pattern. To perform a specific task, the required motor units meet specific demands for force production by activating associated muscle fibers (9).

### Motor Unit Activation

The functional unit of the neuromuscular system is the motor unit. It consists of the motor neuron and the muscle fibers it innervates. Motor units range in size from a few to several hundred muscle fibers. Muscle fibers from different motor units can be anatomically adjacent to each other, and therefore, a muscle fiber may be actively generating force, whereas the adjacent fiber moves passively with no direct neural stimulation. When maximal force is required, all available motor units are activated. Another adaptive mechanism affected by heavy resistance training is the muscle force affected by different motor unit firing rates and/or frequencies.

# Skeletal System

In addition to protecting vital organs, and acting as an important source of nutrients and blood constituents, the primary role of the skeletal system is to provide support for locomotion and movement (45). The skeletal system can be divided into the axial skeleton (skull, vertebral column, and sternum) and the appendicular skeleton (upper and lower extremities). An outer fibrous layer of connective tissue attaches the bone to muscles, deep fascia, and joint capsules. Just beneath the outer layer is a highly vascular inner layer that contains cells for the creation of new bone. The outer and inner layers that cover the bones constitute the periosteum. The periosteum, continuous with tendons and adjacent articulated structures, anchors muscle to bone. Tendons are likewise continuous with the epimysium, the outer layer of connective tissue covering muscle.

## Structure and Function of Joints in Movement

The effective interaction of bone and muscle to produce movement depends somewhat on joint function. Joints are the articulations between bones, and, along with bones and ligaments, they constitute the articular system. Ligaments are tough, fibrous connective tissues that connect one bone to another, whereas tendons connect muscle to bone. Joints are typically classified as fibrous, in which bones are united by fibrous tissue, cartilaginous (with cartilage or a fibrocartilaginous anchor), or synovial, in which a fibrous articular capsule and an inner synovial membrane lining enclose the joint cavity. The cavity is filled with synovial fluid, which provides constant lubrication during human movement to minimize the wearing effects of friction on the cartilaginous covering of the articulating bones. Joints are typically well perfused by numerous arterial branches and are innervated by branches of the nerves supplying the adjacent muscle and overlying skin.

Proprioception is defined as the receipt of information from joints, muscles, and tendons that enables the brain to determine movements and position of the body and its parts. Proprioceptive feedback is an important joint sensation, as is pain, owing to the high density of sensory fibers in the joint capsule. This feedback has obvious importance in regulating human movement and in preventing injury. The degree of movement within a joint is typically called the range of motion (ROM). ROM can be active (AROM), where the range that can be reached by voluntary movement, or passive (PROM), as the range can be achieved by external means (*e.g.*, an examiner or a device). Joints are typically limited in range by the articulations of bones (as in the limitation of elbow extension by the olecranon process of the ulna), ligamentous arrangement, and soft tissue limitations, as occurs in elbow or knee flexion. Movement at one joint may influence the extent of movement at adjacent joints, as a number of muscles and other soft tissue structures cross multiple joints. For example, finger flexion decreases in the presence of wrist flexion because muscles that flex both the wrist and fingers cross multiple joints. More in-depth information about the skeletal system is provided in Chapter 3.

# Neurological System

In the earlier discussion on muscle contraction, the contraction was described as triggered by a nervous impulse of a motor unit. The nervous impulse is released from a motor neuron, which originates from the spinal cord. The spinal cord is a part of the CNS, which helps control all of the peripheral and internal organs. All muscular movements are controlled by the nervous system. To understand the complex control of human movement, understanding neural control is essential.

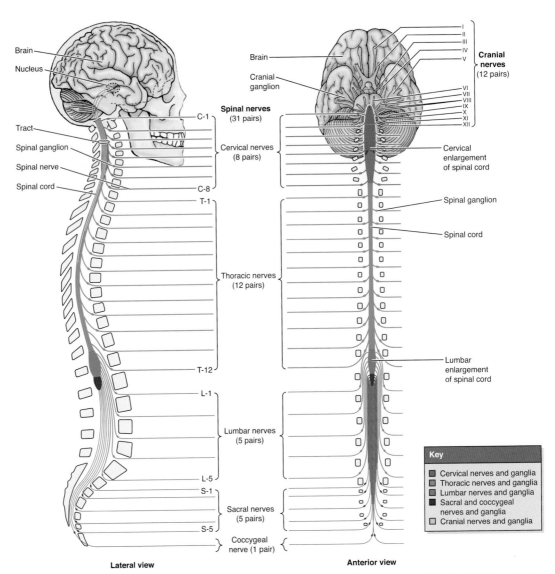

**FIGURE 5.8.** Basic organization of the nervous system. The brain and spinal cord constitute the CNS. A collection of nerve cell bodies in the CNS is a nucleus, and a bundle of nerve fibers connecting neighboring or distant nuclei in the CNS is a tract. The PNS consists of nerve fibers and cell bodies outside the CNS. Peripheral nerves are either cranial or spinal nerves. A collection of nerve cell bodies outside the CNS is a ganglion (*e.g.*, a cranial or spinal ganglion). (From Moore KL, Dalley AF II. *Clinically Oriented Anatomy.* 4th ed. Baltimore [MD]: Lippincott Williams & Wilkins; 1999.)

The nervous system consists of the brain, spinal cord, and peripheral nerves and is divided into the CNS and the peripheral nervous system (PNS). The CNS consists of the brain and spinal cord, whereas the PNS consists of all other peripheral nerves of the voluntary system (Fig. 5.8) (31).

## Central Nervous System

The brain is the most important part of the CNS and is surrounded and protected by the bony skull. The spinal cord is the extension of the brain, which runs along and is surrounded and protected by the vertebral column. The CNS is the body's central control center where sensory stimuli are received, integrated, analyzed, and interpreted, and finally relayed as nerve impulses to muscles and glands for taking action.

## Peripheral Nervous System

The PNS is composed of the cranial nerves associated with the brain and the spinal nerves associated with the spinal cord as well as groups of nerve cell bodies called "ganglia." In other words, the PNS is made up of the nerve cells and their fibers that lie outside the brain and spinal cord (31). The PNS allows the brain and spinal cord to communicate with the rest of the body. There are two types of nerve fibers in the PNS: the afferent, or sensory, fibers and the efferent, or motor, fibers. The sensory nerve fibers are responsible for carrying nerve impulses from sensory receptors in the body to the CNS. Once the received signal is processed and analyzed in the CNS and an action is determined, then motor nerve fibers are called to convey the nerve signal from the CNS to the effectors, either the muscles or other organs. The PNS can be subdivided into two functional branches: the somatic nervous system and the visceral nervous system. Both systems are composed of an afferent division (sending feedback to the CNS to adjust responses) and an efferent division (sending signals out to the body). The somatic nervous system primarily regulates the voluntary contraction of the skeletal muscles, whereas the visceral system involves the motor activities that control internal organs such as the smooth (involuntary) muscles, cardiac muscle, and glands of the skin and viscera. The latter is also referred to as the ANS.

## Autonomic Nervous System

The ANS regulates visceral activities such as HR, digestion, breathing, and the secretion of hormones. These activities normally are operated subconsciously and continue to function throughout life. However, they can also be altered to a certain limit consciously. These activities can be carried out even if the organs are deprived of innervation by the ANS. The ANS includes two pathways, the sympathetic pathway and the parasympathetic pathway, which complement each other. The sympathetic pathway stimulates visceral activities under stressful (or alarming) conditions, which results in acceleration of metabolism, HR, and breathing and adrenal hormone release. Exercise can be viewed as a stressful stimulus to the body that triggers the sympathetic pathway for generating more energy and muscular force. When the stressful stimulus subsides, the parasympathetic pathway brings the visceral activities back to normal, for example, decreasing HR and breathing, relaxing the muscles, and increasing gastrointestinal activities. The parasympathetic pathway helps conserve and restore body resources.

## Neuromuscular Control

The information transmitted and relayed by the sensory and motor nerves is in a form of electrical energy referred to as the "nerve impulse." The sensory stimulation received through vision or touching is transmitted to the CNS. A motor command is then released after the integration and decision making of the motor cortex of the brain. A nerve pulse is then transmitted to the targeted muscles through an efferent neuron for activating muscle contraction. The functional unit of the neuromuscular system is the motor unit (35). It consists of the motor neuron and the muscle fibers it innervates. When maximal force is required, all available motor units are activated. Another adaptive mechanism affected by heavy resistance training is the muscle force affected by different motor unit firing rates and frequencies (35).

Motor unit activation is also influenced by the size principle. This principle is based on the observed relationship between motor unit twitch force and recruitment threshold. Specifically, motor units are recruited in order according to recruitment thresholds and firing rates, resulting in a continuum of voluntary force. Whereas type I motor units are the smallest and possess the lowest recruitment thresholds, type IIa and IIx motor units are larger in size and have higher activation thresholds. Therefore, as force requirements of an activity increase, the recruitment order progresses from type I to IIa to IIx motor units. Thus, most muscles contain a range of motor units (type I and

II fibers), and force production can span wide levels. Maximal force production requires not only the recruitment of all motor units, including high-threshold motor units, but also recruitment at a sufficiently high firing rate. It has been hypothesized that untrained individuals cannot voluntarily recruit the highest threshold motor units or maximally activate muscles. Furthermore, electrical stimulation has been shown to be more effective in eliciting gains in untrained muscle or injury rehabilitation scenarios, suggesting further inability to activate all available motor units. Thus, training adaptation develops the ability to recruit a greater percentage of motor units when required.

## Muscle Spindle and Golgi Tendon Organs

Other than the motor unit, muscular contraction is also affected by specialized sensory receptors in the muscles and tendons that are sensitive to stretch, tension, and pressure. These receptors are termed "proprioceptors." A sensory receptor called a "muscle spindle" is sensitive to the stretch of a muscle and is embedded within the muscle fiber. Anytime the muscle is stretched or shortened, the spindle is also stretched or shortened. The muscle spindles provide sensory information regarding the changes and rate of change in the length and tension of muscle fibers. Their main function is to respond to stretch of a muscle and, through reflex action, to initiate a stronger muscle action to reduce this stretch (35). This is known as the "stretch reflex." In contrast to the muscle spindles, the Golgi tendon organs are another type of specialized proprioceptor that attaches to the tendons near the junction of the muscle (Fig. 5.9). These receptors detect differences in the tension generated by active muscle rather than muscle length. When excessive tension is detected by the Golgi tendon organs, a continuous reflex inhibition signal is fired to prevent the muscle from contracting. Hence, the Golgi tendon organs serve as a protective sensory system to prevent muscle injury resulting from overcontraction.

**FIGURE 5.9.** Structure of the Golgi tendon organ. (From Premkumar K. *The Massage Connection: Anatomy and Physiology*. 3rd ed. Baltimore [MD]: Lippincott Williams & Wilkins; 2011, with permission.)

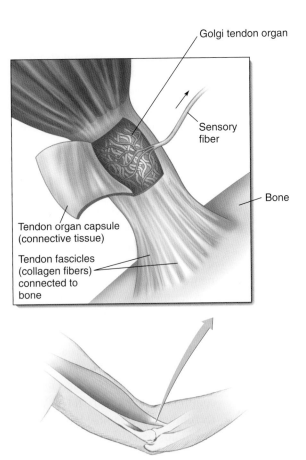

# Exercise System Adaptations: Strength, Cardiovascular

Long-term exercise training is important to overall health and physical fitness. A well-designed exercise training program leads to long-term physiological changes (adaptation), including improvements in muscular strength and endurance, cardiovascular function, musculoskeletal flexibility, and changes in body composition. These improvements allow for the enhancement of athletic performance, increased function to engage in leisure-time physical activity and perform activities of daily living more comfortably, and maintain functional independence later in life.

## Resistance Training

Resistance training is an effective exercise modality to improve muscular strength and endurance. Strength improves when a load greater than what one is accustomed is applied to the muscle fiber and its contractile proteins over a period. The tension required for strength gain is about 60%–80% of the muscle's maximum force; however, a range of 75%–90% of one repetition maximum (1-RM) is recommended for optimizing strength gains (18). For improvements to take place, the resistance applied against a muscle must be large enough to impose a demand on the body system, thus creating an "overload" of the muscle. This is the so-called overload principle and can be accomplished by modifying the number of repetitions, the amount of resistance, or the number of sets. The amount of overload required depends on the individual's current level of muscular fitness. Hypertrophy, or the increase in muscular size, is thought to occur through the remodeling of proteins within the muscle cell and an increase in the number of myofibrils (25). Hypertrophy is the most prominent adaptation seen with resistance training (25). However, changes to the muscle fibers are not the only adaptations seen with resistance training. Tendons, ligaments, and the muscles' surrounding tissue also undergo hypertrophy and strengthening in order to withstand the greater amount of forces produced by the hypertrophied muscle (11,33).

Strength training also improves aerobic enzyme systems. Increases in aerobic enzyme activity have been reported from resistance training (7,12,17). Moreover, increases in oxidative enzymes have been demonstrated to be higher in type IIa fibers than in type IIx fibers. The increase in oxidative metabolism of muscles after long-term strength training is also associated with increases in capillary supply and the concentration of cellular mitochondria. Capillaries per unit area and per fiber are significantly increased in response to varying types of heavy resistance training (such as a combination of concentric and eccentric resistance exercise). Increased capillary density may facilitate performance of low-intensity weight training by increasing blood supply to active muscle. It also increases the ability to remove lactate and thereby improves the ability to tolerate training under highly acidic conditions. All of these changes promote oxygen delivery and use within the muscle fiber, thereby improving muscular endurance (18).

Part of the strength gain resulting from strength training is attributed to changes in the nervous system. This is especially true during the early stages of strength training. Training tends to reduce the neuromuscular inhibition in both the CNS and proprioceptors (*e.g.*, Golgi tendon organs). Other neural factors include the increased neural drive to muscle, increased synchronization of motor units, and increased activation of the contractile apparatus.

## Cardiovascular Exercise

Physical inactivity is now classified as a major contributing risk factor for heart disease, with a similar impact to that of elevated blood cholesterol level, cigarette smoking, and hypertension (43). Moreover, longitudinal studies have shown that higher levels of aerobic fitness are associated with lower mortality from heart disease even after statistical adjustments for age, coronary risk factors, and family history of heart disease (6). These findings and other recent reports in persons with and without heart disease have confirmed an inverse association between aerobic capacity and cardiovascular mortality (5).

Endurance exercise training increases functional capacity and provides relief of symptoms in many clients with coronary artery disease (CAD). This is particularly important because most clients with clinically manifest CAD have a subnormal functional capacity (50%–70% of those of similar age and sex), and some may be limited by symptoms at relatively low levels of exertion. Improvement in function appears to be mediated by increased central and/or peripheral oxygen transport and supply, whereas relief of angina pectoris (*i.e.*, chest pain/discomfort) may result from increased myocardial oxygen supply, decreased oxygen demand, or both.

Most exercise studies on healthy subjects demonstrate 20% ($\pm10\%$) increases in aerobic capacity ($\dot{V}O_{2max}$), with the greatest relative improvements among the most unfit (43). Because a fixed submaximal work rate has a relatively constant aerobic requirement, the physically trained individual works at a lower percentage of $\dot{V}O_{2max}$, with greater reserve after exercise training. Enhanced oxygen transport, particularly increased maximal SV and cardiac output, have traditionally been regarded as the primary mechanism underlying the increase in $\dot{V}O_{2max}$ with training.

The effects of long-term exercise training on the ANS act to reduce myocardial demands at rest and during exercise. A lower HR during submaximal exercise after endurance training may be attributed to an intracardiac mechanism (an effect directly on the myocardium, *e.g.*, increased SV during submaximal work) or an extracardiac mechanism (*e.g.*, alterations in trained skeletal muscle) or both. The result is a reduced HR and SBP at rest and at any fixed oxygen uptake or submaximal work rate.

The increased oxidative capacity of trained skeletal muscle appears to offer a distinct hemodynamic advantage. Lactic acid production and muscle blood flow are decreased at a fixed external workload, whereas submaximal $\dot{Q}$ and oxygen uptake are unchanged or slightly reduced. As a result, there are compensatory increases in a-$\bar{v}O_2$ difference at submaximal and maximal exercise. All of this means that at submaximal exercise levels, the cardiovascular system functions more effectively, and at maximal exercise a greater power output can be achieved.

## Overall Changes

The HR response plays a critical role in the delivery of oxygen to working skeletal muscle. The resting HR decreases by approximately 10–15 bpm as a result of cardiovascular training (21). SV will increase both at rest and during exercise up to a point, as a result of long-term cardiovascular training. $\dot{Q}$ will increase during exercise but will not change significantly at rest in endurance trained individuals. The a-$\bar{v}O_2$ difference increases with long-term cardiovascular training, particularly near-maximal exertion. Both resting SBP and DBP may decrease (if elevated consistently before starting regular cardiovascular training) with long-term cardiovascular training. Resting lactate levels remain relatively unchanged with long-term cardiovascular training (4). As a result of proper cardiovascular training, less lactic acid will be produced at submaximal workloads during exercise (16). For responses to aerobic conditioning in untrained individuals, see Table 5.1.

## Sex-Specific Improvement

The salutary effects of chronic endurance training in men are well documented (Table 5.2). Numerous studies now provide ample data on $\dot{V}O_{2max}$, cardiovascular hemodynamics, body composition, and blood lipids as well as changes with physical conditioning of middle-aged and older women. The results demonstrate that women with and without CAD respond to aerobic training in much the same way as men when subjected to comparable programs in terms of frequency, intensity, and duration of exercise (1). Improvement is negatively correlated with age, habitual physical activity, and initial $\dot{V}O_{2max}$ (which is generally lower in women than in men) and positively

| Table 5.1 | Physiological Adaptations to Aerobic Conditioning in Untrained Individuals | | | |
|---|---|---|---|---|
| | | | Physiologic Response | |
| **Variable** | **Unit of Measure** | | **Submaximal Effort** | **Maximal Effort** |
| $\dot{V}O_{2max}$ | $mL \cdot kg^{-1} \cdot min^{-1}$ | | ↔ | ↑ |
| Resting heart rate | bpm | | ↓ | ↑ |
| Exercise heart rate | bpm | | ↓ | ↑ |
| Maximum heart rate | bpm | | ↔ | ↔ |
| a-$\bar{v}O_2$ difference | $mL\ O_2 \cdot 100\ mL\ blood^{-1}$ | | ↑ | ↑ |
| Maximum minute ventilation | $L \cdot min^{-1}$ | | ↓ | ↑ |
| Stroke volume | $mL \cdot beat^{-1}$ | | ↓ | ↑ |
| Cardiac output | $L \cdot min^{-1}$ | | ↓ | ↑ |
| Blood volume | L | | ↑ | ↑ |
| Systolic blood pressure | mm Hg | | ↓ | ↔ or ↑ |
| Blood lactate | $mL \cdot 100\ mL\ blood^{-1}$ | | ↓ | ↑ |
| Oxidative capacity of skeletal muscle | Multiple variables[a] | | ↓ | ↑ |

[a]Represents increase in skeletal muscle mitochondrial number and size, capillary density, and/or oxidative enzymes.
↑, increase; ↓, decrease; ↔, no change.

| Table 5.2 | Benefits of Increasing Cardiorespiratory Activities and/or Improving Cardiorespiratory Fitness[a] |
|---|---|

**Improved cardiorespiratory function:**

- Increased maximal oxygen uptake
- Increased maximal $\dot{Q}$ and SV
- Increased capillary density in skeletal muscle
- Increased mitochondrial density
- Increased lactate threshold
- Lower HR and BP at a fixed submaximal work rate
- Lower myocardial oxygen demand at a fixed submaximal work rate
- Lower minute ventilation at a fixed submaximal work rate

**Improved immune function:**

Improved glucose tolerance and insulin sensitivity

Improved work, recreational, and sports performance

Decreased fatigue in daily activities

**Decreased risk of the following:**

- Mortality from all causes
- Coronary artery disease
- Cancer (colon, perhaps breast and prostate)
- Hypertension
- Noninsulin-dependent diabetes mellitus
- Osteoporosis
- Anxiety
- Depression

**Improved blood lipid profile:**

- Decreased triglycerides
- Increased high-density lipoprotein cholesterol
- Decreased postprandial lipemia

Improved body composition

Enhanced sense of well-being

[a]Many of the health benefits accrue from physical activity may have relatively little effect on increasing cardiorespiratory fitness (41).

correlated with conditioning frequency, intensity, and duration (19). There are, however, large differences between individuals in the effects of physical conditioning independent of age, initial capacity, or conditioning program. These individual variations in response to aerobic exercise training may result from childhood patterns of activity, state of conditioning at the initiation of the program, or degree of physiological aging. Body compositional differences in trainability may also play an important role with respect to the results of physical conditioning. Obese women demonstrate lower aerobic capacity (per kilogram body weight), altered cardiovascular hemodynamics, and elevated serum lipids than leaner women (20). This initial varied profile may serve to modify the outcome of an aerobic conditioning program with respect to the magnitude of quantitative change.

## SUMMARY

The purpose of this chapter was to introduce the Personal Trainer to the basic concepts of exercise physiology. The topics in this chapter are not all inclusive due to length limitations not because other areas of exercise physiology are not important. Emphasis is placed on cardiovascular and pulmonary physiology, musculoskeletal function, and adaptations to training because the Personal Trainer may encounter these more often. However, endocrine, metabolic, and other body functions are also important; thus, it is recommended that as new issues with individual clients arise, Personal Trainers should seek out additional references that can assist in understanding the conditions and how the body functions under conditions of physical stress. This proactive approach to learning a client's condition will assist the Personal Trainer to develop safe and effective exercise program for their clients.

# REFERENCES

1. Ades PA, Waldmann ML, Polk DM, Coflesky JT. Referral patterns and exercise response in the rehabilitation of female coronary patients aged greater than or equal to 62 years. *Am J Cardiol.* 1992;69(17):1422–5.

2. Alman RE, Sloniger MA. Cardiorespiratory and health-related physical fitness assessments. In: Swain DP, editor. *ACSM's Resource Manual for Guidelines for Exercise Testing and Prescription.* 7th ed. Baltimore (MD): Wolters Kluwer Health/Lippincott Williams & Williams; 2014. p. 335–54.

3. American College of Sports Medicine. *ACSM's Guidelines for Exercise Testing and Prescription.* 10th ed. Philadelphia (PA): Wolters Kluwer; 2018.

4. Astrand PO, Rodahl K, Dahl HA, Stromme SB. *Textbook of Work Physiology: Physiological Bases of Exercise.* 4th ed. Champaign (IL): Human Kinetics; 2003. 656 p.

5. Blair SN, Kampert JB, Kohl HW, et al. Influences of cardio-respiratory fitness and other precursors on cardiovascular disease and all-cause mortality in men and women. *JAMA.* 1996;276(3):205–10.

6. Blair SN, Kohl HW, Paffenbarger RS, Clark DG, Cooper KH, Gibbons LW. Physical fitness and all-cause mortality. A prospective study of healthy men and women. *JAMA.* 1989; 262(17):2395–401.

7. Bloomer RJ, Goldfarb AH. Anaerobic exercise and oxidative stress: a review. *Can J Appl Physiol.* 2004;29(3):245–63.

8. Brooke MH, Kaiser KK. Muscle fiber types: how many and what kind? *Arch Neurol.* 1970;23(4):369–79.

9. Caiozzo VJ. The muscular system: structural and functional plasticity. In: Farrell PA, Joyner MJ, Caiozzo VJ, editors. *ACSM's Advanced Exercise Physiology.* 2nd ed. Baltimore (MD): Wolters Kluwer Health/Lippincott Williams & Williams; 2012. p. 117–51.

10. Comess KA, Fenster PE. Clinical implications of the blood pressure response to exercise. *Cardiology.* 1981;68(4): 233–44.

11. Conroy B, Earle RW. Bone, muscle, and connective tissue adaptations to physical activity. In: Baechle TR, Earle RW, editors. *Essentials of Strength Training and Conditioning.* Champaign (IL): Human Kinetics; 2000. p. 57–72.

12. Costill DL, Coyle EF, Fink WF, Lesmes GR, Witzmann FA. Adaptations in skeletal muscle following strength training. *J Appl Physiol.* 1979;46(1):96–9.

13. Coyle EF, Feiring DC, Rotkis TC, et al. Specificity of power improvements through slow and fast isokinetic training. *J Appl Physiol.* 1981;51(6):1437–42.

14. Dehn M, Mullins CB. Physiologic effects and importance of exercise in patients with coronary heart disease. *J Cardiovasc Med.* 1977;2:365–87.

15. DiNubile NA. Strength training. *Clin Sports Med.* 1991; 10(1):33–62.

16. Emter CA, Laughlin MH. Adaptations to cardiorespiratory exercise training. In: Swain DP, editor. *ACSM's Resource Manual for Guidelines for Exercise Testing and Prescription.* 7th ed. Baltimore (MD): Wolters Kluwer Health/Lippincott Williams & Williams; 2014. p. 496–510.

17. Exner GU, Staudte HW, Pette D. Isometric training of rats — effects upon fast and slow muscle and modification by an anabolic hormone (nandrolone decanoate). I. Female rats. *Pflugers Arch.* 1973;345(1):1–14.

18. Fleck SJ, Kraemer WJ. *Designing Resistance Training Programs.* 4th ed. Champaign (IL): Human Kinetics; 2014. 520 p.

19. Franklin BA, Bonzheim K, Berg T. Gender differences in rehabilitation. In: Julian DG, Wenger NK, editors. *Women and Heart Disease.* London (United Kingdom): Martin Dunitz; 1997. p. 151–71.

20. Franklin B, Buskirk E, Hodgson J, Gahagan H, Kollias J, Mendez J. Effects of physical conditioning on cardiorespiratory function, body composition and serum lipids in relatively normal-weight and obese middle-aged women. *Int J Obes.* 1979;3(2):97–109.

21. Frick MH, Elovainio RO, Somer T. The mechanism of bradycardia evoked by physical training. *Cardiologia.* 1967;51(1):46–54.

22. Gellish RL, Goslin BR, Olson RE, McDonald A, Russi GD, Moudgil VK. Longitudinal modeling of the relationship between age and maximal heart rate. *Med Sci Sports Exerc.* 2007;39(5):822–9.

23. Gladden LB. A lactatic perspective on metabolism. *Med Sci Sports Exerc.* 2008;40(3):477–85.

24. Gladden LB. Muscle as a consumer of lactate. *Med Sci Sports Exerc.* 2000;32(4):764–71.

25. Goldberg A, Etlinger J, Goldspink L, Jablecki C. Mechanism of work-induced hypertrophy of skeletal muscle. *Med Sci Sports Exerc.* 1975;7:248–61.

26. Hogan MC, Gladden LB, Kurdak SS, Poole DC. Increased [lactate] in working dog muscle reduces tension development independent of pH. *Med Sci Sports Exerc.* 1995;27(3):371–7.

27. Karvonen MJ, Kentala E, Mustala O. The effects of training on heart rate: a longitudinal study. *Ann Med Exp Biol Fenn.* 1957;35(3):307–15.

28. Lenfant C, Chobanian AV, Jones DW, Roccella EJ. Seventh report of the Joint National Committee on the Prevention, Detection, Evaluation, and Treatment of High Blood Pressure (JNC 7): resetting the hypertension sails. *Hypertension.* 2003;41(6):1178–9.

29. Lin KJ, Edelman, ER, Strichartz G, Lilly LS. Basic cardiac structure and function. In: Lilly LS, editor. *Pathophysiology of Heart Disease.* Baltimore (MD): Lippincott Williams & Wilkins; 2011. p. 1–27.

30. MacRae HS, Dennis SC, Bosch AN, Noakes TD. Effects of training on lactate production and removal during progressive exercise in humans. *J Appl Physiol.* 1992;72(5):1649–56.

31. Marieb EN, Hoehn KN. *Human Anatomy and Physiology.* 8th ed. San Francisco (CA): Benjamin-Cummings Publishing Company; 2009.

32. McArdle WD, Katch FI, Katch VL. *Exercise Physiology.* 8th ed. Baltimore (MD): Wolters Kluwer Health/Lippincott Williams & Williams; 2014. 1088 p.

33. Michna H, Hartmann G. Adaptation of tendon collagen to exercise. *Int Orthop.* 1989;13(3):161–5.

34. Mitchell JH, Blomqvist G. Maximal oxygen uptake. *N Engl J Med.* 1971;284(18):1018–22.

35. Moritani T. Motor unit and motoneurone excitability during explosive movement. In: Komi PV, editor. *Strength and Power in Sport.* 2nd ed. Oxford (United Kingdom): Blackwell Science; 2003. p. 27–49.

36. Naughton J, Haider R. Methods of exercise testing. In: Naughton JP, Hellerstein HK, Mohler IC, editors. *Exercise Testing and Exercise Training in Coronary Heart Disease.* New York (NY): Academic Press; 1973. p. 79.

37. Proske U, Morgan DL. Muscle damage from eccentric exercise: mechanism, mechanical signs, adaptation and clinical applications. *J Physiol.* 2001;537(Pt 2):333–45.

38. Saltin B, Gollnick PD. Skeletal muscle adaptability: significance for metabolism and performance. In: Peachey LD, Adrian RH, Geiger SR, editors. *Handbook of Physiology.* Bethesda (MD): American Physiological Society; 1983. p. 555–631.

39. Smeltzer SC, Bare BG, Hinkle JL, Cheever KH. *Brunner and Suddarth's Textbook of Medical-Surgical Nursing.* 12th ed. Philadelphia (PA): Lippincott Williams & Wilkins; 2010. 2240 p.

40. Stanish WD, Rubinovich RM, Curwin S. Eccentric exercise in chronic tendinitis. *Clin Orthop Relat Res.* 1986;208:65–8.

41. Sumida KD, Urdiales JH, Donovan CM. Enhanced gluconeogenesis from lactate in perfused livers after endurance training. *J Appl Physiol.* 1993;74(2):782–7.

42. Triplett NT. Structure and function of body systems. In: Haff GG, Triplett NT, editors. *Essentials of Strength and Conditioning.* 4th ed. Champaign (IL): Human Kinetics; 2016. p. 2–17.

43. U.S. Department of Health and Human Services. *Physical Activity Guidelines Advisory Committee Report, 2008.* Washington (DC): U.S. Department of Health and Human Services; 2008. 61 p.

44. Vrbová G. Influence of activity on some characteristic properties of slow and fast mammalian muscles. *Exerc Sport Sci Rev.* 1979;7(1):181–213.

45. Zernicke RF, Wohl GR, LaMonthe JM. The skeletal-articular system. In: Tipton CM, editor. *ACSM's Advanced Exercise Physiology.* Baltimore (MD): Lippincott Williams & Wilkins; 2009. p. 95–111.

# 6

# Nutrition and Human Performance

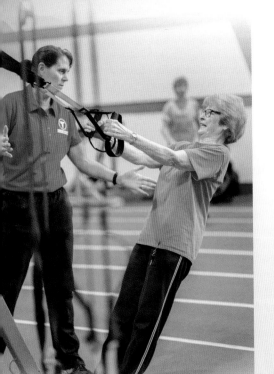

## OBJECTIVES

**Personal Trainers should be able to:**

- Understand the functions of the three energy substrates (carbohydrate, protein, and fat) in health and performance.

- Know the role of vitamins and minerals in health and performance.

- Understand the importance of hydration in maintaining health and achieving optimal performance.

- Know the essential elements of energy balance as related to weight management, body composition, and performance.

- Understand issues related to nutrient supplementation and strategies for discerning the circumstances under which specific supplements may be appropriate.

- Understand practical issues related to eating for performance, including travel, the precompetition meal, during-competition nourishment, and postcompetition replenishment.

## INTRODUCTION

Nutrition and athletic performance are closely linked, making it unlikely to experience success with a physical training program that has no integrated nutrition strategy. Personal Trainers who recommend the use of nutrition strategies to achieve an ideal weight or body composition should bear in mind the impact this strategy could have on physical performance and should consider that certain strategies may predispose clients to disease and injury.

An improvement in client conditioning cannot be realized by focusing only on time spent in training to improve flexibility, endurance, and/or power. The adjunct nutritional strategies clients should follow before arriving at the pool or gym, the foods and drinks they consume immediately following exercise and after they go home, and what they do to ensure an optimal flow of fluid and energy into their muscles are all critical to improving power and endurance, sustaining concentration, and optimizing performance. Failure to consider nutrition as an integral component of the skills training and/or conditioning program will increase health risks and result in poor performance-improvement rates. Well-nourished clients do better, recover more quickly from soreness and injuries, and derive more performance-improving benefits from long and strenuous training sessions. Therefore, Personal Trainers should help clients match the dynamics of exercise with a supportive nutrition strategy.

> Well-nourished clients do better, recover more quickly from soreness and injuries, and derive more performance-improving benefits from long and strenuous training sessions.

Scientific information exists on the relationship between good nutrition and exercise performance, but the massive quantities of misinformation on nutrition makes it difficult for Personal Trainers to know when and what to eat before practice and competition; the foods that will best sustain energy levels; the best drinks and foods to consume before, during, and after exercise; how to balance an optimal energy intake with an ideal body composition; and how to make certain that the intake of nutrients matches nutrient needs. These and other issues are covered in this chapter with the aim of helping the Personal Trainer assist their clients in understanding the key nutritional strategies that are related to improving exercise performance while sustaining good health.

## Scope of Practice

Personal Trainers should be aware that, in most states, the profession of dietetics is regulated by law. The practice of dietetics is typically performed by a Registered Dietitian who has the academic degree and proper certifications or licenses to provide clinically relevant individually specific meal plans or diet plans and to provide medical nutrition therapy for individuals suffering from specific diseases. The Personal Trainer must respect these professionals by always seeking out their assistance when governed by laws. Typically, Personal Trainers do not develop or provide meal/diet plans for clients, particularly when malignancy is involved, because this activity falls within the scope of practice for Registered Dietitians. Personal Trainers can, and should, recognize when it is appropriate to refer clients to a Registered Dietitian. Personal Trainers should locate Registered Dietitian(s) and establish a referral system or network.

**FIGURE 6.1.** Scope of practice.

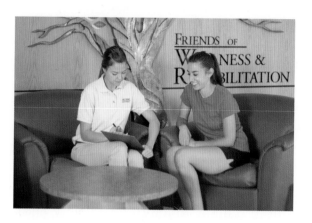

Typically, Personal Trainers do not develop or provide meal/diet plans for clients, particularly when malignancy is involved, because this activity falls within the scope of practice for Registered Dietitians.

Although laws typically have been written to protect the scope of practice for dietitians, the specific scope of practice for Personal Trainers regarding nutrition is not as clear. However, it appears that Personal Trainers can teach the fundamentals of nutrition to clients (as outlined in this chapter) and to also assist with a weight loss program that would include both calorically modified diets and exercise (Fig. 6.1). Personal Trainers should also be aware of, and be able to recognize, patterns of disordered eating and make the appropriate referral to a health care practitioner who has the experience necessary to treat these conditions. Personal Trainers are urged to investigate any and all laws pertaining to the practice of dietetics in their local area.

 ## Essential Nutritional Concepts

Nutrients give metabolically active tissues, including muscles, organs, and bones, the energy needed for work, tissue repair, and tissue development. Well-nourished clients have better disease resistance and enhanced cardiovascular function, are more likely to grow normally and build needed muscle and skeletal tissue, and will heal well if they are injured. For clients to be healthy and successful, they must consider nutritional needs as important as the skills/performance training.

### Nutrients

There are six classes of nutrients: carbohydrates, proteins, fats, vitamins, minerals, and water. Clients should not be taught to think of any individual nutrient as more important than any other nutrient; rather, the focus should be on nutrient balance, which is critical to good health and performance. With the help of a Personal Trainer, clients should try to find the appropriate balance between all the nutrients because too much or too little of any single nutrient increases the risk of poor health and/or performance problems. For example, too little iron intake could lead to poor endurance and a lower ability to burn fat, whereas too much protein might increase urine production and increase the risk of dehydration. The best strategy for maintaining a nutrient balance is to eat a wide variety of foods, regularly consume fresh fruits and vegetables, and avoid a monotonous intake of the same few foods day after day (Fig. 6.2). Consumption of a wide variety of foods will ensure optimal nutrient exposure. No single food has all the nutrients a person needs to stay healthy, so eating a wide variety of foods helps people know that all the needed nutrients are available to them. An added benefit of eating a wide variety of foods is avoidance of potential nutrient toxicities that may result from an excess consumption of potentially toxic food components. Easily available and inexpensive nutrient supplements dramatically increase

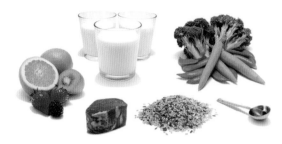

**FIGURE 6.2.** Nutrients that provide energy: oil, grains, legumes, meats, fruits, fruit juices, and vegetables. (Thomas DT, Erdman KA, Burke LM. American College of Sports Medicine joint position statement. Nutrition and athletic performance. *Med Sci Sports Exerc.* 2016;48[3]:543–68.)

the possibility of nutrient toxicities. The common belief that "if a little bit of a nutrient is good, and then more must be better" is wrong. Providing more nutrients than the body can use does not provide a benefit; it forces cells into using valuable energy resources to excrete the surplus, with the additional risk of developing toxicity reactions and/or nutrient insensitivities.

There is a great deal of nutritional misinformation on television and in popular magazines, making it difficult for people to make the right nutritional decisions. Many believe people (particularly celebrities) who sell nutritional supplements despite the lack of credible scientific evidence for what they're selling. Part of the problem is that the "placebo effect" is at play with nutrition (*i.e.,* if you believe that something will work, it will actually work despite the lack of biological reason for the result). Personal Trainers should ask for scientific evidence about whether nutritional products actually work, and when a claim is made, there should be immediate follow-up: "Show me the evidence." Scientific (peer-reviewed) journals are the best source of information. It should be clearly understood that one person's positive experience from taking a substance does not translate into a universal benefit. Claims that sound too good to be true probably are *not* true.

 There are six classes of nutrients: carbohydrates, proteins, fats, vitamins, minerals, and water.

## Nutrients that Provide Energy

Energy nutrients provide fuel for cellular work. Carbohydrates, proteins, and fats (Box 6.1) are considered energy nutrients because they all provide carbon (fuel), which can be "burned" for energy production. Energy nutrients allow us to do muscular work, transfer electrical energy between nerve cells, and help us maintain body temperature at 98.6° F (37° C). Energy is measured in calories, which, in nutrition, are often referred to as kilocalories (kcal) because they represent 1,000 times the calorie unit used in physics. In this chapter, the word "calories" is used synonymously with kilocalories (21).

Exercise results in an increase in the *rate* at which energy is burned. This process is not 100% efficient, so only 20%–40% of the burned energy is converted to mechanical energy, with at least

| Box 6.1 | **Recommended Energy (Calorie) Distribution for Athletes and Physically Active Adults** |
|---|---|

6–10 g (and up to 12 g for extreme and prolonged activities) carbohydrate per kilogram of body weight (45%–65% of total calories)

1.2–2.0 g protein per kilogram of body weight (10%–35% of total calories)

20%–35% of total calories from fat

Adapted from American College of Sports Medicine. Joint position statement: nutrition and athletic performance. American College of Sports Medicine, American Dietetic Association, and Dietitians of Canada. *Med Sci Sports Exer.* 2000;32(12):2130–2145, and American College of Sports Medicine. American College of Sports Medicine position stand. Nutrition and athletic performance. *Med Sci Sports Exer.* 2009;41(3):709–31.

60% of the energy lost as heat. This extra heat causes body temperature to rise, which requires an increase in the sweat rate as a means of cooling down body temperature. Therefore, the two essential components of sports nutrition that Personal Trainers should focus on are the following:

1. Finding ways to provide enough extra energy at the right time to satisfy the additional energy needs of physical activity
2. Finding ways to provide enough fluid at the right time to maintain body water and replace the fluid that was lost as sweat

## Meeting Energy Needs for Optimal Weight and Body Composition

The relationship between weight and energy (*i.e.*, caloric) intake is relatively simple: If a person gains (by eating) more energy than is expended, the excess energy is stored, and body weight will increase. Consumption of lesser energy than a person burns results in the utilization of some body tissues to satisfy the need of energy, and body weight will drop. Consistently, consuming too little energy will burn enough lean mass (muscles) that the *rate* at which calories are burned (called the "metabolic rate") will decrease. The result of a lower metabolic rate is usually higher body weight (from more body fat) because of a diminished ability to burn the energy that is consumed. Therefore, maintaining an energy-balanced state or deviating from it only slightly is an important strategy for both body weight and body composition maintenance (Fig. 6.3). Clients wishing to increase muscle mass should perform exercises needed to enlarge muscle mass and slightly increase (by 300–400 kcal) daily caloric intake. Clients wishing to decrease body fat should make only subtle decreases (no more than 300–400 kcal, depending on body size) in daily energy intake while maintaining a vigorous conditioning schedule to maintain muscle mass.

For athletic competitors, lower weight results in lower activity-related resistance, and all sports have resistance associated with them. Skaters must overcome the resistance of a skate blade going over the ice, cyclists must cope with air resistance, power lifters have the resistance from weights, and divers and gymnasts experience resistance as they tumble through the air. Sports performance is related to the ability of the athlete to overcome resistance (or drag) and the ability to sustain power output by overcoming this resistance on repeated bouts for long distances (19). Although these two factors (overcoming resistance and sustaining power output) are clearly related to performance, they are perceived by many athletes to be in conflict — a fact that causes many athletes problems with satisfying energy needs.

**FIGURE 6.3.** Meeting energy needs for optimal weight and body composition: fitness exercise class.

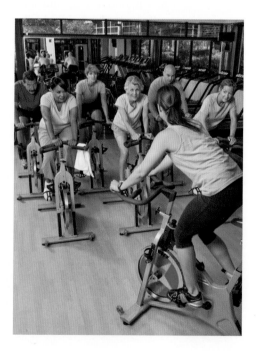

Consistently, consuming too little energy will burn enough of your lean mass (muscles) that the *rate* at which calories are burned (called the "metabolic rate") will decrease.

Athletes often view their ability to overcome resistance or drag with their ability to carry lots of muscle and relatively little fat. As fat mass does little to contribute to sports performance and may contribute to drag, this makes lots of sense. However, the *strategy* that athletes often adopt to reduce fat mass and maximize muscle mass is to follow a "diet" by dramatically lowering total energy intake. This dieting strategy is counterproductive because it restricts the intake of energy that is needed to sustain power output and may result in a lowering of muscle mass.

Herein lies the dilemma: How can clients maximize their ability to sustain power output while, at the same time, reduce body fat percentage? A number of studies suggest that the answer may lie in consuming small but frequent meals to stay in better energy balance throughout the day (12,17). Energy balance has typically been assessed in 24-hour units (12,17). That is, if a person consumes 3,000 kcal and burns 3,000 kcal during a day, he or she is in "energy balance." However, what happens *during* the day to achieve a state of energy balance makes a difference (12). If most of the day is spent in an energy-deficit state (*i.e.*, more calories are burned than consumed) but then huge meal is eaten at the end of the day to satisfy energy needs, a person still might be in energy balance at the end of the day. However, it appears that people who do this have different outcomes than those who maintain an energy-balanced state throughout the day. Eating small but frequent meals has the following benefits (6,11,13,15,17,18,20,21,24):

- Maintenance of metabolic rate
- Lower body fat and lower weight on higher caloric intakes
- Better glucose tolerance and lower insulin response (making it less likely that fats will be produced from the foods you eat)
- Lower stress hormone production
- Better maintenance of muscle mass
- Improved physical performance

Surveys have suggested that people (particularly athletes) tend to delay eating until the end of the day, and many experience severe energy deficits earlier in the day (particularly on days when they train hard and need the energy the most!). Problems with energy deficits include the following (6,8):

- Difficulty maintaining carbohydrate stores (this would impede endurance in high-intensity activities)
- Problems maintaining lean (muscle) mass
- Lower metabolic rate
- Difficulty meeting nutrient needs (foods carry both energy *and* other nutrients)
- Increased risk of injury (undernourished athletes may develop mental and muscular fatigue that, in some sports, would predispose them to injury)
- Missed opportunities to aid muscle recovery

Maintaining energy balance throughout the day by consuming small but frequent meals *during* the day is an excellent strategy for minimizing these problems.

## Carbohydrate

The word *carbohydrate* is often referred to if it is a single compound. In fact, carbohydrates come in many different forms that have different nutritional outcomes. Some carbohydrates are digestible, whereas others are not; some are considered "complex," whereas others are "simple"; and some carbohydrates contain soluble fiber, whereas others contain insoluble fiber (Fig. 6.4). The basic form of carbohydrate energy for human nutrition is the simple sugar glucose, and our bodies make a complex carbohydrate called glycogen, which is the storage form of glucose (Tables 6.1–6.3). Carbohydrate recommendations range from 3 to 12 g per kilogram body weight with the amount dependent on the total daily expenditure, sex, activity, and environmental conditions (1).

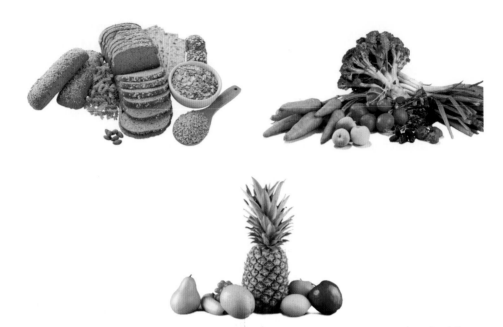

**FIGURE 6.4.** Carbohydrate foods — fruits, vegetables, grains (cereals, pasta, etc.), and potatoes.

| Table 6.1 | Quick Facts about Carbohydrates |
|---|---|
| Minimum intake | 50–100 g · d$^{-1}$ (200–400 kcal) needed to avoid ketosis |
| Average U.S. intake | 200–300 g · d$^{-1}$ (800–1,200 kcal) |
| Recommended fiber intake | 20–30 g · d$^{-1}$ or more |
| Average U.S. fiber intake | 10–15 g · d$^{-1}$ |
| Recommended intake of carbohydrate as percentage of total caloric intake | 55% of total calories; up to 65% of total calories for athletes |
| Good sources of carbohydrate | Grains, legumes, seeds, pasta, fruits, vegetables, etc. |

| Table 6.2 | Examples of Good High-Carbohydrate Snacks | |
|---|---|---|
| Apple | Fruit cup | Orange juice |
| Bagel | Fruit smoothie | Popcorn |
| Baked corn chips | Energy bar | Rice |
| Baked potato | Grapes | Saltine crackers |
| Banana | Mashed potatoes | Spaghetti |
| Beans | Mixed berries | Whole-wheat toast |
| English muffin | Oatmeal | |

| Table 6.3 | Common High-Carbohydrate Foods | |
|---|---|---|
| **Food** | **Calories from Carbohydrate (%)** | **Total Calories** |
| Sugar (1 tbsp) | 100 | 48 |
| Pretzel sticks (10 small) | 100 | 8 |
| Maple syrup (1 tbsp) | 100 | 64 |
| Cranberry juice (1 cup) | 100 | 152 |
| Cola, regular (12 oz) | 100 | 164 |
| Apples (1 med) | 100 | 84 |
| Apricot juice (1 cup) | 97 | 148 |
| Sugar frosted flakes cereal (1 oz) | 96 | 108 |
| Raisins (1 cup) | 94 | 489 |
| Orange (1 raw) | 94 | 64 |
| Rice, white (1 cup) | 93 | 216 |
| Orange juice (1 cup) | 93 | 112 |
| Sweet potatoes (1 med) | 93 | 120 |
| Corn flakes cereal (1 oz) | 92 | 104 |
| Potato, baked (1 med) | 91 | 224 |
| Banana (1 raw) | 89 | 121 |
| Carrots (1 raw) | 88 | 32 |
| Potato, mashed with milk (1 cup) | 86 | 173 |
| Tomato sauce (1 cup) | 86 | 84 |
| Cantaloupe (1/2 melon) | 84 | 105 |
| Tomato (1 raw) | 83 | 24 |
| Green beans (1 cup) | 83 | 48 |
| Spaghetti (1 cup cooked) | 82 | 157 |
| Yogurt, low-fat fruit flavored (8 oz) | 75 | 230 |
| Bread, wheat (1 slice) | 74 | 65 |
| Bread, oatmeal (1 slice) | 74 | 65 |
| Beans (1 cup) | 70 | 217 |
| Broccoli (1 spear) | 58 | 69 |

Adapted from U.S. Department of Agriculture, Nutrient Data Laboratory, Agricultural Research Service. *USDA National Nutrient Database for Standard Reference Release 28*. Washington, DC: Government Printing Office; 2015.

## Functions of Carbohydrate

Carbohydrates have a number of functions in the body, including the following:

- *Providing energy* ($4 \text{ kcal} \cdot \text{g}^{-1}$). Carbohydrate is the preferred fuel for the body, and it is a quick energy source.
- *Protein sparing.* This is an often-overlooked, yet very important, function of carbohydrates. Because carbohydrate (glucose) is a preferred fuel, providing enough carbohydrate to meet most energy needs preserves (*i.e.,* "spares") protein from being broken down and used as a source of energy.
- *Oxidation of fat.* It has been said that "fats burn in a carbohydrate flame." That is, to burn fats efficiently and completely, some carbohydrates are needed.
- *Acting as a part of other compounds.* Carbohydrates are essential components of other compounds essential in human nutrition.
- *Storing energy.* Carbohydrate is stored as glycogen, which is an excellent storage form because it can be easily converted back to glucose and used for energy.

## Types of Carbohydrate

Carbohydrates come in a number of forms:

- *Simple carbohydrates (sugars).* These are sugars such as glucose, fructose (typically found in fruits and vegetables), galactose (one of the sugars in milk), sucrose (table sugar), lactose (milk sugar), and maltose (grain sugar).
- *Polysaccharides.* These are carbohydrates that contain many molecules of connected sugars. Polysaccharides can be digestible (starch, dextrins, and glycogen) or indigestible (cellulose, hemicellulose, pectin, gums, and mucilages). Dietary fiber is a carbohydrate that cannot be digested but is useful in the diet because it may lower fat and cholesterol absorption, improves blood sugar control, and may reduce the risk of colon cancer and heart disease.

Should the focus of a client's diet be carbohydrate, protein, or fat? Many studies show that *carbohydrates are the limiting energy substrate.* That is, when carbohydrates run out, people typically reach a point of exhaustion. For this reason, people should consume carbohydrates 3–12 g per kilogram of body weight per day, depending on the desired intensity and duration of the exercise (1). Please note that the distribution of carbohydrate, protein, and fat was previously expressed as a percent of total calories (*e.g.,* 60% of total calories from carbohydrate was the common recommendation). However, because high energy intakes can easily satisfy carbohydrate needs at a significantly lower proportion of total calories, it is now recommended that energy substrate distribution be expressed in grams per kilogram. Because the body's storage capacity for carbohydrates is relatively limited, carbohydrates should be provided throughout the day in small, frequent meals. A key reason for the small/frequent meal recommendation is to sustain blood sugar (glucose), which is the primary fuel for the central nervous system (brain). If the brain receives insufficient glucose, mental fatigue will result, and mental fatigue leads to muscle fatigue. Blood glucose level reaches its peak approximately 1 hour after a meal and is back to premeal levels about 2 hours after (2). This strongly suggests that meal frequency should be approximately every 3 hours to avoid the mental and muscle fatigue that could result from low blood sugar level. To be more specific regarding carbohydrate consumption per body weight, a 75-kg (165-lb) person would need to consume between 225 g (900 kcal) and 900 g (3,600 kcal) per day from carbohydrate alone. Ultimately, the amount of carbohydrate needed is associated with the intensity and duration of physical activity, gender, and the environmental conditions (cold, humid, hot, etc.) (1).

Different activities have different carbohydrate requirements per unit of time. For instance, when walking at a brisk pace, 17% of the fuel comes from carbohydrate; when jogging at a medium pace, approximately 50% of the fuel comes from carbohydrate; and when running at a very fast

By consuming a high-carbohydrate diet and carbohydrate-containing sports beverages, a client can improve energy reserves and enhance performance of repeated bouts of high-intensity activity.

pace, approximately 72% of the fuel comes from carbohydrate (24). However, because the length of time spent in these activities is usually much different (you can walk at a brisk pace much longer than you can run flat out), the total carbohydrate requirement may be similar when calculated over the total time invested in the activity.

A single 30-second bout of high-intensity activity could reduce muscle carbohydrate (glycogen) storage by more than 25%. By consuming a high-carbohydrate diet and carbohydrate-containing sports beverages, a client can improve energy reserves and enhance performance of repeated bouts of high-intensity activity.

### The Glycemic Index

The glycemic index is a measure of how different consumed carbohydrate foods affect the blood sugar level. Foods are compared with the ingestion of glucose, which has an index value of 100. Foods with a lower glycemic index help maintain blood sugar, avoid an excessive insulin response that can encourage the production of fat, and keep people feeling better longer (25). Although the glycemic index (Table 6.4) is a useful guide, Personal Trainers should be aware that

| Table 6.4 | High, Medium, and Low Glycemic Index Foods | |
|---|---|---|
| **High Glycemic Index (>85)** | **Medium Glycemic Index (60–85)** | **Low Glycemic Index (<60)** |
| Glucose | All-bran cereal | Fructose |
| Sucrose | Banana | Apple |
| Maple syrup | Grapes | Applesauce |
| Corn syrup | Oatmeal | Cherries |
| Honey | Orange juice | Kidney beans |
| Bagel | Pasta | Navy beans |
| Candy | Rice | Chick-peas |
| Corn flakes | Whole grain rye bread | Lentils |
| Carrots | Yams | Dates |
| Crackers | Corn | Figs |
| Molasses | Baked beans | Peaches |
| Potatoes | Potato chips | Plums |
| Raisins | | Ice cream |
| White bread | | Milk |
| Whole wheat bread | | Yogurt |
| Sodas (nondiet) | | Tomato soup |
| Sports drinks | | |

Adapted from Rankin JW. *Glycemic Index and Exercise Metabolism*. Barrington (IL): Gatorade Sports Science Institute, Sports Science Exchange, Publication no. 64; 1997:10(1).

| Table 6.5 | Quick Facts for Protein |
|---|---|
| Recommended intakes | Infants: 2.2 g · kg$^{-1}$ of body weight<br>Children: 1.0–1.6 g · kg$^{-1}$ of body weight<br>Adults: 0.8 g · kg$^{-1}$ of body weight<br>Adult athletes: 1.2–1.7 g · kg$^{-1}$ of body weight (17) |
| Recommended intake of protein | 10%–35% of total calories |
| Good sources of protein | Meat, poultry, fish, yogurt, eggs, milk; combinations of legumes (beans and dried peas) with cereal grains |

Foods with a lower glycemic index help maintain blood sugar, avoid an excessive insulin response that can encourage the production of fat, and keep people feeling better longer.

different people have different responses to food. For instance, people who exercise regularly are much more tolerant of foods with a high glycemic index than are people who rarely exercise (23). Young people must meet the combined energy needs of growth, exercise, and tissue maintenance and so will have a higher requirement for calories per unit of body weight (and therefore carbohydrate) than will adult athletes. Athletes interested in lowering either weight or body fat levels should consider focusing on foods with a medium to low glycemic index.

## Protein

Proteins are complex compounds that consist of different connected amino acids, which uniquely contain nitrogen. Proteins in the body are constantly changing, with new proteins being made and old ones broken down. Growth hormone, androgen, insulin, and thyroid hormone are anabolic hormones (i.e., they cause new protein to be produced). Cortisone, hydrocortisone, and thyroxin are catabolic hormones (i.e., they influence the breakdown of proteins).

The protein requirement for physically active people is about double that for nonathletes (Table 6.5). The nonathlete (average) adult's requirement for protein is 0.8 g per kilogram of body weight, whereas the adult athlete requirement for protein ranges between 1.2 and 1.7 g per kilogram of body weight. An athlete who weighs 180 lb (about 82 kg) would require between 98 and 140 g of protein per day (22). At 4 kcal · g$^{-1}$, this is between 492 and 656 kcal from protein per day (Fig. 6.5). Most athletes far exceed this amount of protein just from the

**FIGURE 6.5.** Protein foods — meats, poultry, dairy (cheese, milk, yogurt), and legumes.

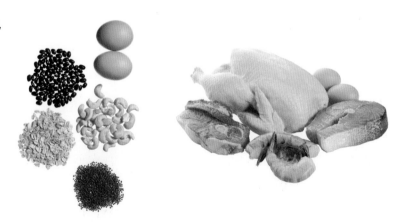

| Table 6.6 | Examples of Good High-Protein Snacks | |
|---|---|---|
| Cheese | | Tuna sandwich |
| Chicken | | Hamburger |
| Cooked beef, lamb, or pork strips | | Soy burger |
| Milk | | Cottage cheese |
| Yogurt | | Turkey sandwich |

foods they consume. Consider that the protein in a hamburger, a chicken fillet sandwich, and one cup of milk combined provides more than half the total daily protein requirement for a 180-lb (82-kg) athlete (Table 6.6). A total energy intake sufficient to allow the anabolic utilization of protein, and not burned to satisfy the energy requirement, is needed to sustain optimal performance (1).

### Functions of Protein

Proteins have a number of functions in the body, including the following:

- *Enzyme and protein synthesis.* There are hundreds of unique tissues and enzymes that are proteins.
- *Transportation of nutrients to the right places.* Proteins make "smart" carriers, enabling nutrients to go to the right tissues.
- *A source of energy.* The carbon in protein provides the same amount of energy per unit of weight as carbohydrates ($4 \text{ kcal} \cdot \text{g}^{-1}$).
- *Hormone production.* Hormones control many chemical activities in the body, and these are made of unique proteins. For instance, testosterone (male hormone) is an important tissue-building hormone.
- *Fluid balance.* Protein helps control the fluid balance between the blood and surrounding tissues. This helps people maintain blood volume and sweat rates during physical activity.
- *Acid–base balance.* Proteins can make an acidic environment less acidic and an alkaline environment less alkaline. High-intensity activity can increase cellular acidity (through lactate buildup), which protein can help buffer.
- *Growth and tissue maintenance.* Protein is needed to build and maintain tissue. This is one reason why the protein requirement for growing children can be double that of adults and slightly higher for athletes (27).
- *Synthesis of nonprotein, nitrogen-containing compounds.* Phosphocreatine is a high-energy, nitrogen-containing compound that can quickly release energy over a short duration for quick-burst activities (Box 6.2).

### Box 6.2    Supplementation with Creatine Monohydrate

Research has shown that creatine monohydrate supplementation may improve performance in repeated high-intensity activities, particularly in athletes with marginal caloric intakes. However, the data on the safety of creatine monohydrate supplementation is incomplete and not clear. A safer strategy would be to ensure that people have adequate calorie and protein intakes.

## Protein Quality

Protein quality is determined by the presence (or absence) of essential amino acids and their distribution. It is "essential" to take in these amino acids from food because the body is not capable of manufacturing them. Examples of foods containing protein with all the essential amino acids in a desirable ratio include meats, eggs, milk, cheese, and fish. Nonessential amino acids can be manufactured (synthesized) in the body, so it is not "essential" to consume foods that contain them. Most foods contain both nonessential and essential amino acids, but it is the presence of a comprehensive set of essential amino acids that makes a high-quality protein.

People frequently take protein supplements, but these may contain proteins with an incomplete set of essential amino acids, making the supplements low in quality and, even if they do deliver a high-quality protein, they tend to be expensive. The best protein supplement would be a few pieces of steak or fish or an egg. Vegetarians can ensure optimal protein quality by combining cereal grains (rice, wheat, and oats) with legumes (dried beans or peas). Vegetarians are clearly at more risk for inadequate protein intake because the best source of high-quality protein is foods of animal origin (*i.e.*, meat and fish). However, with some good dietary planning, vegetarians can consume enough high-quality protein.

> Most foods contain both nonessential and essential amino acids, but it is the presence of a comprehensive set of essential amino acids that makes a high-quality protein.

Protein is the focus of many diets (Table 6.7), but there is a tendency to consume too much of it (10). Studies have found that people do best with protein intakes that supply approximately 1.2–2.0 g of protein per kilogram of body weight. For a 75-kg (165-lb) person, that amounts to no more than

| Table 6.7 | Foods High in Protein | |
|---|---|---|
| Food | Calories from Protein (%) | Total Calories |
| Tuna, canned in water (3 oz) | 93 | 129 |
| Shrimp, canned (3 oz) | 87 | 97 |
| Chicken, roasted, breast (3 oz) | 80 | 185 |
| Turkey, roasted light meat (3 oz) | 79 | 127 |
| Crab meat, canned (1 cup) | 75 | 123 |
| Chicken, roasted, drumstick (1.6 oz) | 73 | 66 |
| Clams, raw (3 oz) | 72 | 61 |
| Salmon, baked (3 oz) | 65 | 129 |
| Turkey, roasted dark meat (3 oz) | 64 | 150 |
| Beef steak, broiled (5 oz) | 62 | 284 |
| Halibut, broiled, with butter (3 oz) | 60 | 134 |
| Lamb, leg, roasted, lean (2.6 oz) | 60 | 134 |
| Salmon, canned (3 oz) | 60 | 113 |
| Pork, roasted (5 oz) | 53 | 304 |
| Cheese, cheddar (1 oz) | 26 | 109 |
| Peanut butter (1 tbsp) | 19 | 104 |

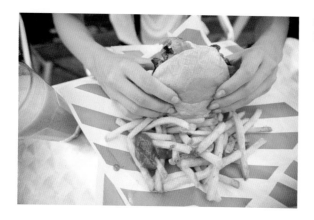

**FIGURE 6.6.** Fat foods — oil, butter, margarine, bacon, and fried foods.

150 g (600 kcal) of protein per day (1). Athletes doing intense endurance training or strength-trained athletes may require protein at the upper range of the recommended intake level (1.4–2.0 g · kg$^{-1}$).

Although protein isn't the best fuel for physical activity, it is a fuel that can help satisfy energy needs if other fuels (*i.e.*, carbohydrate and fat) are inadequate. During an energy restriction, where energy availability is limited, protein in excess of the Recommended Dietary Allowance (RDA) (but below the safe upper limit) may help to support the maintenance of lean mass by providing a source of energy. However, under such energy restrictions, it should be understood that the primary use of protein will be to support the need for energy rather than to sustain or increase the lean mass. There is no question that energy needs must be satisfied before considering the best way to distribute carbohydrate, protein, and fat.

## Fat

Many people misconceive that higher fat intakes can enhance athletic performance. The generally accepted healthy range of fat intake for physically active people is between 20% and 35% of total daily calories (Fig. 6.6). For someone consuming 2,500 kcal per day, this amounts to no more than 875 kcal per day as fat (about 97 g of fat). Although this is considered the accepted healthy limit, people typically will do better with fat intakes that are no higher than 25% of daily calories. This level of intake will provide more room in the diet for needed carbohydrates (Tables 6.8 and 6.9).

The generally accepted healthy limit for fat intake is no more than 30% of total daily calories.

| Table 6.8 | Fats |
|---|---|
| Recommended intakes | Fat intake should provide between 20% and 35% of total calories. |
| Essential fatty acid | Linoleic acid (and α-linoleic acid) is the essential fatty acid and must be provided in consumed foods; this fatty acid is found in corn, sunflower, peanut, and soy oils. |
| Carrier of vitamins | Fat is the carrier of the fat-soluble vitamins: vitamins A, D, E, and K. |
| Calorie-dense nutrient | Fats provide more than twice the calories, per equal weight, of carbohydrate and protein (9 vs. 4 kcal · g$^{-1}$). |
| Cholesterol–fat relationship | High fat intakes (in particular saturated fats) are the main culprit for increasing circulating blood cholesterol levels. |
| Food sources | Oil, butter, margarine, fatty meats, fried foods, prepared meats (sausage, bacon, salami), and "whole-milk" dairy products |

| Table 6.9 | Percent Fat Calories from Common Foods | |
|---|---|---|
| **Food** | **Calories from Fat (%)** | **Total Calories** |
| Butter (1 tbsp) | 100 | 99 |
| Margarine (1 tbsp) | 100 | 99 |
| Mayonnaise (1 tbsp) | 100 | 99 |
| Corn oil (1 tbsp) | 100 | 126 |
| Vegetable shortening (1 tbsp) | 100 | 117 |
| Olive oil (1 tbsp) | 100 | 126 |
| Blue cheese salad dressing (1 tbsp) | 90 | 80 |
| Cream cheese (1 oz) | 88 | 102 |
| 1,000 island salad dressing (1 tbsp) | 87 | 62 |
| Sour cream (1 tbsp) | 87 | 31 |
| Sausage, Brown 'N Serve (1 link) | 85 | 53 |
| Brazil nuts (1 oz) | 84 | 203 |
| Hazelnuts (1 cup) | 83 | 780 |
| Hotdog (1) | 83 | 141 |
| Cream, Half & Half (1 tbsp) | 82 | 22 |
| Bologna (2 slices) | 80 | 180 |
| Coconut, raw, shredded (1 cup) | 80 | 303 |
| Almonds, whole (1 oz) | 74 | 183 |
| Cheddar cheese (1 oz) | 74 | 109 |
| Feta cheese (1 oz) | 73 | 74 |
| Blue cheese (1 oz) | 72 | 100 |
| Avocado (1 whole) | 65 | 371 |
| Donuts, plain (1) | 50 | 216 |
| Milk, whole (1 cup) | 49 | 148 |
| Chicken, fried breast (1 breast) | 46 | 354 |
| Milk, 2% (1 cup) | 36 | 125 |
| Milk, 1% (1 cup) | 25 | 107 |

### Functions of Fat

Fat has a number of important functions in the body:

- *Fat is a source of energy.* Fat provides 9 kcal · g$^{-1}$ (compared with 4 kcal · g$^{-1}$ from both carbohydrates and proteins).
- *Fat provides insulation from extreme temperatures.*
- *Cushion against concussive forces.* Fat protects organs against sudden concussive forces, such as a fall or a solid "hit" in football.
- *Satiety control.* Fat, because it stays in the stomach longer than other energy nutrients, makes people feel fuller longer.
- *Fat gives food flavor.*
- *Fat carries essential nutrients.* Make sure that your clients get the necessary fat-soluble vitamins (A, D, E, and K) and essential fatty acids, which are found in vegetable and cereal oils.

### Classifications and Definitions of Fat

- *Fats and oils.* Fats are solid at room temperature and usually contain a high proportion of saturated fatty acids; oils are liquid at room temperature and typically (there are notable exceptions) contain a high proportion of unsaturated fatty acids.
- *Triglycerides, diglycerides, and monoglycerides.* Triglycerides are the most common form of dietary fats and oils, whereas diglycerides and monoglycerides are less prevalent but still commonly present in the food supply.
- *Short-chain, medium-chain, and long-chain fatty acids.* The most common dietary fatty acids are long-chain, containing 14 or more carbon atoms. Medium-chain triglycerides (MCT oil), containing 8–12 carbon atoms, have received some attention recently as an effective supplement for increasing caloric intake in athletes. Although MCT oil may hold some promise in this area, it has not been adequately tested. Short-chain fatty acids contain six carbon atoms or less.
- *Polyunsaturated fatty acids.* These fatty acids have a tendency to lower blood cholesterol level. The good thing about these fats is that they are typically associated with lots of vitamin E (found in vegetable and cereal oil, such as corn oil), which many people need.
- *Monounsaturated fatty acids.* These fatty acids tend to lower blood cholesterol level while maintaining high-density lipoprotein (good) cholesterol (found in olive oil and canola oil).
- *Saturated fatty acids.* These fatty acids tend to increase serum cholesterol (found in meats and dairy products).
- *Low-density lipoproteins.* This is the major carrier of cholesterol and other lipids in the blood.
- *High-density lipoproteins.* These lipoproteins carry lipids away from storage and to the liver for metabolism and/or excretion. Because they are associated with removal of cholesterol, they are considered "good cholesterol."

For a 75-kg (165-lb) person consuming a 3,000-kcal diet, approximately 750 kcal would come from fat if fat contributed about 25% of total calories. Because fats provide 9 kcal · g$^{-1}$, this amounts to between approximately 83 g of fat per day. There has been a great deal of attention given to high-fat, high-protein, low-carbohydrate diets recently, but there is no evidence that these diets are useful for enhancing athletic performance (1). One such popular diet is the "Zone" diet. Cheuvront (10) described the Zone as a low-carbohydrate diet (in both relative and absolute terms). For instance, a male marathoner weighing 64 kg with 7.5% body fat would, following the Zone, have a 1,734-kcal intake, whereas his predicted caloric requirement is more than 3,200 kcal. This is a calorically deficient diet by any standard. It is, therefore, quite true that people on the Zone would lose weight because it is an energy-deficient intake. However, your clients must meet energy requirements to sustain power output, so any severely energy-deficient diet, such as the Zone (whether it is high fat, high protein, or high carbohydrate), is not recommended for optimizing athletic performance.

## Vitamins and Minerals

Vitamins are substances that help essential body reactions take place. The best strategy to make certain that an adequate amount of all the vitamins is consumed is to eat a wide variety of foods and consume plenty of fresh fruits and vegetables daily. Some vitamins are water-soluble, whereas others are fat-soluble. See Tables 6.10 through 6.12 for a summary of major vitamins and minerals. Remember that nutrient balance is a key to optimal nutrition, so people should avoid single-nutrient supplementation unless this has been specifically recommended by a physician to treat an existing nutrient deficiency disease (7). If a nutrient supplement is warranted because of an obviously poor-quality food intake, people should try a multivitamin, multimineral supplement that provides no more than 100% of the Dietary Reference Intakes (DRI) for each nutrient. The scientific literature suggests that vitamin and mineral deficiencies are uncommon for most people. When deficiencies exist, they are most likely for vitamin $B_6$ and other B-complex vitamins, iron, and calcium, especially when caloric intake is too low to meet energy demands (5).

> The best strategy to make certain that an adequate amount of all the vitamins is consumed is to eat a wide variety of foods and consume plenty of fresh fruits and vegetables daily.

| Table 6.10 | Water-Soluble Vitamins | | |
|---|---|---|---|
| **Vitamin and Adult Requirement** | **Functions** | **Deficiency/Toxicity** | **Food Sources** |
| Vitamin C (also called L-ascorbate) 75–90 mg · $d^{-1}$ | ■ Antioxidant ■ Collagen formation ■ Iron absorption ■ Carnitine synthesis ■ Norepinephrine synthesis Athletic performance: conflicting study results; as antioxidant, may be useful in alleviating muscle soreness and in aiding muscle recovery | Deficiency: scurvy, bleeding gums, fatigue, muscle pain, easy bruising, depression, sudden death | Fresh fruits and vegetables, particularly high in citrus fruits and cherries |
| Thiamin (also called vitamin $B_1$) 1.1–1.2 mg · $d^{-1}$ | ■ Oxidation of carbohydrates ■ Nerve conduction Athletic performance: conflicting study results | Deficiency: beriberi (heart disease, weight loss, neurological failure) | Seeds, legumes, pork, and enriched/fortified grains and cereals |
| Riboflavin (also called vitamin $B_2$) 1.1–1.3 mg · $d^{-1}$ | ■ Oxidation of carbohydrates and fats ■ Normal eye function ■ Healthy skin Athletic performance: low-level supplement may be desirable for athletes involved in low-intensity, high-endurance sports | Deficiency: swollen tongue, sensitivity to light, cracked lips, fatigue | Milk, liver, and whole and enriched grains and cereals |
| Niacin 14–16 mg · $d^{-1}$ | ■ Oxidation of carbohydrates and fats ■ Electron transport (energy reactions) Athletic performance: conflicting study results | Deficiency: pellagra (diarrhea, dermatitis, dementia) | Amino acid tryptophan (60:1 conversion ratio), and enriched grains and cereals |

| Table 6.11 | Fat-Soluble Vitamins | | |
| --- | --- | --- | --- |
| **Vitamin and Adult Requirement** | **Functions** | **Deficiency/Toxicity** | **Food Sources** |
| Vitamin A (retinol) ~1,000 retinol equivalents 700–900 mg · d$^{-1}$ (This vitamin is potentially highly toxic if taken in large amounts.) | ■ Vision<br>■ Growth<br>■ Reproduction<br>■ Immune function<br>■ Healthy skin<br>Athletic performance: no evidence that supplementation aids performance | Deficiency: night blindness, eye disease, growth failure, unhealthy skin, susceptibility to infections<br>Toxicity: headache, vomiting, hair loss, bone abnormalities, liver damage, death | Fish liver oils, liver, butter, vitamin A + D– added milk, egg yolk Pro-vitamin A (β-carotene) in dark-green leafy vegetables yellow vegetables and fruits, and fortified margarines |
| Vitamin D (ergocalciferol and cholecalciferol) Requirement difficult to establish because of variations in sunlight exposure 5 mg · d$^{-1}$ (This vitamin is extremely toxic taken in high amounts.) | ■ Calcium absorption<br>■ Phosphorus absorption<br>■ Mineralization of bone<br>Athletic performance: no studies | Deficiency: rickets in children, osteomalacia in adults, poor bone mineralization<br>Toxicity (this is the most toxic of the vitamins): renal damage, cardiovascular damage, high blood calcium, calcium deposits in soft tissues | Fish liver oils, fortified (A and D) milk, skin synthesis with exposure to light; small amounts found in butter, liver, egg yolk, and canned salmon and sardines |
| Vitamin E (α-tocopherol) 15 mg · d$^{-1}$ | ■ Powerful antioxidant<br>■ Involved in immune function<br>Athletic performance: antioxidant properties may be useful in preventing oxidative damage | Deficiency: premature breakdown of red blood cells, anemia in infants, easy peroxidative damage of cells | Vegetable oils, green leafy vegetables, nuts, legumes (foods of animal origin are *not* good sources) and/or in muscle recovery |
| Vitamin K (phylloquinone K$_1$, menaquinone, menadione) 90–120 mg · d$^{-1}$ | Involved in blood clotting (referred to as the antihemorrhagic vitamin) | Deficiency: longer clotting time | Green leafy vegetables and intestinal bacterial synthesis |

Adapted from Manore M, Thompson J. *Sports Nutrition for Health and Performance*. Champaign (IL): Human Kinetics; 2000; Williams MH. *Nutrition for Health, Fitness & Sport*. 6th ed. Boston (MA): McGraw-Hill; 2002; and Benardot D. *Nutrition for Serious Athletes: An Advanced Guide to Foods, Fluids, and Supplements for Training and Performance*. Champaign (IL): Human Kinetics; 2000.

## Water-Soluble Vitamins

Water-soluble vitamins, which include vitamins B and C, are vitamins for which the body has limited storage capacity. These vitamins are typically associated with carbohydrate foods, such as fresh fruits, breads and cereals, and vegetables. The B vitamins are needed for the metabolism of carbohydrates, proteins, and fats and so are critical to the higher energy requirements of athletes (4). Luckily, good-quality foods that are high in carbohydrates are typically also foods that provide B vitamins (*e.g.*, enriched breads, enriched cereals, and pasta) (4).

| Table 6.12 | Minerals | | |
|---|---|---|---|
| **Minerals and Adult Requirement** | **Functions** | **Deficiency/Toxicity** | **Food Sources** |
| Calcium 1,500 mg · d$^{-1}$ | ▪ Structure of bones and teeth<br>▪ Blood coagulation<br>▪ Nerve impulse transmission<br>▪ Muscle contraction<br>▪ Acid–base control<br>Athletic performance: particularly critical in athletes to ensure adequate bone density to reduce the risk of stress fractures | Deficiency: reduced bone density, osteoporosis, stress fractures | Milk and other dairy foods, dark green leafy vegetables, canned fish (with bones), calcium-fortified orange juice |
| Phosphorus 700 mg · d$^{-1}$ | ▪ Structure of bones and teeth<br>▪ Component of adenosine tri-phosphate (ATP) and other energy-yielding compounds<br>▪ Part of many vitamin B coenzymes<br>▪ Part of DNA and RNA<br>▪ Acid–base control | Deficiency (rare) may occur with large, long-term intakes of magnesium-containing antacids | Meats, cereals, grains, and dairy products |
| Iron 8 mg · d$^{-1}$ (with 18 mg · d$^{-1}$ for women between 19 and 50 yr of age) | ▪ Involved in oxygen trans-fer to cells (hemoglobin in blood; myoglobin in muscle)<br>▪ In numerous oxidative enzymes<br>Athletic performance: commonly inadequate in athletes, resulting in poor performance and other health problems | Deficiency: microcytic anemia, leading to weakness, loss of energy, easy fatigue (This is the most common mineral deficiency.) | Most absorbable iron: meats, poultry, fish, egg yolk<br>Less absorbable iron: dark-green vegetables, legumes, peaches, apricots, prunes, raisins |
| Zinc 8–11 mg · d$^{-1}$ | ▪ Immune system<br>▪ Wound healing<br>▪ In more than 70 enzymes in-volved in energy metabolism | Deficiency: growth retardation, poor wound healing, frequent infections, muscle weakness | Seafood, organ meat, meat, wheat germ, yeast (Most plant foods are not good sources.) |
| Magnesium 320–420 mg · d$^{-1}$ | ▪ Energy metabolism of carbo-hydrate and fat<br>▪ Protein synthesis<br>▪ Water balance<br>▪ Muscle contractions | Deficiency: muscle weakness | Available in many foods, but highest in meats, whole-grain cereals, seeds, and legumes |

Adapted from Manore M, Thompson J. *Sports Nutrition for Health and Performance*. Champaign (IL): Human Kinetics; 2000; Williams MH. *Nutrition for Health, Fitness & Sport*. 6th ed. Boston (MA): McGraw-Hill; 2002; and Benardot D. *Nutrition for Serious Athletes: An Advanced Guide to Foods, Fluids, and Supplements for Training and Performance*. Champaign (IL): Human Kinetics; 2000.

Vitamin C is a water-soluble vitamin that is often the focus of supplements taken by most people. Although vitamin C is critical to good health, people should be reminded that the DRI for vitamin C is only 75–90 mg and that level is 2 standard deviations above the average human requirement. Most supplements contain between 250 and 500 mg of vitamin C or more, providing a good deal more than is needed. On top of the vitamin C intake from foods, which is typically well above the DRI for this vitamin, supplementation makes it easy for people to get too much. Although the potential toxicity of vitamin C is relatively low, even an excess of this relatively nontoxic vitamin can increase the risk of kidney stones. People should be encouraged to have a balanced exposure to all the vitamins, a strategy that will help encourage good health and avoid problems associated with excess intake and deficiencies.

### Fat-Soluble Vitamins

Fat-soluble vitamins are those vitamins that are delivered with fats and oils. For instance, milk is fortified with the fat-soluble vitamins A and D, which are in the fat component (cream) of the milk. Vegetable and cereal oils are excellent sources of vitamin E, an important antioxidant that can help protect cells from becoming damaged through oxidation. This is important because physical activity increases the amount of oxygen pulled into cells, thereby increasing the risk for oxidative damage.

Supplements of vitamins A and D should be taken only under the advice of a physician because of their high potential toxicity. Other vitamins such as vitamin $B_6$ have also been shown to produce toxicity if taken in excess. As a general rule, it is generally better to derive vitamins through the consumption of a wide variety of foods rather than supplements, as supplementation may more easily result in toxicity and may also give individuals the wrong impression that a good quality diet is unnecessary because supplements are consumed.

## Minerals

Minerals are inorganic substances that are involved in water balance, nerve impulse stimulation, acid–base balance, and energy reactions (see Table 6.12). Iron and zinc are critically important for energy metabolism but are also among the nutrients of which people may not be consuming enough. This is particularly true of vegetarians because the best source of these minerals is red meat.

The most common nutrient deficiency in most industrialized countries is a deficiency in iron. Because of the prevalence of this deficiency, people (especially females) should periodically have a blood test to determine iron status. This test should include an assessment of hemoglobin, hematocrit, and ferritin. An assessment of iron status is particularly important for vegetarians or people who are on weight loss diets.

Calcium is important for the skeletal maintenance and repair, for muscle contraction, and for normal blood clotting. Vitamin D is essential for calcium absorption, so athletes who do the majority of their training indoors and who are in weight-restricted and/or subjectively scored sports where appearance is important (*e.g.*, skating, gymnastics, and diving), where energy intake is often restricted, may be at risk for vitamin D, calcium, and energy intakes. This combination may place female athletes at risk of developing amenorrhea and higher bone fracture risk (1).

Iron deficiency is a common nutrient deficiency in industrialized countries.

## Fluid and Hydration

Water carries nutrients to cells and carries waste products away from cells. It serves as a body lubricant and, through sweat, helps maintain body temperature. Lean tissue (muscles and organs) is more than 70% water, and about 60% of total body weight is water (29). A failure to supply sufficient water is more likely to cause quick death than a failure to supply any other single nutrient.

Water is lost through breathing (breath is moist), the skin (this happens even if there is no obvious "sweat"), urine, sweat, and feces. It is critically important to consume sufficient fluid to

**FIGURE 6.7.** Fluid and hydration.

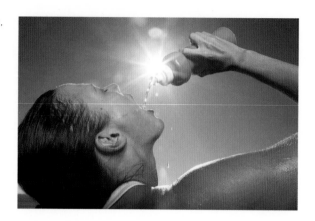

maintain body water stores, yet most people rarely stay optimally hydrated (Fig. 6.7). In fact, many people commonly wait until they become extremely thirsty (indicating a state of dehydration) before they consume fluids. Weight stability, before and after exercise, is a good indication that water needs have been met during an exercise program. People who experience significant weight (*i.e.*, water) loss during practice should learn how to drink more fluid to stabilize weight because a 2% body weight loss is associated with reduced performance (16).

## Meeting Fluid Needs

A key to athletic success is *avoidance* of a state of underhydration. This is not as easy as it may seem because many people rely on "thirst" as the alarm bell for when to drink. Thirst, however, is a delayed sensation that does not occur until the person has already lost 1–2 L of fluid. Because of this, people should learn to consume fluids on a fixed time interval rather than relying on thirst for when to drink. Staying optimally hydrated and fueled during exercise has multiple benefits, including the following (22):

> People may benefit from consuming fluids on a fixed time interval rather than relying on thirst to indicate when to drink.

- A less pronounced increase in heart rate
- A less pronounced increase in core body temperature
- Improvement in cardiac stroke volume and cardiac output
- Improvement in skin blood flow (enabling better sweat rates and improved cooling)
- Maintenance of better blood volume
- A reduction in net muscle glycogen usage (improving endurance)

Fluid intake recommendations are as follows (1,14):

- Drink as much as needed to match sweat losses.
- Do not rely on thirst as a stimulus to drink (the thirst sensation will occur only after 1–2 L [1%–2% of body weight] has already been lost).
- Checking urine color can be helpful to detect hydration. Urine should have a clear, pale yellow color.
- Sweat rates are often 0.3–2.4 L per hour, and it is difficult to consume and absorb enough fluid to match these losses.
- Consumption of large volumes of fluid increases the risk of gastrointestinal distress, thereby affecting performance.
- Ingestion of large volumes of dilute, low- (or no-) sodium fluid may increase the risk of hyponatremia.
- If left on their own, athletes will often develop dehydration even when there are sufficient fluids nearby for them to consume.
- To ensure better athlete compliance, fluids should be cool, should taste good, and should be readily available.

## Fluid Consumption Guidelines

The American College of Sports Medicine guidelines are useful for avoiding dehydration, but the type of fluids consumed is also important for achieving optimal performance (1). In general, studies have shown that a 6%–8% carbohydrate solution that also contains between 100 and 200 mg sodium per cup, such as that found in many sports beverages, is ideal from the standpoint of gastric emptying and intestinal absorption, for reducing mental and physical fatigue during both stop-and-go sports and endurance sports, for encouraging drinking during physical activity, and for improving performance. Studies comparing 6%–8% carbohydrate solutions with water and solution with higher carbohydrate concentrations have consistently found that the lower carbohydrate solutions are best (1).

## Water versus Sports Drinks

There are clear advantages of sports drinks over water for most exercising adults (9).

- Water provides no flavor or electrolytes, which cause people to want to drink. Beverages that make people *want* to drink help them stay well hydrated. Studies show that people drink 25% more sports drink than water, and young children will drink 90% more sports beverage than water (3,14,28).
- Water has no energy, whereas sports beverages contain carbohydrate. The carbohydrate helps provide muscles with needed fuel to avoid early fatigue and poor performance.
- The sodium provided by sports beverages helps maintain blood volume, a factor that is critical to maintaining sweat rates and performance. Sweat contains sodium, which water alone does not replace (Table 6.13).

| **Table 6.13** | **Warning Signs of Dehydration, Heat Exhaustion, and Heat Stroke: What to Do?** |
|---|---|
| Dehydration with loss of energy and performance | Drink carbohydrate- and electrolyte-containing sports drinks; avoid beverages with carbonation, which can cause gastrointestinal distress. |
| Dehydration with muscle cramps | Immediately stop exercising and massage the cramping muscle(s); consuming a sports beverage that contains sodium may help relieve the cramp. |
| Heat exhaustion with dizziness, light-headedness, and cold, clammy skin | Immediately replace fluids while in a cool, shaded area until the dizziness passes; stretching may improve circulation and prevent fainting; lying with the legs elevated will improve blood circulation to the head, thereby alleviating the dizziness. |
| Heat exhaustion with nausea/headaches | Rest in a cool place until the nausea passes; drinking fluids to rehydrate is critical; lying down may help relieve headaches. |
| Heat stroke with high body temperature and dry skin | Immediately get out of the heat and seek immediate medical treatment; feeling chilly with arms tingling and with goose bumps means skin circulation has shut down and heat stroke is imminent; this is an extremely serious condition that must be immediately treated. |
| Heat stroke with confusion or unconsciousness | Confusion strongly suggests, and unconsciousness confirms, heat stroke. This is a medical emergency that calls for fast cooling with ice baths or any other available means to lower body temperature. |

Adapted from Casa DJ, Armstrong LE, Hillman SK, et al. National Athletic Trainers' Association position statement: fluid replacement for athletes. *J Athl Train.* 2000;35(2):212–24.

# Dietary Supplements and Ergogenic Aids

Dietary supplements are concentrated sources of vitamins, minerals, and energy substrates that are taken to "supplement" the nutrients derived from foods. Ergogenic aids are substances that enhance a person's athletic ability, through either improvement in power or enhanced endurance. The terms *dietary supplements* and *ergogenic aids* often are used interchangeably, but they are not the same (Fig. 6.8).

> Ergogenic aids are substances that enhance a person's athletic ability, through either improvement in power or enhanced endurance.

### Dietary Supplements

Dietary supplements may be used to conveniently intervene in a known dietary deficiency, whereas ergogenic aids are often taken for the sole purpose of improved performance whether or not there is a known deficiency. It is common, for instance, for people with iron deficiency anemia to be prescribed iron supplements to help them complement the iron they are getting from the food they eat and build up their iron stores. The proven effectiveness for many nutritional supplements, in the face of a nutrient deficiency disorder, has been demonstrated in numerous clinical trials. However, there is no evidence that it is useful or warranted to take high doses of dietary supplements in the absence of a known nutrient deficiency. An example of the overuse of dietary supplements is protein and/or amino acids (the building blocks of protein). In fact, excess nutrients may cause toxicity or, at the very least, create the need to expel the excess nutrients. People wishing to take a nutrient supplement without the diagnosis of a specific nutrient deficiency should limit their intake to multivitamin, multimineral supplements that provide no more than 100% of the recommended daily allowances.

### Ergogenic Aids

Ergogenic aids, on the other hand, have typically not been tested for either effectiveness or safety. There is also some concern that up to 20% of ergogenic aids may contain substances that are not listed on the label and are considered banned by the World Anti-Doping Agency and other athletic organizations. Athletes are taking a high risk unless the supplements/ergogenic aids they take have been tested by independent groups (1). There are two ergogenic aids that have been clearly shown to improve a person's capacity to perform better: carbohydrates and water. With the exception of these, there is little consistent evidence to suggest that other substances touted as having an "ergogenic benefit" actually do anything to improve performance (Table 6.14). When ergogenic aids do work, it is usually because they help meet energy or nutritional requirements as a result of poor

**FIGURE 6.8.** Dietary supplements and ergogenic aids.

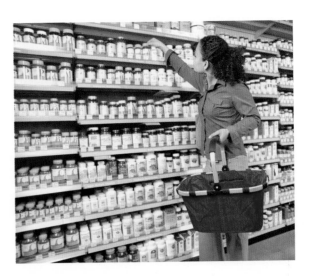

| Table 6.14 | Samples of Products Commonly Sold as Ergogenic Aids |
|---|---|
| **Supplement** | **Facts** |
| Androstenedione | Advertised as useful for increasing muscular strength and size. It is a hormone that is used to synthesize the hormone testosterone. (Testosterone is a male anabolic steroid hormone that is known to aid in the development of muscle mass.) There may be negative side effects (increased body hair and cancer are established problems) similar to those of testosterone, but studies on efficacy and safety have not been published. This substance is banned by the IOC, IPC, NCAA, USOC, NFL, and NHL. |
| Caffeine | Advertised as useful for improving endurance by enabling more effective fat metabolism during exercise. It is a central nervous system stimulant but has a reduced dose effect (people adapt to it, so increasingly higher doses are needed to obtain an ergogenic benefit). In high doses, caffeine may have a diuretic effect, thereby increasing the chance for dehydration. Although in the past caffeine was on the banned substance list by the IOC, it was removed from this list early in 2004. |
| Creatine | Creatine is synthesized from three amino acids and is part of phosphocreatine, which is a fuel used anaerobically to initiate high-intensity activity. However, stored phosphocreatine suffices to support activity for only several seconds and must be resynthesized for use in similar subsequent activities. It is hypothesized that supplemental creatine aids in this resynthesis, and some studies have shown that creatine supplementation is effective in maintaining strength/power for repeated bouts of short-duration, high-intensity activities. However, creatine supplementation is associated with weight increases (from muscle or water or both), and studies have not evaluated its effectiveness in athletes who are known to be consuming sufficient energy. In addition, the safety of creatine supplementation has not been adequately studied. |
| Ephedrine | This is a central nervous system stimulant that is sold over the counter as a decongestant. Its use is banned by the NCAA and the IOC, and it has undesirable side effects when taken in frequent and/or large doses. (The U.S. Food and Drug Administration recommends a maximum of no more than 8 mg per dose provided three times daily for a maximum of 7 d when used as a decongestant.) The side effects associated with ephedrine include increased heart rate, increased blood pressure, and nervousness, all of which are associated with strokes, seizures, and heart attacks. Caffeine consumption appears to increase the effect of ephedrine. It is theorized that ephedrine improves athletic performance and reduces body weight. Its chemical similarity to amphetamine suggests that it may lower appetite and thus have an impact on weight, but there is no evidence that it improves athletic performance. |
| Ginseng | There are numerous claims for ginseng, ranging from a cure for all ills to improving energy to enhancing immune function. However, it has been difficult to do athletic performance studies with ginseng because concentrations of the active ingredient(s) vary widely within and between brands. Therefore, there is no good evidence to support supplemental ginseng as an ergogenic substance. Luckily, it also appears that ginseng consumption has little risk of producing negative side effects, with the possible exception of causing insomnia in some subjects. |
| L-Carnitine | This is a substance produced by the body and used to transport fat into cell mitochondria so it can be used as energy. It is theorized that taking carnitine supplements will increase the amount of fat that is moved into mitochondria, thereby increasing the total amount of fat burned and helping reduce body fat levels. There is no solid evidence that supplementary carnitine has this effect. |

*(continued)*

| Table 6.14 | Samples of Products Commonly Sold as Ergogenic Aids (continued) |
|---|---|
| **Supplement** | **Facts** |
| Medium-chain triglycerides (MCT oil) | MCT oil is sold as a substance that can improve muscular development and increase the loss of body fat by increasing metabolic rate. Although there is no evidence of these effects, MCT oil may be an effective means of increasing total caloric intake in athletes with high-energy requirements who are having difficulty meeting energy needs. It is metabolized more like a carbohydrate than a fat but has a higher energy density than carbohydrates. Large intakes may be associated with gastrointestinal disturbances. |
| ω-3 Fatty acids (fish oils, canola oils) | It is hypothesized that ω-3 fatty acids stimulate the production of growth hormone (somatotrophin), thereby enhancing the potential for muscular development. It is well established that ω-3 fatty acids reduce red-cell stickiness, thereby reducing the chance for a blood clot leading to a heart attack. ω-3 Fatty acids are also associated with a reduced inflammatory response in tissues through the production of specific prostaglandins. One of these prostaglandins (E1) may be associated with the production of growth hormone. Although supplemental intake of ω-3 fatty acids may not be warranted, there is sufficient evidence of some beneficial effects that athletes should consider consuming cold-water fish (salmon, tuna) twice weekly. |
| Pyruvic acid (pyruvate) | Pyruvate is produced from carbohydrates as a result of anaerobic metabolism and is a principal fuel leading into aerobic metabolism. It has been hypothesized, therefore, that supplemental pyruvate will enhance aerobic metabolism and promote fat loss. However, because carbohydrate intake adequately satisfies the entire need for pyruvate, it makes little sense that supplementation of pyruvate will improve performance. |

IPC, International Paralympic Committee; IOC, International Olympic Committee; NCAA, National Collegiate Athletic Association; USOC, United States Olympic Committee; NFL, National Football League; NHL, National Hockey League.
Adapted from Manore M, Thompson J. *Sports Nutrition for Health and Performance*. Champaign (IL): Human Kinetics; 2000; Williams MH. *Nutrition for Health, Fitness & Sport*. 6th ed. Boston (MA): McGraw-Hill; 2002; and Benardot D. *Nutrition for Serious Athletes: An Advanced Guide to Foods, Fluids, and Supplements for Training and Performance*. Champaign (IL): Human Kinetics; 2000.

eating behaviors. It is clearly healthier and less costly to eat better foods than to rely on substances that are often of unknown origin and unknown quality and untested for safety or effectiveness.

## Special Conditions

There are certain conditions that may require special nutritional attention. These include physical activity in environmental extremes (very hot, humid, cold, or high altitude environments) and vegetarianism (1).

Dehydration risk is high in extremely hot and humid environments because it is difficult to evaporate sweat into an environment that is already hot and humid. Sweat becomes ineffective as a way of dissipating heat, causing a greater volume of sweat to be produced in the body's attempt to control body temperature. As a result, exercise in hot and humid environments greatly increases dehydration and heat illness risk. Specific to young athletes, they typically have fewer sweat glands and can produce less sweat per gland and therefore are likely to be at even greater risk of developing serious heat illness. Regardless, care should be taken that athletes, of any age, remain well hydrated and are frequently checked for signs of heat illness.

Dehydration risk is also high in cold weather environments because there are greater respiratory losses of water, and the clothing worn makes heat dissipation difficult, causing an increase in the sweat production. Athletes in cold weather conditions may not be as aware of the possibility of dehydration as athletes exercising in hot weather environments, making it necessary to remind them of the importance of drinking fluids in frequent intervals. High-altitude environments also tend to be cold environments, but they carry the additional problem of causing diuresis as well, particularly at altitudes greater than 2,500 m. It has been estimated that a total of 3–4 L of fluid per day would be required to maintain normal hydration in athletes who are exercising at high altitude.

Vegetarian athletes are perfectly capable of satisfying their nutritional requirements, but they should do so with the knowledge that it is more difficult to obtain satisfactory levels of, in particular, calcium, iron, zinc, protein, vitamin $B_{12}$, and energy. The more liberal the vegetarian intake (*i.e.*, ovo-vegetarians who consume eggs; or lacto-ovo-vegetarians who consume eggs and dairy products), the easier it is to satisfy total energy and nutrient needs. Vegetarian athletes should make certain that their intakes fully satisfy their needs by either consulting a Registered Dietitian, by requesting that their physician periodically perform blood tests to determine whether at-risk nutrients are at satisfactory levels, by periodically doing a food intake assessment of nutrients consumed, or through a combination of these.

## Practical Considerations

### One Day before a Competition

Although athletes often focus on the food consumed immediately before competition, it is actually important to start preparing in advance. Suggested considerations for the day prior to competition include the following:

- Avoid high-fat foods such as fried food, chips, cake, and chocolate.
- Eat a good breakfast (*e.g.*, toast, oatmeal, cereal, milk, and fruit).
- Have sandwiches, rolls, pasta, or rice for lunch (Fig. 6.9).
- Have rice, pasta, noodles, or potatoes plus vegetables and lean meat, chicken, or fish for dinner and yogurt and fruit for dessert.
- Eat a carbohydrate snack at dinner.
- Drink an extra 16 oz (475 mL) of fluid throughout the day.

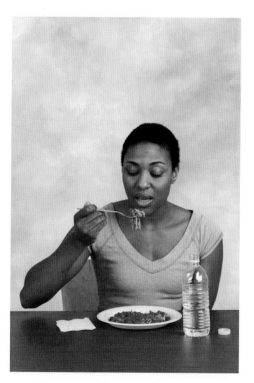

**FIGURE 6.9.** One day before competition, athletes should focus on foods that are relatively high in carbohydrate and relatively low in fat. Foods should be consumed in small, frequent meals rather than a single large meal.

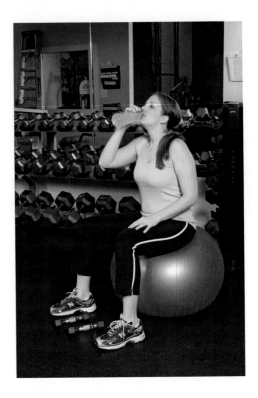

**FIGURE 6.10.** Immediately before exercise or competition, an athlete sipping on sports beverage.

## Immediately before Exercise or Competition

The pre-exercise meal should focus on providing carbohydrates and fluids. Ideally, people should consume a high-carbohydrate, low-fat meal 3–4 hours before exercising or competition. Light-carbohydrate snacks (*e.g.*, crackers) and carbohydrate-containing beverages can be consumed after the meal and before exercise, provided that large amounts are not consumed at one time (Fig. 6.10). Carbohydrate intake associated with performance enhancement ranges from 1 to 4 g $\cdot$ kg$^{-1}$, with timing, amount, and food choices suited to the individual, consumed 1–4 hours prior to exercise (1). There are several goals for the pre-exercise meal, including the following (4):

- Making certain that athletes obtain sufficient energy to see them through as much of the exercise bout as possible
- Preventing feelings of hunger (hungry people may be letting blood sugar get low, which is not a good way to start an exercise bout)
- Consuming enough fluids to begin exercise in a fully hydrated state
- Consuming only familiar foods
- Avoiding foods high in fiber or foods that cause gas (*e.g.*, broccoli, cauliflower)
- Drinking 5–7 mL per kilogram of body weight (2–3 mL $\cdot$ lb$^{-1}$) of water or sports beverage at least 4 hours before practice or competition
- Drinking an additional 7–10 oz (200–300 mL) of fluid 10–20 minutes before practice or competition

## During Exercise or Competition

Depending on the nature and duration of the exercise, consumption of carbohydrates may or may not have a significant impact on performance. During very brief exercise (<45 min), consumption of carbohydrates is not needed. However, with more sustained and higher intensity exercise (45–75 min), small amounts of carbohydrates, including utilizing a mouth rinse tech-

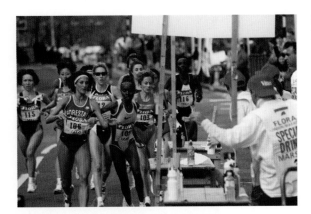

**FIGURE 6.11.** During competition, athletes grabbing drinks at fluid station during a race (marathon).

nique, are beneficial to performance. Evidence suggests that frequent contact of carbohydrate with the mouth can stimulate the brain and central nervous system to enhance perceptions of well-being leading to performance enhancements. For long-duration activities (1–2.5 hr) that allow for consumption of solid foods (*e.g.*, cycling, cross-country skiing), some people prefer to periodically consume bananas, breads, and other easy-to-digest carbohydrate foods. If solid foods are consumed, there should still be ample consumption of carbohydrate-containing beverages (Fig. 6.11). The carbohydrate target should be approximately $30–60 \text{ g} \cdot \text{hr}^{-1}$. For anything over 2.5 hours in duration (*e.g.*, ultra-endurance exercise), a carbohydrate target of up to $90 \text{ g} \cdot \text{hr}^{-1}$ is recommended. Drink 28–40 oz of fluid (sports beverages containing a 6%–8% carbohydrate solution and electrolytes are preferred) per hour. This corresponds to about 7–10 oz (200–300 mL) every 10–15 minutes, but this amount may need to be adjusted on the basis of body size, sweat rate, exercise intensity, and environmental conditions (Box 6.3) (1). This level of intake has been shown to improve time to fatigue in endurance activities. Two main goals are to avoid dehydration and to avoid the mental and muscular fatigue that can be caused by inadequate carbohydrate (4).

## After Exercise or Competition

When and what is consumed following exercise depends on the time and intensity of the exercise session (1). Consuming 1.0–1.2 g carbohydrate per kilogram during the first 4–6 hours after completion of exercise is associated with enhance muscle glycogen recovery. Muscles are receptive to replacing stored glycogen following exercise because of a higher level of the enzyme (glycogen synthetase) that can enhance the conversion of carbohydrate to stored glycogen. This strategy amounts to consuming carbohydrates between 200 and 400 kcal immediately following activity and then an additional 200–300 kcal within the next several hours (Fig. 6.12). People who have difficulty eating foods immediately following exhaustive exercise should try high-carbohydrate liquid supplements (4). Some examples of high-carbohydrate foods are included in Table 6.15.

| Box 6.3 | Practical Suggestion for Assessing Fluid Intake during Exercise |
|---|---|

Weigh an athlete before and after exercise. Weight loss indicates a less than optimal hydration state. Approximately 1 pint (about 600 mL) of fluid should be consumed for each pound (0.45 kg) of body weight lost during exercise.

**FIGURE 6.12.** Rehydrating and eating an energy bar after exercise.

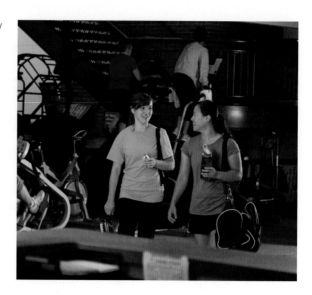

After exercise, people should drink at least 20 oz (600 mL) of fluid per pound of body weight that was lost during the exercise session (26). This should be consumed within 2 hours of finishing the practice or competition, with the goal of returning body weight to near pre-exercise weight before the next exercise bout.

## Eating on the Road

Although it may take a little more effort to maintain a proper diet while traveling, it is well worth the effort. These suggestions should help your clients maintain a diet that will keep up their level (11).

1. Pack nutrient-dense foods. Examples include sports bars, dried fruits, granola bars, bagels, and canned tuna.
2. Pick up some basic foods once you arrive at your destination. Examples include fresh fruits and vegetables, applesauce, cheese, breads, and soups.
3. If eating out, order lower fat items or items listed as "healthier" options from the menu. The following are some general guidelines.

| Table 6.15 | Examples of High-Carbohydrate Foods | |
|---|---|---|
| Food | Calories | Carbohydrate (%) |
| 1 Bagel | 165 | 76 |
| 2 Slices of bread | 135 | 81 |
| 1 Gatorade energy bar | 250 | 75 |
| 1 Cup of plain pasta | 215 | 81 |
| 3 Cups of popcorn | 70 | 79 |
| 1 Baked potato | 100 | 88 |
| 1 Apple | 80 | 100 |
| 1 Orange | 65 | 100 |
| 1 Cup of vegetable juice | 55 | 93 |

### Breakfast

- Order pancakes, French toast, muffins, toast, cereal, fruit, and juices.
- Request toast, pancakes, etc., be served without butter or margarine. Use syrup or jam but no butter or margarine to keep carbohydrate high and fat to a minimum.
- Choose low-fat dairy products (*e.g.*, skim or 1% milk, low-fat yogurt, low-fat cheese).
- Cold cereal can be a good breakfast or snack that can be taken with you.

### Lunch

- On sandwiches, look for lower fat meats such as turkey and chicken. Request it without the spread (*e.g.*, mayo, special sauce).
- Choose foods that are broiled, baked, microwaved, steamed, or boiled rather than fried.
- Salad bars are good options, but avoid the high fat additions like olives, fried croutons, nuts, and seeds.
- Baked potatoes, which are high in carbohydrates, are also good options but ordered with butter and sauces "on the side."
- Soups and crackers can be good low-fat meals; stay away from cream soups.
- Juices, low-fat milk, and low-fat milk shakes are a more nutritious choice than soda pop.

### Dinner

- Order high-carbohydrate foods such as pasta, baked potatoes, rice, breads, vegetables, salad bars, and fruits.
- Eat thick crust pizzas with low-fat toppings such as green peppers, mushrooms, Canadian bacon, and onions. Avoid fatty meats such as pepperoni or sausage, extra cheese, and olives.
- Eat breads without butter or margarine — use jelly instead. Ask for salads with dressing "on the side" so that you can add minimal amounts yourself. Ask for low-fat salad dressings.

### Snacks

Have snacks such as whole-grain breads, muffins, bagels, tortillas, fruit, fruit breads, low-fat crackers, pretzels, unbuttered popcorn, oatmeal raisin cookies, fig bars, animal crackers, fruit juice, carrot sticks, cherry tomatoes, breakfast cereal, canned liquid meals, and dried and fresh fruits.

### Don't Forget about Fluids

To prevent dehydration, you should keep well hydrated at all times, even on the road, by drinking frequently before, during, and after exercise. Drink plenty of water, even when ordering other beverages. Consider bringing a water bottle or squeeze bottle that can be refilled at a water fountain. In addition, limit caffeinated or alcoholic beverages as these are diuretics and cause fluid loss.

##  Understanding a Food Label (From the U.S. Food and Drug Administration, Center for Food Safety and Applied Nutrition)

Food labels can help you understand the nutritional content of a food by serving size. Each food label contains basic information on food components that should be consumed in more limited quantities, such as total fat, saturated fat, cholesterol, and sodium, and also has information on nutrients that people generally need more of, such as dietary fiber, vitamin C, calcium, and iron.

## Serving Size

Each food label contains basic information on food components that have the potential of being bad for you, such as total fat, saturated fat, cholesterol, and sodium, and also has information on nutrients that people generally need more of, such as dietary fiber, vitamin C, calcium, and iron.

The serving size listed is different for each type of food to make it easier for people to understand. A typical serving size is in familiar serving size units, such as cups or pieces, and also includes the weight of the serving size in grams. In the example given here (Fig. 6.13), the serving size is 1 cup, which for this food has a weight of 228 g. You can also see that the label indicates that there are two servings (*i.e.*, 2 cups) in the container.

## Calories

The unit of measure for energy in a food is "calories," and the total calories provided by a single serving (*i.e.*, 1 cup) of this food is 250. Because it is unhealthy for humans to chronically consume more than 30% of total calories from fat, the food label also indicates the percent of total calories from fat provided by one serving of food, which in this case is 18%. A person may not make a decision to eat or avoid a food based on this value, but by understanding if the food is relatively low or high in fat, individuals can make logical decisions about the other foods consumed.

## Percent of Daily Value

Each of the nutrients on a label has a recommended "daily value" (DV). A DV of 100% represents the recommended upper limit for total fat, saturated fat, cholesterol, and sodium, whereas 100% of total carbohydrate and dietary fiber represents the recommended minimum intake. However, please note that the DV is based on percentage of a nutrient that would be delivered with a 2,000-kcal diet. Many people, particularly those who are physically active, consume diets that are much higher than 2,000 kcal. Therefore, the % DV must be considered in the context of the total calories consumed. Typically, 5% DV or less is considered low and 20% DV or more is considered high. Using the label in Figure 6.13, consuming one serving of this food would provide 18% of the DV for fat, which is OK. However, if a person were to consume the entire package content, which has the two servings, the % DV would be 36%, which is considered high for a single food. Put simply, a 36% DV for fat means that the other foods consumed on the same day should be much lower in fat to avoid exceeding a % DV of 100% for fat. The easiest way to use the % DV is to compare foods that are similar in order to see which foods have the lowest fat content or the highest nutrient content.

The % DV can be used to determine the relative content of the nutrients listed on the label. The same rules would apply, but in this case, look for foods that are relatively high (*i.e.*, a % DV of 20 or better) in nutrient concentration. For food substances that do not have a % DV, such as *trans* fats and sugar, use the label to compare similar products when making a purchasing decision for similar products. In general, try to avoid foods that contain *trans* fats, and limit the intake of sugars.

 **Frequently Asked Nutrition Questions**

## Should I Take Protein Supplements?

Protein supplements are popular in most sports, at most athletic levels — from beginners to elite athletes — regardless of the goals of the people taking them. Some people take protein supplements to lose weight, some to gain weight, some to gain muscle, some to make them stronger, and some to increase endurance. Actually, humans are incapable of using protein for

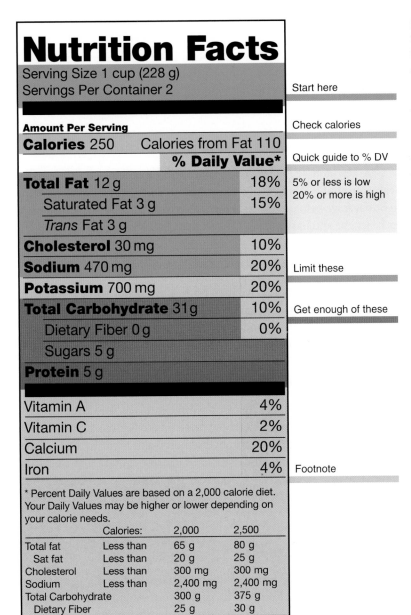

## Nutrition Facts

Serving Size 1 cup (228 g)
Servings Per Container 2

| **Amount Per Serving** | | |
|---|---|---|
| **Calories** 250 | Calories from Fat 110 | |
| | | **% Daily Value*** |
| **Total Fat** 12 g | | 18% |
| Saturated Fat 3 g | | 15% |
| Trans Fat 3 g | | |
| **Cholesterol** 30 mg | | 10% |
| **Sodium** 470 mg | | 20% |
| **Potassium** 700 mg | | 20% |
| **Total Carbohydrate** 31 g | | 10% |
| Dietary Fiber 0 g | | 0% |
| Sugars 5 g | | |
| **Protein** 5 g | | |
| Vitamin A | | 4% |
| Vitamin C | | 2% |
| Calcium | | 20% |
| Iron | | 4% |

\* Percent Daily Values are based on a 2,000 calorie diet.
Your Daily Values may be higher or lower depending on
your calorie needs.

| | Calories: | 2,000 | 2,500 |
|---|---|---|---|
| Total fat | Less than | 65 g | 80 g |
| Sat fat | Less than | 20 g | 25 g |
| Cholesterol | Less than | 300 mg | 300 mg |
| Sodium | Less than | 2,400 mg | 2,400 mg |
| Total Carbohydrate | | 300 g | 375 g |
| Dietary Fiber | | 25 g | 30 g |

Start here

Check calories

Quick guide to % DV

5% or less is low
20% or more is high

Limit these

Get enough of these

Footnote

**FIGURE 6.13.** The food label (for more information on how to read a food label, visit the following Web site: http://www.fda.gov/Food/IngredientsPackagingLabeling/LabelingNutrition/ucm274593.htm). (Reprinted from U.S. Department of Health and Human Services. *A Healthier You* [Internet]. Washington [DC]: U.S. Department of Health and Human Services. Available from: www.health.gov/dietaryguidelines/dga2005/healthieryou/html/tips_food_label.html.)

anabolic (tissue-building) purposes above the level of approximately 1.5 g of protein per kilogram of body weight. Protein taken in excess of this amount is either burned as a source of energy (calories) or stored as fat. Neither of the latter two options is particularly good because people rarely wish to put on additional fat weight, and getting rid of excess nitrogenous waste can make you dehydrated.

## What about Creatine?

Creatine monohydrate supplements have been shown to help maintain power on repeated bouts of high-intensity activity. However, this benefit may be as a result of an inadequate caloric intake in the tested subjects. As creatine monohydrate use has never been tested for safety (there is beginning evidence that taking supplements may alter the body's synthesis of creatine), it makes sense to avoid taking creatine but begin making certain that energy (calorie) consumption matches need. A good strategy for doing this is to eat small, frequent meals high in carbohydrates.

## Should I Consume Sports Drinks or Does Water Work Just as Well?

Sports drinks contain carbohydrate and electrolytes that are useful in maintaining water and energy balance. Studies of endurance athletes, athletes in stop-and-go sports, and athletes in power sports all show that consumption of sports drinks during practice and competition does a better job of enhancing athletic performance than water alone.

## Should I Stay Away from Caffeinated Beverages before a Workout?

People adapt to caffeine, so if you are accustomed to having a cup of coffee or a caffeine-containing cola, there should be no problem with consuming it before a workout. You should never increase the consumption of a caffeinated food or beverage before exercise above a level to which you are accustomed. This would likely increase your heart rate and have a diuretic effect that could make you dehydrated.

## Should I Skip Lunch If I'm Trying to Lower My Body Fat Level?

Skipping meals is one of the biggest reasons people have high body fat levels. If you are trying to lose body fat, your goal should be to maintain blood sugar levels through the consumption of small, frequent meals. Skipping a meal will cause you to produce excess insulin the next time you eat, which will make *more* fat than if you ate more frequently.

## Will a High-Protein, Low-Carbohydrate Diet Help Me Lose Weight?

There is nothing in the literature to suggest that lowering carbohydrate intake is useful for improving exercise performance. On the contrary, inadequate carbohydrate intake is almost always associated with reduced performance. High-protein, low-carbohydrate diets are typically low-calorie diets — the reason for the weight loss. However, dramatic reductions in caloric intake almost always result in a rebounding of weight. The best strategy for weight loss is to consume a little less than is currently needed to maintain current weight (say, about 300 kcal less) and to eat small, frequent meals to maintain blood sugar levels.

## Should I Eat or Drink Anything during Exercise?

Maintaining a constant flow of carbohydrates to muscles and maintaining blood sugar during competition is an important strategy for success. Your clients should consider sipping on a sports beverage during competition to achieve this result. If there are long breaks during an exercise workout, then consuming a carbohydrate snack (*e.g.*, crackers, bread) might be acceptable provided that fluid is also consumed.

## I'm a Profuse Sweater and Occasionally Get Serious Cramps. Is There Anything I Should Be Doing to Avoid this Problem?

Cramps are typically associated with dehydration and sodium loss. Try making certain that sufficient sodium-containing fluids (*i.e.*, sports beverages) are consumed during practice and competition. Unless you have a history of high blood pressure, you should also consider adding a small amount of salt to the food you eat, following with plenty of water.

## How Can I Tell if I'm Dehydrated?

The easiest way to tell is that your urine will be dark, and there won't be very much of it. Light-colored or clear urine is a sign of adequate hydration, whereas dark urine suggests dehydration. It takes time to rehydrate, so avoiding dehydration is the appropriate strategy.

## SUMMARY

This important chapter on nutrition is not intended to establish the Personal Trainer as a nutritionist or dietitian. There are laws in most states and around the world that protect this important discipline. The intent of this chapter is to make the Personal Trainer aware of certain nutrition-related questions that may come up in a typical training session. The Personal Trainer should be aware of the extent of information that can be distributed to clients and when it might be necessary to refer the client to a licensed dietitian. Both disciplines are encouraged to work together when a client has nutrition-related questions and is in need of a special diet for a medical condition or for a balanced weight loss program. Equally important is for the dietitian to understand the scope of practice for Personal Trainers. A team approach with the Personal Trainer prescribing exercise and the dietitian prescribing nutritional strategies is the recommended method to treating a client with nutrition issues. In general, athletic trainers should be aware that athletes have higher needs for energy and fluids. The intake of foods and fluids occur at times that are closely linked to physiological need and do not inhibit or interfere with physical activity. Both severe hunger and thirst should be avoided through readily available foods and beverages, the consumption of which should occur within the context of a well-planned and integral part of the athletic endeavor.

## REFERENCES

1. American College of Sports Medicine, American Dietetic Association, Dietitians of Canada. Joint position stand. Nutrition and athletic performance. *Med Sci Sports Exerc.* 2016;48(3):543–68.

2. American Diabetes Association. Postprandial blood glucose. *Diabetes Care.* 2001;24(4):775–8.

3. Bar-Or O, Wilk B. Water and electrolyte replenishment in the exercising child. *Int J Sport Nutr.* 1996;6(2):93–9.

4. Benardot D. *Advanced Sports Nutrition.* Champaign (IL): Human Kinetics; 2006. 352 p.

5. Benardot D. *Nutrition for Serious Athletes: An Advanced Guide to Foods, Fluids, and Supplements for Training and Performance.* Champaign (IL): Human Kinetics; 2000. 352 p.

6. Benardot D. Timing of energy and fluid intake: new concepts for weight control and hydration. *ACSMs Health Fit J.* 2007;11(4):13–19.

7. Benardot D, Clarkson P, Coleman E, Manore M. *Can Vitamin Supplements Improve Sports Performance?* Barrington (IL): Gatorade Sports Science Institute; 2001; 6 p.

8. Benardot D, Martin DE, Thompson WR. Maintaining energy balance: a key for effective physical conditioning. *Am J Med Sports.* 2002;4(1):25–30, 40.

9. Casa DJ, Armstrong LE, Hillman SK, et al. National Athletic Trainers' Association position statement: fluid replacement for athletes. *J Athl Train.* 2000;35(2):212–24.

10. Cheuvront SN. The "Zone" diet and athletic performance. *Sports Med.* 1999;27:213–28.

11. Department of Nutritional Sciences, Cooperative Extension, The University of Arizona. *Eating on the Road* [Internet]. 2002 [cited 2017 Mar]. Available from: http://www.umassathletics.com/documents/2014/8/6/DSWF_Eating_On_The_Road.pdf

12. Deutz B, Benardot D, Martin D, Cody M. Relationship between energy deficits and body composition in elite female gymnasts and runners. *Med Sci Sports Exerc.* 2000;32(3):659–68.

13. Fabry P, Hejl Z, Fodor J, Braun T, Zvolankova K. The frequency of meals: its relation to overweight, hypercholesterolaemia, and decreased glucose-tolerance. *Lancet.* 1964;2(7360):614–5.

14. Gatorade Sports Science Institute. *Fluids 2000: Sports Drinks vs. Water.* Barrington (IL): Sports Science Center Topics; 2000.

15. Hawley JA, Burke LM. Meal frequency and physical performance. *Br J Nutr.* 1997;77(suppl 1):S91–103.

16. Horswill CA. Effective fluid replacement. *Int J Sports Nutr.* 1998;8(2):175–95.

17. Iwao S, Mori K, Sato Y. Effects of meal frequency on body composition during weight control in boxers. *Scand J Med Sci Sports.* 1996;6(5):265–72.

18. Jenkins DJ, Wolever TM, Vuksan V, et al. Nibbling versus gorging: metabolic advantages of increased meal frequency. *N Engl J Med.* 1989;321:929–34.

19. Lamb DR. *Basic Principles for Improving Sport Performance.* Barrington (IL): Gatorade Sports Science Institute, Sports Science Exchange; 1995.

20. LeBlanc J, Mercier I, Nadeau A. Components of postprandial thermogenesis in relation to meal frequency in humans. *Can J Physiol Pharmacol.* 1993;71(12):879–83.

21. Luke A, Schoeller DA. Basal metabolic rate, fat-free mass, and body cell mass during energy restriction. *Metabolism.* 1992;41(12):450–6.

22. Manore M, Thompson J. *Sports Nutrition for Health and Performance.* Champaign (IL): Human Kinetics; 2000. 536 p.

23. McArdle W, Katch F, Katch V. *Sports & Exercise Nutrition*. Philadelphia (PA): Lippincott Williams & Wilkins; 1999. 704 p.

24. Metzner HL, Lamphiear DE, Wheeler NC, Larkin FA. The relationship between frequency of eating and adiposity in adult men and women in the Tecumseh Community Health Study. *Am J Clin Nutr*. 1977;30:712–15.

25. Rankin JW. *Glycemic Index and Exercise Metabolism*. Barrington (IL): Gatorade Sports Science Institute, Sports Science Exchange, Publication no. 64; 1997:10(1).

26. Romijn JA, Coyle EF, Sidossis LS, et al. Regulation of endogenous fat and carbohydrate metabolism in rela-

tion to exercise intensity and duration. *Am J Physiol*. 1993;265(12):E380–91.

27. USDA Nutrient Data Laboratory, Agricultural Research Service. *USDA National Nutrient Database for Standard Reference Release 28*. Washington (DC): Government Printing Office; 2015.

28. Wilk B, Bar-Or O. Effect of drink flavor and NaCl on voluntary drinking and hydration in boys exercising in the heat. *J Appl Physiol*. 1996;80:1112–7.

29. Williams MH. *Nutrition for Health, Fitness and Sport*. 6th ed. Boston (MA): McGraw-Hill; 2002. 688 p.

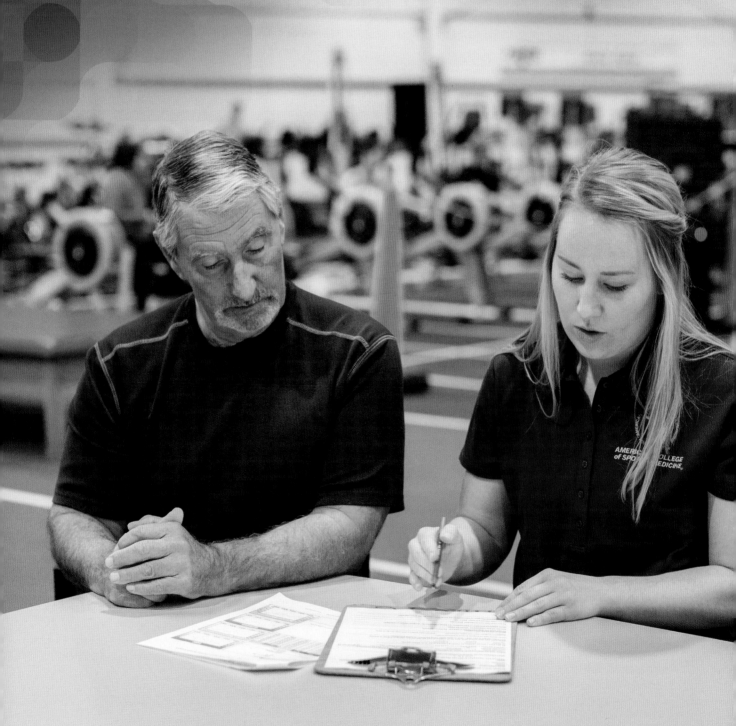

# Theories of Behavior Change

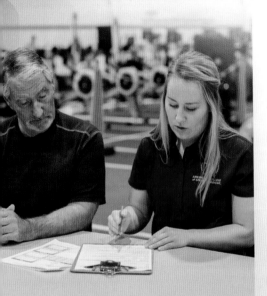

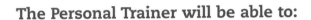

**The Personal Trainer will be able to:**

- List reasons why it is important to use theory to guide behavior change.

- Describe ways to use theories of behavior change to develop programs addressing a variety of lifestyle changes.

- Explain the role that self-efficacy, self-monitoring, goal setting, and feedback play in behavior change.

- Describe the main ideas, important tools, strengths, and limitations of theories discussed in this chapter: self-efficacy theory, attribution theory, transtheoretical model, health belief model, theory of planned behavior, social cognitive theory, goal setting theory, small changes model, and socioecological model.

- Discuss and design tailored interventions for clients using relevant elements of theory.

# INTRODUCTION

Although most Personal Trainers would be immediately encouraged by Joan's eagerness to begin and her insight into her own situation, working with this client will be challenging (Case Study 7.1). Several factors about Joan's case are characteristic of many clients who seek professional assistance with behavior change, particularly for weight management. First, Joan has slowly gained weight over the years and is currently classified as obese. She has high cholesterol, and because of her weight and family history, she is at an increased risk of type 2 diabetes. Second, Joan has made numerous attempts to lose weight on her own without long-term success. She has been able to lose weight but not maintain weight loss. She also has high expectations about the amount of weight to be lost within her self-imposed time frame. Finally, the demands of being a nurse and the irregularity of her work schedule impose additional challenges. Although many clients approach Personal Trainers ready and willing to make significant changes, often, the challenges of behavior change prevent clients from being successful long term. How can a Personal Trainer help Joan achieve sustainable behavior change that will result in maintained weight loss and improvements in health?

## Case Study 7.1

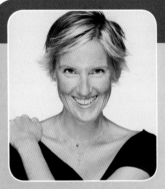

### Wedding Weight Worries

Joan is a 43-year-old nurse and mother of two children, ages 19 and 21 years. A friend of hers recommended that she hire a Personal Trainer. Joan reports that she was never overweight when growing up, although her sister was "heavy-set" as far back as she can remember. Joan recalls that she had trouble losing the baby weight that she gained during her first pregnancy and that she has been gaining weight a little at a time over the years.

Last year, Joan attended her 25th high school reunion and felt ashamed by her weight, after which she vowed to herself that she would become healthier. Over the last year, she has tried several different diets on her own, all without lasting success. Even though she was able to lose 10–15 lb with each new dieting attempt, she has been unable to stick to her plans for longer term and thus could not keep the weight off. She reports that she enjoys exercise but that she often finds herself eating more on days when she works out and eventually loses the motivation and energy to find time in her chaotic schedule to get to the gym. After gaining back the weight from her last diet, Joan realized it was time to seek professional intervention.

Currently, Joan has high cholesterol and is concerned about a family history of type 2 diabetes. Her current body mass index (BMI) is 31 (height = 65 in; weight = 185 lb). Her self-stated goal is to lose 25 lb before her son's wedding, 2 months from tomorrow. Joan is eager to get started, and you immediately appreciate her enthusiasm, motivation, and insight.

### QUESTIONS FOR CONSIDERATION

What else would you want to know about Joan? Knowing that she has tried and failed previously, what advice could you give her to help her future efforts? What types of exercises would you suggest and why? How would you progress her program over the next 4–6 weeks?

# The Challenge of Behavior Change

With over 35% of men and 40% of women in the United States listed with a BMI $>30.0 \text{ kg} \cdot \text{m}^{-2}$, it is clear that change is needed (20). However, changing behavior is one of the most challenging endeavors that one could undertake. At some point, everyone has probably tried to change a behavior. Maybe it involved giving up a bad habit or making a new year's resolution to eat healthy, start to recycle, or volunteer more time. Most likely, there has been a lack of success with one or more of these attempts at behavior change. Why is behavior so difficult to change?

> Changing behavior is challenging because so many factors play an important role — readiness for change, motivation, ability, perceived self-efficacy, and even situational factors such as scheduling or peer influence.

Changing behavior is challenging because so many factors play an important role — readiness for change, motivation, ability, perceived self-efficacy, and even situational factors such as scheduling or peer influence. In addition, behaviors that have been a part of one's life for a significant amount of time have likely been reinforced and maintained by one's environment. To make matters more complex, researchers have yet to reach a consensus regarding the way that all of these factors interact to produce behavior or behavior change. This chapter will provide a description of the most prominent behavior-change theories as well as possible applications of these theories for Personal Trainers.

Because of the significant health implications of overweight and obesity (11), weight management interventions that target dietary behavior and physical activity have been the focus of much research (Box 7.1). These interventions vary by modality (*i.e.*, telephone, Internet, in person), setting (*i.e.*, workplace, clinic, health center, physician, church), format (*i.e.*, individual, group), and regimen (*i.e.*, recommended dietary restriction and energy expenditure). Findings offer support for these various interventions as a successful means of helping participants attain improvements in dietary behavior and physical activity in the short term (19). Traditional behavioral weight loss programs, which encourage reduced caloric intake accompanied by increased caloric expenditure, typically result in a loss of 10% of initial body weight (13), an amount associated with a reduction of related health risks (23). Unfortunately, long-term findings suggest that participants who successfully complete behavioral weight management programs will gain two-thirds of their weight back within the first year following completion and almost all of it before 5-year follow-up (27). These findings indicate that even when participants are successful in initial behavior change, they may be unable to maintain changes after intervention.

Although few studies have examined the maintenance of health behaviors independent of weight outcomes, Fjeldsoe and colleagues (19) reviewed studies of behavior change that included at least a 3-month after assessment. Interventions included in the review targeted diet, physical activity, or both. Of the interventions included, 90% demonstrated differences in treatment and control groups at the end of the intervention. At the follow-up assessment (3 or more months postintervention), 38% maintained differences between groups on all out-

| Box 7.1 | Did You Know? |
| --- | --- |

- Among overweight/obese adults who successfully lose 10% of their initial body weight, 33.5% will regain their weight within the first year (56).
- Within 5 years, approximately 95% of people regain their weight just below baseline (27).
- Those who do not meet public health recommendations for physical activity are twice as likely to regain weight as those who do meet recommendations (56).

| Box 7.2 | **Definition of Terms** |
|---------|-------------------------|

**Construct:** An abstract variable that serves to explain a concept, or acts as a link to explain the observed relations between independent and dependent variables.

**Control and treatment groups:** A control group is a group or condition with which the effects of the experimental procedure or test condition are to be compared. The treatment group, or experimental group, is a group or condition in which the subjects are assigned the experimental treatment (*e.g.*, they undergo an intervention). It is important to include both a control and a treatment group in experimental studies to ensure that the effect of the treatment was genuine and not because of a placebo effect.

**Empirical:** Information obtained from observation or measurement using experimentation.

**Intervention:** An intervention is action taken or a treatment program developed to help someone change his or her behavior. Physical activity interventions attempt to offer programming and information that will help participants increase their physical activity.

**Mediator:** A mediator is a condition, state, or other factor that is presumed to intervene between the independent variable and the outcome. In other words, a mediator is some event or manipulation that has to happen in order for behavior to change. For example, in physical activity promotion, goal setting may be a mediator that is taught

as a part of an intervention to facilitate behavior change.

**Meta-analysis:** A meta-analysis summarizes the results of several similar studies by combining results to generate an overall effect size. The effect size examines the strength of the effect of X on Y.

**Moderator:** A moderator is a condition or variable (*e.g.*, age, gender) that alters or changes the relationship between X and Y by affecting the strength or direction of the results of an intervention. A statistical adjustment (*i.e.*, covariate) can be identified to minimize the impact of the moderator on a statistical analysis.

**Randomization:** Randomization, or random assignment, is the random allocation of sampling units (*e.g.*, participants) to conditions. This technique is considered the gold standard for designing experimental studies. If participants are randomly assigned, it is more likely that the results are due to the treatment and not because a biased sample was used.

**Wait-list control group:** A control group in which the subjects wait to receive the experimental treatment until after it has been administered to and found effective in the experimental group. This group serves as a control group for a period of time comparable to the experimental period. Once the experimental group is finished, this wait-list control group receives the intervention.

*Source*: Rosenthal R, Rosnow RL. *Essentials of Behavioral Research: Methods and Data Analysis*. 3rd ed. New York (NY): McGraw-Hill; 2008.

comes and 72% maintained differences by group on at least one outcome. Results such as these support the notion that although interventions have been successfully developed to result in initial health behavior change, behavior-change maintenance may be a more challenging feat. Thus, the following question remains: How can behavior-change interventions be improved to provide long-term success?

There is currently an overabundance of available interventions targeted at individuals trying to lose weight. Although it is important to remember that every individual is unique and may require different intervention components in order to succeed, using data- or evidence-based research to inform treatment provides insight into which intervention components are most consistently associated with successful behavior change. Personal Trainers and other health providers should refer current literature to determine which interventions are validated and thus most likely to be effective for a given client (see Box 7.2 for commonly used terms).

# Why Is Theory Important?

A theory is a framework that describes how and why behavior changes for a given population in a particular setting. Grounding interventions in theory is important because instead of simply stating that an intervention should include several random components, which makes it difficult to discern which components contributed to any behavior change, the inclusion of theory provides a foundation to understand how individual factors within an intervention influence behavior (49). Because there are currently over 70 behavior-change techniques identified in the literature (21), teasing apart these individual techniques is important for understanding how an intervention works.

For example, imagine that an exercise intervention for a client proves to be very successful. This intervention includes a number of different techniques, including goal setting, daily positive affirmations, problem solving, and a financial incentive. Because this intervention was so successful, it will be utilized again; however, can the most effective techniques from this intervention be specifically identified? Which techniques did not help to improve behavior? How did these techniques help the client? Did certain techniques succeed in altering specific behaviors? Should this intervention help all clients or certain subpopulations of clients? These are important questions that theory can help to answer.

Theory is also important in that it allows for replicable, sustainable, and generalizable interventions (31). The aforementioned intervention may be so successful that others want to utilize it as well. In order to assure that trainers utilize the intervention properly with an appropriate population, theory should be used to guide its application. If this intervention can be replicated many times with successful results across many populations and settings, then the intervention is said to be generalizable and it has strong empirical support.

Importantly, research has illustrated that theory-driven interventions are, in fact, more effective than those that are not, even if they appear to function on the same principles. Consider two strong examples. In one study, researchers completed a randomized experimental study that compared two walking programs with different levels of theoretical fidelity. Theoretical fidelity is defined as "the level of precision in replicating theory-based recommendations" (50). In other words, the high fidelity group followed theory, whereas the other group utilized the same techniques but did not use theory to guide the procedures. In this study, the high-fidelity group (using elements from social cognitive theory discussed later in the chapter) did twice as well as the low-fidelity group at the 1-mile walk test, reported greater satisfaction with the program, achieved their goals more often, and had more positive expectations, illustrating the importance of utilizing interventions strongly supported by theory.

Another example directly related to personal training was a study that assessed 59 male and female adults who were overweight or obese and wanted to lose weight (36). Participants were randomized to one of three groups for 16 weeks: (a) personal training 2 days a week plus a 20-minute weekly educational meeting with a nutritionist who utilized an educational behavior-change program from the U.S. Department of Agriculture (USDA), (b) personal training 2 days a week plus a weekly 20-minute theory-driven behavior-change meeting with a lifestyle coach (using the small changes model of behavior change discussed later in the chapter), or (c) a wait-list control group. The main goal was to match both of the treatment groups on the amount of time spent meeting so that the only difference was what was done during that 20-minute meeting each week (*i.e.*, one group received an educational behavior-change program, and the other group received a theory-based behavior-change program). Results at the 4-month mark showed that compared with the wait-list control group (who gained weight), the participants who received the theory-driven intervention lost over four times as much weight as the educational behavior-change group—and they kept it off at a 3-month follow-up visit (month 7; Fig. 7.1). Submax fitness and

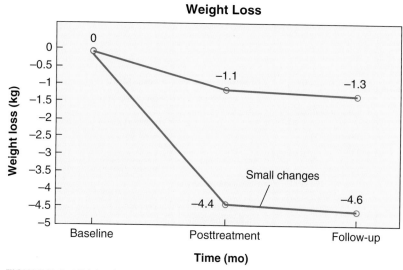

**FIGURE 7.1.** Weight change between two personal training programs with or without theory. (From Lutes LD, Winett RA, Barger SD, et al. Small changes in nutrition and physical activity promotes weight loss and maintenance: 3-month evidence from the ASPIRE randomized trial. *Ann Behav Med*. 2008;35:351–7, with permission.)

strength testing confirmed that both groups exhibited exactly the same improvements in strength and aerobic fitness across treatment. Results from this study made it clear that if weight loss and maintenance are goals of a behavior-change program, using theory to plan and implement an intervention is more effective than simply providing education.

Theory allows us to better understand what is known and what is yet to be learned. The systematic testing of theory allows for identification of new behavior-change constructs and replacement of elements of an intervention that are not as effective.

Finally, theory allows us to better understand what is known and what is yet to be learned. The systematic testing of theory allows for identification of new behavior-change constructs and replacement of elements of an intervention that are not as effective. Ultimately, theories are made to evolve and can be constantly improved. Rival theories may provide evidence for alternatives to an approach that can lead to more significant behavior change. Considering this, these authors agree that "nothing is more practical than a good theory" (49). In the rest of the chapter, six popular theories currently identified in the physical activity literature will be explained. Many of these theories gained prominence in areas other than physical activity research (*e.g.*, smoking cessation and screening behaviors) and have been adapted to address the special concerns related to increasing physical activity.

## The Transtheoretical Model

The first of six theories that will be explained is the transtheoretical model (TTM). The TTM, first used to examine smoking cessation, is an integrative model that was developed using constructs from other known theories such as the social learning theory and the social cognitive theory (which will be presented later in this chapter). Researchers such as Andrea Dunn and Bess Marcus adapted the model to specifically address how it can be applied to physical activity research as physical activity is viewed as a behavior.

The TTM states that individuals' behaviors are based on their readiness or stage of change. Figure 7.2 presents the five stages of change. As a Personal Trainer, you have probably noticed that

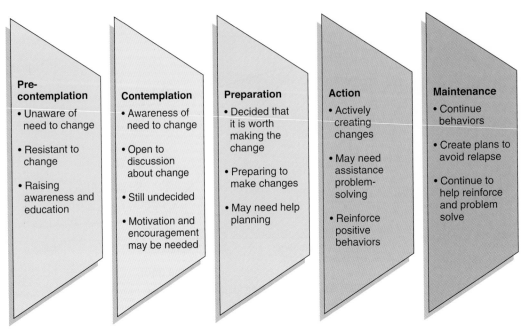

**FIGURE 7.2.** The stages of change from the transtheoretical model.

each of your clients may be at various degrees of readiness to change, and that this tends to predict his or her ability to change. If this is the case, then you already understand part of the foundation of the TTM (46).

1. *Precontemplation*: The client is not intending to take action toward change and is not considering benefits of change at this time.
2. *Contemplation*: The client is considering the negative consequences of their behavior and is considering changes within the next 6 months.
3. *Preparation*: The client has developed a plan of action toward behavior change and will be making changes in the immediate future (next 30 days).
4. *Action*: The client is actively making behavior changes (regularly active for less than 6 months).
5. *Maintenance*: The client has been actively maintaining the changes made during the action stage, the new behaviors have been established for 6 months or more, and the client is now working to prevent relapse.

Once a stage of change is identified with a client, applying the processes of change, can help him or her move to more advanced stages of change. There are 10 processes of change, which can be cognitive or behavioral. The processes of change will help progress clients through the stages of change. Typically, the cognitive processes are applied in the earlier stages of change, and the behavioral processes are applied in the later stages of change. Examples of cognitive processes of change, which are effectively used in the precontemplation, contemplation, and preparation stages include increasing awareness about the problems related to sedentary behavior (consciousness raising), assessing how being active or inactive affects a person's life (environmental reevaluation), evaluating oneself as an active person or couch potato (self-reevaluation), or helping clients identify moments of emotion related to physical activity (dramatic relief; see Case Study 7.2 for an example). Examples of behavioral processes of change, which are most effectively used in the action and maintenance stages, include removing cues for sedentary behavior (stimulus control), finding support for active behaviors (helping relationships), and reinforcing positive behaviors (reinforcement management). Any and all of these processes of change are encouraged during the maintenance phase of TTM (42). Some examples for using the processes of change tools with the stages of change (45,46) are provided in Table 7.1.

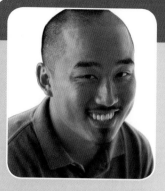

## Case Study 7.2

### Helping John Identify a Moment of Dramatic Relief

John has been really busy lately, and it is starting to affect his motivation for exercise. He had a recent situation where his little girl wanted him to play outside with her and he kept feeling overheated and out of breath. His weight played a role in his ability to play with his daughter.

### QUESTIONS FOR CONSIDERATION

What questions could you ask John to help him identify a moment of dramatic relief? Can you think of things you could discuss that would help him reidentify his priorities and get his exercise program back on track?

Naturally, as clients move through the stages of change, as they develop different perspectives on behavior, and as they build change-related skills and experiences, their self-efficacy increases. Self-efficacy refers to the client's belief in his or her ability to succeed and is an important component of behavior-change success. Clients with higher self-efficacy have a greater level of confidence and belief in change and are more likely to engage in successful behaviors. This increase promotes further progression and change.

| Table 7.1 | Strategies for Combining Stages of Change and Processes of Change | |
|---|---|
| **Processes of Change** | **Appropriate Stage for Use** |
| **Cognitive Strategies** | |
| Consciousness raising (increasing awareness) | Precontemplation, contemplation, preparation |
| Dramatic relief (understanding emotions) | Precontemplation, contemplation, preparation |
| Environmental reevaluation (aware of impact on others) | Precontemplation, contemplation, preparation |
| Self-reevaluation (creating a new self-image) | Precontemplation, contemplation, preparation |
| Social liberation processes (support from others) | Precontemplation, contemplation, preparation |
| **Behavioral Strategies** | |
| Self-liberation (make a commitment to self) | Preparation, action, maintenance |
| Counter conditioning (using substitutes) | Preparation, action, maintenance |
| Helping relationships (finding support, trust, acceptance) | Action, maintenance |
| Reinforcement management (using rewards) | Action, maintenance |
| Stimulus control (managing the environment positively) | Action, maintenance |

Data from Prochaska JO, Velicer WF. The transtheoretical model of health behavior change. *Am J Health Promot.* 1997;12(1):38–48.

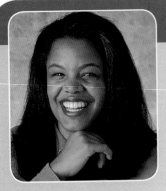

## Case Study 7.3

### Helping a Client Assess the Pros and Cons of Healthy Behaviors (a Decisional Balance Exercise)

Wendy works hard and often has to work late. This interferes with her ability to cook healthy dinners for her family, and in her fast-paced world, exercise is an even lower priority. On the other hand, she has high blood pressure and knows that her best strategy for lowering her blood pressure and helping her family stay healthy is taking the time to cook balanced meals and building exercise into her day.

### QUESTIONS FOR CONSIDERATION

What types of questions would you ask Wendy to help her determine ways in which she could build exercise and healthy eating into her day? How would you help her discuss the pros and cons of changing her current behaviors? (Remember to make your questions and responses as nonjudgmental as possible.)

As evident in the stages of change, clients may not always be ready to change. There may be a level of uncertainty in deciding to see a Personal Trainer or make other changes. This is why the TTM also uses a decisional balance tool. This allows the client to assess the importance of the "pros" and "cons" of behavior change and work through any ambiguity (see Case Study 7.3). This technique is designed to reinforce the reasons why behavior change is important while recognizing, appreciating, and ultimately working through the challenges that the client faces. It is important to give adequate time and respect to the challenges, or "cons" of behavior change; after all, increasing physical activity is difficult, and the client will appreciate that the trainer recognizes real challenges instead of downplaying them. Conversely, by ignoring these challenges, a trainer may never help the client work through the core of his or her unhealthy behaviors.

Often, after a client in precontemplation or contemplation assesses his or her decisional balance, a conclusion is reached that behavior change is worth the challenges. It is important for the client to come to this conclusion him- or herself and take ownership of this goal, instead of having it "forced" on them by a trainer. An example of a simple decisional balance is offered below in Figure 7.3.

**Decisional Balance for Health Changes**

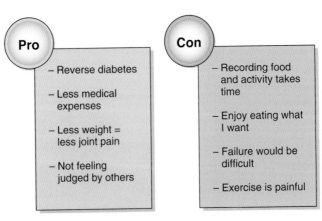

**FIGURE 7.3.** Decisional balance.

| Box 7.3 | Tips for Avoiding Arguments and Reducing Resistance |
| --- | --- |

- **Listen.** Simply repeat what you heard the person say. Avoid getting ahead of the priorities and needs expressed by the participant.
  - *"What I hear you saying is that you're stressed and increasing your exercise is not a priority right now."*

- **Make it hypothetical.** If you've encountered resistance regarding a particular issue, make the topic less threatening by turning it into a hypothetical scenario. Get the participant back to voicing the positive side of the argument for change. This will allow them to hear themselves make the arguments for change.
  - *"Suppose you made a change and are looking back on it now. How did it happen?"*

- **Acknowledge the resistance.** This may allow the participant to clarify his or her desires, which you steamrolled over in your haste to get commitment to a goal.
  - *"Sounds like talking about increasing your steps is not something you want to do."*
  - *"You have doubts that this program will work for you."*

- **Emphasize personal choice and control.** Remind them that what they do is up to them. Instead of directing clients or telling them what to do, collaborate on solutions.
  - *"It sounds like finding time to eat in the morning is hard when you are taking care of the kids. What ideas do you have for trying to solve this?"*
  - *"While I was planning on focusing on upper body today, it sounds like you also really want to work on cardio. What would be most helpful to focus on today?"*

- **Emphasize success.** Always assist clients to see the positives in what they are doing. It will help increase their confidence and understand that they can be successful.
  - *"On the 1–10 scale, you said your level of motivation was 5. Why a 5 and not something lower like a 1 or 2?"*

- **Acknowledge ambivalence.** Validate client's feelings and show that you understand.
  - *"On one hand, you really value the convenience, taste, and low cost of fast food, but on the other, you're afraid if you don't stop eating this food every day that it will kill you."*

- **Match the participant's readiness.** Mismatched interventions are only fuel for resistance. Action-oriented solutions are meaningless to someone who is only contemplating change!

Personal Trainers may have a tendency to advise clients how to change. However, unsolicited advice often puts the client on the defensive and increases resistance. Ironically, defensive clients are likely to argue for the reasons why they should *not* change! Furthermore, research shows that the more a client resists, the less likely he or she is to change (39). For some tips on how to best assist a client in working through resistance without increasing defensiveness, see Box 7.3.

Consider Case Study 7.1, Wedding Weight Worries, what stage did you choose for Joan? Upon presenting at your fitness facility, Joan had made a plan to seek your services to help her get into a structured exercise routine; she seems likely to be making changes in the immediate future. Therefore, she is in the preparation stage (Box 7.4). Note that Joan has likely been in each of these stages at some point, as is common with clients trying to achieve health behavior change. Her current stage is important in helping to guide intervention.

When beginning an intervention with Joan using TTM, it is important to assess her stage of readiness and complete a decisional balance exercise. Because Joan is in the preparation/action stage, it is important to help her increase her commitment to change by utilizing consciousness raising, dramatic relief, and self-reevaluation processes tools. Joan will also benefit from utilizing volitional strategies to help her develop a concrete plan and problem solving skills to make her goals attainable. You may consider helping Joan develop concrete goals, track her progress, and offer positive feedback.

| Box 7.4 | Apply: Wedding Weight Worries |
|---|---|

Take a moment and think back to the example of Joan in Case Study 7.1. What stage of change do you think Joan is in? Consider the following:

■ Is she intending to change or not yet?
■ Has she decided to change in the immediate future?
■ Does she have a plan?
■ Is she already making changes?

Although TTM proves to be promising, research provides mixed results regarding its effectiveness at changing physical activity. However, a meta-analysis by Hutchinson and colleagues (26) suggests that this may be because most research that claims to use the TTM does not actually utilize the complete theoretical model of change. Many studies use only parts of the theory or only cite the stages of change. However, classifying the client into a stage of change does not lead to behavior change; it is the specific processes of change utilized as a result of understanding a client's stage of change that help clients increase their physical activity. In fact, in the meta-analysis by Hutchinson and colleagues (26), only 29% of the studies reviewed utilized all dimensions of the TTM. This does not necessarily mean that full TTM-based interventions are more effective than those that use an incomplete TTM. Of the 17 interventions that did not utilize the complete TTM, 71% showed significant short-term physical activity change (26). Unfortunately, TTM did not appear to result in long-term physical activity change consistently across either group of studies, suggesting that TTM may be improved on to increase long-term success. That is why many researchers believe that considering all available theories and using them in combination, when warranted, can be even more powerful. Theories such as the health belief model (HBM), discussed next, have often been used as a foundation for or contribution to other theories.

##  The Health Belief Model

Like the TTM, the HBM (Table 7.2) (51) is a widely used theoretical approach. Developed in the 1950s, this model has been used to increase health screening behaviors, and it suggests that the main predictors of behavior change are (a) the perceived seriousness of a potential health problem (*e.g.,* hypokinetic disease) related to the behavior (*e.g.,* physical inactivity), (b) one's susceptibility to potential health consequences, and (c) the perceived benefit or belief that making the suggested behavior changes will result in decreased risk of consequences (48). Clients must believe any perceived barriers are outweighed by benefits, and they must have the confidence in their ability to perform an action (2). According to the client, the cost of changing behavior should be relevant and worth the risk reduction it offers. You may have worked with clients who have said that they are exercising now because heart disease runs in their family and they are trying to avoid developing the disease themselves. This trend is also evident in research. For example, a study on 143 older women found that understanding health risks and exercise benefits led to more physical activity, whereas being unsure of health risks and exercise benefits led to increased likelihood of avoiding physical activity (44).

> Clients must believe any perceived barriers are outweighed by benefits, and they must have the confidence in their ability to perform an action (2). According to the client, the cost of changing behavior should be relevant and worth the risk reduction it offers.

The HBM has also been shown to be effective in intervention studies. One intervention targeting a group of African American breast cancer survivors offered eight weekly HBM sessions that focused on increasing the participants' perceived susceptibility and severity of breast cancer

| Table 7.2 | Health Belief Model Constructs and Strategies | |
|---|---|---|
| **Construct** | **Exercise-Specific Definition** | **Change Strategy** |
| Perceived susceptibility | Beliefs about the chances of getting a disease/condition if do not exercise | ▪ Explain risk information based on current activity, family history, other behaviors, etc. |
| Perceived severity | Beliefs about the seriousness/consequences of disease/condition as a result of inactivity | ▪ Refer individual to medically valid information about disease.<br>▪ Discuss different treatment options, outcomes, and costs. |
| Perceived benefits | Beliefs about the effectiveness of exercising to reduce susceptibility and/or severity | ▪ Provide information on benefits of exercise to preventing/treating condition or disease.<br>▪ Provide information regarding all of the other potential benefits of exercise (*e.g.*, quality of life, mental health). |
| Perceived barriers | Beliefs about the direct and indirect costs associated with exercise | ▪ Discuss Ex $R_x$ options to minimize burden.<br>▪ Provide information on different low-cost activity choices. |
| Cues to action | Factors that activate the change process and get someone to start exercising | ▪ Help individual look for potential cues.<br>▪ Ask the individual what it would take for him or her to get started. |
| Self-efficacy | Confidence in ability to exercise | ▪ Assess level of confidence for different types of activity.<br>▪ Use self-efficacy building techniques to enhance exercise confidence. |

Ex $R_x$, exercise prescription.
Data from Rosenstock IM, Strecher VJ, Becker MH. Social learning theory and the health belief model. *Health Educ Q.* 1988;15(2):175–83

(57). During this time, participants were asked to record daily step counts using a pedometer and make weekly step goals. These women were able to significantly increase steps (baseline steps/day = 4,791, final steps/day = 8,297, $p <.001$) and decrease weight ($p = .005$). Moreover, these results continued during a 3-month follow-up. Although these results support using the HBM, this particular population may have a greater understanding of risks and benefits because they have experienced cancer and thus have an understanding of the health risks involved in sedentary behaviors.

Unfortunately, there are some limitations to the HBM. A recent meta-analysis of 18 studies (including a total of 2,702 participants) found that although benefits and barriers to behavior change were predictors of intervention success, they were overall weak predictors (10). The author ultimately recommended not using HBM in behavior-change interventions due to these modest results. Although this review did not evaluate physical activity interventions, it does offer valuable information for future theoretical work and questions: Will HBM be effective for a physical activity-specific intervention?

Fortunately, theories are meant to be improved, and research on the HBM has allowed for better understanding of the underlying impact of health beliefs. For example, a recent study illustrates that the relationship between health belief constructs (perceived seriousness and susceptibility) and behavior is mediated by one's affective state (30). In other words, a client's emotional state and feelings related to physical activity may play an important role in behavior change and may be added to the HBM. Researchers have presented this alternative HBM as the behavioral affective associations model (BAAM) (30).

To apply the HBM to Joan's case, Joan will be more likely to engage in long-term physical activity if she recognizes and understands her risk of illness associated with a sedentary lifestyle, accepts that this risk is serious, and believes that engaging in a physical activity and nutrition intervention will reduce this risk. Because of this, it is important to allow Joan to explore her beliefs about the implications of her weight status, sedentary lifestyle, and disease risk and to offer Joan some education regarding these issues and how physical activity can reduce these risks. Joan may also benefit from the use of external and verbal cues to help remind her of these risks and benefits. Helping Joan process feelings toward exercise as well as helping her cope with negative feelings and teaching her to have more positive thoughts regarding her activity habits may help change her perspective of physical activity.

In summary, the HBM can be beneficial particularly for clients who have clear, identified health risks and have high intentions and motivations to change. However, feeling intention and motivation toward change is not always enough to elicit actual behavior change, as is evident with the theory of planned behavior.

## Theory of Planned Behavior

The theory of planned behavior (TPB; Fig. 7.4), which was developed from the theory of reasoned action, has been used extensively in advertising, public relations campaigns, and more recently in health behavior-change efforts. The TPB suggests that intention to engage in a behavior will ultimately result in that behavior, and a client's level of intent is shaped by his or her attitudes toward the behavior (how helpful and enjoyable the behavior is perceived to be), subjective norms (social pressure), and perceived behavioral control (self-efficacy and controllability) (1,6). Consider Yolanda's case presented in Case Study 7.4.

If TPB is applied to Yolanda's case, then Yolanda is likely to engage in successful behavior change because she enjoys physical activity (she used to play on a sports team), she still has friends who pursue activity, and she feels that she can reverse her blood pressure through activity. In other words, her attitudes, subjective norms, and perceived control are predictive of change. By using TPB, you may encourage her to remember past successes (however small) and record current successes to increase the number of mastery experiences thus bolstering self-efficacy, provide fun

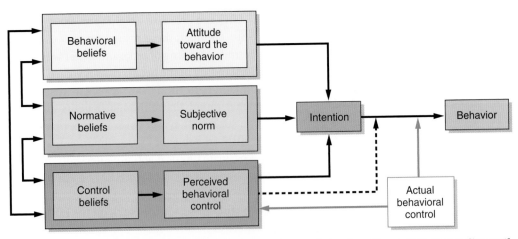

**FIGURE 7.4.** The theory of planned behavior. (Reprinted with permission from Ajzen I. *TPB diagram* [Internet]. [cited 2011 Jun 15]. Available from: http://people.umass.edu/aizen/tpb.diag.html)

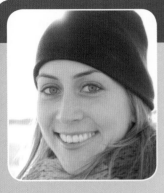

## Case Study 7.4

### Sedentary Secretary

Yolanda is a 30-year-old woman who is interested in increasing her physical activity and muscle tone. She reports that she played softball in college and stayed fairly active, but now that she is out of school and works as a secretary, sitting behind a desk all day, she has struggled to maintain physical activity. Although she still has several friends who play in a recreational softball league, she has not found time to join them. Recently, her doctor diagnosed her with high blood pressure, which is what finally led her to hire a Personal Trainer.

### QUESTIONS FOR CONSIDERATION

How could the TPB be applied to Yolanda's case? Are there ways you could change her attitudes, subjective norms, and perceived control? Can you encourage Yolanda, the former athlete, to remember her past successes and make note of current successes to increase self-efficacy and create a fun, group atmosphere that might be socially enticing?

alternative activities catered to the individual to improve attitude, and create a group-based intervention format so that she experiences additional positive social pressure.

Although TPB has been effective in behavior modification related to smoking, alcohol abuse, and eating habits (6), it remains to be seen whether the TPB can promote increased physical activity on its own. It seems that although TPB can significantly increase one's intention to exercise, this may not necessarily translate into actual behavior change. In a study utilizing pedometers, TPB predicted significant improvements in intention to walk but did not result in step count change (55). Furthermore, in one intervention targeting adolescents, TPB explained 43% of the variance in self-reported physical activity, but only 13% of activity measured on an accelerometer (37). One explanation may be that TPB only focuses on purposeful, structured activity and not daily lifestyle activity increases, which are what most objective measurements of physical activity measure. Despite doubts, in a meta-analysis of 185 studies, TPB did predict physical activity, although it accounted for 39% of intention and only 27% of behavior (4). This suggests that people's intentions regarding activity change may not be in line with actual behaviors. It has been referred to as an intention–behavior gap (35). Some researchers suggest that this intention–behavior gap may occur because behavior change has both motivational and volitional components (24). Thus, researchers have introduced a new construct to TPB: implementation intention.

Implementation intention has been added to the TPB model to account for the volitional component of behavior change. Implementation intention utilizes skills that increase the likelihood that intentions are acted on. These skills include problem solving, goal setting, coping with challenges, and recording progress (5,15). Research shows that implementation intention, in addition to TPB, leads to significant behavior change above and beyond that gained by TPB alone (5,15).

Research also shows that the ability to self-monitor may be a particularly important construct within implementation intention. In one of a two-part series of studies, researchers sealed pedometers (to prevent participants from seeing their step counts) in order to determine whether TPB constructs could predict activity change (52). Although TPB predicted change in several of its theoretical constructs, it ultimately did not predict actual step counts. Interestingly, there was also no correlation between actual step counts and self-reported walking. This study suggests that an important aspect of physical activity interventions is feedback; without seeing the pedometer values, participants were not able to determine their own activity levels. Furthermore, using this feedback to set future goals may be an important component to TPB treatments along with implementation intention. Both of these constructs may encourage participants to walk more. Using different theoretical constructs within TPB could help bridge the intention–behavior gap and help clients achieve their goals. One theory that may help bridge this gap is social cognitive theory, described in more detail in the following section.

# Social Cognitive Theory

Bandura's social cognitive theory (SCT) is perhaps the most commonly used theory in behavior change today and is based on the HBM discussed previously (7). Personal Trainers may already be using SCT techniques with clients, even if they have not learned about this theory. Although SCT does not emphasize perceived susceptibility as much as HBM, it adds several important constructs that are important for predicting behavior change. SCT states that outcome expectations (*i.e.*, what you think will happen as a result of your new behavior) and self-efficacy (*i.e.*, situation-specific self-confidence) are the most important factors in behavior change. These factors are further divided into environment (both physical and social), personal/individual (emotions, thoughts), and behavior (one's skills and abilities, past experiences) all of which that may shape expectancies (22,48) (Fig. 7.5). Notice in Figure 7.5 both personal factors and environmental factors lead to the behavior. The behavior can be either positive or negative depending on the influence from the other two factors. Thus, behavior may be shaped by observational learning, reinforcement and incentives, and coping skills.

SCT stands apart from other theories in that it puts great emphasis on a client's thoughts and feelings, thus emphasizes behavior at the interpersonal level. Proponents of SCT believe that clients actively shape their lives by thinking, feeling, reflecting, and observing themselves (Fig. 7.6).

If clients repeatedly think that they are unable to improve their weight status or that they are a "failure," they will not have positive outcome expectations (Box 7.5), will feel incompetent, and have a negative attitude toward exercise. In turn, they will be more likely to drop out of an exercise program. Furthermore, unrealistic thoughts are also not helpful to a client. For example, consider Mark (Case Study 7.5).

If Mark continues to think that he can lose 20 lb in just 2 weeks in addition to toning his whole body, then he is setting himself up for failure. Because these types of thoughts and feelings are not helpful, it is the trainer's task to help the client identify them. These thoughts should be replaced with realistic ideas to break this negative cycle and increase likelihood for success by improving the client's self-efficacy and outcome expectations. Surrounding clients with cues, social support, and

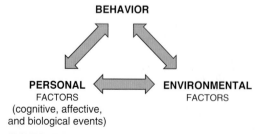

**FIGURE 7.5.** Basis of social cognitive theory. (Reprinted with permission from Ajzen I. *TPB Diagram* [Internet]. Amherst [MA]: University of Massachusetts. Available from: http://people.umass.edu/aizen/tpb.diag .html.)

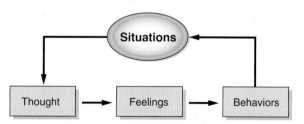

**FIGURE 7.6.** Thoughts, feelings, and behaviors. (Reprinted with permission from Bandura A. *Social Foundations of Thought and Action: A Social Cognitive Theory.* Englewood Cliffs [NJ]: Prentice Hall; 1986.)

| Box 7.5 | The Power of Thoughts |
|---|---|

One's thoughts are very powerful — they can shape feelings and behaviors. Kind, realistic thoughts as a part of one's self-talk promote confidence to make positive lifestyle changes. In contrast, beating oneself up with negative thoughts reduces the confidence needed to make changes. These are called thought traps.

For example, a person who always tells himself he is fat may feel depressed and hopeless. He may then decide to give up on physical activity and healthy eating. Negative thoughts can result in a vicious cycle of self-defeat. Because of this, you may choose to use SCT techniques to help your client break the cycle and replace bad thoughts with more realistic ones.

education can enrich their environment and also promote further behavior change. In other words, a supportive environment increases self-efficacy and confidence, which in turn affects behaviors.

To apply SCT to Joan, if she is confident that she can meet goals, overcome challenges, and improve her health, then she will be able to succeed in her behavior change. Thus, teaching Joan skills and self-maintenance techniques (*i.e.*, self-monitoring and planning), highlighting her successes, and offering her coping and problem-solving skills will increase her self-efficacy. Focusing on how she accomplished past successes and encouraging rewards (such as positive praise and nonfood-based self-rewards) will increase her expectancies for success.

SCT applied to Mark might look different compared to Joan. Although Joan has had success with past attempts at weight management, Mark has not. In Mark's example, place greater emphasis

## Case Study 7.5

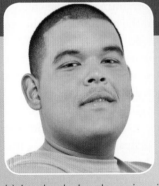

### Mad for Muscles

Mark is an 18-year-old high school graduate who just moved to your area to begin college. He reports that he has been overweight since elementary school. He was never athletic or good at sports, and as a result, he acquired more sedentary hobbies such as video games, computer games, and social networking. Mark was often teased and bullied for his weight in school and was never chosen for any sports teams. Thus, he has always avoided sports or other physical activity. He has several close friends from high school who also enjoy video games and computer games.

Mark tells you that he has tried several popular diets and that he and his friends typically eat junk food when they hang out. Mark notes that if he suggests something active instead of their usual video games or computer games, his friends may laugh at him. As a result, Mark has not had much success with behavior change. Mark is hoping that this will be his opportunity to a start fresh since he moved to start college. He'd like to lose weight and make new friends, including a girlfriend.

Currently, Mark has a BMI of 38 (height = 70 in; weight = 265 lb). His self-stated goal is to lose about 20 lb before classes start (in 2 wk) and to "get buff" in order to "be attractive" to women and go on dates. Mark is eager to lose weight but seems hesitant about the structure and discipline it may require.

### QUESTIONS FOR CONSIDERATION

What past experiences has Mark experienced that challenge him when trying to exercise? What types of thoughts and feelings might Mark be experiencing related to exercise? How does Mark's environment help or hinder his efforts? How might Mark become more supported socially and emotionally as he tries to exercise?

on building self-efficacy to change behavior, especially in the initial stages. Mark will benefit from learning self-maintenance techniques and problem-solving skills to help him manage challenges and experience success that he can build on to bolster self-efficacy. In addition, Mark will need assistance discovering enjoyable physical activities. For example, taking Mark's love for video games and pairing it with exercise (such as an interactive video game) may be the perfect way for him to be active while doing something he enjoys.

SCT has been supported by a number of research studies. One particularly noteworthy study illustrated that a 52-week online SCT intervention assessing 272 participants resulted in improvements in physical activity and physical activity related self-efficacy and self-regulation (3). Furthermore, social support, self-efficacy, outcome expectations, and self-regulation led to better results and are closely related to SCT constructs. SCT addresses goal setting — the main focus of the goal-setting theoretical model which is described next.

## Goal Setting Theory

Although goal setting is a common construct within several theoretical models, some consider goal setting a theoretical orientation of its own merit (16,18). Research on goal setting theory (GST) suggests that four different mechanisms play a role in goal-related behavior change (32):

1. Goals direct attention and energy toward desired behaviors
2. Goals lead to greater effort
3. Goals extend the time and energy devoted to a desired behavior
4. Goals increase the use of goal-relevant skills

The success of goal setting is moderated or affected by the level of commitment to the change; the importance of the goal, self-efficacy, feedback on goal progress; and the attainment of the appropriate skill level to achieve the goal.

> The success of goal setting is moderated or affected by the level of commitment to the change.

Research in GST has provided an understanding of the type of health goals that are most effective. Research shows that individuals who develop self-selected goals are more likely to be successful than those who have goals determined from an outside source (32) (Box 7.6). This may be because intrinsic motivation is lower when goals are set without the client's input (54). As health professionals, it is tempting to push clients to certain standards or behaviors believed to be optimal. Instead, set up clients for success by collaborating with them and working within their lifestyles when setting goals.

Research also illustrates that specific goals are much more effective than asking clients to "do their best." Setting an ambiguous goal does not provide the client with a concrete performance level or behavior for which to strive. In fact, when clients are asked to "do their best," they do not perform as well as when they select a specific goal (32). Help clients avoid this goal setting trap by encouraging them to develop a way to track and measure specific behaviors. For example, a goal of "walking more" is not a specific or measurable goal and it leaves the client without much guidance. Instead, set a goal such as "acquire 1,000 more steps a day by walking

---

**Box 7.6      Client-Centered Care**

When clients become collaborators in making decisions that affect their lifestyle, they are more likely to follow through with the treatment plan. It is essential to actively listen and validate the client's feelings. It takes practice to resist the urge to "be an expert" and try to "fix" the client. The Personal Trainer's job is to help the clients fix themselves.

around the office building at lunch." This goal is more measurable, can be tracked with a motion sensor (such as a pedometer, accelerometer, or mobile app), and provides specific feedback to guide the client's behaviors. Furthermore, if this goal is not achieved, the client may be able to pinpoint the barriers to behavior change more accurately. Specific strategies for helping clients set effective goals will be discussed in detail in a subsequent section of this chapter. In the following section, a novel model that includes goal setting in combination with elements from other theories is described.

## The Small Changes Model

Small changes model (SCM), a new model, utilizes several elements from other theories within its framework (35). SCM provides a new approach to behavior change that has been successfully utilized in nutrition-based and physical activity–based interventions. SCM is unlike more traditional physical activity theoretical interventions (14,34,36) (Fig. 7.7). First, SCM client goals are relative to baseline activity in order to help the client make realistic, attainable changes. For example, if a client is only exercising once a month, exercising every day may be a large and unrealistic goal to attain. Instead, the SCM client could slowly increase his or her number of workout sessions to a level that is realistic and maintainable as a lifestyle change.

SCM allows clients to make small behavioral changes. The belief is that clients will maintain smaller behavior changes more easily and will continue to build on them over time. For example, research shows that although weight loss is more gradual in SCM programs than in more traditional programs, weight loss continues to occur at 3, 6, and 9 months after treatment; in contrast, clients from more traditional programs often regain weight at these time points (14,34,36).

Another aspect to SCM is that clients select their own goals (Box 7.7). This allows them to take ownership, thereby increasing their self-efficacy. Finally, because research shows that self-monitoring

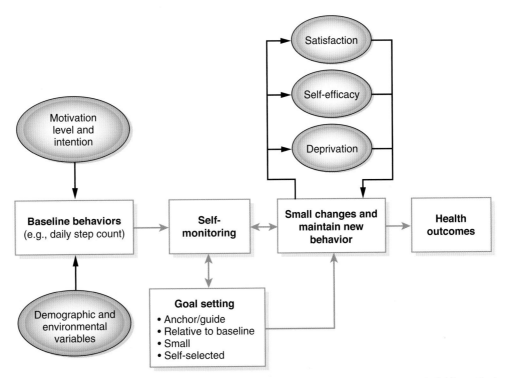

**FIGURE 7.7.** Small changes model. (Reprinted with permission from Lutes LD, Steinbaugh E. Theoretical models for pedometer use in physical activity interventions. *Phys Ther Rev.* 2010;15[3]:143–53.)

## Box 7.7   Remember: Goals Should Be "SMALL"

**S:** Self-selected. Your goals should be your own. Choose goals that fit into your life and only change behaviors that you are willing to negotiate. Remember, being realistic, not idealistic, is key.

**M:** Measurable. Develop a concrete way to track your goal. Consider the question, "How will I know when my goal has been met?"

**A:** Action-oriented. How are you going to achieve your goals? Having an action plan allows you to complete the steps needed to make your goals a reality.

**L:** Linked to your life. Goals are best achieved if they work within your lifestyle and match your challenges and strengths. Are your goals designed to fit you and your everyday life?

**L:** Long-term. Because you want to be healthy for life, any changes you consider should be something you could see yourself doing for the rest of your life. Create lifestyle-related goals that you feel confident you can maintain.

is one of the key factors in behavior change, clients are asked to monitor their own behaviors to assist with goal setting, problem solving, feedback, and self-reward. Cognitive behavioral therapy, which emphasizes the role of thinking in our behavior, is also utilized to help clients address thoughts that may impact feelings and behaviors related to their goals.

To apply SCM to Joan's case, ask Joan to complete a 1-week baseline record of her activity during which she will not try to change her behaviors. After 1 week, this baseline record would be used to learn about what Joan typically eats and how active she is from day to day. Because Joan has experienced initial success in the past, she will have some idea of what works for her, and she will select goals based on these reflections, with guidance from her Personal Trainer. Goals should be small, specific, and should fit into her lifestyle. Joan should self-monitor her daily activity and slowly build on her goals.

Although the components of intervention would be similar for Mark, how do you think his intervention would be different? For starters, his baseline levels of activity and eating habits differ from Joan's. Mark has not had success in the past with health behavior change and thus will need more guidance with goal setting and strategies for reaching goals. It is especially important for his goals to be realistic and specific so that he can experience success and self-efficacy necessary to ensure that he is able to maintain and build on his changes. Most likely, the Personal Trainer's main challenge with Mark will be helping to guide his goals. Furthermore, both Mark and Joan will benefit from problem-solving training, affective coping skills, and cognitive restructuring. Thus, it is important to remember that although each theory can be applied to various clients, each client's unique factors and situation will require the Personal Trainer to apply knowledge and skills to tailor interventions to fit the client's needs. Moreover, it is important to note that even though initial studies using the SCM have shown some potential for long-term behavior change with regard to weight management, this theory is new and more research is needed. In particular, little is known about its effectiveness in individuals with high-risk medical conditions (*e.g.*, cancer, heart disease, morbid obesity) or individuals with less developed abilities to make informed choices (*e.g.*, young children).

> It is important to remember that although each theory can be applied to various clients, each client's unique factors and situation will require the Personal Trainer to apply knowledge and skills to tailor interventions to fit the client's needs.

In addition to unique personal factors, such as the ones discussed in the SCM, environmental factors also influence behavior. Even the best interventions can be supported or thwarted by the environment; therefore, researchers have developed an approach called the socioecological model (SEM).

## Socioecological Model

When developing a theoretical approach to physical activity intervention, it is important to view a client not as a single independent entity but as someone within a larger social framework and infrastructure. Health behaviors are shaped not only by individual decisions but also by environmental influences. The SEM addresses this relationship: Behaviors are shaped by interpersonal interactions, the surrounding environment, community, policy, and law (29) (Fig. 7.8). For example, Joan wants to make several healthy behavior changes. The environment in which she lives will strongly impact her goals, barriers, and behaviors. For example, is Joan's neighborhood safe to walk? Are there sidewalks available? Is Joan utilizing an assistance program to purchase food that limits purchase options? Is she the primary food provider in the home? Do her familial duties limit her free time? Does she have social support? All of these factors will impact Joan's behaviors and cause potential barriers to her goals if left unaddressed.

As a Personal Trainer, you may choose to address these interactions by creating an eco-map with your client that may highlight some barriers and supports (Fig. 7.9). Eco-maps are drawings that highlight both positive and negative connections between the client and his or her environment (28). By completing a map together, you may be able to build rapport with your client, increase awareness, plan for challenges, embrace support, promote self-reflection, and identify areas of improvement. Think of the eco-map as a tool that helps clients share their story so that a Personal Trainer may in turn help them make changes that fit within their life contexts. To make an eco-map, the client and Personal Trainer will draw a diagram. Even though the Personal Trainer may show the client an example, ultimately the client should be responsible for completing the writing and designing of the map in order to feel in control of the process. The Personal Trainer or client may designate different styles of arrows to designate different types of relationships (see examples in Fig. 7.9). Remember, relationships are a two-way interaction; what may be helpful to one member of a relationship may not be for another. Also, the Personal Trainer should remember to include structural supports as well. Is there a recreation center nearby? This may go in the eco-map. This should be a collaborative activity in which the client explores these relationships. The Personal Trainer may then ask, "How can we change the map

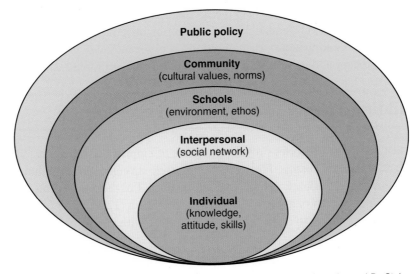

**FIGURE 7.8.** Socioecological model. (Adapted with permission from Lutes LD, Steinbaugh E. Theoretical models for pedometer use in physical activity interventions. *Phys Ther Rev.* 2010;15[3]:143–53.)

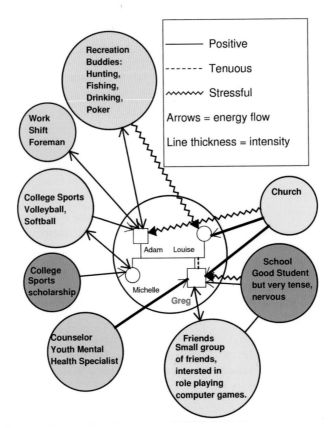

**FIGURE 7.9.** Sample eco-map. (Adapted with permission from Kennedy V. Ecomaps. *MAI Review.* 2010;3:1–12.)

to help you receive the support you need to make your changes successful?" For a more detailed discussion of eco-maps, see Kennedy's review (28).

Various theories of behavior change have been discussed in this chapter. Each has its unique contributions, strengths, and limitations as well as similarities with other theories. These theories help us to understand or explain behavior in the clients in which the Personal Trainer may work. Using these theories may help the Personal Trainer build trust and rapport, express empathy, bolster listening skills, and reflect on spoken or unspoken behaviors. They also assist the Personal Trainer in asking appropriate questions in order to devise goals. For a review of the highlights of each theory and its relative strengths and weaknesses (Table 7.3).

 **Building Theory Intro Intervention**

The described theories provide a number of empirically supported, valuable tools to help clients with behavior change. For instance, research strongly supports the use of self-monitoring, goal setting, and feedback as tools that effectively aid participants in increasing physical activity when included as part of a physical activity intervention (17,43). The following section reviews some of these techniques to make them easier to utilize with clients in the future.

## Self-Monitoring

Self-monitoring refers to the practice of tracking one's own behavior for the dual purpose of increasing awareness and monitoring progress. This process can take many forms. For example, self-monitoring may mean writing exercise in a planner, getting on the scale weekly, entering food

| Table 7.3 | Comparison of the Behavior-Change Theories | | |
|---|---|---|---|
| **Main Idea** | **Important Tools** | **Strengths** | **Limitations** |
| **Transtheoretical Model of Change (TTM)** | | | |
| Change is based on one's readiness to change. Clients can moved through change stages using the processes of change. Personal Trainers should begin working with the client in their current stage. | Decisional balance Processes of change (*e.g.*, self-liberation, reinforcement management, dramatic relief) Self-efficacy and confidence in change "Rolling with resistance" | Helps those at all stages of readiness (no required readiness); Reduces friction (client and Personal Trainer) | Research shows mixed results May be more effective for some behaviors than others |
| **Health Belief Model (HBM)** | | | |
| Behavior change is predicted by one's feeling of susceptibility to health consequences, the perceived seriousness of the consequences, and the belief that making changes will reduce the risk. | Explore health concerns and vulnerability Education Identify barriers and benefits to change Use of external cues to remind client of risks and benefits | Clients have a greater understanding of health. | May not be as effective for clients who do not have identified health risks |
| **Theory of Planned Behavior (TPB)** | | | |
| The intention to make behavior change leads to change. If a client has a positive attitude about change, feels that it is enjoyable, has feelings of controllability and self-efficacy, and recognizes that the social network values change, he or she will be more likely to change. | Enhance self-efficacy Explore attitudes related to change Introduce enjoyable activities Utilize group activities or buddy systems Help identify and engage social support | TPB treatments significantly increase intention. | "Intention–behavior gap"; intention does not always lead to behavior. |
| **Social Cognitive Theory (SCT)** | | | |
| Outcome expectations and self-efficacy are the most important factors to behavior change. The physical and social environment is key. One's skill set, reinforcement and incentives, coping skills, experiences, and thoughts and feelings determine change. | Utilize role models Self-monitoring, planning, and problem solving Increase social support Skill development, self-efficacy Utilize environmental cues and reinforcements Break thought chains (stop negative thoughts, feelings and behaviors) Recognize past successes | Considers client's environment, thoughts, and feelings toward behavior change | Many factors to consider in one treatment program |

*(continued)*

| Table 7.3 | Comparison of the Behavior-Change Theories (continued) | | |
| --- | --- | --- | --- |
| Main Idea | Important Tools | Strengths | Limitations |
| **Goal Setting Theory (GST)** | | | |
| Setting goals leads to behavior change. Particularly, setting goals that are specific, manageable, attainable, realistic, and time-specific lead to behavior-change success. Also important to change is self-efficacy, feedback, skill level, and the perceived importance of the goal. | Self-directed goals<br>Utilize recording and monitoring tools<br>Problem-solving skills<br>Feedback<br>Allow client to express reasons to change<br>Review past successful goals and "what worked"<br>Regular goal setting | Gives clients a concrete plan for change<br>May be utilized within other theories | May not address factors such as thoughts, emotions, and environment |
| **Small Changes Model** | | | |
| Behavior change is achieved through setting realistic, maintainable goals that are small, relative to baseline activity, and cumulative. Combines components such as goal setting, feedback, and self-monitoring to yield achievement of initial goals and increases in self-efficacy to further behavior change. | Self-selected goals<br>Goals are relative to baseline<br>Goals are small<br>Utilize monitoring tools and feedback<br>Problem-solving skills<br>Goals are linked to lifestyle and maintainable across time. | Promotes gradual and cumulative behavior change while increasing self-efficacy | New theory with only a handful of studies to date. Moreover, little is known about its effectiveness for certain groups of people. |
| **Socioecological Theory** | | | |
| Behavior change is a result of not only the individual factors but also the social structure, environment, community, policy, and law. | Address barriers and highlight supports<br>Create an eco-map<br>Work with social network, teachers, bosses, political leaders, and city planners to affect change<br>Help clients explore and ask for social support<br>Implement cues in the environment for change<br>Allow clients to share cultural and community practices | Recognizes that clients are affected by their greater environment | The environmental structure (including community, policy, and law) can be very difficult to change and change is slow at best. |

intake into a tracking Web site, or wearing an accelerometer. Self-monitoring plays an important role in physical activity intervention. In fact, a recent meta-regression including 122 research studies and 44,000 participants concluded that self-monitoring was the most influential predictor of successful behavior change for physical activity (38). Researchers found that interventions including self-monitoring with at least one other technique (intention formation, goal setting, feedback, review of goals) were more effective than those that did not. Similarly, a meta-analysis of physical activity interventions concluded that interventions that utilized self-monitoring demonstrated significantly larger effect sizes than those that did not include self-monitoring (12). In other words, interventions that include self-monitoring exert a larger influence on physical activity behavior than interventions that do not. Self-monitoring is an important tool in increasing physical activity because its use increases client awareness of behavior, offers accountability, provides information for the Personal Trainer on the client's behavior outside of meetings, allows for goal setting and tracking progress, provides an opportunity for feedback, and is a skill that a client can use on their own, after intervention.

### The Use of Physical Activity Trackers and Mobile Apps

One of the drawbacks of self-monitoring is that it is often subjective. In other words, it involves the client's self-report and "best guess" of the amount of activity completed. Although one might assume that clients would not intentionally misrepresent their behavior, there are many reasons why they might intentionally or unintentionally misreport their behavior. For example, clients may not be diligent about recording behavior and then try to remember all of their behavior just before coming in to meet with a Personal Trainer. This can lead to inaccurate recall of behavior. In addition, clients may overestimate the amount of time or distance they exercised. It is important to keep in mind the emotions that clients may have in response to being overweight or "out of shape." Some clients may misrepresent behavior because of shame about their actual behavior or out of a desire to impress or please their Personal Trainer. Physical activity trackers such as pedometers, mobile apps provide a less subjective measure of physical activity by tracking daily steps and distance. However, this requires clients to remember to wear these devices regularly and be willing to use creativity when finding places to wear them (especially for women).

Another drawback of self-monitoring is that if clients are forgetful or perceive self-monitoring as a burden, they may not continue to utilize it. Although it is important to include self-monitoring as a part of physical activity intervention, clients will not benefit from self-monitoring unless they utilize it! In a study to determine factors contributing to increases in physical activity, researchers examined several adherence variables and found that individuals who were compliant with self-monitoring tasks were more likely to meet physical activity guidelines at the end of the 6-month follow-up than those who were not adherent (25). In another study of factors contributing to behavioral change, researchers discovered that participants who consistently self-monitor activity using an exercise diary significantly increased their activity and lost more weight than those who were inconsistent in their self-monitoring behavior (9). For these reasons, it is imperative that Personal Trainers discuss the importance of self-monitoring with clients upon introducing it as part of treatment. However, be careful to not assume that more means better. This discussion should include what behaviors, foods, or patterns that the patient would find most helpful to help them begin their behavior-change journey. In addition, it is always good to discuss potential barriers to effective self-monitoring as well as brainstorming ways to overcome potential barriers to using problem-solving strategies.

## Goal Setting

As previously discussed, another important component of successful physical activity intervention and behavior change is goal setting. The current literature on physical activity behavior change suggests that goal setting is an important tool to promote increased and maintained activity (17,41,53). Goal setting can be used in the short term not only to initiate behavior change but also to plan ahead for obstacles and set goals for realistic long-term outcomes. Researchers examining the impact of setting goals applied to physical activity concluded that goal setting improves performance by (a) increasing effort, persistence, attention, and motivation and (b) facilitating progress toward long-term goals (33).

Goals are typically more effective if they are client-selected. Clients will take more ownership of goals that they have chosen for themselves. Does it seem more likely that an individual would commit to a goal that someone else has suggested or one that they have chosen for themselves? Most likely, an individual would feel more committed to a goal they have chosen for themselves. Goals that are accepted and embraced by clients are more likely to alter behavior (33). As a Personal Trainer, how can you allow clients to set their own goals while ensuring they choose effective ones? You can teach your client the important components of an effective goal and then help them to mold their goals into more effective ones. The important components of an effective goal are discussed subsequently.

### SMART Goals

> SMART goals are specific, measurable, achievable (or action-oriented), realistic, and time-oriented.

In order for a goal to be effective, there are several factors that should be taken into account. SMALL goals were described previously. Another prominent tool that can help Personal Trainers and clients to remember effective goal-setting strategies is the acronym: SMART (8). SMART goals are specific, measurable, achievable (or action-oriented), realistic, and time-oriented (see example in Box 7.8). Specific goals target a specific behavior and include a detailed plan; making a behavior plan is more

---

### Box 7.8 Apply: Wedding Weight Worries, Part 2

With the aspects of SMART goals in mind, assess your understanding and practice utilizing SMART goals with Joan.

In your second meeting with Joan, you introduce goal setting and discuss how to set SMART goals. After some thought and discussion, Joan decides that her first goal (in addition to exercising with you Monday, Wednesday, and Friday at the gym) is to exercise on her own 2 days during the upcoming week. Her plan is to walk her dog on Tuesday and Saturday.

- Do you think this is a SMART goal?
- Most goals will be SMART in some ways but could use improvement in other ways. How could Joan's goal be improved? Ask yourself:
  - Is it specific? Is it measurable?
  - Is it action-oriented?
  - Is it realistic?
  - How about time-oriented?
- Be sure to affirm the parts of Joan's goal that are SMART. You could say something like:
  - "That is a great start! It seems specific, measurable, action-oriented, realistic, and time-oriented! Can you think of any ways that we could make it more specific (or other component)?"
- Joan's goal includes the what, when, and with whom but could include a time or distance as well as a location. Does she plan to walk around her neighborhood or drive to the park?

After further discussion, Joan decides that her goal for the upcoming week is to walk her dog on Tuesday and Saturday. On Tuesday, she will walk twice around her block in her neighborhood, and on Saturday, she will drive to the park and walk for 30 min. She also has a rain plan to walk through the grocery store. Be sure to commend Joan for setting a SMART goal and make sure that she has a way to remember it and record the outcome for next session.

likely to be implemented than a broad or vague goal. Measurable goals are more effective than those that are difficult to quantify. Achievable goals are those that can be achieved and are action-oriented because they target behaviors as opposed to outcomes, leaving no uncertainty about goal achievement. Goals that are challenging but achievable are more likely to lead to behavior change and maintenance than unrealistic goals (41). SMART goals include a time frame and are relatively short-term in order to allow for feedback and modification if necessary. Personal trainers should use clinical judgment and past experience to assist clients in setting realistic goals. Understanding how to set SMART goals will help you as a Personal Trainer to teach your client an effective tool, which they can use after intervention to assist them in maintaining behavior change. For more information on SMART goals, refer to Chapter 8.

## Feedback

Feedback is often defined as two-way communication between two or more parties. Personal Trainers need to keep this in mind so that they do not impose their views without taking the views of the client into consideration. Physical activity interventions often combine goal setting and self-monitoring with feedback. Essentially, this is because goal setting allows for feedback in the same way that self-monitoring allows for goal setting. Consider Mark's example. How can Mark set goals related to his amount, frequency, duration, or intensity of exercise if he does not keep track of what, when, and how much exercise he achieves? In addition, it is much easier to provide feedback to Mark regarding his progress if you have a physical record of his exercise and whether or not he met his goals. Similarly, setting goals would not be of much use to Mark without keeping record to determine if he met his goals and then receiving feedback, whether positive or negative, or both. Research on goal setting has shown this to be true — feedback about progress is necessary for goal setting to be an effective part of physical activity intervention (33). More information regarding feedback is provided in Chapter 9.

> Feedback not only is necessary for effective goal setting but has also been labeled an important component of physical activity behavior change.

Feedback not only is necessary for effective goal setting but has also been labeled an important component of physical activity behavior change. In a study to determine factors involved in behavior change, researchers found that both telephone and print feedback increased the likelihood of physical activity behavior change (40). In a recent study, researchers found that after providing in-person group weight management using small changes, a 6-month telephone follow-up period with a feedback component resulted in continued to lose weight across the follow program — almost doubling their weight loss (34). Therefore, not all contact has to be in person to be effective. Personal Trainers should remember to utilize the telephone, e-mail, or texting as an effective alternative resource for providing feedback. It is important to find the most preferred way (besides in-person feedback) your client expects and likes.

Needless to say, feedback will vary between individuals based on goals, progress, and other circumstantial factors. For this reason, it is necessary to tailor interventions to each individual's needs. In a small intensive study, trainers delivered a physical activity intervention including goal setting, self-monitoring, and feedback to participants, allowing modifications to the intervention in order to accommodate client preferences (17). At the end of the intervention, all participants significantly increased physical activity regardless of differences in intervention. Tailoring an intervention to a client's current level of motivation will increase long-term adherence to behavioral change. In other words, modifying an intervention to meet a client at their current motivational level will increase the likelihood that they will maintain their physical activity behavioral change across time. Beyond individual preferences and differences in motivation level, clients will differ by current level of activity, physical fitness, and situational or environmental factors like access to facilities, scheduling challenges, and social support.

## Customizing to a Population

Although many studies describe the efficacy of interventions tailored to special populations like the elderly, children, those with physical limitations such as arthritis, and various cultures, a discussion of each of these is beyond the scope of this chapter. However, it is important for Personal Trainers to understand each client's unique needs based on any combination of factors relating to age, physical ability, gender, culture, or other individual factor as well as being open to modifications based on preference or perceived need. Whereas the Personal Trainer is the expert in physical activity, clients are experts on themselves. Sometimes, tailoring to meet a client's need or preference may not seem the best or may go against the Personal Trainer's beliefs. In such cases, Personal Trainers should carefully consider the pros and cons of including such preferences from a health/fitness as well as relational perspective, using experience and expertise to guide clients to a compromise that both the client and Personal Trainer can feel comfortable implementing.

## Rapport

One of the most fundamental components of a successful intervention is rapport. Rapport refers to a sense of trust, respect, or confidence, which a client holds for his or her Personal Trainer. Experts say that rapport with a client is the first step to behavior change and adherence (47). Often, rapport building is the first task of a Personal Trainer, preceding other interventions. Although a client may have initial respect for you as a Personal Trainer because of the title, respect and confidence is earned based on your skill and prescribed intervention. For ideas on how to build rapport, consider the following:

- Be sure to display/communicate your credentials.
- Confirm your professionalism by dressing and acting professionally.
- Highlight things that you have in common such as likes, dislikes, or experiences (show that the two of you relate to each other).
- Affirm any client strengths that you have noted.
- Empathize with their struggles/feelings.
- Self-disclosure: Share relevant struggles you have had in the past, take sincere interest in your client — people can detect insincerity.
- Nonverbal cues: Have good eye contact, open posture, and appropriate facial expressions.
- Remain nonjudgmental and open-minded.
- Be a mindful and active listener and remain present in the moment.
- Offer explanations for the components of intervention.
- Continuously ask your client how they feel about the information you are providing them throughout the session.

 **Lessons Learned**

Although there is no prescription guaranteed to help a client to achieve and maintain physical activity behavior change, the discussed theories and their components have been empirically tested and shown to increase the likelihood of success. At the same time, Personal Trainers must be wary of presuming that what works for one client will work for every other client. As such, it is important to be flexible and open-minded, with a willingness to tailor interventions to each client's unique needs. The task of the Personal Trainer is to incorporate empirically supported components of physical activity change into each client's intervention in the way that will most benefit that particular client. Consider the examples in Case Studies 7.6 and 7.7.

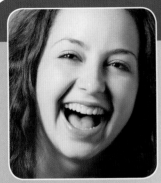

## Case Study 7.6

### Overweight Sedentary Teenager

Sydney is a 16-year-old girl who is overweight and inactive. Her physician has strongly suggested that she actively try to lose some weight because of the concern that her family has a history of type 2 diabetes and heart disease. Sydney tells you that she spends most of her free time listening to music, watching movies with friends, or reading a book. She plays clarinet in the school band but has never liked sports. In the initial meeting, she is timid and appears self-conscious but is amenable to your suggestions. She admits that although she is "not good" at sports or exercise, she is a highly self-motivated person and is driven to accomplish goals and finish what she starts.

#### QUESTIONS FOR CONSIDERATION

What questions would you ask Sydney to learn more about her potential for physical activity? What types of physical activity do you think she would like? How would you use goal setting and feedback to help Sydney reach her goals?

Case Studies 7.6 and 7.7 illustrate the variation in referral reasons and client factors. Recognizing these differences can help Personal Trainers to tailor interventions to each client's needs. Although both Sydney and Michael will benefit from goal setting and feedback, the style with which feedback is successfully and effectively delivered will likely vary between the two cases. In addition, Personal Trainers will need to utilize different strategies with Sydney and Michael in order to develop rapport. For example, talking with Sydney about playing clarinet in her high school band will most likely build rapport; however, that same discussion may not get very far with Michael. What are some other ways in which the interventions for Sydney and Michael might differ?

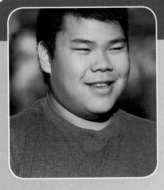

## Case Study 7.7

### Overweight Active Teenager

Michael is a 17-year-old boy who is overweight but muscular. He reports that he plays football and is active at practice but also has a big appetite. He is seeking the assistance of a Personal Trainer because his coach wants him to shave time off of his quarter mile over the summer. He also needs help improving his cardiovascular fitness and sticking to his routine. In the initial meeting, Michael is jovial and a little sarcastic. He says, "I am competitive but lazy."

#### QUESTIONS FOR CONSIDERATION

What questions would you ask Michael to learn more about what motivates him for physical activity? What types of physical activity or exercise do you think he would like? How would you use goal setting and feedback to help Michael reach her goals?

Michael will need more accountability than some because of his self-reported tendency to not complete tasks. Also, there may be additional challenges that Michael is facing besides his reported "laziness." Explore whether "laziness" may be a cover for issues such as anxiety, pain, etc. Michael may also respond well to challenge and competition — even if it is with himself and his past performance. Measurable, short-term goals and self-monitoring will be especially useful for Michael and should be emphasized. On the other hand, Sydney will need specific feedback in order to learn how to exercise in a way that is effective for her. Time and extra care will need to be spent building rapport so that she believes and trusts in the intervention and in herself. Attending to Sydney's past successes will help to build self-efficacy, and allowing her to choose her own activities will give her ownership of something she previously "did not like." Self-monitoring will likely be an effective tool for Sydney because she is conscientious and will likely be good at recording, which will build feelings of self-efficacy. Goal setting will also vary, based on each client's unique short- and long-term goals as well as situational constraints, like schedule, family situation, influence of friends, or access to facilities. What are some additional ways in which a Personal Trainer would tailor an intervention differently for Sydney or Michael?

## SUMMARY

As one can easily gather after reading this chapter, there are many different theories of behavior change, each with its own unique strengths and weaknesses. Although there is some overlap across theories, each represents a unique foundation and combination of principles and components (for a review, refer to Table 7.2). Although research exists to support various theories, it is up to the Personal Trainer to interpret empirical support and use expertise combined with the skills discussed within this chapter to decide which principles or components to apply with each individual client based on his or her unique needs and situational factors.

## REFERENCES

1. Ajzen I. The theory of planned behavior. *Organ Behav Hum Decis Process*. 1991;50:179–211.
2. American College of Sports Medicine. *ACSM's Guidelines for Exercise Testing and Prescription*. 10th ed. Philadelphia (PA): Wolters Kluwer; 2018.
3. Anderson-Bill ES, Winett RA, Wojcik JR, Winett SG. Web-based guide to health: relationship of theoretical variables to change in physical activity, nutrition, and weight at 16-months. *J Med Internet Res*. 2011;13(1):e27.
4. Armitage CJ, Connor M. Efficacy of the theory of planned behavior: a meta-analytic review. *Br J Soc Psychol*. 2001;40:471–99.
5. Armitage CJ, Sprigg CA. The roles of behavioral and implementation intentions in changing physical activity in young children with low socioeconomic status. *J Sport Exerc Psychol*. 2010;32:359–76.
6. Baban A, Craciun C. Changing health-risk behaviors: a review of theory and evidence-based interventions in health psychology. *J Cog Behav Psych*. 2007;7(1):45–67.
7. Bandura A. *Social Foundations of Thought and Action: A Social Cognitive Theory*. Englewood Cliffs (NJ): Prentice-Hall; 1986. 544 p.
8. Bovend'Eerdt TJH, Botell RE, Wade DT. Writing SMART rehabilitation goals and achieving goal attainment scaling: a practical guide. *Clin Rehabil*. 2009;23:352–61.
9. Carels RA, Darby LA, Rydin S, Douglass OM, Cacciapaglia HM, O'Brien WH. The relationship between self-monitoring, outcome expectancies, difficulties with eating and exercise, and physical activity and weight loss treatment outcomes. *Ann Behav Med*. 2005;30(3):182–90.
10. Carpenter CJ. A meta-analysis of the effectiveness of health belief model variables in predicting behavior. *Health Commun*. 2010;25(8):661–9.
11. Centers for Disease Control and Prevention. Health Consequences of Obesity [Internet]. Atlanta (GA): Centers for Disease Control and Prevention; [cited 2017 Feb 6]. Available from: https://www.cdc.gov/obesity/adult/causes.html
12. Conn VS, Valentine JC, Cooper HM. Interventions to increase physical activity among aging adults: a meta-analysis. *Ann Behav Med*. 2002;24(3):190–200.
13. Cooper Z, Fairburn CG. Cognitive-behavioral treatment of obesity. In: Wadden T, Stunkard A, editors. *Handbook of Obesity Treatment*. New York (NY): Guilford Press; 2002. p. 465–79.
14. Damshroder L, Lutes LD, Goodrich D, Gillon L, Lowery J. A small-change approach delivered via telephone promotes weight loss in veterans: results from the ASPIRE-VA pilot study. *Patient Educ Couns*. 2010;79(20):262–6.
15. Darker CD, French DP, Eves FF, Sniehotta FF. An intervention to promote walking amongst the general population

based on an "extended" theory of planned behaviour: a waiting list randomised controlled trial. *Psychol Health.* 2010; 25(1):71–88.

16. Dishman RK, Vandenberg RJ, Motl RW, Wilson MG, Dejoy DM. Does relations between goal setting, theory-based correlates of goal setting and increases in physical activity during a workplace trial. *Health Educ Res.* 2009;25(4):620–31.

17. Donaldson JM, Normand MP. Using goal setting, self-monitoring, and feedback to increase calorie expenditure in obese adults. *Behav Intervent.* 2009;24:73–83.

18. Estabrooks PA, Nelson CC, Xu S, et al. Frequency and behavioral outcomes of goal choices in the self-management of diabetes. *Diabetes Educ.* 2005;31(3):391–400.

19. Fjeldsoe B, Neuhaus M, Winkler E, Eakin E. Systematic review of maintenance of behavior change following physical activity and dietary interventions. *Health Psychol.* 2011;30(1):99–109.

20. Flegal KM, Kruszon-Moron D, Carroll MD, Fryar CD, Ogden CL. Trends in obesity among adults in the United States, 2005 to 2014. *JAMA.* 2016;315:2284–91.

21. Francis J, Michie S, Johnston M, Hardeman W, Eccles M. How do behaviour change techniques map on to psychological constructs? Results of a consensus process. *Psychol Health.* 2005;20:83–4.

22. Glanz K, Lewis FM, Rimmer BK, editors. *Health Behavior and Health Education: Theory, Research, and Practice.* 2nd ed. San Francisco (CA): John Wiley and Sons; 1997. 496 p.

23. Goldstein DJ. Beneficial health effects of modest weight loss. *Int J Obes Relat Metab Disord.* 1992;16:397–415.

24. Gollwitzer PM. Goal achievement: the role of intentions. *Eur Rev Soc Psychol.* 1993;4:141–85.

25. Heesch KC, Masse LC, Dunn AL, Frankowski RF, Dolan Mullen P. Does adherence to a lifestyle physical activity intervention predict changes in physical activity? *J Behav Med.* 2003;26(4):333–48.

26. Hutchinson AJ, Breckon JD, Johnston LH. Physical activity behavior change interventions based on the transtheoretical model: a systematic review. *Health Educ Behav.* 2009;36:829–45.

27. Institute of Medicine. *Weighing the Options: Criteria for Evaluating Weight-Management Programs.* Washington (DC): National Academy Press; 1995. 296 p.

28. Kennedy V. Ecomaps. *MAI Review.* 2010;3:1–12.

29. Kirk A, De Feo P. Strategies to enhance compliance to physical activity for patients with insulin resistance. *Appl Physiol Nutr Metab.* 2007;32(3):549–56.

30. Kiviniemi MT, Voss-Humke AM, Seifert AL. How do I feel about the behavior? The interplay of affective associations with behaviors and cognitive beliefs as influences on physical activity behavior. *Health Psychol.* 2007;26(6):152–8.

31. Lippke S, Ziegelman JP. Theory-based health behavior change: developing, testing, and applying theories for evidence-based interventions. *Applied Psychol.* 2008;57(4):698–716.

32. Locke EA, Latham GP. Building a practically useful theory of goal setting and task motivation. A 35-year odyssey. *American Psychol.* 2002;57(9):705–17.

33. Locke EA, Latham GP. The application of goal setting to sports. *Int J Sport Psychol.* 1985;7:205–22.

34. Lutes LD, Daiss S, Barger SD, Read M, Steinbaugh E, Winett RW. A small changes approach promotes initial and continued weight loss with a phone-based follow-up: 9-month results from ASPIRE II. *Am J Health Promot.* 2012; 26:235–8.

35. Lutes LD, Steinbaugh E. Theoretical models for pedometer use in physical activity interventions. *Physical Therapy Reviews.* 2010;15(3):143–53.

36. Lutes LD, Winett RA, Barger SD, et al. Small changes in nutrition and physical activity promotes weight loss and maintenance: 3-month evidence from the ASPIRE randomized trial. *Ann Behav Med.* 2008;35:351–7.

37. Maddison R, Hoorn SV, Jiang Y, et al. The environment and physical activity: the influence of psychosocial, perceived, and built environmental factors. *Int J Behav Nutr Phys Act.* 2009;6(19):1–11.

38. Michie S, Abraham C, Whittington C, McAteer J, Gupta S. Effective techniques in healthy eating and physical activity interventions: a meta-regression. *Health Psychol.* 2009;28(6):690–701.

39. Miller WR, Benefield RG, Tonigan JS. Enhancing motivation for change in problem drinking: a controlled comparison of two therapist styles. *J Consult Clin Psychol.* 1993; 61(3):455–61.

40. Napolitano MA, Papandonatos GD, Lewis BA, et al. Mediators of physical activity behavior change: a multivariate approach. *Health Psychol.* 2008;27(4):409–18.

41. Nigg CR, Borrelli B, Maddock J, Dishman RK. A theory of physical activity maintenance. *Applied Psychol.* 2008;57(4): 544–60.

42. Nigg CR, Geller KS, Motl RW, Horwath CC, Wertin KK, Dishman RK. A research agenda to examine the efficacy and relevance of the transtheoretical model for physical activity behavior. *Psychol Sport Exerc.* 2011;12:7–12.

43. Normand M. Increasing physical activity through self-monitoring, goal setting, and feedback. *Behav Intervent.* 2008;23:227–36.

44. O'Brien Cousins S. "My heart couldn't take it": older women's beliefs about exercise benefits and risks. *J Gerontol B Psychol Sci Soc Sci.* 2000;55(5):P283–94.

45. Prochaska JO, DiClemente CC. Stages and processes of self-change of smoking: toward an integrative model of change. *J Consult Clin Psychol.* 1983;51(3):390–5.

46. Prochaska JO, Velicer WF. The transtheoretical model of health behavior change. *Am J Health Promot.* 1997;12(1):38–48.

47. Rollnick S, Mason P, Butler C. Health Behavior Change: *A Guide for Practitioners.* London (United Kingdom): Churchill Livingstone; 1999. 240 p.

48. Rosenstock IM, Strecher VJ, Becker MH. Social learning theory and the health belief model. *Health Educ Q.* 1988; 15(2):175–83.

49. Rothman AJ. "Is there nothing more practical than a good theory?" Why innovations and advances in health behavior change will arise if interventions are used to test and refine theory. *Int J Behav Nutr Phys Act.* 2004;1(1):11.

50. Rovniak LS, Hovell MF, Wojcik JR, Winett RA, Martinez-Donate AP. Enhancing theoretical fidelity: an e-mail-based walking program demonstration. *Am J Health Promot.* 2005;20(2):85–95.

51. Ryan RM, Frederick CM, Lepes D, Rubio N, Sheldon KM. Intrinsic motivation and exercise adherence. *Int J Sport Psyc.* 1997;28:335–54.

52. Scott EJ, Eves FF, French DP, Hoppé R. The theory of planned behaviour predicts self-reports of walking, but does not predict step count. *Br J Health Psychol.* 2007;12(4):601–20.

53. Shilts MK, Horowitz M, Townsend MS. Goal setting as a strategy for dietary and physical activity behavior change: a review of the literature. *Am J Health Promot.* 2004;19(2):81–93.

54. Siegert RJ, Taylor WJ. Theoretical aspects of goal-setting and motivation in rehabilitation. *Disabil Rehabil.* 2004;26(1):1–8.

55. Vallance JK, Courneya KS, Taylor LM, Plotnikoff RC, Mackey JR. Development and evaluation of a theory-based physical activity guidebook for breast cancer survivors. *Health Educ Behav.* 2008;35(2):174–89.

56. Weiss EC, Galuska DA, Kettel Khan LK, Gillespie C, Serdula MK. Weight regain in U.S. adults who experienced substantial weight loss, 1999–2002. *Am J Prev Med.* 2007;33(1): 34–40.

57. Wilson DB, Porter JS, Parker G, Kilpatrick, J. Anthropometric changes using a walking intervention in African American breast cancer survivors: a pilot study. *Prev Chronic Dis.* 2005; 2(2):A16.

# Adherence to Exercise: Helping Your Client Stay Active

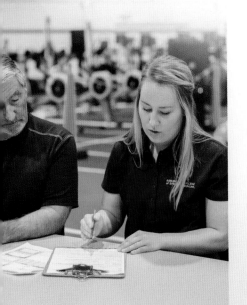

## OBJECTIVES

**Personal Trainers should be able to:**

■ Identify factors that contribute to client adherence to exercise and apply appropriate behavior change strategies to promote adherence among clients.

■ Understand and apply health behavior change models to support and facilitate exercise adherence and apply appropriate strategies to build clients' self-efficacy, motivation, and self-worth related to exercise.

■ Identify barriers to exercise and assist clients in developing strategies to overcome these barriers and avoid relapse.

■ Develop skills to encourage clients to self-regulate their exercise and effectively collaborate with the client to set behavioral goals.

■ Recognize clients' need for social support, create a supportive environment, and teach clients how to access additional forms of support.

■ Identify and apply innovative strategies clients can use to adhere to exercise, such as technology, active transportation, or community-based programs.

# INTRODUCTION

Behavior-change theory, covered in Chapter 7, helped clarify why some people are inactive, others start and stop exercise repeatedly, and still others are able to continue an exercise program indefinitely. This chapter takes behavior-change theory one step further and focuses on tactics to increase client adherence to exercise.

One of the biggest frustrations of Personal Trainers is failing to persuade their clients to adhere to a program that took a significant amount of time to develop. Because the health benefits of regular exercise are often not realized until at least 6 months of continuous participation (1,2), researchers often equate *adherence* with the maintenance stage of the transtheoretical model's (TTM) stages of change (25,43,45,82). Therefore, in this chapter, adherence refers to at least 6 months of continuous participation in exercise.

> Health benefits of regular exercise are often not realized by clients until at least 6 months of continuous participation.

As a Personal Trainer, a large portion of the job is to equip clients with the skills necessary to adhere to exercise. Adherence is important because approximately 50% of people who begin an exercise program drop out within the first 6 months (22). This chapter will focus on identifying factors that contribute to exercise adherence and on designing and implementing strategies that will enhance adherence to exercise. The case studies at the end of this chapter illustrate the factors related to exercise adherence and how strategies can be applied to each client in helping him or her adhere.

Because clients may have different physical, psychological, and environmental obstacles to or reasons for exercise (18,21), understanding the attitudes, values, meanings, and experiences that each client associates with exercise and applying appropriate strategies based on these associations with exercise are extremely important to a client's continued success in an exercise program (68). For example, a client may have no problem scheduling time to exercise but may lack the supportive environment necessary to adhere to exercise, or vice versa. Mastering the ability to "read" clients and teach them to apply strategies to adhere to exercise is critical to the Personal Trainer's ability to help clients succeed. Trainers who are able to master these skills will not only help clients adhere to exercise but will also improve their own reputations as trainers. Table 8.1 identifies numerous factors that may impact adherence, such as outcome expectancy values, major life events, and intensity of exercise (23,82).

> Understanding the attitudes, values, meanings, and experiences clients associate with exercising and then teaching them the appropriate strategies to adhere to exercise based on these factors will contribute to the success of both the client and the Personal Trainer.

Chapter 7 outlined behavior-change theory–based approaches for helping clients adopt exercise, and many of these same approaches used to enhance adoption may help an individual adhere to exercise (24,34). Approaches to promoting exercise adherence that do *not* include theory-based cognitive and behavioral strategies may not be as successful as those rooted in theory (23,34). This section of this chapter discusses three of the strongest theory-based concepts related to exercise adherence: self-efficacy, motivation for exercise, and self-worth (5,82). After these concepts are introduced, strategies to help clients improve their self-efficacy, motivation, and self-worth, and thereby exercise adherence, are discussed. The final section of this chapter introduces additional innovative strategies the Personal Trainer can use to further improve clients' exercise adherence and overall physical activity.

| Table 8.1 | Factors Related to Adherence | |
|---|---|---|
| **Factors Related to Adherence** | **Definition** | **Related** |
| Self-efficacy[a] | Individual's confidence to successfully complete exercise | Perceived barriers, social support |
| Motivation[a] | Extrinsic — exercising for weight loss of appearance<br>Intrinsic — exercising for enjoyment or accomplishment | Social support, self-regulation |
| Self-worth[a] | Satisfaction individuals have with themselves | Self-regulation, perceived barriers, social support |
| Perceived barriers[a] | Numerous factors that impair individual's belief that they can exercise | Self-efficacy, motivation, self-regulation, social support, outcome expectancy values |
| Self-regulation[a] | Strategies for planning, organizing, and managing exercise activities to "stay on track" | Environment |
| Social support[a] | Exchange of aid or assistance among individuals or groups within a social network; includes family support, Personal Trainer support, and support from group dynamics in group-based exercise programs | Self-efficacy, motivation, self-worth |
| Environment[a] | May include access to facilities, weather, neighborhood environment, or where the exercise takes place | Self-efficacy, perceived barriers, self-regulation |
| Self-schemata | Individual's self-image about exercise | |
| Outcome expectancy values | How much the individual values the expected outcome | Self-efficacy |
| Duration and intensity | Length of time spent active and how hard clients work | Self-efficacy, motivation |
| Type of physical activity | The type of physical activity that clients participate in | |
| Major life events | Events in a client's life that impact his or her daily routine (*i.e.*, getting married, death in the family) | Perceived barriers, self-regulation |
| Program tailoring | Having a program that is in accordance with the client's TTM stage of change | |

[a]Discussed in this chapter.

# Self-Efficacy, Motivation, and Self-Worth in Relationship to Exercise Adherence

## Self-Efficacy and Exercise Adherence

Research in physical activity and exercise has identified self-efficacy as one of the most consistent predictors of exercise adherence among adults (46,49,50,57,83). Self-efficacy refers to an individual's confidence in his or her ability to successfully complete a specific behavior (3). Self-efficacy for a specific behavior influences the activities in which that individual chooses to participate. In other words, the higher the self-efficacy, the more effort an individual puts forth toward the activity, and the more persistent he or she is in participating in the behavior — despite barriers and failures (49). When working with clients to build self-efficacy, it is important for the Personal Trainer to understand that self-efficacy may impact clients' abilities to complete tasks (exercise), overcome barriers, and achieve goals. Later in this chapter, strategies to help clients improve their self-efficacy will be discussed. These strategies include teaching clients how to overcome barriers, regulate exercise behaviors, and access social support. These strategies can help clients develop their self-efficacy, motivation for exercise and self-worth, and may, therefore, help them to adhere to exercise (5,82).

> Self-efficacy, a strong predictor of exercise adherence, refers to an individual's confidence in his or her ability to successfully complete a specific task or adhere to a specific behavior.

## Motivation and Exercise Adherence

A client may initially be highly motivated to exercise, but if his or her main goal is to dazzle classmates at a 20-year class reunion, what will continue to motivate him or her after the event is over? When clients are extrinsically motivated, they participate in exercise to achieve external outcomes, such as weight loss and appearance. When clients are intrinsically motivated, they participate in exercise to achieve internal outcomes, such as enjoyment of the activity itself, the feeling of accomplishment after the workout is completed, or the challenge it provides.

Both extrinsic and intrinsic motivations are associated with the self-determination theory (SDT). SDT suggests that certain psychological needs have to be satisfied in order to internalize extrinsic motivation and to become intrinsically motivated. These needs are the following: autonomy (the desire to be responsible for choosing the behavior in which you participate), relatedness (the desire to be connected to others and feel understood by others), and competence (the belief that you are able to complete a specific behavior in order to reach your goal) (19,20). SDT works on a continuum where motivation can range from not have any motivation to being intrinsically motivated. Research has shown that intrinsic motivation and more internalized (*i.e.*, autonomous) forms of extrinsic motivation contribute to exercise adherence (39,73). In other words, clients who personally value and enjoy exercise and find exercise personally challenging are more likely to adhere to exercise (64–66).

In most cases, a client will initially be more extrinsically motivated than intrinsically motivated to participate in exercise. Therefore, strategies that shift individuals' motivations toward intrinsic motivation and autonomy may be essential components of each client's training program (66). Later in this chapter, information is provided relative to encouraging clients to be autonomous, feel connected with others, and improve their competence by teaching strategies for overcoming barriers, setting their own goals, monitoring their exercise, and associating with supportive people and environments. It is important to note, however, that if clients do not value themselves, they may lack the self-efficacy and/or intrinsic motivation to successfully carry out these tasks and ultimately to adhere to exercise. The next section introduces the concept of self-worth and its relationship to self-efficacy, motivation, and exercise adherence.

## Self-Worth and Exercise Adherence

The Personal Trainer can help clients increase their intrinsic motivation for exercise by improving their feelings of autonomy (*e.g.*, letting clients take an active role in designing their exercise plan), relatedness to others (*e.g.*, striving to know clients better by being an empathetic and active listener; see Chapter 9), and competence (*e.g.*, helping clients to slowly and successfully maintain all aspects of their exercise regimen).

Self-worth is often used interchangeably with self-esteem and refers to the satisfaction individuals have with themselves (48). Research provides evidence that exercise and self-worth work interchangeably; that is, increased self-worth leads to increased participation in exercise and vice versa (27,36). Helping a client improve his or her self-worth may be helpful not only for adopting exercise but also for adhering to it long term (38). Therefore, implementing strategies that enhance self-worth at the outset of a client's training is critical to his or her eventual adherence to exercise.

When thinking about how a client can enhance his or her self-worth, it is important for the Personal Trainer to consider principles related to self-efficacy and intrinsic motivation. Not only improvements in self-efficacy may increase self-worth (30,51), but continued improvements to self-worth may also positively impact individuals' self-efficacy. This reciprocal relationship between self-worth and self-efficacy contributes to continued participation in exercise. First, the changes in self-efficacy a client experiences as a result of participating in exercise may also effect changes in self-worth (35,51). In other words, as individuals gain confidence in their ability to exercise on a regular basis, they may feel better about themselves as well. Second, the emotional responses an individual has in relation to his or her participation in exercise may strengthen his or her feelings of self-efficacy for exercise (50). Feeling good about oneself, or increased self-worth, as a result of exercise, successfully overcoming barriers, or achieving exercise-related goals may contribute to an individual's self-efficacy for exercise (38,47,51). These improvements to both factors of adherence are important because clients with enhanced self-worth and self-efficacy often prioritize themselves over other demands in order to participate in exercise and ultimately better adhere to exercise long term (35,38). Similarly, a client's self-worth may also be related to his or her reasons, or motivations, for participating in exercise (69,71). Research suggests that individuals who value themselves and their quality of life more so than weight loss or changes in appearance (*i.e.*, have high levels of self-worth and have intrinsically motivated goals) are more likely to adhere to exercise (27,36,38,69).

Finally, when implementing self-worth–enhancing strategies with clients, it is imperative that Personal Trainers consider their clients' past experiences and values. Self-worth represents the individual's *perception* of how well the self is doing (30); therefore, past, present, and future experiences and values related to exercise will affect how clients feel about themselves. As mentioned previously, clients will have different combinations of obstacles to and reasons for exercise, which may include their self-worth. No general prescription for exercise adherence exists; therefore, the Personal Trainer must learn how to identify clients' obstacles to and reasons for exercise and apply appropriate strategies to improve adherence *on an individual basis*. The rest of this chapter describes various strategies the Personal Trainer can use to directly and indirectly improve clients' exercise adherence by targeting improvements to clients' self-efficacy, motivation, and self-worth.

Self-worth refers to the satisfaction individuals have with themselves and works reciprocally with both self-efficacy and intrinsic motivation to enhance exercise adherence. Self-worth promoting strategies are a critical part of a client's training program and should be implemented throughout the program.

## Strategies for Increasing Exercise Adherence

It is logical that building a client's self-efficacy, motivation (including autonomy, relatedness, and competence), and self-worth may contribute to his or her adherence to exercise. But exactly *how* can the Personal Trainer impact a client's self-efficacy, motivation for exercise, and self-worth? Given

Effective strategies for improving adherence include overcoming barriers to exercise, self-regulating exercise, and accessing social support for exercise.

the relationships among these three factors of adherence, the Personal Trainer can use a multitude of strategies to target any and all of these factors. Three of the most effective strategies Personal Trainers can use to improve clients' adherence include teaching clients how to overcome barriers, regulate exercise behaviors, and access social support. This section outlines (a) these specific theory-based adherence strategies; (b) the strategies' relationships to self-efficacy, motivation for exercise, and/or self-worth; and (c) application of these strategies to the case studies. The tables in this chapter outline additional strategies Personal Trainers can use to help their individual clients adhere to exercise.

## Overcoming Barriers

Barriers are specific to each client and represent individuals' perceived obstacles to exercise (53). Clients may simply not know how to overcome barriers or may have low self-efficacy and/or self-worth for overcoming barriers. Personal Trainers can help their clients overcome barriers to exercise by ensuring clients understand their personal benefits of exercise and perceived barriers to exercise. Using the benefits and barriers each client identifies, the Personal Trainer and client can work together to develop strategies the client can use to overcome each barrier and successfully adhere to exercise. The following sections provide more information on the Personal Trainer's role in helping clients understand their benefits of exercise, their barriers to exercise, and ways to overcome barriers.

### Benefits of Exercise

Individuals who perceive that the benefits of exercise outweigh the barriers to exercise are more likely to continue to exercise (35,37,76). The Personal Trainer may initially teach the client about the physiological and psychological benefits of exercise when clients are adopting exercise. Chapter 13 more thoroughly describes the benefits clients may receive from participation in exercise. When focusing on exercise adherence, the Personal Trainer and his or her client may need to periodically review the client's perceived benefits, as these may change over time (7,45). For example, a client initially focused on exercise for weight loss may begin to understand the emotional benefits, such as increased self-worth or quality of life (14), after participating in exercise for several weeks or months. Although continued acknowledgment of the client's perceived benefits of exercise is important, the focus for clients who are working on adhering to exercise (as opposed to adopting exercise) will primarily be on identifying barriers to continued exercise and developing strategies to overcome these barriers. The Personal Trainer's guidance in relation to overcoming barriers may be crucial to the clients' adherence to exercise.

### Barrier Identification

It is important for the Personal Trainer to note that, like benefits, barriers may differ between clients depending on various factors such as gender, age, weight status, fitness level, and history with exercise. Barriers may be personal, social, or environmental in nature (60) and include obstacles such as a lack of time, motivation, confidence, or social support; family and social expectations; temptations and high-risk situations (*e.g.*, friends inviting a client out for dinner/drinks during scheduled gym time); and an inability to prioritize one's own needs over the needs of others (28,44,55,60). After achieving a better understanding of clients' personal benefits of exercise, the Personal Trainer can not only help clients identify their barriers to exercise but also show them that with some effort and commitment by the client, barriers can be easily overcome. Clients who are able to increase their self-efficacy for overcoming barriers during exercise programs may demonstrate improvements to their self-worth and are more likely to adhere to exercise (38,48,51,83). The following paragraphs outline the three major categories of barriers to exercise — personal, social, and environmental — and strategies the Personal Trainer and his or her clients can use to overcome these barriers.

## Personal Barriers

Personal barriers are individual-level barriers that may be internal or behavioral (76). Examples of personal barriers include lack of time, motivation, knowledge, injury, and extrinsic motivation for exercise. The Personal Trainer can develop strategies with his or her clients to help clients better manage time, assist clients with goal setting to increase enjoyment and motivation, and teach clients about fitness concepts and the benefits of exercise to increase knowledge. The Personal Trainer can also assure clients of his or her fitness credentials and take clients through programs slowly if clients have a fear of injury or are recovering from an injury or illness. Additionally, Personal Trainers can help clients build their self-efficacy and self-worth through intrinsic goal setting and accomplishment of these goals, mastery experiences, social persuasion, and social modeling. Goal setting is discussed in-depth later in this chapter.

First, providing clients with opportunities to successfully complete challenging, but attainable tasks and goals can help them to master experiences, thereby increasing their self-efficacy for exercise. For example, when developing a workout for a client, the Personal Trainer might challenge the client while still considering the client's current fitness level. Performing the task (*e.g.,* the workout) successfully can strengthen a client's self-efficacy; however, the Personal Trainer must also use caution when challenging clients, as failing to master tasks can weaken a client's self-efficacy (3). Second, one of the Personal Trainer's most important roles is often as the client's motivator. Persuading the client to believe that he or she is capable of accomplishing tasks can help the client to build his or her self-efficacy for overcoming barriers, which may also lead to improvements to the client's self-worth. For example, verbally persuading a client that he or she can successfully incorporate exercise into his or her daily routine, despite time barriers, may help the client build confidence to overcome barriers and continue to participate in exercise (3). Finally, providing the client with anecdotal examples of other clients' experiences or the Personal Trainer's own experiences related to overcoming barriers can serve as forms of social modeling that can help clients build their self-efficacy. For example, if a client can relate to someone similar who has successfully overcome barriers, he or she may feel more capable of overcoming his or her barriers, thereby increasing self-efficacy and exercise adherence (3). Specific examples illustrating how the Personal Trainer can utilize goal setting, mastery experiences, social persuasion, and social modeling to help clients build their self-efficacy and self-worth, and overcome personal barriers are located in Table 8.2.

## Social Barriers

Social barriers are barriers that arise in relation to an individual's social network. A social network refers to the group of significant individuals (*e.g.,* close family and friends) in the client's social life (80). Examples of social barriers include caregiving, especially childcare, lack of social support, and sociocultural barriers, such as cultural values regarding gender roles and accepted behaviors. One strategy that Personal Trainers can use is teaching clients home-based exercises or how to engage family members in activity to alleviate barriers related to caregiving. Additionally, understanding what types of social support clients need and teaching them how and where to access this support within or outside of their social networks may help them achieve the support required to adhere to exercise.

| Table 8.2 | Personal, Social, and Environmental Barriers to Exercise |
|---|---|
| **Barrier** | **Strategies to Overcome Barrier** |
| **Personal** | |
| Lack of time | ■ Ask clients to document how they use their time for 1 week and identify areas where they can incorporate exercise.<br>■ Encourage clients to utilize active transportation and make active lifestyle choices (*e.g.*, bike to work, take the stairs).<br>■ Explain to clients that several smaller bouts of exercise (10 min each) can be as effective as one longer bout of exercise.<br>■ Work with the client to help them schedule exercise in their schedules that is realistic. |
| Lack of motivation | ■ Discuss with clients their reasons for hiring a Personal Trainer and for exercising.<br>■ Encourage clients to use self-regulating strategies, such as stimulus control, to make it easier for them to be active.<br>■ Help clients to find activities in which they enjoy participating. |
| Lack of energy | ■ Discuss with clients the benefits of exercise, including increased energy.<br>■ Ask clients what time of day they think they could consistently participate in exercise.<br>■ Discuss clients' diet with them to ensure that they have energy for exercise.<br>■ Encourage clients to employ strategies, such as driving straight to the gym from work. |
| Lack of knowledge about exercise | ■ Utilize "teaching moments" during clients' exercise programs to increase their knowledge of fitness concepts to increase intrinsic motivation by increasing competence. |
| Dislike of sweating or vigorous exercise | ■ Encourage clients to exercise for longer durations at lower intensities.<br>■ Ensure that clients understand that exercising at lower intensities can still provide health benefits.<br>■ Teach clients about the benefits of vigorous exercise.<br>■ Slowly integrate high-intensity exercises into clients' programs to build their intrinsic motivation for vigorous exercise. |
| Physical barriers (*e.g.*, obesity, injury, disease) | ■ Help clients to increase their exercise gradually.<br>■ Provide clients with workouts that do not exacerbate any preexisting or past conditions.<br>■ Discuss with clients the benefits of exercise, as physical barriers may be accompanied by fear.<br>■ Develop goals with clients and discuss with them the plan to achieve these goals. |
| Biological barriers (*e.g.*, puberty, pregnancy, aging) | ■ Understand that certain biological changes may affect clients' current or past participation in exercise. Tailor exercise programs to meet clients' needs and refer to an exercise specialist when necessary.<br>■ Tailor exercise programs to meet the clients' needs and work directly with the client's health care provider.<br>■ Refer to a medical provider when necessary. |

| Table 8.2 | Personal, Social, and Environmental Barriers to Exercise *(continued)* |
|---|---|
| **Barrier** | **Strategies to Overcome Barrier** |
| Poor body image | ▪ Discuss with clients the health and psychological benefits of exercise, as opposed to weight loss/maintenance.<br>▪ Help clients develop goals and rewards not related to weight loss.<br>▪ Encourage clients to recognize qualities they like about themselves, including body and non-body–related attributes.<br>▪ Utilize strategies to build clients' self-worth. |
| Extrinsic motivation | ▪ Clients with extrinsic goals may be discouraged by lack of results or become complacent once extrinsic goals are met. Help clients to develop their intrinsic motivation for exercise.<br>▪ Make clients aware of the long-term effectiveness of intrinsic goals compared to the short-term effectiveness of extrinsic goals, such as weight loss. |
| Past experience(s) with exercise | ▪ Discuss with clients their past experiences (both good and bad) with exercise before starting a training program.<br>▪ Consider each client's past experiences in developing exercise programs to ensure that programs and goals support the development of self-efficacy and self-worth.<br>▪ Concentrate on what successes they had previously had with exercise or a similar behavior change to help increase a level of mastery and self-efficacy. |
| Fear of injury | ▪ Make clients aware of credentials and credentials of related fitness professionals (*e.g.*, group exercise instructors).<br>▪ Communicate with clients throughout the exercise program.<br>▪ Slowly progress clients as their fitness levels increase. |
| **Social** | |
| Family/friend/work obligations | ▪ Encourage clients to have serious discussions with family and close friends to discuss their needs and goals.<br>▪ Teach clients how to access the tangible social support they may need to allay these obligations.<br>▪ Discuss priorities with clients to identify any instances in which obligations are self-imposed (*e.g.*, saying "yes" to everyone who asks). |
| Lack of social support | ▪ Encourage clients to have serious discussions with family and close friends to discuss their needs and goals.<br>▪ Ask clients to identify the social support they need to exercise. Then, discuss various methods of accessing this support.<br>▪ Help clients to identify activities they can do with their friends and family, that is, activities their friends and family enjoy. |
| Culturally inappropriate activities and gender role expectations | ▪ Gender roles can vary by family, age, and culture. Be aware of differences in obligations between men and women. Help clients to develop strategies for overcoming barriers that fit into their lifestyle and belief system. |

*(continued)*

| Table 8.2 | Personal, Social, and Environmental Barriers to Exercise (continued) |
|---|---|
| **Barrier** | **Strategies to Overcome Barrier** |
| **Environmental** | |
| Lack of access to programs or facilities; cost of programs and facilities | ■ Give clients active transport, lifestyle, home, and outdoor activity ideas they can use outside of training sessions.<br>■ Prepare clients to become independent in their exercise behaviors, including teaching them about relapse prevention.<br>■ Help clients become aware of free exercise opportunities within the community.<br>■ Provide clients with the names of exercise DVDs they can use at home. |
| Safety concerns — absence of sidewalks or bike lanes, unsafe neighborhood, heavy traffic | ■ Help clients identify parks or other quiet places in which they can exercise.<br>■ Use strategies for accessing social support to help clients learn how to enlist friends/family to exercise with them.<br>■ Provide clients with a list of affordable home equipment options and provide exercises that can be used with the equipment |
| Bad weather | ■ Teach clients to develop contingency plans so that they have backup plans for each workout.<br>■ Teach clients how to plan for varying weather conditions. Discuss with them the appropriate clothing/apparel they should wear in extreme temperatures. |
| Lack of shower facilities | ■ Provide clients with low-intensity activity options and activities they can do in short bouts. |

### Environmental Barriers

Environmental barriers are physical barriers, often outside of the individual's control, that prevent him or her from being active. Examples of environmental barriers include lack of access to exercise facilities, bad weather, and safety concerns (*e.g.*, absence of sidewalks or bike lanes, crime) (40,60). Providing clients with opportunities to be active outside of the gym, at their homes, or within their daily lifestyles can help them overcome barriers related to lack of access (25). The Personal Trainer can use the self-regulation strategies presented in this chapter to help clients successfully plan for exercise in anticipation of barriers that may upset their exercise plan, such as bad weather. Safety can be a major concern for clients living in all different types of areas (26,40); therefore, the Personal Trainer can help clients find safe walking and cycling routes and structured community-based programs in which they can participate in exercise with other members of their communities. Additional strategies on how the Personal Trainer can help teach clients how to utilize their physical environment to increase their activity instead of viewing the environment as a barrier are provided at the end of this chapter in the "Innovative Strategies to Increase Adherence" section.

Barriers may be personal, social, or environmental. Individuals who are able to increase their self-efficacy for overcoming barriers may be more likely to adhere to exercise. Strategies for overcoming barriers to exercise should be tailored toward each client's specific barriers.

Table 8.2 lists examples of personal, social, and environmental barriers commonly reported by adults and strategies to help clients overcome these barriers. It is important to note that the Personal Trainer can use similar strategies for targeting different types of barriers. For example,

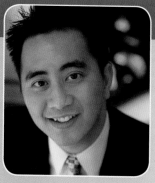

## Case Study 8.1

### Increasing Adherence by Identifying Barriers to Exercise (and Solutions)

Troy recently received a gift certificate for personal training from his mother for Christmas. She thinks that he is getting too heavy and that a Personal Trainer may help him get back into shape. Troy was active in high school and college, playing intramural sports; however, now that he has a full-time job, staying active isn't as easy. Prior to meeting with his Personal Trainer, Troy did not exercise at all and had put on a considerable amount of weight since college. Troy knows he has gained weight, but he's not into going to the gym because he doesn't really enjoy it. Additionally, he is often pressured by his friends to go out for drinks after work, so it's hard for him to stay on track. His mom has been pressuring him to go to the gym to help him find the skills to lose weight.

#### QUESTIONS FOR CONSIDERATION

What types of questions can you ask Troy to learn more about why he has so much trouble adhering to exercise? What barriers do you think play a role in his inability to adhere to exercise? Are there things you can teach him that may help improve his adherence (*e.g.*, identifying time management issues, self-regulation strategies)? Do you think helping him change from extrinsic motivation to intrinsic motivation will help? What strategies can you use to increase his intrinsic motivation?

helping clients to build self-efficacy by mastering experiences may be a strategy used for personal, social, and environmental barriers alike. Creating a similar table with clients may help them identify their individual barriers to exercise and strategies for overcoming these barriers. Barriers to exercise may also change over time within the same client; therefore, periodically using the table to reevaluate barriers with clients may help them develop new strategies for overcoming barriers. The bottom line is that individuals who are able to successfully overcome barriers will develop high self-efficacy for overcoming barriers and become more likely to continue to exercise over time (48). An example of how to help a client overcome barriers to exercise is found in Case Study 8.1.

## Exercise Self-Regulation

Although a client's motivation for exercise is an important predictor of exercise adherence, motivation alone is often not enough to succeed in adhering to exercise (63). Developing additional skills related to exercise self-regulation is necessary to increase exercise adherence. Individuals may *intend* to exercise, but the emergence of barriers and non-exercise–related temptations can make it difficult for them to choose exercise (67). Exercise self-regulation involves strategies for planning, organizing, and managing exercise activities in order to "stay on track." Exercise self-regulation strategies include planning exercise, setting exercise-related goals, self-monitoring exercise behavior, and avoiding relapse (63).

### Planning Exercise

As mentioned earlier, barriers to exercise can be serious inhibitors to exercise adherence. Therefore, in addition to learning strategies for overcoming barriers, clients must learn how to develop a plan for exercise (69). Planning is extremely important because it can help clients get into the habit of exercising regularly, and regular exercise contributes to a simultaneous increase in both self-efficacy and exercise adherence (51,82). Additionally, understanding the client's weekly schedule and commitments and helping them find the best or most realistic days/times to exercise may assist in their exercise adherence.

There are several strategies that can be used to plan for exercise. Specifically, the Personal Trainer can teach clients how to (a) manage their time in order to schedule exercise, (b) develop backup plans in case of unavoidable conflicts, (c) plan their workouts *before* arriving at the gym, (d) implement cues to action to control outside stimuli (*i.e.*, temptations and barriers) and make adherence easier, and (e) identify a variety of ways to be active. Time management is extremely important because clients may tell the Personal Trainer that they do not have enough time for exercise. Asking clients to keep a log of how they spend their time for a day, few days, or an entire week may help them identify areas during the day in which exercise can be incorporated (33). Because life can be unpredictable at times, backup plans are essential to a client's exercise plan. Backup plans make it easier for a client to adhere because plans B and C are in place *before* plan A fails. Additionally, if a client does not have a workout plan before exercising, it may be difficult for him or her to meet exercise goals. The Personal Trainer can help clients understand the importance of having a plan for each workout.

Next, clients can practice stimulus control by putting planned cues to action in place to overcome barriers to exercise. Stimulus control refers to the idea of modifying the client's environment so that it is conducive to making choices that support exercise (18). For example, a client who lacks motivation for exercise might lay his or her exercise clothes out before going to bed at night as a positive cue for exercising. Likewise, a client reporting lack of time as a major barrier to exercise may need help in identifying points during the day when he or she can exercise. It is most important for the Personal Trainer to work with clients to develop specific strategies to control stimuli in order to help them successfully adhere to exercise. Finally, resources can be provided to help clients identify a variety of ways they can become active, such as choosing group fitness classes, enrolling in community programs, registering for events (*e.g.*, a 5-K run), or enlisting friends to exercise with them. Find out what planning strategies each client needs and use the ideas earlier — with other newly developed strategies — to help clients successfully plan exercise.

> Teach clients how to (a) manage their time in order to schedule exercise, (b) develop backup plans in case of unavoidable conflicts, (c) plan their workouts *before* arriving at the gym, (d) control stimuli to make adherence easier, and (e) identify a variety of ways to be active.

### Avoiding Relapse

Chapter 7 described how individuals move through the stages of change within the TTM as they consider exercise behavior. Ideally, individuals move through these stages of behavior change, ultimately reaching maintenance (*i.e.*, adherence) (58). However, even after reaching the maintenance stage of change, psychological factors and high-risk situations, such as expectations of exercise, life events (*e.g.*, births, death in family), holidays, and injuries; decreased social support; and decreased motivation for exercise can impact continued adherence to exercise (6,9,43,81). Factors such as these may cause a lapse (brief period of two or more weeks without exercise) or relapse (complete return to sedentary behavior) in exercise adherence (16). Unfortunately, most adults encounter relapse at some point during their participation in exercise (52). The psychological impact of relapse can negatively influence self-efficacy and self-worth (41). Therefore, talking to clients about relapse *before* it occurs may better prepare them to maintain their participation in exercise (16). Teaching clients that lapses and relapses do not equal failure may not only help them to stay active but may also help them to maintain their self-efficacy and self-worth (45). Understanding the fact that clients may move forward and backward along the TTM is important. Part of the role of the Personal Trainer is being able to provide strategies to prevent any backward slide or relapse in order to assist the client in staying on track with their exercise.

To help clients adhere to exercise and avoid relapse, Personal Trainers may discuss potential situations *before* they occur in order to prepare the client for high-risk situations.

Personal Trainers can help clients commit to an exercise regimen by teaching them the importance of remaining vigilant in their self-regulation of and participation in exercise (45). Discussing expectations for exercise with clients and working with clients to set intrinsic, achievable goals are also important to the improvement of self-efficacy and prevention of relapse (16). Personal Trainers can also ask clients to identify situations that may lead to lapse or relapse and work with clients to develop plans for staying active in these situations. The commitment to exercise the client develops will encourage forming habits related to regular exercise and ultimately limit his or her potential for lapse and/or relapse (45). In addition, if a client plans to discontinue personal training in the near future, the Personal Trainer might discuss how exercise can be continued without his or her help. Utilizing strategies related to self-regulating exercise and overcoming barriers will equip clients with the coping skills they may need to effectively deal with relapse if or when it occurs (43).

### Goal Setting

Goals give action and meaning to behavior, in addition to directing behavior (69). Goal setting must be a collaborative partnership between the Personal Trainer and client. Giving clients the opportunity to make decisions about their goals related to exercise may help them increase their autonomy related to exercise and their competence in goal setting, thus increasing their self-efficacy and helping them to become more intrinsically motivated for exercise. Teaching clients how to properly set goals is especially important if the client's initial motivations for hiring a personal trainer are extrinsically focused (*e.g.*, weight loss, appearance).

A client who focuses on exercising for extrinsic reasons may struggle to adhere to exercise because of lower levels of self-efficacy and self-worth as a result of not meeting extrinsic goals (*e.g.*, not losing the weight they intended to lose) or of losing motivation after meeting extrinsic goals (*e.g.*, losing the weight they intended for a one-time event/reason). Clients often do not know what to do next because they have lost the weight they set out to lose and often fall into relapse because of this extrinsic orientation toward exercise (69). In addition, individuals with extrinsic goals may not value exercise over other intrinsically motivated behaviors or preferred leisure pursuits, such as spending time with family and friends or reading (60,71), and may, therefore, choose other behaviors before exercise. Alternately, a client who is intrinsically motivated to exercise (*i.e.*, enjoyment, feeling good) is more apt to demonstrate improvements to their self-worth and continue exercise participation long term (36,69,82).

The best way for the Personal Trainer to help clients become intrinsically motivated for exercise and set intrinsically motivated goals that will work is to use the SMART goal philosophy (18). The SMART goal philosophy recommends that goals be specific, measureable, achievable, relevant, and time-sensitive (13,60). A goal is specific in that it states *exactly* what the client aims to achieve (*e.g.*, I will participate in a *triathlon*). A goal is measurable in that it can be quantified (*e.g.*, I will run *four times* this week). The achievability of a goal is also related to how realistic the goal is for each particular client. For example, a client with extrinsic motivations for exercise may tell his or her Personal Trainer that he or she wants to lose a significant amount of weight during a short period of time. It is the Personal Trainer's responsibility to educate their clients about realistic goals in order to help clients build and/or maintain their self-efficacy and self-worth toward goal setting. A goal is relevant if it is related to the overall goal set by the client (*e.g.*, I will *run* four times a week to be ready for the *triathlon*). Finally, a goal is time-sensitive in that it has a target end date (*e.g.*, I will participate in a triathlon *in 6 months*). The time-sensitivity of a goal is also related to its achievability (13). The Personal Trainer can help clients understand that reaching exercise-related goals will take time and commitment. Setting SMART goals will help clients more effectively plan and monitor exercise, and, as they develop goal-setting skills, they may feel more autonomous and successful as exercisers (69–71).

Give clients the opportunity to make decisions about their goals related to exercise to help them increase their autonomy related to exercise and their competence in goal setting. Teach clients how to set SMART goals: smart (precise, specific), measurable (quantifiable), achievable (action oriented, what needs done), relevant (realistic, achievable), and time-sensitive (realistic time frame).

The SMART goal philosophy can be applied to the development of both long- and short-term goals. Long-term goals represent the client's overall objective for hiring a Personal Trainer and for exercise, while short-term goals serve as intermediary objectives through which the overall long-term goal can be achieved (45). Each exercise program should include teaching the client to recognize the importance of starting slowly using short-term goals that stay focused on the long-term goal (45). For example, for a client who wishes to participate in a triathlon in 6 months, short-term goals related to the frequency, duration, and intensity of running, cycling, swimming, and resistance training are key to the client's achievement of his or her long-term goal. It is also essential that the Personal Trainer and client periodically reevaluate goals, the client's progress toward goals, and his or her motivations for exercise. With this information in hand, Personal Trainers can modify or refocus short-term goals (and sometimes long-term goals), which is essential for a client's continued progress, achievement of long-term goals, and ultimately adherence (54).

### Self-Monitoring

Monitoring behavior, including the actions and feelings that an individual associates with exercise, can help a client stay on track and adhere to exercise (63). Several tools, including wearable technology, mobile phone applications, the Internet, workout logs, and heart-rate monitors may help clients adhere to exercise (62). Monitoring tools, such as pedometers, show some evidence as motivators for exercise; however, their effectiveness in promoting exercise adherence is equivocal (77).

When working with clients, the Personal Trainer can develop a self-monitoring plan that fits into each client's lifestyle. For example, clients may not be willing to commit to recording their exercise in a workout log, but they may find it easy to work with a mobile phone application in which they can view exercise time, distance traveled or step counts, and average heart rate. Many fitness professionals utilize the Internet to stay connected with clients (79). This not only provides clients with additional social support but also allows them to use online tools, such as blogs and online workout logs, to interact with other clients and monitor their workouts and progress. More information on how to use the Internet to support exercise adherence is provided at the end of this chapter in the "Innovative Strategies to Increase Adherence" section. It is important that the Personal Trainer discuss self-monitoring options with clients to determine which methods of self-monitoring are most appropriate for them. An example of how to use self-monitoring and other self-regulation strategies can be viewed in Case Study 8.2.

Self-regulation allows clients to plan, organize, and manage exercise activities. Setting intrinsically motivated goals with clients may help them adhere to exercise better as compared to setting extrinsically motivated goals. Finding self-monitoring options, such as online workout logs, that work for each client may help them to better self-regulate their exercise.

## Social Support

Social support includes an exchange of aid or assistance among individuals or groups within a social network (80). Research has shown that high levels of social support for exercise lead to higher levels of self-efficacy, which, in turn, lead to increased participation in exercise (63). In fact, like self-efficacy, social support is one of the most consistent predictors of exercise participation (76,80) and can be separated into four types: (a) emotional, (b) tangible, (c) informational, and (d) appraisal. Emotional support refers to encouragement or acceptance from others, especially from one's spouse

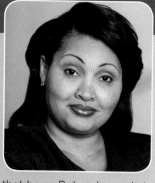

## Case Study 8.2

### Increasing Adherence by Identifying Life Circumstances (Environmental Factors)

Deborah recently went through menopause and is finding that maintaining her weight isn't as easy as it used to be. She often gets down on herself because she isn't happy with her body and the way it looks. Of late, Deborah and her husband have become empty nesters, and Deborah decided to hire a Personal Trainer to help her get in shape. She was hoping that her husband would join with her, but he does not think that he or Deborah needs to change. During the initial stages of Deborah's program, she told the Personal Trainer that her husband does not agree with her decision to hire a Personal Trainer because it costs too much; she also mentioned that sometimes she doesn't exercise because her husband wants her to watch television instead or she gets really busy at work. Deborah had some success initially with weight loss, and she likes group exercise classes, but she is discouraged with how much effort it takes to lose such a small amount of weight.

#### QUESTIONS FOR CONSIDERATION

What factors are playing a role in Deborah's lack of success with her exercise program? What advice can you give her to help increase her adherence to exercise?

### Strategy: Exercise Self-Regulation

Deborah's job (*i.e.*, time and motivation) and lack of social support are serious barriers to her adherence to exercise. Although she *intends* to exercise, she does not have the proper planning tools in place to follow through with her intentions to exercise. Teach Deborah how to plan for exercise. She may need to make a daily schedule, employ strategies such as going straight to the gym after work, or participate in exercise at home or at work some days of the week.

Deborah's self-esteem and poor body image may be discouraging her from exercise. Revisit Deborah's motivations for exercise and encourage her to replace her weight loss goals with goals related to meeting new people, relieving stress, and feeling good.

### Strategy: Social Support

Deborah isn't getting the support she needs to be active from her husband. Consider encouraging Deborah to have a serious conversation with her husband about how important staying active is to her and that she needs his support in order to be successful.

Talk to Deborah about how she can access other sources of social support as well. She mentioned that she enjoyed a group fitness class. Encourage her to introduce herself to the instructor and/or enlist a friend to attend classes with her. Building relationships with the instructor or other participants might give Deborah the accountability she needs to keep attending the class.

or significant other, family, friends, and community; tangible support refers to material aid in order to provide an individual the opportunity to exercise (*e.g.*, shoes or a gym membership); informational support refers to advice or information given in regard to exercise (*e.g.*, a smart phone app that prescribes an exercise plan for a client who travels often); and appraisal support refers to providing the individual with constructive feedback and accepting their beliefs and values (*e.g.*, adjusting a client's exercise plan, such as adding 1 d of resistance training per week, if the client has not progressed toward goals as expected) (80). The Personal Trainer may be responsible for providing the client with all four types of support. One client may need more informational support, whereas another client may need more appraisal support. Understanding a client's social support needs related to exercise will not only prepare the Personal Trainer to effectively provide the support the client needs to adhere to exercise, but it will also help the Personal Trainer guide the client in developing strategies for accessing additional social support outside of the personal training session. Social support beyond the Personal Trainer–client relationship is essential to a client's continued participation in exercise. Strategies that may help clients feel more supported in their participation in exercise include identifying their social support needs, creating a supportive training environment, and teaching the client how to actively access additional social support.

## Social Support Needs

Before teaching clients how to access social support, it is important that they understand what kind of social support they need to adhere to exercise. Table 8.3 includes examples of the different types of social support. Use this table to teach clients about the different types of social support and provide them with examples. For example, emotional support may involve spousal support for taking time to exercise or a friend accompanying a client to the gym. Tangible support may involve help with childcare, household duties, or costs to participate in exercise programs. Informational support may include knowledge and skills the Personal Trainer provides clients or information and referrals from the Personal Trainer regarding something that has been read

| Table 8.3 | Examples of Support |
|---|---|
| **Type of Support** | **Example** |
| Emotional support | ■ Spouse taking a walk with the client<br>■ Friend periodically calling to encourage sticking with a workout program<br>■ Group fitness instructor encouraging your clients attendance in more classes<br>■ Work out partners or buddy systems |
| Tangible support | ■ Spouse offers to cook dinner while your client works out<br>■ Family member offers to watch the kids while your client works out<br>■ Friend offers to pick up your dry cleaning to give your client more time to work out<br>■ Provide reward structures |
| Informational support | ■ E-mails from health Web sites about how to incorporate exercise into your client's life<br>■ Handouts from a personal trainer on new exercise routines<br>■ Magazine subscription that provides your client with monthly information on exercise<br>■ Posters and informational bulletin boards |
| Appraisal support | ■ Spouse who praises your client on the progress your client has made<br>■ Coworkers who give feedback on the changes they have seen in your client<br>■ Provide positive reinforcement and individualized feedback |

Social support is an important predictor of exercise adherence and includes four types: (a) emotional, (b) tangible, (c) informational, and (d) appraisal support. Knowing what kind of support a client needs from the Personal Trainer and from other individuals in their social network is critical to his or her continued participation in exercise.

on the Internet or in a fitness magazine. Appraisal support includes constructive feedback from the Personal Trainer or from significant individuals within a client's social network. Help clients identify which types of support they find the most valuable, which types they currently have, and which types they do not have but need to access in order to adhere to exercise. Research shows that the main source of support for both men and women is their spouse or significant other (35,68); however, clients will certainly come from varying backgrounds. Therefore, knowing and understanding clients' social support needs can help the Personal Trainer and client develop a plan for accessing additional social support if necessary.

## Creating a Supportive Environment

The Personal Trainer is responsible for providing clients with an environment that supports the fulfillment of their needs related to autonomy, relatedness to others, and competence. In order to foster autonomy, Personal Trainers can provide an environment in which clients are given the opportunity to make some of their own decisions in regard to their exercise programs. This collaboration may help a client build autonomy and intrinsic motivation for exercise. Positive reinforcement and rewards system can assist in increasing intrinsic motivation. Furthermore, if clients do not feel understood in relation to their goals, needs, and reactions to successes and failures, the effectiveness of the Personal Trainer, as an exercise leader, may be diminished (19). Clients may lose some of their motivation to exercise and their self-efficacy for exercise due to a lack of relatedness to others. Individuals who work with positive Personal Trainers whom they trust have greater self-efficacy than individuals who are expected to exercise on their own (82). Finally, asking clients to do challenging, but realistic, tasks and exercises within exercise sessions can help them to build competence and self-efficacy for exercise (3,50,82).

## Accessing Social Support

Having social support increases the likelihood of adhering to exercise (80); however, what can be done if a client does not have social support? A client may hire a Personal Trainer because he or she is lacking social support somewhere in his or her life. Clients may need informational support from Personal Trainers because they simply do not know what to do, or they may need emotional support because they lack the motivation to be active on their own. Regardless of their reasons for hiring a Personal Trainer, to ensure that they adhere to exercise, it is essential that they learn *how* to access social support. Teaching clients how to access social support can help them to develop self-efficacy and, ultimately, increase exercise adherence (36,49,50).

A Personal Trainer who provides an environment that fosters clients' autonomy, relatedness to others, and competence may improve their clients' adherence to exercise.

Clients may need to have serious discussions with significant individuals in their social networks (such as spouses or bosses) to make them aware of the importance of exercise in their lives and to express the importance of social support. Clients may need to be counseled as to how to begin such discussions, and Personal Trainers may need to help them identify the support they may need from each individual. Additionally, some of the strategies used for exercise planning, such as joining group fitness classes or enlisting a friend as an exercise partner, can also provide clients with the social support they need to adhere to exercise.

Community programs or sport leagues are an additional avenue clients can use to find support. Many communities have clubs for most active interests, such as walking clubs, running groups, golf leagues, cycling clubs, and volleyball clubs. Additionally, communities offer sport leagues in softball, basketball, soccer, and hockey, to name a few. Utilizing existing programs that are delivered in group settings may provide additional social support. The client's enjoyment of spending time with others may also positively impact adherence (12,17,23,65,74). Online communities and online/mobile supplements to personal training programs are another source of social support that may help clients adhere to exercise, as they are promising approaches for clients with low levels of social support (61). Obviously, the Personal Trainer provides some social support; however, clients should be encouraged to find other resources to help support their exercise adherence. An example of how the Personal Trainer can encourage clients to access additional support can be seen in Case Study 8.2.

> Many clients hire Personal Trainers because they do not have the social support they need to adhere to exercise. Teaching clients *how* to access social support within their social networks or home communities, or even online, may help them to develop self-efficacy and successfully adhere to exercise.

## Innovative Strategies to Increase Adherence

Due to the complexity of factors that contribute to adhering to an exercise program, the Personal Trainer can employ additional innovative strategies to make adhering to exercise easier for their clients. Activities often viewed as distractions from or barriers to exercise can be utilized to support exercise. For example, wearable technology and the Internet have become staples within everyday life and continue to evolve rapidly, making them important avenues for helping clients adhere. Additionally, most people have increasing demands on their time (perhaps one reason why some hire Personal Trainers); therefore, Personal Trainers can help clients to most effectively utilize their time by teaching them how to use their physical environment for exercise. This section introduces two innovative methods, the Internet and the physical environment, to help clients adhere to exercise. However, the Personal Trainer can establish innovative strategies of his or her own based on each client's needs, advances in technology, the community-specific physical environment, or other innovations of which the Personal Trainer is aware.

### Using the Internet to Promote Exercise Adherence

Use of the Internet and mobile technology has grown rapidly worldwide, with 73% of Americans, men and women alike, have a desktop or laptop computer, 68% have a smartphone, and 45% have a tablet (56). More importantly, the Internet has become a significant source of health information among these users (56,79). The Internet can not only be used to support the behavior change strategies discussed in this chapter, such as overcoming barriers, goal setting, self-monitoring, and accessing social support (62,79), but it also provides Personal Trainers the opportunity to provide clients with Web-based interactive tools, refer clients to credible Web sites for additional exercise information, interact with clients remotely between personal training sessions (42), and set up Personal Trainer blogs to which clients can subscribe. More specifically, Personal Trainers can utilize the Internet for online coaching of clients (*e.g.*, via e-mail or chat rooms); to provide peer support and chatting opportunities among clients (*e.g.*, discussion boards, blogs, and chat rooms), video demonstrations

> The Personal Trainer can use the Internet for online coaching of clients and to provide additional support for clients, video demonstrations of exercises, online self-monitoring tools, and newsletters. Personal Trainers are encouraged to creatively utilize innovations in Internet technology to help their clients adhere to exercise.

of exercises, online journaling for clients, and self-monitoring tools (*e.g.*, online exercise/diet logs); and to distribute newsletters to clients (79).

Advancements in wireless technology also provide Personal Trainers with opportunities to reach clients via their mobile phones or tablets. These devices can be used not only for communication with clients but also to provide clients easy access to some of the tools listed earlier, such as exercise tracking tools and videos of exercises. Personal Trainers can talk to their employer about what online features their training facility already provides or can individually develop online opportunities for their clients.

## Using the Physical Environment to Promote Exercise

One often overlooked strategy for adherence is the use of the environment to facilitate exercise. Using the physical environment includes using the surroundings in which clients live, exercise, and interact (15). Two examples of how to use the environment to facilitate exercise are active commuting and exercising outdoors.

### Active Commuting

Active commuting (*i.e.*, cycling or walking to work) is a potential strategy to help clients meet physical activity recommendations and may positively impact their health (8,31,72). Clients who feel time is a barrier may find active commuting to be a feasible option when (a) much of their commuting time is spent in traffic or (b) they are able to add only a minimal amount of time to their commute. Clients who are environmentally conscious may be especially interested in active commuting, as active commuting is seen as a way to improve air quality (78).

Personal Trainers whose clients are interested in active commuting but have not tried it before may need to improve their clients' confidence for overcoming barriers, such as rain, detours, and fatigue (10). When clients feel actively commuting to work is not an option, the Personal Trainer can also suggest cycling or walking to nearby businesses to complete errands or when visiting friends. If clients do not have a bicycle, many cities in the United States are now creating bike share programs where clients, for a small fee, can pick up and drop off a bicycle in different parts of the city (59). Additional strategies the Personal Trainer can encourage the client to utilize to actively use their environment include parking farther away, using the stairs, exiting public transportation a stop earlier than needed, and taking walking breaks at work (26).

> Personal Trainers can encourage clients to utilize the physical environment with the following strategies: actively commuting to work; cycling/walking to complete errands or when visiting friends; or parking farther away, using the stairs, and taking walking breaks at work.

### Exercising Outdoors

In addition to using the environment to actively commute, the Personal Trainer can use the environment to improve clients' enjoyment of exercise. Compared to exercising indoors, being active outdoors in a natural environment may improve mental well-being (75). Creating workouts for clients using the outdoor environment and encouraging clients to exercise on their own outdoors may decrease their feelings of depression, anger, and hostility and/or increase feelings of enjoyment and intention to be active again (4,29,32,75). Exercising outdoors may also give clients a break from the monotony of exercising indoors. To help clients stay motivated for exercise, encourage them to become involved in a variety of activities in different environments (11). Utilizing different environments may also help clients overcome barriers related to time, access to facilities, or lack of money for membership fees.

## SUMMARY

Approaches to promoting exercise adherence that do not include theory-based cognitive and behavioral strategies may not be as successful as those rooted in theory. Adhering to exercise is a difficult process, and clients will need the Personal Trainer's help developing the skills necessary to be successful with exercise. In this chapter, three theory-based concepts that are strongly related to exercise adherence were discussed: self-efficacy, motivation for exercise, and self-worth. In addition, several strategies were introduced that may help improve a clients' self-efficacy, motivation for exercise, and self-worth, all of which may ultimately lead to improved exercise adherence. These strategies include overcoming barriers, self-regulating exercise behaviors, and accessing social support. Through identifying the benefits of and barriers to exercise, clients can be taught how to overcome their barriers. Clients who plan their own exercise, set goals, monitor their exercise behaviors, and avoid relapse will be more autonomous and better able to regulate their own exercise participation. Providing clients with a supportive environment and teaching them how to access additional support may provide the encouragement they need to adhere to exercise. In addition, utilizing innovative strategies, such as the Internet and active commuting, may provide clients with unique tools to maintain exercise. Every client with whom the Personal Trainer works with will have different levels of self-efficacy, motivation for exercise, and self-worth. Clients will also have different values, backgrounds, and perceptions of exercise. Personal Trainers are encouraged to assess the needs of each client to determine what strategies will most effectively help each client successfully adhere to exercise.

## REFERENCES

1. Ainsworth B. Physical activity patterns in women. *Phys Sports Med*. 2000;28(10):25–6.

2. Annesi JJ. Effects of minimal exercise and cognitive behavior modification on adherence, emotion change, self-image, and physical change in obese women. *Percept Mot Skills*. 2000;91(1):322–36.

3. Bandura A. *Social Foundations of Thought and Action: A Social Cognitive Theory*. Englewood Cliffs (NJ): Prentice-Hall; 1986. 617 p.

4. Barton J, Pretty J. What is the best dose of nature and green exercise for improving mental health? A multi-study analysis. *Environ Sci Technol*. 2010;44(10):3947–55.

5. Bauman AE, Sallis JF, Dzewaltowski DA, Owen N. Toward a better understanding of the influences on physical activity: the role of determinants, correlates, causal variables, mediators, moderators, and confounders. *Am J Prev Med*. 2002;23(2 suppl):5–14.

6. Bélisle M, Roskies E, Lévesque JM. Improving adherence to physical activity. *Health Psychol*. 1987;6(2):159–72.

7. Biddle SJH, Mutrie N. *Psychology of Physical Activity: Determinants, Well-Being and Interventions*. New York (NY): Routledge; 2001. 366 p.

8. Brockman R, Fox KR. Physical activity by stealth? The potential health benefits of a workplace transport plan. *Public Health*. 2011;125(4):210–6.

9. Brown WJ, Heesch KC, Miller YD. Life events and changing physical activity patterns in women at different life stages. *Ann Behav Med*. 2009;37(3):294–305.

10. Bruijn GT, Gardner B. Active commuting and habit strength: an interactive and discriminant analyses approach. *Am J Health Promot*. 2011;25(3):e27–36.

11. Burke SM, Carron AV, Eys MA. Physical activity context and university student's propensity to meet the guidelines Centers for Disease Control and Prevention/American College of Sports Medicine. *Med Sci Monit*. 2005;11(4): CR171–6.

12. Carron AV, Hausenblas HA, Mack D. Social influence and exercise: a meta-analysis. *J Sport Exerc Psychol*. 1996; 18(1):1–16.

13. Centers for Disease Control and Prevention. *Evaluation Briefs: Writing SMART Objectives* [Internet]. Atlanta (GA): Centers for Disease Control and Prevention; [cited 2017 Feb 7]. Available from: https://www.cdc.gov/healthyyouth /evaluation/pdf/brief3b.pdf

14. Centers for Disease Control and Prevention, Division of Nutrition, Physical Activity and Obesity, National Center for Chronic Disease Prevention and Health Promotion. *Physical Activity and Health: The Benefits of Physical Activity* [Internet]. Atlanta (GA): Centers for Disease Control and Prevention; [cited 2017 Feb 7]. Accessed from: https://www.cdc.gov/physicalactivity/basics/pa-health/

15. Chiang KC, Seman L, Belza B, Hsin-Chung J. It is our exercise family: experiences of ethnic older adults in a group-based exercise program. *Prev Chronic Dis*. 2008;5(1):A05.

16. Conroy MB, Simkin-Silverman LR, Pettee KK, Hess R, Kuller LH, Kriska AM. Lapses and psychosocial factors

related to physical activity in early postmenopause. *Med Sci Sports Exerc.* 2007;39(10):1858–66.

17. Courneya KS, McAuley E. Cognitive mediators of the social influence-exercise adherence relationship: a test of the theory of planned behavior. *J Behav Med.* 1995;18(5):499–515.

18. Dalle Grave R, Calugi S, Centis E, El Ghoch M, Marchesini G. Cognitive-behavioral strategies to increase the adherence to exercise in the management of obesity. *J Obes.* 2011;2011:348293.

19. Deci E, Ryan R. *Intrinsic Motivation and Self-Determination in Human Behavior.* New York (NY): Plenum Press; 1985. 371 p.

20. Deci EL, Ryan RR. The "what" and "why" of goal pursuits: human needs and the self-determination of behavior. *Psychol Inquiry.* 2000;11(4):227–68.

21. Dishman RK. *Advances in Exercise Adherence.* Champaign (IL): Human Kinetics; 1994. 406 p.

22. Dishman RK. Determinants of participation in physical activity. In: Bouchard C, Shephard RJ, Stephens T, Sutton JR, McPherson BD, editors. *Exercise, Fitness, and Health.* Champaign (IL): Human Kinetics; 1990. p. 75–102.

23. Dishman RK, Buckworth J. Increasing physical activity: a quantitative synthesis. *Med Sci Sports Exerc.* 1996;28(6): 706–19.

24. Donnelly JE, Blair SN, Jakicic JM, Manore MM, Rankin JW, Smith BK. Appropriate physical activity intervention strategies for weight loss and prevention of weight regain for adults. *Med Sci Sports Exerc.* 2009;41(2):459–71.

25. Dunn AL, Andersen RE, Jakicic JM. Lifestyle physical activity interventions: history, short- and long-term effects, and recommendations. *Am J Prev Med.* 1998;15(4):398–412.

26. Dunn AL, Marcus BH, Kampert JB, Garcia ME, Kohl HW, Blair SN. Comparison of lifestyle and structured interventions to increase physical activity and cardiorespiratory fitness: a randomized trial. *JAMA.* 1999;281(4):327–34.

27. Elavsky S. Physical activity, menopause, and quality of life: the role of affect and self-worth across time. *Menopause.* 2009;16(2):265–71.

28. Eyler AA, Matson-Koffman D, Vest JR, et al. Environmental, policy, and cultural factors related to physical activity in a diverse sample of women: the Women's Cardiovascular Health Network Project — introduction and methodology. *Women Health.* 2002;36(2):1–15.

29. Focht BC. Brief walks in outdoor and laboratory environments: effects on affective responses, enjoyment, and intentions to walk for exercise. *Res Q Exerc Sport.* 2009;80(3):611–20.

30. Fox KR. The effects of exercise on self-perceptions and self-esteem. In: Biddle SJH, Fox KR, Boutcher SH, editors. *Physical Activity and Psychological Well-Being.* New York (NY): Routledge; 2000. p. 88–117.

31. Hamer M, Chida Y. Active commuting and cardiovascular risk: a meta-analytic review. *Prev Med.* 2008;46(1):9–13.

32. Harte JL, Eifert GH. The effects of running, environment, and attentional focus on athletes' catecholamine and cortisol levels and mood. *Psychophysiology.* 1995;32(1):49–54.

33. Heesch KC, Mâsse LC. Lack of time for physical activity: perception or reality for African American and Hispanic women? *Women Health.* 2004;39(3):45–62.

34. Hillsdon M, Foster C, Thorogood M. Interventions for promoting physical activity. *Cochrane Database Syst Rev.* 2005;25(1):CD003180.

35. Huberty JL, Ehlers D, Coleman J, Gao Y, Elavsky S. Women bound to be active: differences in long-term physical activity between completers and non-completers of a book club intervention. *J Phys Act Health.* 2013;10:368–78.

36. Huberty JL, Ransdell LB, Sidman C, et al. Explaining long-term exercise adherence in women who complete a structured exercise program. *Res Q Exerc Sport.* 2008;79(3):374–84.

37. Huberty JL, Vener J, Ransdell L, Schulte L, Budd MA, Gao Y. Women bound to be active (years 3 and 4): can a book club help women overcome barriers to physical activity and improve self-worth? *Women Health.* 2010;50(1):88–106.

38. Huberty JL, Vener J, Schulte L, Roberts SM, Stevens B, Ransdell L. Women bound to be active: one year follow-up to an innovative pilot intervention to increase physical activity and self-worth in women. *Women Health.* 2009;49(6):522–39.

39. Ingledew DK, Markland D. The role of motives in exercise participation. *Psychol Health.* 2008;23(7):807–28.

40. King AC, Toobert D, Ahn D, et al. Perceived environments as physical activity correlates and moderators of intervention in five studies. *Am J Health Promot.* 2006;21(1):24–35.

41. Larimer ME, Palmer RS, Marlatt GA. Relapse prevention: an overview of Marlatt's cognitive-behavioral model. *Alcohol Res Health.* 1999;23(2):151–60.

42. Marcus BH, Ciccolo JT, Sciamanna CN. Using electronic/computer interventions to promote physical activity. *Br J Sports Med.* 2009;43(2):102–5.

43. Marcus BH, Dubbert PM, Forsyth LH, et al. Physical activity behavior change: issues in adoption and maintenance. *Health Psychol.* 2000;19(1 suppl):32–41.

44. Marcus BH, Eaton CA, Rossi JS, Harlow LL. Self-efficacy, decision-making and stages of change: an integrative model of physical exercise. *J Appl Soc Psychol.* 1994;24:489–508.

45. Marcus BH, Forsyth LH. *Motivating People to Be Physically Active.* Champaign (IL): Human Kinetics; 2003. 220 p.

46. McAuley E. The role of efficacy cognitions in the prediction of exercise behavior in middle-aged adults. *J Behav Med.* 1992;15(1):65–88.

47. McAuley E, Blissmer B. Self-efficacy determinants and consequences of physical activity. *Exerc Sport Sci Rev.* 2000; 28(2):85–8.

48. McAuley E, Blissmer B, Katula J, Duncan TE, Mihalko SL. Physical activity, self-esteem, and self-efficacy relationships in older adults: a randomized controlled trial. *Ann Behav Med.* 2000;22(2):131–9.

49. McAuley E, Courneya KS, Rudolph DL, Lox CL. Enhancing exercise adherence in middle-aged males and females. *Prev Med.* 1994;23(4):498–506.

50. McAuley E, Jerome GJ, Marquez DX, Elavsky S, Blissmer B. Exercise self-efficacy in older adults: social, affective and behavioral influences. *Ann Behav Med.* 2003;25(1):1–7.

51. McAuley E, Mihalko SL, Bane SM. Exercise and self-esteem in middle-aged adults: multidimensional relationships and physical fitness and self-efficacy influences. *J Behav Med.* 1997;20(1):67–83.

52. Nigg CR, Borrelli B, Maddock J, Dishman RK. A theory of physical activity maintenance. *Appl Psychol Int Rev.* 2008;57(4):544–60.

53. Nigg CR, Riebe D. The transtheoretical model: Research review of exercise behavior and older adults. In: Burban PM,

Riebe D, editors. *Promoting Exercise and Behavior Change in Older Adults: Interventions with the Transtheoretical Model*. New York (NY): Springer; 2002. p. 147–80.

54. Nothwehr F, Yang J. Goal setting frequency and the use of behavioral strategies related to diet and physical activity. *Health Educ Res*. 2007;22(4):532–8.

55. O'Dougherty M, Dallman A, Turcotte L, Patterson J, Napolitano MA, Schmitz KH. Barriers and motivators for strength training among women of color and Caucasian women. *Women Health*. 2008;47(2):41–62.

56. Pew Research Center. Three Technology Revolutions. Washington (DC): Pew Research Center; [cited 2017 Feb 8]. Available from: http://www.pewinternet.org/three-technology-revolutions/

57. Plotnikoff RC, Brez S, Hotz SB. Exercise behavior in a community sample with diabetes: understanding the determinants of exercise behavioral change. *Diabetes Educ*. 2000;26(3):450–9.

58. Prochaska JO, Marcus BH. The transtheoretical model: applications in exercise. In: Dishman RK, editor. *Exercise Adherence II*. Champaign (IL): Human Kinetics; 1994. p. 161–80.

59. Pucher J, Dill J, Handy S. Infrastructure, programs, and policies to increase bicycling: an international review. *Prev Med*. 2010;50(suppl 1):S106–25.

60. Ransdell LB, Dinger MK, Huberty J, Miller KH. *Developing Effective Physical Activity Programs*. Champaign (IL): Human Kinetics; 2009. 199 p.

61. Richardson CR, Buis LR, Janney AW, et al. An online community improves adherence in an Internet-mediated walking program: part 1: results of a randomized controlled trial. *J Med Internet Res*. 2010;12(4):e71.

62. Ritterband LM, Thorndike FP, Cox DJ, Kovatchev BP, Gonder-Frederick LA. A behavior change model for internet interventions. *Ann Behav Med*. 2009;38(1):18–27.

63. Rovniak LS, Anderson ES, Winnett RA, Stephens RA. Social cognitive determinants of physical activity in young adults: a prospective structural equation analysis. *Ann Behav Med*. 2002;24(2):149–56.

64. Ryan RM, Deci EL. Self-determination theory and the promotion and maintenance of sport, exercise, and health. In: Haggar MS, Chatzisarantis NLD, editors. *Intrinsic Motivation and Self-Determination in Exercise and Sport*. Champaign (IL): Human Kinetics; 2007. p. 1–19.

65. Ryan RM, Frederick CM, Lepes D, Rubio N, Sheldon KM. Intrinsic motivation and exercise adherence. *Int J Sport Psychol*. 1997;28:335–54.

66. Ryan RM, Williams GC, Patrick H, Deci EL. Self-determination theory and physical activity: the dynamics of motivation in development and wellness. *Hellenic J Psychol*. 2009;6:107–24.

67. Schwarzer R. Modeling health behavior change: how to predict and modify the adoption and maintenance of health behaviors. *Appl Psychol*. 2008;57(1):1–29.

68. Seefeldt V, Malina RM, Clark MA. Factors affecting levels of physical activity in adults. *Sports Med*. 2002;32(3):143–68.

69. Segar ML, Eccles JS, Richardson CR. Type of physical activity goal influences participation in healthy midlife women. *Womens Health Issues*. 2008;18(4):281–91.

70. Segar M, Jayaratne T, Hanlon J, Richardson C. Fitting fitness into women's lives: effects of a gender-tailored physical activity intervention. *Womens Health Issues*. 2002;12(6):338–47.

71. Segar M, Spruijt-Metz D, Nolen-Hoeksema S. Go figure? Body-shape motives are associated with decreased physical activity participation among midlife women. *Sex Roles*. 2006;54(3):175–87.

72. Shephard, RJ. Is active commuting the answer to population health? *Sports Med*. 2008;38(9):751–8.

73. Silva MN, Vieira PN, Coutinho SR, et al. Using self-determination theory to promote physical activity and weight control: a randomized controlled trial in women. *J Behav Med*. 2010;33(2):110–22.

74. Spink KS, Carron AV. Group cohesion and adherence in exercise classes. *J Sport Exerc Psychol*. 1992;14(1):78–86.

75. Thompson Coon J, Boddy K, Stein K, Whear R, Barton J, Depledge MH. Does participating in physical activity in outdoor natural environments have a greater effect on physical and mental wellbeing than physical activity indoors? A systematic review. *Environ Sci Technol*. 2011;45(5):1761–72.

76. Trost SG, Owen N, Bauman AE, Sallis JF, Brown W. Correlates of adults' participation in physical activity: review and update. *Med Sci Sports Exerc*. 2002;34(12):1996–2001.

77. Tudor-Locke C, Lutes L. Why do pedometers work? *Sports Med*. 2009;39(12):981–93.

78. U.S. Department of Health and Human Services. *Environmental Health*. Washington, DC: [cited 2017 Feb 8]. Available from: https://www.healthypeople.gov/2020/topics-objectives/topic/environmental-health/objectives

79. Vandelanotte C, Spathonis KM, Eakin EG, Owen N. Website-delivered physical activity interventions. *Am J Prev Med*. 2007;33(1):54–64.

80. Vrazel J, Saunders R, Wilcox S. An overview and proposed framework social-environmental influences on the physical-activity behavior of women. *Am J Health Promot*. 2008;23(1):2–12.

81. Wallace LS, Buckworth J. Longitudinal shifts in exercise stages of change in college students. *J Sports Med Phys Fitness*. 2003;43(2):209–12.

82. White JL, Ransdell LB, Vener J, Flohr JA. Factors related to physical activity adherence in women: review and suggestions for future research. *Women Health*. 2005;41(4):123–48.

83. Wilbur J, Vassalo A, Chandler P, McDevitt J, Michaels Miller A. Midlife women's adherence to home-based walking during maintenance. *Nurs Res*. 2005;54(1):33–40.

# Eliciting Positive Perceptions and Behaviors: Coaching Techniques

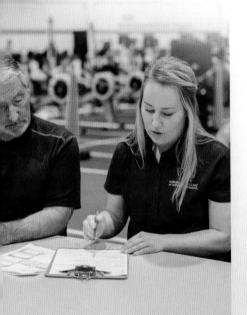

**Personal Trainers should be able to:**

- Describe the Personal Trainer's role in coaching.
- Understand the elements necessary for effective coaching.
- Be aware of verbal and nonverbal client behaviors.
- Provide appropriate responses to client behaviors.
- Understand several techniques used by effective Personal Trainers including
  - Active listening
  - Empathy and nonviolent communication
  - Rapport development
  - Appreciative inquiry
  - Motivational interviewing
  - The 5 As model of behavior change counseling
- Understand the role of self-efficacy, self-esteem, and self-concept in establishing a rapport with clients.
- Identify ways to use technology and alternative Personal Training methods when face-to-face Personal Training is not convenient or possible.
- Recognize that clients have different visual, auditory, and kinesthetic learning styles.

# INTRODUCTION

Personal Trainers take on many roles, including sharing knowledge of training techniques and programs and serving as a friend, confidant, and motivator. They strive to help clients build awareness, set goals, and ultimately find their own solutions to problems and issues. Personal Trainers should not "diagnose" health issues or problems, but instead, they should help clients explore ways to find solutions to the various challenges they will encounter. Personal Trainers also should serve as a resource and conveyor of knowledge. When client needs go beyond the scope of practice for a Personal Trainer, the Personal Trainer should be a resource for appropriate referrals. In order to be the most effective fitness coach, the Personal Trainer should strive to continually develop the skills and competencies covered in this chapter.

## Coaching Techniques

Two of the most essential abilities of a Personal Trainer include strong oral and nonverbal communication. Effective communication skills enable Personal Trainers to apply behavior change theories, or ways to increase adherence and motivation. In order to convey information about these topics to their clients, Personal Trainers should be familiar with coaching techniques. These skills will help Personal Trainers provide social support and professional expertise along with increasing the client's ability to achieve goals and obtain optimal satisfaction and personal fulfillment (8). The ability to connect with a client and effectively communicate with that client will increase the odds of success. Information related to the initial consultation between a Personal Trainer and client is provided in Chapter 10.

Specifically, this chapter will include descriptions and examples of successful strategies that are considered best practices for coaching to elicit positive behavioral outcomes in clients (*e.g.*, active listening, empathy, rapport development, appreciative inquiry, motivational interviewing, and the 5 As model of behavior change counseling). This chapter also addresses the role of client self-esteem, self-concept, and self-efficacy in successfully achieving and maintaining proper health behaviors. This chapter concludes by describing alternative methods of communication that can be used in addition to in-person coaching in order to improve the Personal Trainer's ability to reach and interact with the client.

### Active Listening

Active listening is a communication form that is described as a set of verbal and nonverbal skills necessary for communication in successful family, business, and therapeutic relationships. Active listening can consist of nodding the head, making eye contact, and restating important information.

Active listening also involves clarifying, repeating, and summarizing what the client has said (10,14,20). A Personal Trainer who effectively demonstrates active listening skills possesses unconditional acceptance and unbiased reflection relative to the client's experience. Personal Trainers must understand clients' interpretations of their experiences. The Personal Trainer must not impose personal points of view, experiences, or preconceived notions of the client's situation (52). A Personal Trainer who practices successful active listening will avoid personal interpretation and assumptions and instead ask questions for clarity.

> Active listening involves the listener giving the speaker oral and nonverbal feedback to indicate attention and understanding. The listener accepts what the speaker is saying at face value without inserting personal interpretation.

> ### Box 9.1    For Example: Metaphors
>
> The metaphor, "It's like a walk in the park," to some, may produce images of an easy or invigorating physical activity, performed in a lush green environment that is supportive of healthy social and recreational activities. To others, parks may produce images of abandoned property littered with weeds, garbage, and criminal activities. Also, not everyone can walk even short distances with ease, and so this metaphor also could fill the client with feelings of inadequacy, failure, or resentment.

To be an effective communicator, avoid using slang, metaphors, and other forms of language that might confuse or alienate clients.

There are other strategies that should be considered when employing active listening. A Personal Trainer should refrain from using metaphors (*e.g.*, a figure of speech or a statement in which the literal meaning of the word is quite different from the intent). Although using images, comparisons, and descriptions may be considered by some to be effective strategies to further explain or describe experiences, it is important to recognize that all metaphors are not well understood by all cultures and may have varied meanings between different age, gender, ability, and other diverse groups (Box 9.1). Misunderstandings may result from differences in language styles, vernacular, and popular culture and can be avoided by simply taking all verbal and nonverbal cues from the patient/client without interjecting confusing language or images.

Davidson and Versluys (15) propose four elements of active listening: listening to the spoken statements of the client, observing nonverbal communication, listening to the context of the clients' apprehensions, and listening to the context of the clients' statements that may need to be challenged (Box 9.2). The first element involves listening to the spoken statements of the client which may require the Personal Trainer to reflect on the client's verbal communications. Reflection involves the Personal Trainer carefully paraphrasing what has been communicated without misinterpreting or changing the meaning of what the client said. It is important that the Personal Trainer receive affirmation that the reflection correctly interprets the client's thoughts (Box 9.3).

The second element is observing nonverbal communication which involves paying close attention to the client's facial expressions, eye movements, speech patterns, vocal inflections, posture, and body movements. It has been suggested that many health care professionals, such as physicians and psychologists, identify within a middle class values system, which often produces communication barriers (31,49,50). Does the client who mumbles have poor posture and fails to make eye contact, or is he or she resentful, shy, or simply sleep deprived? If the Personal Trainer is unsure of the meaning of nonverbal communication, it is important to ask the client for clarification and not to simply assume understanding. Some research suggests that clients may feel more positive about the Personal Trainer when he or she appears to be interested, excited, or concerned (25,44). Making eye contact, exhibiting appropriate facial expressions, and taking notes are some ways to demonstrate interest and compassion.

> ### Box 9.2    The Four Elements of Active Listening
>
> - Listening to spoken statements
> - Observing nonverbal cues
> - Understanding contextual anxiety
> - Identifying statements that indicate teaching and learning opportunities

| Box 9.3 | For Example: Interpreting Client's Thoughts |

If a client indicates that she loves the pain and discomfort that accompanies exercise, a Personal Trainer would likely need to gather more information about exactly what the client means. Here, it would be appropriate to learn if the client is describing delayed onset muscle soreness, identifying sensations that she enjoys when pushing her body to perform strenuous activities, recounting a past experience that involved improper training techniques and resulted in pain but was enjoyable to her, or whether the client is simply being sarcastic.

The third element of active listening is listening to the context of a client's apprehensions or anxieties. Many times, a person's verbal communication has two components. The first is the actual meanings of the words the person uses. The second is the person's feelings or attitudes that underlie the content (42) (Box 9.4). The Personal Trainer must try to be sensitive to both the words and the total meaning of the message that the client is attempting to convey. In addition, Personal Trainers must convey that they are trying to understand the client's point of view (42).

The final element of active listening involves listening to the content of a client's statements that may eventually need to be challenged. Clients appreciate having their knowledge respected regardless of their level of education. Using both closed-ended and open-ended questions and reflective active listening statements are ways to learn about the client. In an initial appointment, it may be appropriate for the Personal Trainer to say, "Tell me what you know about exercise or nutrition behavior and health." The Personal Trainer should also ask about hesitations or concerns the client may have about implementing a new nutrition or exercise program. It is important that the Personal Trainer praise the client for the correct information conveyed and then respectfully but completely addresses misinformation or myths that the client discusses during an appointment.

> The client who indicates she loves the pain and discomfort that accompanies exercise could present the opportunity for the Personal Trainer to remind the client that in order for exercise to result in positive outcomes, pain and discomfort are not required.

The client who indicates she loves the pain and discomfort that accompanies exercise could present the opportunity for the Personal Trainer to remind the client that in order for exercise to result in positive outcomes, pain and discomfort are not required. Clients appreciate health and fitness professionals who have a solid, current education and a strong knowledge base and who use language that is honest and easy to understand (26).

Active listening will help the client establish trust and an understanding of the Personal Trainer's roles and responsibilities. During the course of active listening, a Personal Trainer should help the client understand when he or she can assess the problem or when the client will need to be referred to another health care provider (Box 9.5). The Personal Trainer should communicate with the client the role that personal training can take within a larger wellness team that is available to address problems related to physical fitness. Through active listening, the Personal Trainer will learn whether the focus should be motivational, directional, supportive, and/or influential.

| Box 9.4 | For Example: Understanding Apprehensions and Anxieties |

Suppose during an appointment with a Personal Trainer, an obese client says, "I'm here because I want to be healthier." This does not necessarily imply that the client understands the need for weight loss. In fact, in several cultures, being overweight/obese is not only highly acceptable but also considered healthy (56). Instead of saying, "Let's get you on a reasonable exercise and nutrition program to help you lose weight," an appropriate follow-up statement by the Personal Trainer might be "Many people view being healthy in a variety of ways. Help me understand what being healthy means to you."

| Box 9.5 | For Example: Referral to a Health Care Provider |

The Personal Trainer could help a client determine that he avoids physical activity due to a fear of falling. Subsequent tests could reveal that the client has poor balance. The Personal Trainer has assessed one potential cause of low physical activity (a balance problem). As a result, the Personal Trainer could help the client implement a balance training program. However, if balance training does not appropriately address the problem and the client continues to experience frequent falls, the Personal Trainer should refer the client to a primary care provider as there may be other underlying medical issues related to poor balance.

Active listening involves both verbal and nonverbal engagement. The client must receive unconditional attention from the Personal Trainer, who must be nonjudgmental. Learning techniques for asking probing questions (rather than yes/no questions) should deepen the Personal Trainer's understanding of the client's beliefs or feelings. Active listening is important for establishing empathy, and it will help the Personal Trainer and client understand one another's expectation of the relationship they have.

## Empathy

Although active listening is an accepted method of establishing a connection with a client, there is a body of research that suggests this form of communication is more helpful to the listener than to the communicator.

For example, one study (15) assessed the effects of short periods of training on effective communication and found that university psychology students who trained in active listening and other forms of cooperation achieved more successful communication compared with those who did not. First-year master's students who were part of a counselor education program considered themselves to be better counselors after receiving specific active listening training (35). Whether clients who are recipients of active listening appreciate this form of communication is less clear.

> Establishing an emotional connection with the client not only involves active listening but also displaying empathy or a warm responsiveness to the client's needs or concerns.

Several studies have found that although the recipients of active listening found advice resulting from the communication useful, the recipients did not feel that the communicator was empathetic (52). When establishing a connection with a client, it is not only important for the Personal Trainer to be an active listener but also to show empathy.

Empathy is often described as being affective and cognitive. Affective empathy demonstrates the Personal Trainer's ability to respond to the client's emotions with a similar emotion. To be cognitively empathetic indicates the Personal Trainer can intellectually identify with a client's perspective (11). Empathy also has been described as "feeling into" another person's experience (27). The conditions described as being necessary to elicit client change include honesty, mutual respect, effective communication, and warm responsiveness to the client (41). When Personal Trainers consistently demonstrate the aforementioned qualities, they are considered empathetic.

There is a considerable amount of research that suggests that positive client outcomes result from an empathetic counselor/coach (21). A link has been established between client satisfaction, adherence to a plan for behavior change, and the communication style of the person providing counseling or coaching (1). The quality of the relationship between a health professional and client is extremely influential on health outcomes (6). Kim and colleagues (33) showed that empathy significantly influences patient compliance and suggested that a feeling of partnership mediated this response. Empathy may result in the willingness of the Personal Trainer and client to be receptive to each other and evolve into a relationship of accountability, understanding, and success.

| Box 9.6 | For Example: Empathy |
|---------|----------------------|

For example, the Personal Trainer may prescribe rest or a change in exercise regimen for a client who exhibits signs of overtraining. The client may resist for a variety of reasons including exercise addiction, the need for social relationships that only exist in her exercise setting, or the fear of performance decrement that is frequently associated with rest. In this situation, an empathetic Personal Trainer will demonstrate an understanding of and response to the client's needs and feelings and provide constructive advice that will enhance the client's understanding of the problem and solution.

Although empathy may initially appear to be a simple mixture of intellect and emotion, human diversity makes it more complex (18). Gender, age, ability, religion, education, income, and culture may influence empathy. It is not always possible or necessary for Personal Trainers to be able to put themselves in the clients' situation, but it is helpful to make a genuine attempt to try to understand the client's point of view based on the current situation and past experiences. Considerations should be given to personal and professional experiences and social desirability (Box 9.6). Simultaneously, the Personal Trainer should not try to manipulate the client's beliefs. That is, if beliefs of the client prohibit her from consuming certain foods (*e.g.*, vegetarian), the Personal Trainer must work within those restrictions instead of trying to convince the client that certain dietary practices (*e.g.*, no animal protein) produce adverse performance results.

## Developing Rapport

Developing a rapport or positive relationship involves both active listening and demonstrating empathy (19). Rapport development with a client helps the Personal Trainer do a better job of partnering with the client to evaluate and address the problem. To effectively develop rapport, Personal Trainers should develop personal characteristics such as being motivational. Personal Trainers must demonstrate professionalism, confidence, knowledge, skills, and abilities without being condescending to the client. The Personal Trainer also should be compassionate and supportive, respecting the client's similarities and differences. The Personal Trainer should have a sincere desire to learn about a problem and make no assumptions about client expectations, values, influences, or understanding. Instead, the Personal Trainer should motivate the client based on the information shared. Skills mentioned in the previous paragraphs (*e.g.*, verbal and nonverbal communication, and active listening) should be thoroughly developed to help improve rapport. Finally, the Personal Trainer should be attentive to and regularly monitor the progress of both health and performance outcomes and the success of the Personal Trainer-to-client relationship.

When developing a rapport with a client, the Personal Trainer must not only be keenly sensitive to the client but also demonstrate a strong sense of self-awareness. Sometimes, previous experiences should be incorporated into a conversation, and sometimes, they simply do not apply. Personal Trainers should be confident in their ability to address problems while avoiding any preconceived notions about the client (see example in Case Study 9.1).

When this Personal Trainer discusses exercise with Keysha and Sonya, she learns that Sonya has an allergic reaction to sweat; therefore, the reasons for disliking sweat are different for these two women. It is really important to establish rapport and probe further to understand each individual client; it is also important not to assume that what was true for one African American woman is true for all African American women. Once a rapport is established, it is also easier for a client to articulate problems. For example, perhaps a client is adhering to the established exercise program but consistently avoids in-person meetings with the Personal Trainer. When a good rapport is established, it is easier for the client to explain that environmental factors in the exercise room make

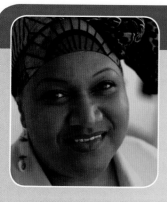

## Case Study 9.1

### Cultural Sensitivity

A Personal Trainer has been training Keysha, an African American woman, who does not like to sweat because she has said it messes up her hair. A second African American woman, Sonya, who also employs the trainer, says she would like to avoid sweating and never mentions her hair.

### QUESTIONS FOR CONSIDERATION

What kinds of questions should the trainer ask these women to ensure that she understands their goals and limitations for exercise? Do you think these women have similar issues? Why or why not? What role might culture have relative to exercise for Keysha and Sonya?

appointments uncomfortable. If possible, the Personal Trainer could then adjust appointment times if other clients or other observers are the source of the client's discomfort. Developing a rapport with the client should make personal training easier and more rewarding.

Even when a strong rapport is developed, it is possible that problems between the Personal Trainer and client will occur. Here, it is important for the Personal Trainer to work with the client to identify the symptoms or source of the problem. Is the Personal Trainer or client the source of the problem? Are the symptoms of the problem physical, emotional, or social? Is the problem caused by a combination of these variables? It is helpful for the Personal Trainer and client to establish awareness of how improvements in the client's health/performance should cause beneficial outcomes that could be coupled with potential casualties (Box 9.7). Communicating about this information and developing trust in order to identify problems and solutions is a necessary component of maintaining rapport with a patient/client.

## Appreciative Inquiry

A fourth skill that Personal Trainers should develop is appreciative inquiry (AI). AI is an approach used for motivating change that focuses on exploring and amplifying strengths. AI is traditionally used in business settings with considerable success in increasing productivity, cooperation,

## Box 9.7    For Example: Rapport

As an outcome of a training program, an athlete improves her performance and wins a starting position on the team. This situation changes the team dynamic and harms teammate social relationships. As a result, the client stops training with the Personal Trainer. In this and similar situations, it is the responsibility of the Personal Trainer to explore how the problem makes the client feel and learn about the experiences that resulted from her problems. What influences did the problem have on the client's personal relationships, psychological health, and/or self-image?

effectiveness, and employee and client satisfaction (12). It can also be applied by Personal Trainers in counseling/coaching situations. The AI framework is based on the belief that organizations or individuals are driven by their focus on and understanding of core values; goals are pursued and realized as a result of the potential positive outcomes. AI involves a process in which each stage is identified by a task and a measurable outcome that is developed from responses to questions asked of the client. AI has five phases of development (5-D): define, discover, dream, design, and deliver (13). These phases are cyclical beginning with defining what is to be learned about the process, discovering what may work best, dreaming of how the plan will work, designing with the client the plan, and delivering the eventual plan using both short- and long-term goals.

The AI approach is used in order for the Personal Trainer and client to work together to define the change process. AI is best used when a client does not have a clear focus; needs support for learning and development; and/or wants to discuss new experiences, values, conditions, or even wishes. With AI, variables or characteristics that can be improved are identified and the client's short- and long-term goals are generated and established. A timeline for progression toward and achievement of goals is determined, and a commitment to positive goals is agreed on. Defining the change process should involve writing down this information so that the Personal Trainer and client can remember what was defined and adhere to the agreements (53).

Discovery involves helping the client identify his or her personal best. This is an inventory that ascertains what is already good in the client's life, how current qualities or situations should be valued and celebrated, and ways in which these qualities can help the client achieve new goals (53) (Box 9.8).

When clients are encouraged to express their beliefs of what they can achieve in the context of the current situation, the Personal Trainer is helping to fulfill that dream. Here, it is important to use positive language such as "I will be able to complete an 8-minute mile," instead of, "I won't be the last one to finish the race." Positive words promote positive attitudes and positive outcomes. This component of AI helps the client describe an ideal self in the short term and long term (53).

Together, the Personal Trainer and client should design a plan. This involves developing actions that support the steps needed to achieve the client's vision. The Personal Trainer is responsible for offering a variety of options to the client while employing active listening to construct an appropriate plan. Again, the Personal Trainer should help the client create short- and long-term goals that are consistent with the client's ideal vision.

Delivery is the last component of AI. Delivery should not be viewed as the final stage of the goal-setting process because the client is encouraged to achieve both short- and long-term goals. It is possible that the client will become complacent or even regresses after the process of AI is complete (see Chapter 8 for information on relapse prevention). For this reason, it is important for the Personal Trainer to help the client develop a plan to sustain the achieved goal and set and reach new goals (53).

## Box 9.8    For Example: Appreciative Inquiry

A client has recently lost his spouse, and his children and grandchildren are concerned about his well-being; his physician has recommended an exercise program in order to improve both physical and psychological health. The Personal Trainer can help him by celebrating the memories of his wife, appreciating the concern of his children, and encouraging him to maintain independence by remaining both physically and socially active through exercise.

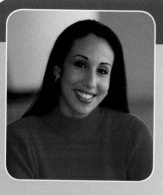

## Case Study 9.2

### Motivational Interviewing

Valerie, who previously had time and energy to work out, says she doesn't have time, energy, or desire to go to the gym because she is exhausted at the end of the day. She doesn't think that walking multiple times during the day or taking the stairs counts as physical activity so she doesn't do those types of things to increase the amount of physical activity in her day.

### QUESTIONS FOR CONSIDERATION

What other questions could you ask Valerie to help her find some answers to her dilemmas (*e.g.*, not having enough time in the day, being exhausted at the end of the day, and thinking that the only "real" exercise is vigorous-intensity exercise)? How would you ask her whether there is another time of day she could exercise? How would you encourage her to increase her level of physical activity above what she is doing now? Give some examples of your exact wording as this is an important facet of motivational interviewing.

## Motivational Interviewing

Motivational interviewing (MI) helps a client commit to changing an unhealthy behavior using more client-centered counseling by combining empathetic counseling and a direct approach to decisive change (40). The overall goal of MI is to resolve any ambivalence from the client, to encourage the client's change talk, and reduce the amount of resistance talk.

Motivational interviewing, another important coaching/counseling technique, involves using Bem's self-perception theory, which suggests that clients are more dedicated to what they hear themselves defend (5).The overall goal of MI is to resolve any ambivalence the from the client, to encourage the client's change talk, and reduce the amount of resistance talk.

Miller and Rollnick (36) suggest that rather than try to implore the client to change her work schedule or quit her job, a more effective strategy would be to avoid confrontation and help the client identify what parts of her life can be changed and the best strategies for her to make those changes. They describe MI as being direct, client-centered counseling that elicits behavior change by helping the client discover and decipher ambivalence. The Personal Trainer encourages the client to talk about what needs to be changed in the context of the client's desires and abilities. In some instances, the client may not recognize the process of behavior change or may not believe that behavior change is necessary or desirable in the current situation (36). In this instance the Personal Trainer should respond with active listening so the client can hear what is being said (Box 9.9).

## Box 9.9    For Example: Motivational Interviewing

A Personal Trainer may ask, "Don't you realize that missing your workouts is the source of your frustration?" A typical response from a client might be "My job is causing me to miss workouts and my boss is the source of my frustration." In this case, the Personal Trainer might rephrase the client's response: "I really need to clearly understand what you are telling me. You are missing your workouts because you work long hours at your job and there's no time to fit in exercise?"

At this point, the Personal Trainer should consider a brief intervention that involves working with the client to explore values and motivations. The Personal Trainer should guide the client to choose whether, when, and how to change. This process involves some directing and more listening. The Personal Trainer should give the client several tools including knowledge, insight, skills, and correct information in order to help elicit behavior change (36).

In MI, external motivation from the Personal Trainer is only intended to inspire a client's intrinsic motivation (see Chapter 8 for a full discussion of developing a clients' intrinsic motivation). If a client demonstrates passiveness, hesitation, or resistance, an immediate intervention or change in strategy is required. Passiveness and resistance indicate that the current MI strategy is not working, potentially because of a difference in views between the Personal Trainer and client (36). Failure of the client to be intrinsically motivated also could result from a lack of understanding due to the miscommunication or even cognitive impairment. It is possible that the Personal Trainer is not identifying problems or barriers in the same context as the client. It also is possible that the client needs a friend, family member, or even a health care provider to help with understanding the information the Personal Trainer is trying to discuss. In this situation, it is necessary for the Personal Trainer to acknowledge the problem, identify its cause, and redirect the client to a path that will facilitate intrinsic motivation.

MI is different from the client-centered counseling technique of active listening because it allows the Personal Trainer to give more direction. MI is appropriate when the client has a need to plan a strategic change. The directive need to change may come from a primary care provider or clinician, the client's spouse or family member, or the client. Because MI only helps identify strategies for successful behavioral change, it is generally combined with other Personal Training strategies mentioned in this chapter (36). Examples of MI are provided in Table 9.1 (2).

| Table 9.1 | Comparison of Motivational Interviewing and Advice Giving | |
|---|---|---|
| | **Motivational Interviewing** | **Advice Giving** |
| Counseling aim | Explore why the individual isn't sure they want to exercise and build his or her motivation to want to change. | Persuade the individual that he or she needs to change and start exercising by providing an Ex R$_x$. |
| Client | Help the individual explore why he or she is inactive, how and he or she might begin exercising, and how exercising is consistent with personal values; use empathy. | Explain that someone who is inactive may be at increased risk for disease (*e.g.*, diabetes mellitus, CVD) |
| Information presentation | Neutrally explain discrepancies between current activity level and recommended levels and allow client to react. | Give the evidence for why being inactive increases the risk of disease. |
| Questioning approach | Open-ended questioning to encourage exploration of thoughts and feelings regarding physical activity | Leading questions to have them "prove" to themselves the risks of their inactivity and why they should be active |
| Dealing with resistance | Use reflection to try to acknowledge their point; resistance is a sign that a new approach is needed; acknowledge that ambivalence to change is normal. | Have counterarguments ready and "correct" any misconceptions. |
| Summarizing | Use their language to summarize both the pros and cons of exercising. | Summarize the dangers of staying inactive and steps they should take to be active. |

CVD, cardiovascular disease; Ex R$_x$, exercise prescription.
Reprinted from American College of Sports Medicine. *ACSM's Guidelines for Exercise Testing and Prescription*. 10th ed. Philadelphia (PA): Wolters Kluwer; 2018.

## The 5 As Model of Behavior Change Counseling

The 5 As model of behavior change counseling is an evidence-based approach used to change a variety of less than desirable health behaviors (23). This model can accompany MI and has been used most frequently in primary care but is appropriate for most health promotion settings (23). The 5 As include assessing, advising, agreeing, assisting, and arranging.

*Assessing* involves measuring the client's beliefs, behaviors, and motivations. A Personal Trainer should *advise* the client based on health risks and behaviors. Next, the Personal Trainer and client can together agree on a set of short-term and long-term realistic goals. Then, the Personal Trainer *assists* the client with anticipating barriers and developing a specific plan to help the client avoid or at least effectively respond to barriers. *Assisting* the client may involve understanding his or her ability, comfort level, and access to available resources. The Personal Trainer may need to assist the client in developing an exercise or other behavior change plan. Finally, assisting may simply involve referring the client to another professional or resource. The final step involves *arranging* subsequent sessions with the client as a method of support. This could involve arranging an appointment with the Personal Trainer or a different provider like a health and fitness professional.

Frequent follow-up contact is an essential part of this behavior change method and can be provided in the form of telephone counseling, support groups, walking clubs, weigh-ins, and/or educational classes. Follow-up contact can either be short-term (1–2 wk after establishing goals) for initial behavior change or twice a month for long-term maintenance of behavior change. It is important that the Personal Trainer receive feedback and frequent updates from the client in order to achieve and maintain behavior change. The 5 As model of behavior change is intended to use the Personal Trainer to strengthen the client's self-management skills until he or she achieves and is able to independently maintain the desired behavior change (51) (Box 9.10).

## Self-Esteem, Self-Concept, and Self-Efficacy

Another important piece of counseling and coaching is being attentive to a client's self-esteem, self-concept, and self-efficacy. Although these concepts are also covered in Chapter 8, they will be discussed briefly here related to the process of Personal Training techniques. Self-esteem represents one's overall view of oneself as a person (32). Self-concept involves one's

---

### Box 9.10 | The 5 As

The 5 As of behavior change counseling are frequently used to guide activities in several types of behavior change programs (23). For example (24):

- A weight management program could consist of the initial identification of overweight and obese patients/clients and referral for advanced assistance if warranted (*advise*).
- An initial interview or survey could include identification of client weight history, current weight-related lifestyle behaviors, weight-related knowledge, self-monitoring, motivation, confidence, and demographic characteristics (*assess*).
- The Personal Trainer and client would identify appropriate weight loss strategies and goals (*agree*).
- Ongoing support would be given from the Personal Trainer as the client worked toward the established goals (*assist*).
- The Personal Trainer would continue to identify opportunities and access to the determined weight loss strategies and resources (*arrange*).

view of one's worthiness and is related to perceived capabilities or skills (37). Self-efficacy is one's estimation of one's personal ability for self-management, goal achievement, and effectiveness or prosperity (3). The difference between self-efficacy and self-concept is that self-efficacy is specific to a certain situation and self-concept is broader. For example, a client could be questioned about her overall value to her volleyball team. Her self-concept places her as a valuable member of the team, whether she is playing or sidelined with an injury and coaching. Her self-efficacy refers to her role as a team leader based on her ability as a setter. Self-esteem, self-concept, and self-efficacy are interrelated yet distinct constructs. Furthermore, these concepts are all important to psychological well-being. In the framework of Personal Training, it is important for the Personal Trainer to understand that these constructs also are related to body image and can be influenced by body changes. These traits also can be potential causes of exercise avoidance if clients are unsure about their ability to commit to, be successful with, or alter health outcomes as a result of behavior change (4,38,45,48).

> It is helpful for the Personal Trainer to identify potential problems that may occur as a result of exercising and then proactively work with the client to arrive at solutions.

If a client is comfortable with his or her current psychological, physical, or disease state, then behavior change could be a threat to his or her current status (Box 9.11). There also are positive psychological reasons for physical activity participation including improved feelings of self-confidence, self-competence, and control of oneself and one's surroundings (43). Other benefits of physical activity include increased opportunities to experience positive social interactions, fun, and enjoyment (46).

It is important to recognize that increased physical activity or exercise can potentially have negative influences on one's quality of life. Some potential negative factors related to physical activity include sweating, body odor, and muscle soreness; additionally, adding exercise could result in a loss of time and increase in injury risk. Other potential negative aspects of exercise that should be addressed include the potential need for resources such as exercise location, space, or money. There are also emotional reasons that a client may not participate in physical activity including fear of embarrassment, failure, or as described in the previous paragraph, threats to personal relationships. It is the responsibility of the Personal Trainer to proactively educate the client about these potential obstacles, together identify those events that are applicable to the client's life, and then proactively create action plans to overcome those barriers and help the client remain physically active.

| Box 9.11 | For Example: Self-Efficacy |
|---|---|

Imagine that your client suffers from chronic back pain. Her husband has taken over the household chores. Her concerned adolescent children now spend more time with her than their peers and have sacrificed several social activities in order to help her. Although your client acknowledges experiencing some guilt around the concessions her family must make for her, she also admits finding enjoyment in being the center of her family's attention. The Personal Trainer should understand that the client is comfortable with her current psychological state and try to encourage her to focus on her desire for good health and independence. It may be helpful for the Personal Trainer to address the client's fear of losing family attention by pointing out other positive benefits to participating in an exercise program to alleviate her back pain. The client could have an improved quality of life not only because of pain reduction but also because of relaxation of muscle tension in other areas of the body, enhanced muscle function to better perform activities of daily living, and improved brain structure and function (47).

# Other Methods of Communication

A Personal Trainer can communicate with clients via phone calls, print materials, e-mail, and other Web-based materials. These forms of communication may be helpful when face-to-face meetings are not convenient or possible.

The previous sections have addressed verbal and nonverbal communication while in the physical presence of the client. There are also situations where the Personal Trainer is not in the presence of the client.

The following paragraphs will describe special considerations when personal training occurs from a distance. To provide additional support to the client between appointments, it is often helpful for the Personal Trainer to use supplemental materials or support.

### Phone Calls

Extra support could occur in the form of phone calls, which simply serve as reminder contacts prior to the initial and/or subsequent appointments. The Personal Trainer may call to remind the client of the day and time that an appointment has been scheduled or check to see how the client is managing prescribed activities. If the Personal Trainer uses phone calls as a support mechanism, it is important to confirm that the client has a phone and that it is okay to be contacted at the provided phone number. When making phone calls to a client, the Personal Trainer should be aware of the need to be respectful of the time of day and the length of the call. The Personal Trainer should also consider privacy issues including whether a discussion can occur in the presence of others or whether/when it is appropriate to leave a detailed message. The Personal Trainer's phone number should be recognizable to the client. For example, many organizational phone lines appear on the caller ID as a number that is different than the number of the phone from which the call is being made. In this situation, the client should be told in advance, what number or organization name will appear on the caller ID, and whether it is possible to return a call to that number. Because the use of caller ID is so prevalent, it also is recommended that the Personal Trainer avoid calling from a personal phone number in order to discourage the client from having unlimited access to the Personal Trainer. The Personal Trainer may also want to consider using a written transcript when making initial calls and reminder messages. This may help to relay information in a complete, clear, and concise manner. Finally, it is important for the Personal Trainer to remember that there may be a prevalence of phone number instability in younger, transient, and low socioeconomic populations. With these groups, it is often helpful to have alternative phone contact information.

### Print Materials

Although electronic communication is widely accepted and popular, the need for print material still exists in some situations. Paper is a useful way to display information in waiting areas. It is also useful when a client is unable to access Web-based material because there is not public Internet access on site, or the client does not have Internet access at home. Print materials are a useful visual aid that can help a client learn, remember, and track progress.

### Using Electronic Media

Web-based materials are also useful visual aids. According to the Pew Research Center (39), nearly 75% of the U.S. adults had broadband Internet at home. The number of people with Internet access in all populations is growing, including older adults. However, although Internet service may be slowing, use of smartphones has increased, and today, nearly 1 in 10 American adults use only a smartphone versus having Internet or broadband service at home (39).

The benefit of using Web-based materials to supplement coaching is that these materials provide an opportunity for the Personal Trainer to direct clients to trusted Web sites for health information. It allows the Personal Trainer to provide the most current information that is most appropriate for each individual. It is always necessary for the Personal Trainer to frequently visit recommended sites because Web addresses and information frequently change or may not be updated in a timely or appropriate manner.

Using electronic media for coaching is a useful way to contact clients who may have limited access to a Personal Trainer because of time, distance, or travel limitations. There are several Web sites available to help a Personal Trainer supplement in-person activities. Additionally, there are several computer Web-based programs that can be purchased to supplement face-to-face business. Again, it is important for the Personal Trainer to thoroughly review and evaluate Web sites and Web-based programs before using them for supplemental support.

Personal Trainers may consider e-mailing educational and support materials to clients. Here, it is important to treat e-mail in the same manner as information shared over the phone, in print, or on the Web. Similar to phone call situations, the Personal Trainer should gain client approval to communicate via e-mail. The client should be informed about what type of information will be sent through e-mail, from whom the e-mail will come, and whether it is possible for the client to respond to the e-mail address from which the information is received. E-mails also should be reviewed for accuracy and appropriate messaging. Finally, e-mail messaging is generally an unsecure form of communication, and it is important for a Personal Trainer to refrain from e-mailing personal health or other information to his or her clients.

As electronic devices become more accessible and user-friendly, the potential opportunities to use these methods of communication for coaching will be enhanced (22). A recent randomized control, lifestyle intervention study compared face-to-face lifestyle modification counseling, telephone counseling, e-mail counseling, and no contact. Internet-based technology was not an effective substitute for human contact (16). The best use of technology may be as a supplemental tool that Personal Trainers use to support behavior change without replacing human interaction.

Videoconference technology also meets this requirement. There have been some successful examples of health counseling through the use of videoconferencing. Dixon and Stahl conducted a randomized controlled trial and showed that patients and physicians were equally satisfied when face-to-face and video-conference visits were compared. The researchers concluded that video conferencing may be an excellent channel for chronic disease care (17). Another study successfully delivered Tai Chi Quan to older adults via videoconference. This intervention was delivered three times per week for 15 weeks and found that participants were able to operate the videoconference. Additionally, fear of falling declined and balance was improved (55). Laflamme and colleagues (34) compared videoconferencing and face-to-face visits to evaluate the medical decisions of physicians and their interactions with residents living in nursing homes. In this study, face-to-face interviews were more effective than videoconferencing, but the physicians found videoconferencing to be a valuable supplementary tool in patient care (34).

Videoconferencing enables the Personal Trainer to not only supervise the client but also demonstrate exercise and other activities without a travel requirement. Personal Trainers may also consider videoconferencing in a group format. Group personal training is likely more cost-effective than one-on-one counseling/coaching (28) and could be a cost-efficient mechanism that improves client outcomes as a result of greater reach, efficacy, adoption, implementation, and maintenance (referred to as RE-AIM) (24). RE-AIM is a model of public health impact that takes into account not just efficacy but also the proportion and characteristics of the population exposed to an intervention and the rates of adoption, implementation, and maintenance of the intervention. Videoconferencing may expand the reach of Personal Training by reducing the need for transportation and lessening the effect of some environmental barriers.

Information technology continues to evolve, become more simplified, and spread at a rapid pace. Widespread broadband and videoconferencing capabilities are likely a matter of time. Primary care visits via videoconferencing are already happening in Boston and Hawaii (17). Physicians and other primary care providers who provide patient care through videoconferencing may have a need to refer their patients to Personal Trainers who provide care and support through distance technology as well.

Similar to the other communication methods, e-coaching can potentially provide increased contact and support when the client and the Personal Trainer are in locations that are not conveniently accessible to one another. When using these methods of communication, special consideration should be given to people with vision, hearing, and cognitive impairments as well as those who speak a primary language that is not English. Special attention also should be paid to ensure that materials are culturally appropriate and easy to understand. There are resources available to make telephone, paper, and electronic forms of communication accessible to these special populations as well (7,9,54).

## SUMMARY

Health coaching provides Personal Trainers a chance to help clients achieve both short- and long-term goals that involve maintenance or improvements in physical condition, physical performance, or general well-being (30). Health coaching occurs through organization and planning that result in a partnership between the Personal Trainer and client. The partnership is ever-evolving, unique to each client and intended to help the client set and achieve goals within his or her own personal context. The role of the Personal Trainer is to provide social support, education, and an appropriate amount of motivation within the framework of the client's desires, abilities, and personal experiences. Health coaching can be delivered in a variety of settings to an extremely diverse population. Special considerations should be made by the Personal Trainer to ensure that the delivery process, method, and location are appropriate for and easily accessible to their clients.

Coaching is a relatively new approach to enhancing client care outside of the traditional health care setting and may be a viable solution to improving overall health and fitness outcomes while reducing overall health care costs (29).

# REFERENCES

1. Ambady N, Koo J, Rosenthal R, Winograd CH. Physical therapists' nonverbal communication predicts geriatric patients' health outcomes. *Psychol Aging.* 2002;17(3):443–52.

2. American College of Sports Medicine. *ACSM's Guidelines for Exercise Testing and Prescription.* 10th ed. Philadelphia (PA): Wolters Kluwer; 2018.

3. Bandura A. The explanatory and predictive scope of self-efficacy theory. *J Soc Clin Psychol.* 1986;4(3):359–73.

4. Baturka N, Hornsby PP, Schorling JB. Clinical implications of body image among rural African-American women. *J Gen Intern Med.* 2000;15(4):235–41.

5. Bem DJ. Self-perception theory. In: Berkowitz L, editor. *Advances in Experimental Social Psychology: Vol. 6.* New York (NY): Academic Press; 1972; p. 1–62.

6. Blasi ZD, Harkness E, Ernst E, Georgiou A, Kleijnen J. Influence of context effects on health outcomes: a systematic review. *Lancet.* 2001;357(9258):757–62.

7. Britner PA, Balcazar FE, Blechman EA, Blinn Pike L, Larose S. Mentoring special youth populations. *J Community Psychol.* 2006;34(6):747–63.

8. Butterworth SW, Linden A, McClay W. Health coaching as an intervention in health management programs. *Dis Manage Health Outcomes.* 2007;15(5):299–307.

9. Chang BL, Bakken S, Brown SS, et al. Bridging the digital divide: reaching vulnerable populations. *J Am Med Inform Assoc.* 2004;11(6):448–57.

10. Comer LB, Drollinger T. Active empathetic listening and selling success: a conceptual framework. *J Personal Selling Sales Manage.* 1999;19(1):15–29.

11. Constantine MG. Social desirability attitudes, sex, and affective and cognitive empathy as predictors of self-reported multicultural counseling competence. *Couns Psychol.* 2000;28(6):857–72.

12. Cooperrider DL, Srivastva S. Appreciative inquiry in organizational life. *Res Org Change Dev.* 1987;1(1):129–69.

13. Cooperrider DL, Whitney DK. *Appreciative Inquiry: A Positive Revolution in Change.* San Francisco (CA): Berrett-Koehler Publishers; 2005. 86 p.

14. Cornelius TL, Alessi G, Shorey RC. The effectiveness of communication skills training with married couples: does the issue discussed matter? *Family J.* 2007;15(2):124–32.

15. Davidson JA, Versluys M. Effects of brief training in cooperation and problem solving on success in conflict resolution. *Peace Conflict.* 1999;5(2):137–48.

16. Digenio AG, Mancuso JP, Gerber RA, Dvorak RV. Comparison of methods for delivering a lifestyle modification program for obese patients: a randomized trial. *Ann Intern Med.* 2009;150(4):255–62.

17. Dixon RF, Stahl JE. A randomized trial of virtual visits in a general medicine practice. *J Telemed Telecare.* 2009; 15(3):115–7.

18. Duan C, Hill CE. The current state of empathy research. *J Counseling Psychol.* 1996;43(3):261–74.

19. Emmons KM, Rollnick S. Motivational interviewing in health care settings. Opportunities and limitations. *Am J Prev Med.* 2001;20(1):68–74.

20. Fassaert T, van Dulmen S, Schellevis F, Bensing J. Active listening in medical consultations: development of the Active Listening Observation Scale (ALOS-global). *Patient Educ Counsel.* 2007;68(3):258–64.

21. Feller CP, Cottone RR. The importance of empathy in the therapeutic alliance. *J Humanistic Counseling Educ Dev.* 2003;42(1):53–61.

22. Glasgow RE, Bull SS, Piette JD, Steiner JF. Interactive behavior change technology: a partial solution to the competing demands of primary care. *Am J Prev Med.* 2004;27(2):80–7.

23. Glasgow RE, Goldstein MG, Ockene JK, Pronk NP. Translating what we have learned into practice: principles and hypotheses for interventions addressing multiple behaviors in primary care. *Am J Prev Med.* 2004;27(suppl 2): 88–101.

24. Glasgow RE, Vogt TM, Boles SM. Evaluating the public health impact of health promotion interventions: the RE-AIM framework. *Am J Public Health.* 1999;89(9):1322–7.

25. Haase RF, Tepper DT. Nonverbal components of empathic communication. *J Couns Psychol.* 1972;19(5):417–24.

26. Harris SR, Templeton E. Who's listening? Experiences of women with breast cancer in communicating with physicians. *Breast J.* 2001;7(6):444–9.

27. Hartley G. Empathy in the counseling process: the role of counselor understanding in client change. *J Humanistic Educ Dev.* 1995;34:13–23.

28. Herman PM, Craig BM, Caspi O. Is complementary and alternative medicine (CAM) cost-effective? A systematic review. *BMC Complement Altern Med.* 2005;5:11.

29. Huffman MH. Health coaching: a fresh approach for improving health outcomes and reducing costs. *AAOHN J.* 2010;58(6):245–50.

30. Huffman MH. Health coaching: a new and exciting technique to enhance patient self-management and improve outcomes. *Home Healthcare Nurse.* 2007;25(4):271–4.

31. Johnson RL, Saha S, Arbelaez JJ, Beach MC, Cooper LA. Racial and ethnic differences in patient perceptions of bias and cultural competence in health care. *J Gen Intern Med.* 2004;19(2):101–10.

32. Judge TA, Bono JE. Relationship of core self-evaluations traits — self-esteem, generalized self-efficacy, locus of control, and emotional stability — with job satisfaction and job performance: a meta-analysis. *J Appl Psychol.* 2001;86(1): 80–92.

33. Kim SS, Kaplowitz S, Johnston MV. The effects of physician empathy on patient satisfaction and compliance. *Eval Health Prof.* 2004;27(3):237–51.

34. Laflamme MR, Wilcox DC, Sullivan J, et al. A pilot study of usefulness of clinician-patient videoconferencing for making routine medical decisions in the nursing home. *J Am Geriatr Soc.* 2005;53(8):1380–5.

35. Levitt DH. Active listening and counselor self-efficacy. *Clin Supervisor.* 2002;20(2):101–15.

36. Miller WR, Rollnick S. Ten things that motivational interviewing is not. *Behav Cogn Psychother.* 2009;37(2):129–40.

37. Pajares F, Miller MD. Role of self-efficacy and self-concept beliefs in mathematical problem solving: a path analysis. *J Educ Psychol.* 1994;86(2):193–203.

38. Perry AC, Rosenblatt EB, Wang X. Physical, behavioral, and body image characteristics in a tri-racial group of adolescent girls. *Obes Res.* 2004;12(10):1670–9.

39. Pew Research Center. Internet/Broadband Fact Sheet [Internet]. Washington (DC): Pew Research Center; [cited 2017 Feb 11]. Available from: http://www.pewinternet.org /fact-sheet/internet-broadband/

40. Resnicow K, Dilorio C, Soet JE, Ernst D, Borrelli B, Hecht J. Motivational interviewing in health promotion: it sounds like something is changing. *Health Psychol.* 2002;21(5): 444–51.

41. Rogers CR. The necessary and sufficient conditions of therapeutic personality change. *J Consult Psychol.* 1957;21(2): 95–103.

42. Rogers CR, Farson RE. Active listening. In: Kolb D, Rubin I, McIntyre J, editors. *Organizational Psychology.* 3rd ed. Englewood Cliffs (NJ): Prentice Hall; 1979; p. 168–80.

43. Ryan MP. The antidepressant effects of physical activity: mediating self-esteem and self-efficacy mechanisms. *Psychol Health.* 2008;23(3):279–307.

44. Sharpley CF, Fairnie E, Tabary-Collins E, Bates R, Lee P. The use of counsellor verbal response modes and client-perceived rapport. *Counselling Psychol Quart.* 2000;13(1):99–116.

45. Sisson BA, Franco SM, Carlin WM, Mitchell CK. Bodyfat analysis and perception of body image. *Clin Pediatr (Phila).* 1997;36(7):415–8.

46. Sonstroem RJ. Attitude testing examining certain psychological correlates of physical activity. *Res Q.* 1974;45(2): 93–103.

47. Sonstroem RJ. Physical self-concept: assessment and external validity. *Exerc Sport Sci Rev.* 1998;26:133–64.

48. Stockton MB, Lanctot JQ, McClanahan BS, et al. Self-perception and body image associations with body mass index among 8–10-year-old African American girls. *J Pediatr Psychol.* 2009;34(10):1144–54.

49. Sue DW, Sue D. Barriers to effective cross-cultural counseling. *J Couns Psychol.* 1977;24(5):420–9.

50. Tervalon M. Components of culture in health for medical students' education. *Acad Med.* 2003;78(6):570–6.

51. Umstattd MR, Moti R, Wilcox S, Saunders R, Watford M. Measuring physical activity self-regulation strategies in older adults. *J Phys Act Health.* 2009;6 (suppl 1):S105–12.

52. Weger H, Castle GR, Emmett MC. Active listening in peer interviews: the influence of message paraphrasing on

perceptions of listening skill. *Int J Listening.* 2010;24(1):34–49.

53. Whitney D, Trosten-Bloom A, Cooperrider D. *The Power of Appreciative Inquiry: A Practical Guide to Positive Change.* 2nd ed. San Francisco (CA): Berrett-Koehler Publishers; 2010. 288 p.

54. Wilcox S, Shumaker SA, Bowen DJ, et al. Promoting adherence and retention to clinical trials in special populations: a women's health initiative workshop. *Controlled Clin Trials.* 2001;22(3):279–89.

55. Wu G, Keyes LM. Group tele-exercise for improving balance in elders. *Telemed J E Health.* 2006;12(5):561–70.

56. Yancey AK, Simon PA, McCarthy WJ, Lightstone AS, Fielding JE. Ethnic and sex variations in overweight self-perception: relationship to sedentariness. *Obesity (Silver Spring).* 2006;14(6):980–8.

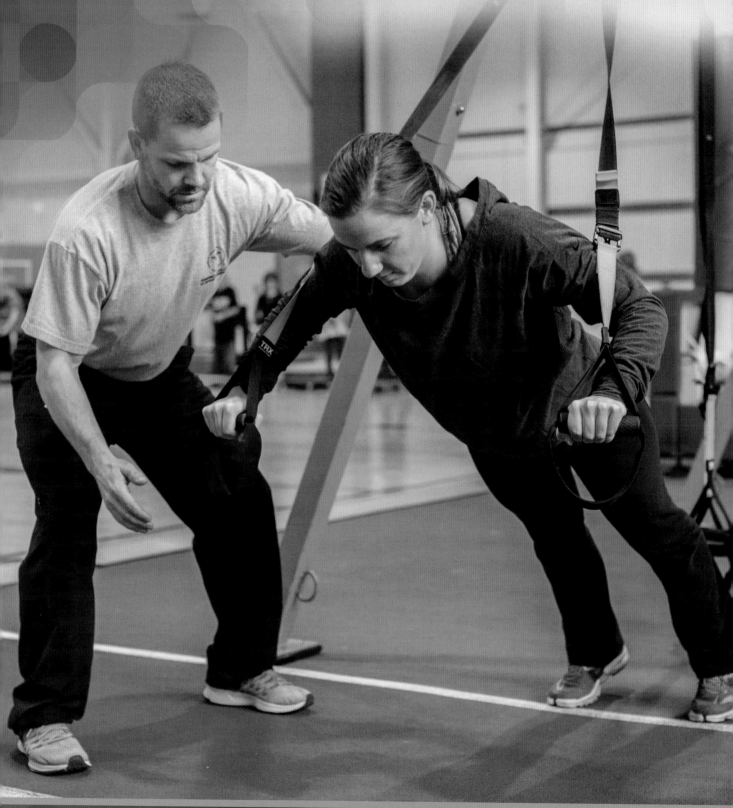

PART **IV** Initial Client
Screening

# 10 The Initial Client Consultation

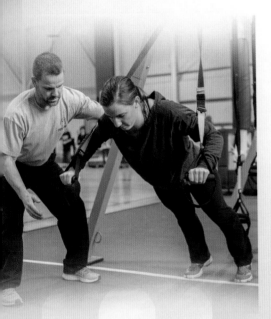

## OBJECTIVES
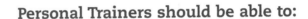

**Personal Trainers should be able to:**

- Learn the attributes of relationship marketing and how it pertains to the initial and ongoing appointments with the client.

- Understand the critical attributes for providing exceptional customer service and hospitality.

- Learn the nonverbal communication skills needed to successfully engage the client during any appointment.

- Become familiar with client-centered approach to health and fitness coaching.

- Understand the elements and value of the initial client contact as a precursor to the initial client consultation.

- Understand the components and preparation for the initial client consultation, how to structure the appointment, and the precedence it sets for the duration of the client–Personal Trainer relationship.

- Learn strategies for recommending and selling appropriate personal training packages and obtaining client commitment.

## INTRODUCTION

Within the initial client consultation, the Personal Trainer establishes precedence for the type of working relationship that will ensue. Therefore, it is critical that a sound foundation is built to facilitate a trusting, respectful, and mutually rewarding professional relationship. This chapter is designed to expose the Personal Trainer to both behavioral and business aspects of communication that should be utilized in the initial meeting with the client and beyond. Specific attributes for the initial client contact and initial client consultation are detailed, along with the rationale for why these appointments are structured in a systematic and comprehensive manner. There are likely program and process differences between Personal Trainers who work in a commercial club, private gym, or corporate fitness facility, yet there are more commonalities that exist in the profession. Although the chapter is written to address universal professional themes, at times differentiating between settings, each Personal Trainer is encouraged to adapt the content accordingly to the work environment and the relationship built with the client.

 ## Aspects of Successful Client Relations

The profession of personal training is centered on a strong relationship between the client and the Personal Trainer. Although relationship dynamics vary from client to client, there are some behaviors that the Personal Trainer should exhibit as a foundation for business development. For example, customer service and hospitality are essential to demonstrate continuously to garner client trust and respect. Incorporating relationship marketing concepts will further enhance the Personal Trainer's communication style and assist in conveying to the client that the relationship is of extraordinary value and importance. In addition, being aware of nonverbal communication skills and using a client-centered approach to coaching are important.

> The Personal Trainer can and should create a strong framework for attracting and retaining long-lasting client–Personal Trainer relationships.

### Customer Service and Hospitality

Personal Trainers, similar to a variety of health care providers, are in the service management industry. Clients seek out a Personal Trainer because they desire a service that will assist and guide them in a direction that is compatible with their health and fitness goals. Similar to those who seek out a clergy member to assist with spiritual goals, or call on a financial advisor to guide in monetary matters, people will seek out the services of a Personal Trainer. The Personal Trainer should recognize this entrusted opportunity — to guide and to make a direct positive impact on another person's life — as an honor and a special privilege. Author and restauranteur Danny Meyer firmly espouses that it takes both great customer service and hospitality to rise to the top of any service field, and that distinguishing between the two is critical for success (9).

Meyer refers to customer service as the delivery of technical processes or preplanned behaviors that are to be performed in a certain manner toward the client. In other words, these actions can be described as a monologue between the business provider and the customer (9). Customer service is exhibited by simply delivering a standard of service that meets the client's needs and expectations. However, it should be noted that clients do not seek or expect mediocre service (7). Therefore, it is recommended that the Personal Trainer continually perform at a higher level than expected to accommodate the discerning client. Examples of exceptional customer service include the following:

- Courtesy call 24-48 hours prior to meeting
- Be on time, or early, for appointments.
- Be 100% prepared for all appointments.
- Respond to phone, text, and e-mail messages promptly and courteously.
- Demonstrate organization and reliability and always follow up on what has been promised.
- Provide fitness training programs that are based on science or credible resources.
- Answer client's questions concisely and accurately within the scope of practice.
- Refer clients to appropriate professionals when the issue is outside of the scope of practice.
- Listen to client concerns, respond with sincerity, and solicit feedback.
- Speak respectfully to the client and of others.
- Dress appropriately and professionally.

A commitment to customer service should be a consistent practice to establish the Personal Trainer's reputation as a business professional. Consistently performing these actions will undoubtedly make an impression on the client and set the groundwork for a successful personal training business.

The principle of hospitality is also centered in customer service (7); however, it takes the concept a step further by providing a "holistic approach to meeting customers' needs within the context of a personal relationship and experience." Where customer service focuses on meeting the client's rational needs and expectations, hospitality also addresses the client's emotional needs by demonstrating graciousness, caring, and thoughtfulness (9). This emotional element is what creates an "experience" and establishes true client loyalty.

Although most commonly associated with the hotel or restaurant industry, hospitality is a focal point for companies in the health and fitness industry as well (3). One such fitness management company sees caring and serving the client so vital that it is stated as one of four operating missions of the organization. In conjunction, the company offers a hospitality-based employee training program that has proven to be a distinguishing factor among competitors and is a key component in attracting and retaining world-class clients. Addressing hospitality outside of the hotel and restaurant industry, a business consultant who assists organizations in enhancing their customer experience aptly titled a recent article "No Matter What Business You're in, You're in the Hospitality Business" (3).

By many definitions, hospitality is centered on the intangible and emotionally driven behaviors that demonstrate to the clients that they are special and cared for by the Personal Trainer. Where customer service is a monologue, hospitality is a dialogue, conveying that the client's needs are the priority in an interactive communication (9). Warmth, friendliness, kindness, and the instinct to want to do the right thing for the client are ultimately at the core of hospitality. These emotional skills are difficult to find in individuals, and even more difficult to train, but if demonstrated can pay big dividends. Exhibiting hospitality often equates to clients thoroughly enjoying themselves, and as a result, they yearn to have the experience again and will share it with others. The net result of sharing with others, known as word-of-mouth advertising, cannot be understated, as it leads to client loyalty and referrals that are paramount to the success of a Personal Trainer in business.

> Hospitality is centered on the intangible and emotionally driven behaviors that demonstrate to the clients that they are special and cared for by the Personal Trainer.

According to Meyer (9), professionals who create a hospitality experience typically possess the following traits:

- *Optimistic warmth*: genuine kindness, thoughtfulness, and a sense that the glass is always half full
- *Intelligence*: open-mindedness and an insatiable curiosity to learn

- *Work ethic*: a natural tendency to do something as well as possible
- *Empathy*: an awareness of, care for, and connection to how others feel and how the individual's actions affect others
- *Self-awareness and integrity*: understanding what makes a person tick and a natural inclination to be accountable for doing the right thing

A Personal Trainer possessing the aforementioned traits will innately be able to exhibit the following examples of hospitality:

- Greet the client with an appropriately firm handshake, authentic smile, and eye contact.
- Convey that the client's best interest is in mind under any circumstance.
- Address client requests and do what is possible to make them happen.
- At the end of a session, sincerely thank the client for his or her time.
- Make follow-up calls/e-mails to see how the client feels after a personal training session.
- Send a handwritten card to thank the client after an initial appointment or when a significant goal has been reached.
- Search for opportunities to go above and beyond what is expected.

The Personal Trainer should strive to embrace and exhibit both customer service and hospitality. Establishing a habit of providing consistent and reliable service, as well as taking the extra steps to demonstrate to the clients that they are cared for, will make an indelible impression. Many clients are more interested in knowing how much the Personal Trainer cares than in knowing how much the Personal Trainer knows. Conveying this will allow the Personal Trainer to experience not only the joy of giving and the pride that accompanies it but certainly the rewards of client satisfaction and allegiance as well.

## Relationship Marketing

The principle of marketing is central to any successful business and incorporates many of the concepts from customer service and hospitality. Considered a future trend in marketing, relationship marketing is a vital component in the service industry and encourages thinking and acting like the customer to secure and retain a trusting and loyal long-term relationship (7). Although similar, hospitality and relationship marketing are not mutually exclusive and actually should be carried out simultaneously. The primary goal of marketing is to bring the buyer (client) and the seller (Personal Trainer) together, the strategies of which are worthy of the Personal Trainer's attention leading into the initial client consultation.

What differentiates this new paradigm of relationship marketing from conventional marketing is that first, a personal relationship with the customer should take precedence, and sales will follow; and second, retaining existing clients should take precedence over seeking new customers (Box 10.1). In contrast, traditional marketing places great emphasis on the constant hunt for new sales to new customers. Although traditional marketing has its place in the business of personal training, relationship marketing concepts certainly have notable implications for the Personal Trainer as well.

---

**Box 10.1    Principle of Relationship Marketing**

- A personal relationship with the customer should take precedence, and sales will follow.
- Retaining existing clients should take precedence over seeking new customers.

Adapted from Kandampully JA. *Services Management: The New Paradigm in Hospitality*. Upper Saddle River (NJ): Pearson Education; 2007.

Relating to the client will facilitate a mutual desire to have a trusting, loyal, and long-lasting working relationship.

The first premise of relationship marketing is to emphasize the personal relationship with the client, which is supported by the idea that customers have a deep desire to trust the business provider and are inherently loyal (7,8). Customers have also been found to be loyal to those who trust them, so it is crucial that the Personal Trainer interact with the client in a way that reinforces this trust. As a result, the Personal Trainer will be rewarded with the client's desire to maintain the working relationship. On the other hand, even though clients resist changing business providers, as is the case with dentists or doctors, they will seek another provider if this trust is abused (7,8). Relating to the client will facilitate a mutual desire to have a trusting, loyal, and long-lasting working relationship.

The second premise of relationship marketing is to focus on retaining existing clients as opposed to only seeking new clients. Research indicates that retained customers are very profitable over time for reasons including increased purchases, referrals, and lower operating costs (to maintain existing clients vs. marketing for new clients). It is common for businesses to lose an average of 15%–20% of its customers each year; however, businesses can double their growth if those customer losses are cut in half (13). Additionally, traditional business research estimates that attracting a new client costs five times more than keeping an existing one (4,6). As such, it is in the best interest of the Personal Trainer to survey departing clients in order to understand the reasons for leaving. If the factors are controllable, the Personal Trainer should take action with existing clients to minimize these defections in the future.

The Personal Trainer should pay close attention to relationship marketing as a means to success. Favorable word-of-mouth advertising, perhaps the most cost-effective marketing strategy in business, has the opportunity to flourish if the Personal Trainer is meeting expectations and nurturing the client relationship. Furthermore, when the broader business concepts of customer service, hospitality, and relationship marketing are integrated, the Personal Trainer will be better equipped to face the challenges that inherently exist in the business world. Considering that 25%–50% of business operating costs stem from poor service, or not performing up to par the first time, it behooves the Personal Trainer to be attentive to the facets that enhance service quality right from the start (6). When putting these conceptual tools into action prior to and during the first client meeting, the Personal Trainer will have a greater capacity to not only survive but excel in attracting and retaining clients as well.

## The Power of Nonverbal Communication

Because the client–Personal Trainer relationship is crucial for success, every facet of relationship building is important and the spoken word is only part of the communication puzzle. Much can be learned about people by observing their nonverbal cues, because most people are not good at concealing emotions (11). In some cases, watching nonverbal cues is believed to be more reliable and essential to understanding another person than listening to speech (11). For example, if there seems to be a discrepancy between one's speech and body language, the listener will likely place more value in the body language of the communicator. Therefore, knowledge of body language is invaluable for success in both personal and professional relationships. Not only can a Personal Trainer learn to become a more effective nonverbal communicator, but learning these cues will enhance the ability to understand the client as well.

Watching nonverbal cues is believed to be more reliable and essential to understanding another person than listening to speech.

Body language such as posture, eye contact, and facial expressions speak volumes about an individual's thoughts and emotional state. For example, posture and stance are strong indicators of how engaged a person is in a job and if he or she believes in the product or service being sold. Simply observing a person's stance can quickly determine energy, confidence, and sense of power in a position (10). Facial expressions may provide the best body language clues, though. In particular, a person is said to lack sincerity or truthfulness if there is a contradiction between words and facial expressions. Additionally, facial expressions from emotional responses come and go quickly; therefore, a person who holds an expression for an extended period of time may not be exhibiting a genuine emotion (12).

Although a powerful tool, interpreting body language is a science that has evolved over time and still holds some disagreement among experts. For example, it has been thought that people who stand while holding their hands behind their back exude power; however, it has also been found that observers think these people are untrustworthy. Additionally, individuals who are unable to make eye contact have been thought to be lying, yet this can also be interpreted as nervousness (11). Nonetheless, it may be helpful to "study" your client, as cultural differences may effect the interpretation of body language. For example, in some cultures, direct eye contact may be interpreted as rude, emphasizing the importance of understanding the client's background.

These and other body language distinctions can be used to provide the Personal Training client with tailored customer service and hospitality. For example, the Personal Trainer should be observant of the client when the client is walking into the facility, office, or on the exercise floor. Upon meeting, if the client has slouching posture, crossed arms, and shifty eye contact, this may indicate nervousness and insecurity. The Personal Trainer should take extra steps to maintain a warm and patient demeanor while explaining what to expect during the meeting and give the client opportunities to express concern or ask questions. In another scenario, if the client's facial expression indicates confusion while hesitantly performing a new exercise, he or she may not verbalize the need for assistance. In response, the Personal Trainer should take the initiative to demonstrate the exercise again, reiterate movement cues, and provide positive reinforcement of what the client is doing correctly to increase confidence of the skill.

On the other hand, the Personal Trainer must be aware that his or her nonverbal communication is being observed and equally has an impact. For example, imagine a client enthusiastically describing how he or she felt after the last training session while the Personal Trainer is leaning against the exercise machine looking off in another direction. How would this make the client feel? Similarly, imagine a client performing an exercise and inquiring if the movement is being done correctly, only to discover that the Personal Trainer is preoccupied with watching television. How would this make the client feel? Apathy and divided attention are not attributes of customer service, hospitality, or the client-centered approach and should be avoided at all costs, or trust will diminish. The Personal Trainer must exercise self-awareness at all times when working with clients to ensure that positive nonverbal communication is being expressed. Accordingly, cell phones and other personal communication devices should be left off the exercise training floor such that your first priority is the client with whom you are working.

Exhibiting positive body language can certainly be a powerful business tool. Consider that the actions a businessperson exhibits within the first 15 seconds of walking into a room will likely make or break a sale even before talking begins (10). Regardless of the type of business, this kind of influence is very valuable and has been shown to be a function of a person's body language attractiveness. With all else being equal, those who have attractive body language tend to be more successful. Below are some behaviors that increase one's body language attractiveness and can improve nonverbal communication skills (10):

- *Appearance and physique*: Maintain good hygiene along with a healthy and fit appearance. Clothing colors are also influential. For example, these are the specific messages that some colors can convey: red (power, danger, force, passion), orange (excitement, encouragement), yellow (happiness, energy, intelligence), green (harmony, safety), blue (trust, confidence, peace), purple (luxury, creativity), white (safe, purity), and black (power, mystery, aggressive, unsafe) (5). Depending upon the kind of message the Personal Trainer wants to convey to a client on any particular day, uniform colors can have a powerful influence on the relationship with the client.
- *Eye contact*: The more frequent eye contact the better, although staring for more than a few seconds at a time can be uncomfortable for the client and may be construed as flirtatious. Frequent blinking conveys a wandering mind or one that wants to interrupt; therefore, blink less.

- *Facial expressions*: Smile often and appear interested. Widening the eyes and raising eyebrows express interest and surprise. On the contrary, narrowing the eyes or lowering the eyebrows can mean disgust, anger, or sadness.
- *Head movements*: Keep chin up and nod "yes" to show interest.
- *Gestures*: Be expressive with hands and body movements without exaggeration.
- *Posture*: Sit and stand erect and lean forward to show interest. Leaning back is perceived as informal. Keep arms and legs uncrossed to convey a secure and welcoming demeanor.
- *Proximity and orientation*: Be as close as possible without crowding the client. A comfortable range is between 1.5 and 4 ft (0.46 and 1.22 m), yet it is important to read the client's body language and adjust accordingly.
- *Timing and synchronization*: Speed up activities but not to the point of ineffectiveness.
- *Nonverbal aspects of speech*: Balance the need to listen with the need to talk. Letting the client do the talking can often lead to them providing information that otherwise might have been missed. Having the Personal Trainer control the conversation with proper questioning can allow the client to talk and feel valued while the Personal Trainer absorbs information.

These categories of behavior increase the attractiveness of a person to others, which can assist in enhancing communication between two people. In short, possessing enthusiasm can quickly lead to all the behaviors listed without consciously having to focus on each point. Conscious awareness can not only enhance the Personal Trainer's ability to exhibit these traits but also improve the ability to identify them in others.

## The Client-Centered Approach to Coaching

In conjunction with exhibiting acts of customer service and hospitality, there are motivational and behavioral change coaching skills that will further enhance the client–trainer relationship if taken into account. These fundamental skills will increase the trainer's understanding of the client in a collaborative framework; therefore, increase the trainer's ability to affect behavior change. Referred to as the "client-centered approach," the motivational interviewing skills of rapport building, exhibiting empathy, and active listening are central to keeping the client's perspective at the forefront (2). Although this style of relationship building takes more time in the initial client consultation and beyond, the partnership approach will likely yield more positive results. For example, when used by physicians, the results include higher client satisfaction and improved compliance along with reduced concerns and physical symptoms (15). Contrary to the style of many Personal Trainers, this approach does not encourage giving unsolicited advice. Although it is beneficial under some circumstances, Rollnick and colleagues (14) found that advice giving can hinder behavior change because it can be perceived as condescending and undermines the client's intelligence and sense of independence. Telling a client what to do may lead to resentment, so it is important for the Personal Trainer to think twice before attempting an unwelcome verbal monologue of directions. Clearly, a client seeks a Personal Trainer for motivation and advice, but the way in which it is done should be considered, and the client-centered approach provides the context for such communication. Therefore, adopting a motivational interviewing method, which is both collaborative and directive, will enhance intrinsic motivation toward healthy behavior change.

> Referred to as the "client-centered approach," the motivational interviewing skills of rapport building, exhibiting empathy, and active listening are central to keeping the client's perspective at the forefront (2).

### Rapport Building

The first element of the client-centered approach is establishing rapport, which is developed by building a trusting and respectful relationship with the client. Starting the working relationship

| Box 10.2 | Summary of Client-Centered Techniques |
|---|---|

- Ask simple, open-ended questions (*i.e.*, questions that elicit details instead of yes-or-no responses).
- Listen and encourage with verbal and nonverbal prompts.
- Clarify and summarize. Check your understanding of what the client said and check to see whether the client understood what you said.
- Use reflective listening. This involves making statements that aim to bridge the gap between what the client is saying and the meaning behind the statements.

From Rollnick S, Mason P, Butler C. *Health Behavior Change. A Guide for Practitioners.* New York (NY): Churchill Livingstone; 1999. p. 225.

in this manner is critical and can readily be accomplished by asking open-ended questions (Box 10.2). For example, simply asking the client to describe a typical day will give the Personal Trainer information that may be useful in guiding the client to more healthful eating or exercise habits (14). For this type of rapport building to be effective, the Personal Trainer must keep in mind that open-ended questions are meant to gather information rather than be an interrogation. Asking simple noninvasive questions can help the Personal Trainer get a better understanding of the client. This process should take approximately 3–5 minutes and can start by simply asking, "Can you tell me about a recent typical day for you from beginning to end, so I can get a clearer picture of what it looks like?" or "The last time you worked out, what did you like or dislike about it?" If the clients feel that they are being judged, they will be less likely to elaborate, so it is important to allow the clients to speak freely without interrupting to point out problem areas. Ideally, the Personal Trainer will be speaking 10%–15% of the time and be focused on pacing the conversation, asking the clients to elaborate when necessary (14).

### Exhibiting Empathy

Another way of establishing rapport is to demonstrate empathy by earnestly listening and expressing understanding. Individuals often feel a kinship with others who can relate to them or who have had similar experiences. One way of demonstrating empathy is to listen, repeat what was said, and clarify what was said in the form of a question (2). As an example, a client may volunteer information about his or her exercise habits over the years and state that he or she is reluctant to get in shape for fear of experiencing more injuries. In this case, the Personal Trainer may ask, "So that I understand you, fear of injuries has kept you from engaging in a regular exercise routine. Is that correct?" Paraphrasing, rather than just repeating the client's words, reaffirms to the client, the Personal Trainer was listening intently and understands.

### Active Listening

Attempting to understand the underlying meaning of what a client is saying is referred to as active listening. Although requiring more skill and practice, this technique further enhances rapport and demonstrates empathy through the use of reflective statements (2). Using the example earlier, the Personal Trainer may say, "It sounds like you are hesitant to exercise regularly at this time (reflective statement). Many people are hesitant to exercise after an injury (empathetic statement). Can you tell me about your specific concerns (open-ended question)?" This nonjudgmental style of communication tells the client that the Personal Trainer understands the emotions that the client may be experiencing, while providing an additional opportunity for the Personal Trainer to learn more

---

## Box 10.3    Indicators that the Client-Centered Approach Is Being Used

- The Personal Trainer is speaking slowly.
- The client is talking more than the Personal Trainer.
- The client is talking about behavior change.
- The Personal Trainer is listening intently and directing the conversation when appropriate.
- The client appears to be making realizations and connections not previously considered.

From Rollnick S, Mason P, Butler C. *Health Behavior Change. A Guide for Practitioners.* New York (NY): Churchill Livingstone; 1999. p. 225.

---

about the client while keeping the conversation focused on important distinctions. This process will help garner mutual trust, enhance the client's self-awareness, and provide the Personal Trainer with more insight as to what will help facilitate healthful behavior change.

Building rapport, exhibiting empathy, and listening actively will help build an effective communication bridge between the client and the Personal Trainer. A summary of the three motivational interviewing techniques can be seen in Box 10.2, whereas Box 10.3 lists the indicators that the client-centered approach is being used. Additional guidance on various motivation and behavioral modification tools can also be found in Chapter 8.

# Preceding the Initial Client Consultation

## Generating Clients

Certainly, one of the pressing issues in any business is attracting new customers or clients. Some Personal Trainers may have the luxury of working in a facility where clients are continually being referred, in which case the Personal Trainer has to focus only on client retention, utilizing concepts stated previously. However, in many cases, the responsibility is on the Personal Trainer to not only retain clients but seek and secure new ones as well. Following are the strategies to generate new clients that can be applied to corporate, private, or commercial club settings.

### Word-of-Mouth Advertising

One of the most cost-effective and powerful methods of marketing is word-of-mouth referrals from satisfied clients. Oftentimes, these referrals will be unsolicited without any effort needed on behalf of the Personal Trainer. On the other hand, the Personal Trainer may also want to express to existing clients that new clients are desired and that referrals are appreciated. In this case, the Personal Trainer may want to advertise a client referral program in which the existing client receives a complimentary fitness assessment or receives a discount on future sessions for each referred new client.

### Fitness Floor Exposure

Personal Trainers working with clients on the floor are a walking advertisement of their style and services. For this reason, it is important to consistently exhibit professionalism and provide focused attention while training an existing client. Potential clients will likely not be attracted to Personal Trainers who appear distracted, disinterested, or not respectful of the client being trained. However, keeping an approachable disposition and making friendly eye contact with other members between exercises are certainly encouraged. If not working with a client, Personal Trainers may want to walk the fitness floor and make themselves available for questions, which may lead to more interest and personal training inquiries. Examples such as wearing a shirt that has the words, "Personal Trainer" largely displayed can assist in distinguishing the Personal Trainer from other staff or setting up a demonstration table in the front lobby can help bring exposure to the services they provide. The more exposure a Personal Trainer has with members increases their chances of parlaying that into personal training.

## Complimentary Consultations

Although some may be of the opinion that offering free services devalues a service overall, occasionally marketing complimentary initial client consultations may be a strategy that can differentiate one Personal Trainer or club over another and lead to more clients.

## Front Desk Contacts

Depending on the size of the club and member inquiry process, the front desk staff or receptionist may be the first individual to field a question about personal training services. The process may dictate that staff refer member inquiries to the Personal Trainer directly or to a Personal Training Director first. In either case, it is important for the Personal Trainer to develop a strong working relationship with the "gatekeeper" staff and routinely communicate if new clients are desired. Stating availability, training style, and desired client special populations of interest may also be valuable reminders to the staff. Brochures and promotional flyers should also be displayed at a front desk or central location whenever possible with particular attention given to design and layout because it is a professional reflection on the Personal Trainer.

## Professional Networking and Referrals

Personal Trainers should be part of an integrated community network of mutually referring health care professionals including, but not limited to, doctors (medical, chiropractic, naturopathic), physical therapists, certified athletic trainers, exercise physiologists, massage therapists, acupuncturists, wellness coaches, and registered dietitians. Retail fitness, nutrition, and health food stores, as well as local service professionals such as real estate and insurance agents and accountants, are viable referral sources. The Personal Trainer may want to join a professional networking group to facilitate these relationships in the community or make personal office visits and ask whether it is possible to display business cards or brochures while providing referrals in return.

## Internet and Social Media Marketing

Increasing the number of exposure points will certainly enhance the consistency of new client interest, and in today's economy, Internet presence is paramount. It appears that all population demographics are increasingly using the Internet to obtain information and to socially connect; therefore, it is recommended that the Personal Trainer possess a personal Web site, utilize the club's Web site, or be active on one of the variety of social network sites. Creating and maintaining a Web site blog is also recommended, which may help not only attract but retain clients by facilitating a continual dialogue. Web site content should highlight areas of expertise and training style and include client success stories or testimonials with relevant images (be sure prior permission is obtained, for confidentiality protection). In addition, utilizing other social media sites such as Facebook, YouTube, Twitter, or Instagram may be other outlets to increase exposure. These sites can be used to share positive status updates, special events, or incentives for clients and potential clients. However, if these sites are used, it is important to keep them as professional sites and not use any personal accounts.

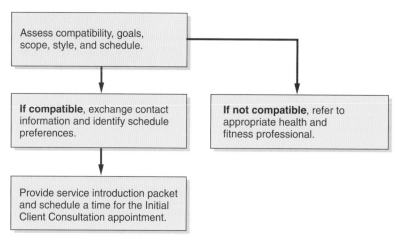

**FIGURE 10.1.** Initial client contact process.

## Initial Client Contact

It is advisable that the Personal Trainer have a process to screen and take new clients. Not only will this assist the Personal Trainer in gathering and organizing critical information about a potential client but, perhaps, more importantly, it is the first opportunity to make an impression on the client by demonstrating organization, care, and professionalism. A flowchart of the recommended initial client-contact process is shown in Figure 10.1. This process may occur in person, over the phone, or via e-mail. Regardless of the communication method, great care should be taken to ensure that all elements of customer service, hospitality, and the client-centered approach are being incorporated when interfacing with the client (Fig. 10.2).

### Initial Client-Contact Process

A more detailed description of the initial client-contact process (see Fig. 10.1) is outlined as follows:

- Assess compatibility and refer as needed.
- Discuss the client's health and fitness goals and any relevant health conditions/limitations and ensure experience and scope are sufficient to meet the client's needs.
- Discuss experience, training style, and educational background and ensure that it is both adequate and appealing to the client.
- State the fee structure and ensure that it is agreeable to the client.

**FIGURE 10.2.** Greeting a client.

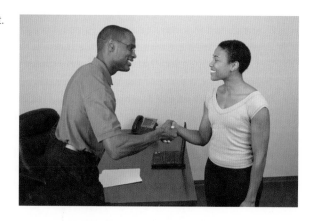

- Discuss the client's schedule preferences and assess compatibility for ongoing appointments.
- Refer to an alternate Personal Trainer or other health care professional if goals and interests are not compatible or if outside scope of practice or expertise (see Chapter 11 for detailed guidance on the professional referral process).
- Exchange contact information.
  - Exchange phone numbers and e-mail addresses while identifying the preferred method of communication.
- Schedule the initial client consultation.
  - Schedule a mutually agreeable appointment for the initial client consultation if there is clear compatibility and interest between both parties to proceed.
  - Explain clearly what to expect and how to prepare for the initial client consultation in terms of appropriate dress, nutrition and hydration preparation, avoiding significant exertion prior, and what the appointment will include.
- Provide a service introduction packet.
  - Critical contents of the packet are intended to be returned prior to the next appointment and may include the following: Health/Medical History Evaluation Form, Medical Clearance Form if necessary (see Chapter 11 for sample forms), and Informed Consent. Additionally, the Client–Personal Trainer Agreement (see "Components of the Consultation" section) should be given to the client to be completed and returned at the next appointment. These forms may be distributed in hard copy directly or soft copy forms can be sent electronically to the client based on preference. The Personal Trainer will instruct the client to complete the forms and return them at the next meeting.
  - Provide additional information on a Web site dedicated to the service introduction, which may contain supporting marketing materials such as client testimonials, health care professional endorsements, and Personal Trainer publications or press clippings.
  - Contents of the packet intended for review may include a business card, Personal Trainer bio and welcome letter, facility brochure, and training services pricing structure.

### Client Intake Form

The aforementioned process should be used in conjunction with the client intake form, which is used to obtain the critical client contact information (Fig. 10.3).

### Preparing for the Initial Client Consultation

The initial client contact is the precursor to the initial client consultation and is a valuable springboard for the next meeting when set up correctly. First, it is important that the Personal Trainer remind the client the day and time of the next meeting and the time allotted for the appointment. Next, it should be clearly articulated what the next appointment will include, the recommended attire, necessary equipment, and if a hydration bottle is needed. The client should also be reminded to complete and return the necessary forms and to contact the Personal Trainer if any questions or concerns arise. The Personal Trainer should take exceptional care in departing with the new client by making eye contact and shaking hands, walking the client to the door, and then thanking the client by name while genuinely expressing that the next visit is eagerly awaited. Ideally, if the Personal Trainer exhibits traits of outstanding customer service, hospitality, and relationship building in this initial meeting, the client will be motivated and inspired to return for the next visit.

> The Personal Trainer should take exceptional care in departing with the new client by making eye contact and shaking hands, walking the client to the door, and then thanking the client by name while genuinely expressing that the next visit is eagerly awaited.

## New Client Intake Form

**Contact Information**

Date: _____ _____ Phone _____ In-Person

Name:

_____

Address:

_____

Preferred method of contact:

_____ Phone (home): _____

_____ Phone (cell): _____

_____ Email: _____

Training Schedule Interest (circle all that apply):

| Sunday | Monday | Tuesday | Wednesday | Thursday | Friday | Saturday | Sunday |
|--------|--------|---------|-----------|----------|--------|----------|--------|
| am | am | am | am | am | am | am | am |
| midday | midday | midday | midday | midday | midday | midday | midday |
| pm | pm | pm | pm | pm | pm | pm | pm |

**Health and Fitness Information**

General Health and Fitness Goals (check all that apply):

☐ strength                    ☐ disease management

☐ endurance                   ☐ stress management

☐ sport performance           ☐ weight management

☐ physical appearance         ☐ energy/vitality

Health or other Fitness Professional(s) treating client:

_____

_____

Medical Considerations/Limitations:

_____

_____

MD Release Form Needed: _____ Yes _____ No

MD Name/Phone Contact (if necessary):

_____

**Action Items**

Referral to Health of Fitness Professional: _____ Yes _____ No

Referral:

_____

*If compatible:*

MD Release Form (if necessary) Date Sent: _____ Rec'd: _____

Initial Client Consultation Date: _____

Service Introduction Packet Delivered: _____ In-Person _____ Email _____ Mail

Comments:

_____

_____

**FIGURE 10.3.** Example of a new client intake form.

# Initial Client Consultation

Up to this point, much of the groundwork has been laid in preparation for the initial client consultation. Indeed, some of the most important work in a Personal Trainer's profession is in establishing rapport, creating a comfortable and welcoming environment, and inspiring motivation in a client. What remains are the more technical elements that a consultation may include.

## Consultation Location and Confidentiality

Of utmost importance is the location of the client consultation, as it sets the tone for information sharing and relationship building. The Personal Trainer must view this experience through the eyes of a new client and create a hospitable and private environment accordingly. Discussion of personal and confidential health information must be held in the strictest confidence and taken seriously. Additionally, it is common for new clients to feel uneasy about themselves and their health and fitness status and a fitness center environment may exacerbate those insecurities. Although not all clients will externally exhibit such sensitivities, it is best to err conservatively. Therefore, creating a welcoming and nonjudgmental atmosphere in a private space should be a priority.

Specifically, the consultation and assessment should be in an enclosed room or remote space within the facility, so that verbal communication is not clearly discernible to other clients. The space should be free from distracting background noise or music, along with any visual distractions that could hinder a focused conversation between client and Personal Trainer. The area should be clean and organized, comfortably accommodate two to four chairs, and have a desk or table wide enough for the Personal Trainer to review or explain documents. The area should have good lighting and proper ventilation. In accordance with American College of Sports Medicine (ACSM) recommendations, the assessment area should maintain a comfortable temperature between 68° F and 72° F (20° C and 22° C), with humidity below 60% (1). If it is not possible to have a separate room to conduct the initial consultation, sitting with the client facing away from other clients may be advisable to maximize privacy and prevent voices from carrying.

## Introduction and Consultation Agenda Review

As previously discussed, the Personal Trainer should warmly welcome the client upon first sight with a handshake and smile and engage in light conversation to put the client at ease. Next, the Personal Trainer should lead the client to the private consultation area and review the sequence and content of the initial client consultation. Even though the Personal Trainer has previously outlined the process in the initial client contact, it is recommended that a step-by-step review of the process again be provided at this point. For example, the Personal Trainer may say:

> I'm very glad that you have taken this step toward enhancing your health and fitness and I'm eager for us to get started. First, I'd like to outline what this appointment will include so that you know what to expect and to see if you have any questions or concerns. Does that sound alright with you?

If concerns are expressed, address them and then continue.

> We will begin by reviewing the paperwork that you were asked to complete (Personal Trainer–Client Agreement, Health/Medical History Evaluation Form [and/or Physical Activity Readiness Questionnaire], Informed Consent, and Medical Clearance Form as needed). Then, I'd like to hear more about your health and fitness goals and interests. This will help me get to know you better and help us determine which fitness assessments we should perform. Finally, we will conduct the fitness assessments, discuss the results, and discuss an action plan together. Do you have any questions before we begin?

Not only does clearly defining the structure of the appointment lessen anxiety, but it provides an opportunity for the client to express concerns or feelings about performing a given part of the assessment. For example, a client may be uncomfortable with the prospect of a caliper body-fat composition test if self-conscious about a weight problem. This provides the Personal Trainer an opportunity to empathize with the client and modify or eliminate a test as appropriate. If a client expresses any trepidation about a test, the Personal Trainer should immediately honor the request without any pressure. During this trust-building time, the benefit of expressing understanding will far outweigh the cost of convincing a client to do something with which he or she is uncomfortable.

## Components of the Consultation

Once the stage has been set for the appointment, the Personal Trainer can continue with carrying out the key components of the consultation. This includes reviewing the documents that were given to the client during the initial client contact. Ideally, the client will have already completed the forms so that more time can be spent on getting to know the client, performing assessments, and goal setting; otherwise, it is important to note that these elements may be provided over the course of one or two appointments, depending on the time availability and appointment structure of the Personal Trainer's club or facility. Either way, the following elements should be included.

### Personal Trainer–Client Agreement

It is very important to review expectations between the client and the Personal Trainer before joining in a business relationship. For example, cancelled or no-show appointments have financial ramifications for both parties, and so ensuring mutual understanding is critical from the start. The document can be adapted to include other essential business expectations (Fig. 10.4). Be sure to retain a copy of this document for yourself and give a copy to the client.

### Health/Medical History Evaluation Form and/or PAR-Q

Discussing the client's current health status and history is imperative in getting to know his or her areas for improvement as well as limitations. This information will further assist the Personal Trainer in assessing risk and whether a Physical Activity Readiness Questionnaire (PAR-Q) and/or Medical Clearance Form is necessary to proceed (see Chapter 11 for more detailed guidance on the use of a Health/Medical History Evaluation Form and/or PAR-Q).

### Medical Clearance Form

If determined through the use of the Health/Medical History Evaluation or PAR-Q that the client should see a physician before starting either a moderate- or high-intensity exercise routine, it is imperative to have this document signed by both the client and the physician. It may provide important restriction information that should be taken into account during program testing and design (see Chapter 11 for more detailed guidance on the use of a medical clearance form).

### Informed Consent

From an ethical and legal perspective, it is important that the client understand the risks and benefits of performing assessments and engaging in a guided exercise program. Reviewing the informed consent verbally with the client at the onset allows opportunities for inquiries, serves as a document of understanding, and should be signed by the client (see Chapter 11 for more detailed guidance on the use of an informed consent).

The Personal Trainer should ask additional questions about the client's goals to get more specific responses as well as timelines that the client seeks for achievement.

### Client Goals

Using the information from the client intake form (see Fig. 10.3) as a guide, the Personal Trainer should ask additional questions about the client's goals to get more specific responses as well as timelines that the client seeks for achievement. Motivational interviewing techniques will help to facilitate intrinsically motivated goals from a collaborative discussion (see Chapter 8 for more detailed guidance on goal setting).

**Personal Training Client Agreement**

I, _____, have read and agree to the following:
(Client's Name-Please Print)

• Appointments will be scheduled directly through my assigned Personal Trainer and can be scheduled on days and times that are mutually agreed upon.

• I have exchanged contact information with my Personal Trainer and have indicated my preference for being contacted. I understand that the facility staff is not authorized to give out my Personal Trainer's personal contact information.

• I may not bring an outside Personal Trainer into the facility to train with me.

• Private personal training sessions are one hour.

• I understand that I am expected to arrive for my appointments on time, dressed and ready to train. If I arrive late for my appointment, I understand that my training session will end at the previously scheduled time.

• Cancellation Policy: I understand that appointments must be cancelled by contacting my Personal Trainer directly, within 24 hours of my scheduled time, in order to avoid being charged for the full session.

• No Show Policy: I understand that if I do not show up for my scheduled training session, I will be charged for the full session.

• In the event that my Personal Trainer fails to contact me within 24 hours of our scheduled session, or does not show up, he/she will schedule an additional session at no cost to me.

• I understand that I may communicate any customer service issue and/or acknowledge excellent performance to the Facility Manager.

Client Signature: _____   Date: _____

Personal Trainer (Print): _____   Date: _____

**FIGURE 10.4.** Example of personal training client agreement. (Adapted from Plus One Health Management, Inc., New York [NY]: 2008, with permission.)

## Health and Fitness Assessment

Once any health limitations or restrictions are ascertained and goals identified from the aforementioned process, it is time to perform the fitness assessment. Even though a general overview of the tests to be performed is explained at the beginning of the consultation (Fig 10.5), it is advised to thoroughly explain and demonstrate each assessment immediately prior to it being performed to further minimize any anxiety or confusion that the client may have. Selecting and explaining tests that emphasize a balanced program is important and may include resting heart rate and blood pressure as well as body composition, cardiovascular fitness, strength, endurance, range of motion, and anthropometric and postural measures (see Chapter 12 for more detailed guidance on health and fitness assessments).

**FIGURE 10.5.** Client consultation.

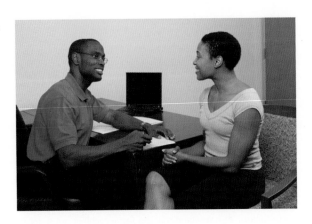

### Assessment Results and Action Plan

Upon the completion of any assessment, most clients are eager to receive the results. If the results can be given immediately after the tests, it enables the client and the Personal Trainer to begin taking action toward mutually identified goals. It is important to share the results in a positive manner, emphasizing that the results are a baseline with which to measure progress over time. Based on the results, a referral to a physician or other health care professional may be needed for a medical release. In this case, the Personal Trainer should print the findings on the form so that the client can deliver the information to the health care professional to review.

## Recommending Appropriate Personal Training Packages

At this time, based on the findings of the assessment and verbalized goals, the Personal Trainer should detail a recommended action plan for training with the client. The appointment frequency and number of sessions purchased should be determined by the client's needs and goals. For example, if an experienced client wants to learn new exercise movements to supplement his or her current routine of 4 days per week, then the Personal Trainer likely should recommend meeting only once a week. On the other hand, a new client who is unfamiliar with exercise not only needs to learn how to perform exercise movements safely and with good form but may also need assistance in establishing an exercise habit. In this case, to facilitate learning and encourage an active lifestyle, the Personal Trainer may want to suggest training two to four times per week for 4–16 weeks. This will help the client begin to perfect and memorize the movement patterns and build the foundation for habitual exercise.

Unfortunately, a problem occurs when the beginning exerciser purchases too few sessions. As a result, the sessions occur so infrequently that the client does not have the opportunity to memorize and perform the movement patterns correctly. The disappointed client then feels that the Personal Trainer or training itself is not successful. For this reason, the Personal Trainer must be clear with the client at the beginning and recommend the exercise program that the client needs to succeed. Otherwise, it does the client a disservice if the Personal Trainer is making recommendations solely on monetary concerns versus what will help the client reach individual goals. Thus, the importance of clarity when recommending personal training packages during the initial client consultation becomes apparent and will ultimately help the Personal Trainer succeed in being truthful and realistic about progress.

## Obtaining Client Commitment

Obtaining client commitment through the act of purchasing a package of training sessions can be an act fraught with anxiety for many Personal Trainers. Making recommendations is one part of the equation, yet "landing the sale" is another aspect that does not always come easily. Ideally, the selling process at this point of the initial client consultation should be a positive one for both parties. After developing rapport during the initial client contact, along with a thoughtful, caring, and educational approach to the initial client consultation, the client's purchase of a personal training package will be a natural step in the process of obtaining exercise and fitness training.

> After developing rapport during the initial client contact, along with a thoughtful, caring, and educational approach to the initial client consultation, the client's purchase of a personal training package will be a natural step in the process of obtaining exercise and fitness training.

The Personal Trainer should keep in mind that the client needs the help of a personal training professional and that this is the primary reason that the client has sought out personal training services. The Personal Trainer should focus the client's attention on the service, instruction, motivation, guidance, enthusiasm, safety, and education that he or she will receive from the personal training experience. The Personal Trainer may also remind the client of the value of personal training by the increased sense of self-esteem and the benefits of feeling healthier and being in better shape to actively enjoy life.

One approach to the sale of training sessions is to review the personal training packages that the facility offers and to point out the most commonly purchased package by clients and why. For example, the Personal Trainer can tell the client that most of beginning training clients purchase package A and train 2 days per week. The Personal Trainer could ask, "Would you like to purchase that package?" or "How would you like to proceed?" This approach can help move the client toward purchasing a package of sessions. Common objections to personal training package purchases may arise from the client because of money, time, procrastination, and/or other conflicts. Thus, the Personal Trainer should be prepared to respond and anticipate possible objections. It is important to remember that pressuring a client into an exercise program to which he or she is not willing or is unable to commit could be a pitfall rather than a success story for both the client and the Personal Trainer. On the contrary, the Personal Trainer should maintain a positive attitude, relax and listen to what the client has to say, and then evaluate the objection and respond with empathy and truthfulness.

When the client commits, the Personal Trainer should not act surprised with the sale but rather show appreciation by thanking the client and have the client review and sign all required agreements or contracts. If a commitment is not obtained from the client, the Personal Trainer should maintain a positive perspective and remember that not everyone is going to seek services after the initial client consultation. Demonstrating professionalism, the Personal Trainer should recommend other sources to the client to enhance health and fitness. Based on this customer-focused behavior, the client may likely refer friends or family members or decide to give personal training another chance in the future.

## Leading into the Next Client Appointment

Ideally, throughout both the initial client contact and consultation, the Personal Trainer will have exhibited outstanding customer service and hospitality, along with positive nonverbal communication. In addition, behaviors to enhance the concepts of relationship marketing and the client-centered approach to coaching should have been conscientiously demonstrated.

After the initial client consultation is complete, all the necessary paperwork has been reviewed and a goal-setting action plan has been discussed, the next appointment should be confirmed. At that time, the Personal Trainer should express gratitude to the client for his or her time and display eagerness for the next visit. As a token of hospitality, the Personal Trainer should send a follow-up note or phone call to the client to compliment him or her on the successful step toward health and fitness while reminding the client of the next appointment and how to prepare.

> The Personal Trainer should express gratitude to the client for his or her time and display eagerness for the next visit.

As was discussed in the "Relationship Marketing" section, it is important for businesses to continually evaluate success in order to minimize the percentage of "defections" or those clients who do not return. Appropriately at this time, the Personal Trainer should reevaluate how the meeting went. Whether it ended in a large package purchase or not, the Personal Trainer should spend time mentally reviewing and then write down the positives and negatives that occurred in the consultation. The Personal Trainer should work on the areas of communication skills or approach that may need improvement. All these actions combined will certainly help facilitate a successful beginning to a long-lasting client relationship and set the standard for future client interactions.

## SUMMARY

There are several points of client contact leading up to the initial client consultation appointment that set the groundwork for a successful client–Personal Trainer relationship. This includes contact when attempting to generate new clients, the initial client contact when identifying compatibility, and the initial client consultation itself. Every stage of the relationship is critical, so attention to detail should be paid to effective communication throughout the process. Demonstrating exceptional customer service, hospitality, and positive nonverbal cues from the onset not only communicates pride in professionalism but speaks to the respect and high regard placed in the client as well. Furthermore, a focus on relationship marketing coupled with a client-centered approach engenders trust between the parties. Finally, the Personal Trainer should demonstrate professionalism during the initial client consultation by using appropriate information-gathering tools and testing protocols while communicating skillfully about health and fitness results and the respective personal training action plan.

# REFERENCES

1. American College of Sports Medicine. *ACSM's Guidelines for Exercise Testing and Prescription*. 10th ed. Philadelphia (PA): Wolters Kluwer; 2018.

2. American College of Sports Medicine. *ACSM's Resource Manual for Guidelines for Exercise Testing and Prescription*. 6th ed. Baltimore (MD): Lippincott Williams & Wilkins; 2010. 868 p.

3. Capek F. No matter what business you're in, you're in the hospitality business. *Customer Innovations — Driving Profitable Growth* [Internet]. [cited 2017 Feb 14]. Available from: http://customerinnovations.wordpress.com/2007/11/14/no-matter-what-business-youre-in-youre-in-the-hospitality-business/

4. Gummesson E. Making relationship marketing operational. *Int J Serv Industry Manag*. 1994;5(5):5–20.

5. Hagen S. *The Everything Body Language Book: Master the Art of Nonverbal Communication to Succeed in Work, Love, and Life*. Cincinnati (OH): Adams Media Publishing; 2008. 289 p.

6. Holmund M, Kock S. Relationship marketing: the importance of customer-perceived service quality in retail banking. *Serv Ind J*. 1996;16(3):287–304.

7. Kandampully JA. *Services Management: The New Paradigm in Hospitality*. Upper Saddle River (NJ): Pearson Education, Inc.; 2007. 378 p.

8. Kandampully J. Service quality to service loyalty: a relationship which goes beyond customer services. *Total Qual Manag*. 1998;9(6):431–43.

9. Meyer D. *Setting the Table: The Transforming Power of Hospitality in Business*. New York (NY): HarperCollins Publishers; 2006. 320 p.

10. Morgan N. Are you standing in the way of your own success. In: *The Results-Driven Manager: Face-to-Face Communications for Clarity and Impact*. Boston (MA): Harvard Business School Publishing; 2004. p. 82–5.

11. Morgan N. The truth behind the smile and other myths. In: *The Results-Driven Manager: Face-to-Face Communications for Clarity and Impact*. Boston (MA): Harvard Business School Publishing; 2004. p. 73–81.

12. Morgan N. What your face reveals and conceals. In: *The Results-Driven Manager: Face-to-Face Communications for Clarity and Impact*. Boston (MA): Harvard Business School Publishing Corporation; 2004. p. 86–94.

13. Reichheld FF, Sasser WE Jr. Zero defections: quality comes to services. *Harv Bus Rev*. 1990:105–11.

14. Rollnick S, Mason P, Butler C. *Health Behavior Change. A Guide for Practitioners*. New York (NY): Churchill Livingstone; 1999. 225 p.

15. Stewart M, Brown JB, Weston WW, et al. *Patient-Centered Medicine: Transforming the Clinical Method*. 2nd ed. Abingdon (United Kingdom): Radcliffe Medical Press Ltd.; 2003. 360 p.

# 11

# Preparticipation Physical Activity Screening Guidelines

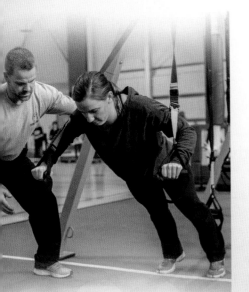

## OBJECTIVES

**Personal Trainers should be able to:**

- Understand the process and outcomes of the American College of Sports Medicine (ACSM) Preparticipation Physical Activity Screening.

- Explore the importance of and issues with preparticipation physical activity screening as well as to investigate the various tools that may be used including the Physical Activity Readiness Questionnaire for Everyone (PAR-Q+) and a health history questionnaire.

- Determine course of action with a client once their risk has been established.

- Discuss the concept of absolute and relative contraindications to exercise testing.

# INTRODUCTION

Ever since the increased promotion of physical activity in modern times, there has been an emphasis on preparticipation physical activity screening to ensure that the risks of an increased physical activity do not outweigh the benefits of this healthy behavior (6). The process of preparticipation physical activity screening has been increasingly professionalized over the years since its introduction. The American College of Sports Medicine (ACSM) is perhaps the best known organization in the area of preparticipation physical activity screening in the United States. The ACSM formally titled this process *risk stratification* in the 1990's in ACSM's *Guidelines for Exercise Testing and Prescription, Fourth Edition* (GETP) publication. This process was retitled *risk classification* in 2013 (3). With the release of 10th edition of GETP in 2017, there were some substantial changes to the preparticipation physical activity screening process including the elimination of the *risk stratification/classification* terminology (including low-, moderate-, and high-risk strata) and the nonuse of adding/subtracting ACSM risk factor thresholds for overall risk. This will be discussed further in this chapter.

The preparticipation physical activity screening process is also intimately tied to the contraindications for graded exercise testing discussed later in this chapter. This chapter will explore the preparticipation physical activity screening concept so the ACSM Certified Exercise Physiologist[SM] (EP-C) and Certified Personal Trainer (CPT) can make informed decisions about the readiness of an individual to undertake a physically active lifestyle.

## Importance of Preparticipation Physical Activity Screening

In order to reduce the likelihood of occurrence of any untoward or unwanted event(s) during a physical activity program, it is prudent to conduct some form of preparticipation physical activity screening on a client (24). Preparticipation physical activity screening, along with cardiovascular risk factor assessment discussed later in this chapter, may also be the first step in a health-related physical fitness assessment. Preparticipation physical activity screening involves gathering and analyzing demographic and health-related information on a client along with some medical/health assessments such as the presence of signs and symptoms in order to aid decision making on a client's physical activity future (3). The preparticipation physical activity screening is a dynamic process in that it may vary in its scope and components depending on the client's needs from a medical/health standpoint (*e.g.*, the client has some form of cardiovascular, metabolic, and/or renal disease, abbreviated as CMR) as well as the presence of signs and symptoms suggestive of CMR disease (*e.g.*, chest pain of an ischemic nature) and their physical activity program goals (they currently participate in moderate physical activity for the past 3 months).

The following is a partial list of the reasons why it is important to first screen clients for participation in physical activity programs (3,17):

- To identify those with medical contraindications (exclusion criteria) for performing physical activity
- To identify those who should receive a medical/physical evaluation/exam and clearance prior to performing a physical activity program
- To identify those who should participate in a medically supervised physical activity program
- To identify those with other health/medical concerns (*i.e.*, orthopedic injuries, *etc.*)

## History of Preparticipation Physical Activity Screening

There are several national and international organizations that have made suggestions about just what these preparticipation physical activity screening guidelines should be including the ACSM (1,2,11,28). However, it is helpful to remember that these are just guidelines or suggestions. The prudent EP-C or CPT should devise a preparticipation physical activity screening scheme that best meets the needs of their client(s) and environment(s).

For instance, the U.S. Surgeon General in the 1996 report on *Physical Activity and Health* stated that (24)

> Previously inactive men over age 40, women over age 50, and people at high risk for CVD [CVD is an abbreviation for cardiovascular disease] should first consult a physician before embarking on a program of vigorous physical activity to which they are unaccustomed. People with disease should be evaluated by a physician first. . . .

In addition, a summary of the "cautions" listed on many pieces of exercise equipment as well as in exercise books and videos is to

- "First consult your physician before starting an exercise program."
- "This is especially important for
    - Men ≥45 years old; women ≥55 years old
    - Those who are going to perform vigorous physical activity
    - And for those who are new to exercise or are unaccustomed to exercise"

There is one major set of formal screening guidelines for individuals who wish to embark on a physical activity program. This set comes from the ACSM. The ACSM has published this set in their popular and often revised text, *ACSM's GETP* starting with their 4th edition in 1991. Several other professional organizations including the American Heart Association (AHA) have also published and revised their own set of preparticipation physical activity screening guidelines. The AHA guidelines were published most recently in their journal *Circulation* in 2001 (3,11).

As stated earlier, the ACSM, through its GETP text, has addressed preparticipation physical activity screening (3). In the past, the ACSM has listed these preparticipation physical activity screening guidelines often under the moniker, "Risk Stratification." Through the first eight editions (although risk stratification did not appear formally in the first three editions) of the GETP, there have been several revisions made to this risk stratification section. The ninth edition of the GETP terms this process as *risk classification*. The recent (2017) 10th edition of GETP has put forth major changes to the preparticipation physical activity screening process (3). We would categorize the revisions made to the GETP preparticipation physical activity screening process as mostly an elimination of the "strata" or levels used in risk classification as well as the elimination of the use of the ACSM risk factor thresholds for the process. In the place of the ACSM risk factor thresholds is the dependence on the physical activity history of the participant as well as the presence of CMR disease and the presence of signs and symptoms suggestive of CMR disease (3).

## Levels of Screening

According to the ACSM, there are two basic approaches to preparticipation physical activity screening (3). One of these approaches can be performed by the individual wishing to become more physically active without direct input from an exercise professional (self-guided screening). Although the other approach involves interaction with an exercise professional such as an EP-C or CPT (professionally supervised screening). These two levels of screening are not mutually exclusive; for instance, an individual may first use the self-guided method before seeking an EP-C or CPT for professional guidance in preparticipation screening.

## Self-Guided Screening

Self-guided approaches to preparticipation physical activity screening have been suggested by many organizations from the ACSM to the AHA as a minimum or starting point for the individual who wishes to increase his or her physical activity (3). The Physical Activity Readiness Questionnaire for Everyone (PAR-Q+) has been suggested for use in self-guided screening and is discussed next.

### Physical Activity Readiness Questionnaire+

The Health History Questionnaire (HHQ) is generally thought of as being a comprehensive assessment of a client's medical and health history. Because the HHQ can be more information than is needed in some situations, the Physical Activity Readiness Questionnaire, or PAR-Q, was developed in Canada to be simpler in both scope and use (26). The original PAR-Q contains seven YES/NO questions that have been found to be both readable and understandable for an individual to answer. The PAR-Q was designed to screen out those clients from not participating in physical activities that may be too strenuous for them. The PAR-Q has been recommended as a minimal standard for entry into moderate-intensity exercise programs. Thus, the PAR-Q may be considered a useful tool for individuals to gauge their own "medical" readiness to participate in physical activity programs (3). However, since the PAR-Q may be best used to screen those who are at high risk for exercise and thus may need a medical exam, it may not be as effective in screening low- to moderate-risk individuals (28). Thus, the PAR-Q has recently morphed into the PAR-Q+ with some word changes among the seven YES/NO questions to better classify all individuals (3) (Fig. 11.1).

Thus, at the minimum, a prudent EP-C or CPT should consider suggesting to their clients that they fill out a PAR-Q+ prior to participation in any self-guided physical activity program (3,32).

The PAR-Q has been found to be a useful tool (26). In one article by de Oliveira Luz and colleagues (9), the PAR-Q was found to have a high (89%) sensitivity (producing many true positives) for picking up potential medical conditions that might impact an individual's exercise responses in older subjects. However, it should be noted that the specificity (or true negatives) of the PAR-Q in this subject pool was estimated at 42% (9). Thus, the PAR-Q may be quite good at detecting potential problems in clients before they occur in an exercise setting, but the form may also wrongly identify clients as having a potential problem when on further evaluation, there is no need for concern. This may not be a bad situation as the form errors of the side of caution. The prudent EP-C or CPT may therefore need to intervene in such cases as well as involve further health care professionals.

Because there are some potential problems noted with the PAR-Q as far as its ability to discern if an individual's potential adverse medical condition might impact his or her exercise response, the PAR-Q+ was developed. However, the PAR-Q+ is a very recent development and thus statistics related to the PAR-Q+ effectiveness are not yet available. It has been suggested by Jamnik and colleagues (16) that a qualified health/fitness professional (EP-C or CPT) may, using ACSM preparticipation physical activity screening process perform a thorough screening process.

### ePARmed-X+Physician Clearance Follow-Up Questionnaire

The ePARmed-X+Physician Clearance Follow-Up Questionnaire was developed also in Canada as a tool that a physician can use to refer individuals to a professionally supervised physical activity program and make recommendations for that program. This form was designed to be used in those cases where a YES answer on one of the seven questions in the PAR-Q+ necessitates further medical clearance using the self-guided method. It is also worth noting, that not while required, the ePARmed-X+Physician Clearance Follow-Up Questionnaire (Fig. 11.2) could be used for medical clearance in a professionally supervised preparticipation physical activity screening.

# 2015 PAR-Q+

### The Physical Activity Readiness Questionnaire for Everyone

The health benefits of regular physical activity are clear; more people should engage in physical activity every day of the week. Participating in physical activity is very safe for MOST people. This questionnaire will tell you whether it is necessary for you to seek further advice from your doctor OR a qualified exercise professional before becoming more physically active.

## GENERAL HEALTH QUESTIONS

| Please read the 7 questions below carefully and answer each one honestly: check YES or NO. | YES | NO |
|---|---|---|
| 1) Has your doctor ever said that you have a heart condition ☐ OR high blood pressure ☐? | ☐ | ☐ |
| 2) Do you feel pain in your chest at rest, during your daily activities of living, **OR** when you do physical activity? | ☐ | ☐ |
| 3) Do you lose balance because of dizziness **OR** have you lost consciousness in the last 12 months? Please answer **NO** if your dizziness was associated with over-breathing (including during vigorous exercise). | ☐ | ☐ |
| 4) Have you ever been diagnosed with another chronic medical condition (other than heart disease or high blood pressure)? **PLEASE LIST CONDITION(S) HERE:** _____ | ☐ | ☐ |
| 5) Are you currently taking prescribed medications for a chronic medical condition? **PLEASE LIST CONDITION(S) AND MEDICATIONS HERE:** _____ | ☐ | ☐ |
| 6) Do you currently have (or have had within the past 12 months) a bone, joint, or soft tissue (muscle, ligament, or tendon) problem that could be made worse by becoming more physically active? Please answer **NO** if you had a problem in the past, but it *does not limit your current ability* to be physically active. **PLEASE LIST CONDITION(S) HERE:** _____ | ☐ | ☐ |
| 7) Has your doctor ever said that you should only do medically supervised physical activity? | ☐ | ☐ |

☑ **If you answered NO to all of the questions above, you are cleared for physical activity.**
**Go to Page 4 to sign the PARTICIPANT DECLARATION. You do not need to complete Pages 2 and 3.**

▶ Start becoming much more physically active – start slowly and build up gradually.

▶ Follow International Physical Activity Guidelines for your age (www.who.int/dietphysicalactivity/en/).

▶ You may take part in a health and fitness appraisal.

▶ If you are over the age of 45 yr and **NOT** accustomed to regular vigorous to maximal effort exercise, consult a qualified exercise professional before engaging in this intensity of exercise.

▶ If you have any further questions, contact a qualified exercise professional.

⬤ **If you answered YES to one or more of the questions above, COMPLETE PAGES 2 AND 3.**

⚠ **Delay becoming more active if:**

✓ You have a temporary illness such as a cold or fever; it is best to wait until you feel better.

✓ You are pregnant - talk to your health care practitioner, your physician, a qualified exercise professional, and/or complete the ePARmed-X+ at **www.eparmedx.com** before becoming more physically active.

✓ Your health changes - answer the questions on Pages 2 and 3 of this document and/or talk to your doctor or a qualified exercise professional before continuing with any physical activity program.

**OSHF**
Ontario Society for Health and Fitness

**FIGURE 11.1.** Physical Activity Readiness Questionnaire for Everyone (PAR-Q+). (Reprinted from Warburton DER, Jamnik VK, Bredin SSD, et al. Executive summary: The Physical Activity Readiness Questionnaire [PAR-Q+] and Electronic Physical Activity Readiness Medical Examination [ePAR-MED-X]. *Heath Fitness J Can.* 2011;4[3]:24–5c, with permission.) (*continued*)

# 2015 PAR-Q+

### FOLLOW-UP QUESTIONS ABOUT YOUR MEDICAL CONDITION(S)

**1.    Do you have Arthritis, Osteoporosis, or Back Problems?**

If the above condition(s) is/are present, answer questions 1a-1c        If **NO** ☐ go to question 2

| | | |
|---|---|---|
| 1a. | Do you have difficulty controlling your condition with medications or other physician-prescribed therapies? (Answer **NO** if you are not currently taking medications or other treatments) | YES☐ NO☐ |
| 1b. | Do you have joint problems causing pain, a recent fracture or fracture caused by osteoporosis or cancer, displaced vertebra (e.g., spondylolisthesis), and/or spondylolysis/pars defect (a crack in the bony ring on the back of the spinal column)? | YES☐ NO☐ |
| 1c. | Have you had steroid injections or taken steroid tablets regularly for more than 3 months? | YES☐ NO☐ |

**2.    Do you have Cancer of any kind?**

If the above condition(s) is/are present, answer questions 2a-2b        If **NO** ☐ go to question 3

| | | |
|---|---|---|
| 2a. | Does your cancer diagnosis include any of the following types: lung/bronchogenic, multiple myeloma (cancer of plasma cells), head, and neck? | YES☐ NO☐ |
| 2b. | Are you currently receiving cancer therapy (such as chemotheraphy or radiotherapy)? | YES☐ NO☐ |

**3.    Do you have a Heart or Cardiovascular Condition?** *This includes Coronary Artery Disease, Heart Failure, Diagnosed Abnormality of Heart Rhythm*

If the above condition(s) is/are present, answer questions 3a-3d        If **NO** ☐ go to question 4

| | | |
|---|---|---|
| 3a. | Do you have difficulty controlling your condition with medications or other physician-prescribed therapies? (Answer **NO** if you are not currently taking medications or other treatments) | YES☐ NO☐ |
| 3b. | Do you have an irregular heart beat that requires medical management? (e.g., atrial fibrillation, premature ventricular contraction) | YES☐ NO☐ |
| 3c. | Do you have chronic heart failure? | YES☐ NO☐ |
| 3d. | Do you have diagnosed coronary artery (cardiovascular) disease and have not participated in regular physical activity in the last 2 months? | YES☐ NO☐ |

**4.    Do you have High Blood Pressure?**

If the above condition(s) is/are present, answer questions 4a-4b        If **NO** ☐ go to question 5

| | | |
|---|---|---|
| 4a. | Do you have difficulty controlling your condition with medications or other physician-prescribed therapies? (Answer **NO** if you are not currently taking medications or other treatments) | YES☐ NO☐ |
| 4b. | Do you have a resting blood pressure equal to or greater than 160/90 mmHg with or without medication? (Answer **YES** if you do not know your resting blood pressure) | YES☐ NO☐ |

**5.    Do you have any Metabolic Conditions?** *This includes Type 1 Diabetes, Type 2 Diabetes, Pre-Diabetes*

If the above condition(s) is/are present, answer questions 5a-5e        If **NO** ☐ go to question 6

| | | |
|---|---|---|
| 5a. | Do you often have difficulty controlling your blood sugar levels with foods, medications, or other physician-prescribed therapies? | YES☐ NO☐ |
| 5b. | Do you often suffer from signs and symptoms of low blood sugar (hypoglycemia) following exercise and/or during activities of daily living? Signs of hypoglycemia may include shakiness, nervousness, unusual irritability, abnormal sweating, dizziness or light-headedness, mental confusion, difficulty speaking, weakness, or sleepiness. | YES☐ NO☐ |
| 5c. | Do you have any signs or symptoms of diabetes complications such as heart or vascular disease and/or complications affecting your eyes, kidneys, **OR** the sensation in your toes and feet? | YES☐ NO☐ |
| 5d. | Do you have other metabolic conditions (such as current pregnancy-related diabetes, chronic kidney disease, or liver problems)? | YES☐ NO☐ |
| 5e. | Are you planning to engage in what for you is unusually high (or vigorous) intensity exercise in the near future? | YES☐ NO☐ |

**FIGURE 11.1.** *(continued)*

# 2015 PAR-Q+

**6.     Do you have any Mental Health Problems or Learning Difficulties?** *This includes Alzheimer's, Dementia, Depression, Anxiety Disorder, Eating Disorder, Psychotic Disorder, Intellectual Disability, Down Syndrome*

If the above condition(s) is/are present, answer questions 6a-6b          If **NO** ☐ go to question 7

| | | |
|---|---|---|
| 6a. | Do you have difficulty controlling your condition with medications or other physician-prescribed therapies? (Answer **NO** if you are not currently taking medications or other treatments) | YES☐ NO☐ |
| 6b. | Do you **ALSO** have back problems affecting nerves or muscles? | YES☐ NO☐ |

**7.     Do you have a Respiratory Disease?** *This includes Chronic Obstructive Pulmonary Disease, Asthma, Pulmonary High Blood Pressure*

If the above condition(s) is/are present, answer questions 7a-7d          If **NO** ☐ go to question 8

| | | |
|---|---|---|
| 7a. | Do you have difficulty controlling your condition with medications or other physician-prescribed therapies? (Answer **NO** if you are not currently taking medications or other treatments) | YES☐ NO☐ |
| 7b. | Has your doctor ever said your blood oxygen level is low at rest or during exercise and/or that you require supplemental oxygen therapy? | YES☐ NO☐ |
| 7c. | If asthmatic, do you currently have symptoms of chest tightness, wheezing, laboured breathing, consistent cough (more than 2 days/week), or have you used your rescue medication more than twice in the last week? | YES☐ NO☐ |
| 7d. | Has your doctor ever said you have high blood pressure in the blood vessels of your lungs? | YES☐ NO☐ |

**8.     Do you have a Spinal Cord Injury?** *This includes Tetraplegia and Paraplegia*

If the above condition(s) is/are present, answer questions 8a-8c          If **NO** ☐ go to question 9

| | | |
|---|---|---|
| 8a. | Do you have difficulty controlling your condition with medications or other physician-prescribed therapies? (Answer **NO** if you are not currently taking medications or other treatments) | YES☐ NO☐ |
| 8b. | Do you commonly exhibit low resting blood pressure significant enough to cause dizziness, light-headedness, and/or fainting? | YES☐ NO☐ |
| 8c. | Has your physician indicated that you exhibit sudden bouts of high blood pressure (known as Autonomic Dysreflexia)? | YES☐ NO☐ |

**9.     Have you had a Stroke?** *This includes Transient Ischemic Attack (TIA) or Cerebrovascular Event*

If the above condition(s) is/are present, answer questions 9a-9c          If **NO** ☐ go to question 10

| | | |
|---|---|---|
| 9a. | Do you have difficulty controlling your condition with medications or other physician-prescribed therapies? (Answer **NO** if you are not currently taking medications or other treatments) | YES☐ NO☐ |
| 9b. | Do you have any impairment in walking or mobility? | YES☐ NO☐ |
| 9c. | Have you experienced a stroke or impairment in nerves or muscles in the past 6 months? | YES☐ NO☐ |

**10.     Do you have any other medical condition not listed above or do you have two or more medical conditions?**

If you have other medical conditions, answer questions 10a-10c          If **NO** ☐ read the Page 4 recommendations

| | | |
|---|---|---|
| 10a. | Have you experienced a blackout, fainted, or lost consciousness as a result of a head injury within the last 12 months **OR** have you had a diagnosed concussion within the last 12 months? | YES☐ NO☐ |
| 10b. | Do you have a medical condition that is not listed (such as epilepsy, neurological conditions, kidney problems)? | YES☐ NO☐ |
| 10c. | Do you currently live with two or more medical conditions? | YES☐ NO☐ |

**PLEASE LIST YOUR MEDICAL CONDITION(S) AND ANY RELATED MEDICATIONS HERE:** _____

_____

_____

## GO to Page 4 for recommendations about your current medical condition(s) and sign the PARTICIPANT DECLARATION.

Copyright © 2015 PAR-Q+ Collaboration  3 / 4
01-01-2015

**FIGURE 11.1.** (*continued*)

# 2015 PAR-Q+

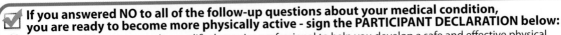

☑ **If you answered NO to all of the follow-up questions about your medical condition, you are ready to become more physically active - sign the PARTICIPANT DECLARATION below:**

▶ It is advised that you consult a qualified exercise professional to help you develop a safe and effective physical activity plan to meet your health needs.

▶ You are encouraged to start slowly and build up gradually - 20 to 60 minutes of low to moderate intensity exercise, 3-5 days per week including aerobic and muscle strengthening exercises.

▶ As you progress, you should aim to accumulate 150 minutes or more of moderate intensity physical activity per week.

▶ If you are over the age of 45 yr and **NOT** accustomed to regular vigorous to maximal effort exercise, consult a qualified exercise professional before engaging in this intensity of exercise.

⬤ **If you answered YES to one or more of the follow-up questions** about your medical condition:

You should seek further information before becoming more physically active or engaging in a fitness appraisal. You should complete the specially designed online screening and exercise recommendations program - the **ePARmed-X+ at www.eparmedx.com** and/or visit a qualified exercise professional to work through the ePARmed-X+ and for further information.

⚠ **Delay becoming more active if:**

✓ You have a temporary illness such as a cold or fever; it is best to wait until you feel better.

✓ You are pregnant - talk to your health care practitioner, your physician, a qualified exercise professional, and/or complete the ePARmed-X+ **at www.eparmedx.com** before becoming more physically active.

✓ Your health changes -  talk to your doctor or qualified exercise professional before continuing with any physical activity program.

⬤ You are encouraged to photocopy the PAR-Q+. You must use the entire questionnaire and NO changes are permitted.
⬤ The authors, the PAR-Q+ Collaboration, partner organizations, and their agents assume no liability for persons who undertake physical activity and/or make use of the PAR-Q+ or ePARmed-X+. If in doubt after completing the questionnaire, consult your doctor prior to physical activity.

## PARTICIPANT DECLARATION

⬤ All persons who have completed the PAR-Q+ please read and sign the declaration below.

⬤ If you are less than the legal age required for consent or require the assent of a care provider, your parent, guardian or care provider must also sign this form.

*I, the undersigned, have read, understood to my full satisfaction and completed this questionnaire. I acknowledge that this physical activity clearance is valid for a maximum of 12 months from the date it is completed and becomes invalid if my condition changes. I also acknowledge that a Trustee (such as my employer, community/fitness centre, health care provider, or other designate) may retain a copy of this form for their records. In these instances, the Trustee will be required to adhere to local, national, and international guidelines regarding the storage of personal health information ensuring that the Trustee maintains the privacy of the information and does not misuse or wrongfully disclose such information.*

NAME _____     DATE _____

SIGNATURE _____     WITNESS _____

SIGNATURE OF PARENT/GUARDIAN/CARE PROVIDER _____

————— **For more information, please contact** —————
**www.eparmedx.com**
**Email: eparmedx@gmail.com**

**Citation for PAR-Q+**
Warburton DER, Jamnik VK, Bredin SSD, and Gledhill N on behalf of the PAR-Q+ Collaboration.
The Physical Activity Readiness Questionnaire for Everyone (PAR-Q+) and Electronic Physical Activity
Readiness Medical Examination (ePARmed-X+). Health & Fitness Journal of Canada 4(2):3-23, 2011.

**Key References**
1. Jamnik VK, Warburton DER, Makarski J, McKenzie DC, Shephard RJ, Stone J, and Gledhill N. Enhancing the effectiveness of clearance for physical activity participation; background and overall process. APNM 36(S1):S3-S13, 2011.
2. Warburton DER, Gledhill N, Jamnik VK, Bredin SSD, McKenzie DC, Stone J, Charlesworth S, and Shephard RJ. Evidence-based risk assessment and recommendations for physical activity clearance; Consensus Document. APNM 36(S1):S266-s298, 2011.

The PAR-Q+ was created using the evidence-based AGREE process (1) by the PAR-Q+ Collaboration chaired by Dr. Darren E. R. Warburton with Dr. Norman Gledhill, Dr. Veronica Jamnik, and Dr. Donald C. McKenzie (2). Production of this document has been made possible through financial contributions from the Public Health Agency of Canada and the BC Ministry of Health Services. The views expressed herein do not necessarily represent the views of the Public Health Agency of Canada or the BC Ministry of Health Services.

**OSHF**
Ontario Society for Health and Fitness

**FIGURE 11.1.** (*continued*)

# ePARmed-X+ Physician Clearance Follow-Up

This form is separated into three main sections:

A) Background information regarding the PAR-Q+ and ePARmed-X+ clearance process,
B) A brief history and demographic information regarding the participant, and
C) The physician's recommendations regarding the participant becoming more physically active.

At the end of this process, the participant is recommended to take this signed clearance form to a qualified exercise professional or other healthcare professional (as recommended in the ePARmed-X+) before becoming <u>more</u> physically active or engaging in a fitness appraisal.

## A BACKGROUND INFORMATION REGARDING THE PAR-Q+ AND ePARmed-X+ CLEARANCE PROCESS

The ePARmed-X+ is an easy to follow interactive program ([www.eparmedx.com](www.eparmedx.com)) that can be used to determine an individual's readiness for increased physical activity participation or a fitness appraisal. The ePARmed-X+ supplements the paper and online versions of the new Physical Activity Readiness Questionnaire for Everyone (PAR-Q+).

Individuals who use the ePARmed-X+ have had a positive response to the PAR-Q+, or have been directed to the online program by a qualified exercise professional or another healthcare professional, owing to his/her current medical condition. At the end of the ePARmed-X+, it is possible that the participant is advised to consult a physician to discuss the various options regarding becoming <u>more</u> physically active. In this instance, the participant will be required to receive medical clearance for physical activity from a physician. Until this medical clearance is received, the participant is restricted to low intensity physical activity participation.

This document serves to assist both the participant and physician in the physical activity clearance process.

## B PERSONAL INFORMATION

NAME: _____    SEX: ☐ M or ☐ F

ADDRESS: _____    BIRTHDATE (mm/dd/yy): _____
_____
_____

TELEPHONE: _____    HEALTH/MEDICAL NUMBER: _____

**REASON FOR REFERRAL (SELECT ALL THAT APPLY):**

☐ QUALIFIED EXERCISE PROFESSIONAL REFERRAL
☐ HEALTH CARE PROFESSIONAL REFERRAL
☐ ePARmed-X+ RECOMMENDATION

**FIGURE 11.2.** ePARmed-X+ Physician Clearance Follow-Up Questionnaire+. (Reprinted from Warburton DER, Jamnik VK, Bredin SSD, et al. Executive summary: The Physical Activity Readiness Questionnaire [PAR-Q+] and Electronic Physical Activity Readiness Medical Examination [ePAR-MED-X]. *Heath Fitness J Can.* 2011;4[3]:24–5c, with permission.) (*continued*) ePARmed-X+ Online

## C ePARmed-X+ PHYSICAL ACTIVITY READINESS PHYSICIAN REFERRAL FORM

Based on the current review of the health status of ______________________________(name)
I recommend the following course of action:

- ☐ The participant should avoid engaging in physical activity at this time.
- ☐ The participant should engage in only a medically supervised physical activity/exercise program involving the supervision of a qualified exercise professional (or other appropriately trained health care professional) and overseen by a physician.
- ☐ The participant is cleared for intensity and mode appropriate physical activity/exercise training under the supervision of a qualified exercise professional.
- ☐ The participant is cleared for intensity and mode appropriate physical activity/exercise training with limited supervision (i.e., unrestricted physical activity).

The following precautions should be taken when prescribing exercise for the aforementioned participant:

- With the avoidance of: ______________________________
- With the inclusion of: ______________________________

**NAME OF PHYSICIAN**: ______________________________

ADDRESS: ______________________________

TELEPHONE: ______________________________

**Date of Medical Clearance (mm/dd/yy)**: ______________________________

**PHYSICIAN/CLINIC STAMP AND SIGNATURE**

NOTE: This physical activity/exercise clearance is valid for a period of six months from the date it is completed and becomes invalid if the medical condition of the above named participant changes/worsens.

Version: September 7, 2014 Page 2 of 2 

**FIGURE 11.2.** *(continued)*

# Professionally Supervised Screening

Self-analysis of risk for physical activity is important with the large number of individuals who are currently not physically active but hopefully will become more active soon perhaps by self-guidance. Thus, they will need to, or should, use some means to determine their physical readiness, like the PAR-Q+. However, many individuals will seek the knowledge and guidance of an EP-C or CPT for this service. Professional readiness, under the guidance of an EP-C or CPT, may involve collecting a health history on an individual (and possibly medical clearance, if warranted) while following the ACSM preparticipation physical activity process (3). The EP-C or CPT may be involved in professional screening at the "lower" levels of risk, whereas professionals such as the ACSM Certified Clinical Exercise Physiologist® (CEP) will be more likely involved with individuals at a higher risk. In the following section, we discuss the HHQ as well as the medical evaluation/clearance.

## Health History Questionnaire

Some form of an HHQ is necessary to use with a client to establish his or her medical/health risks for participation in a physical activity program (13,28). The HHQ, along with other medical/health data, is also used in the process of preparticipation physical activity screening. The HHQ should be tailored to fit the needs of the program as far as asking for the specific information needed from a client. In general, the HHQ should minimally assess a client's (3)

- Family history of CMR disease
- Personal history of various diseases and illnesses including CMR disease
- Surgical history
- Past and present health behaviors/habits (such as history of cigarette smoking and physical activity)
- Current use of various drugs/medications
- Specific history of various signs and symptoms suggested of CMR disease among other things

The current edition of the GETP contains a more detailed list of the specifics of the health and medical evaluations (including desirable laboratory tests) (3). Again, the prudent EP-C or CPT should tailor the HHQ to their client's specific needs. A sample HHQ is included in this chapter (Fig. 11.3).

## Medical Examination/Clearance

A medical examination led by a physician (or other qualified health care professional) may also be necessary or desirable to help evaluate the health and/or medical status of your client prior to a physical activity program. The suggested components of this medical examination can be found in the most current edition of the GETP (3). In addition to a medical examination, it may be desirable to perform some routine laboratory assessments (*i.e.*, fasting blood cholesterol and/or resting blood pressure) on your client prior to physical activity programming (28). Clients who are at a higher risk for exercise complications may need (it is recommended) a medical clearance prior to participation in a physical activity program.

## Preparticipation Physical Activity Screening Process

The process for screening prior to participation in a physical activity program has been altered significantly from past iterations of this process from the ACSM (3). Essentially, only three items need to be considered to complete the process, as is spelled out in Figure 11.4. Perhaps the first item to consider in the process is the individual's past physical activity history. The individual can be queried about his or her physical activity history using the HHQ and/or by questioning. Next, the individual should be evaluated for the presence of known CMR disease. This, too, can be assessed using the HHQ and/or by questioning. Finally, in the process is the assessment of the individual's presence of signs and symptoms that can be suggestive of CMR disease. The ACSM in its recent GETP provides a form for the assessment of all three of these components of the process. This form can be found in Figure 11.5.

## HEALTH HISTORY QUESTIONNAIRE

NAME_____AGE_____DATE_____DATE OF BIRTH_____
　　　　First　　　　M.I.　　　　Last　　　　　　　　day/month/yr　　　　　　　day/month/yr

ADDRESS_____
　　　　　　Street　　　　　　　　　　　　　　City/State/Zip

TELEPHONE (home)_____(business)_____(cell)_____

OCCUPATION_____PLACE OF EMPLOYMENT_____

MARITAL STATUS: (circle one)　　　SINGLE　　　MARRIED　　　DIVORCED　　　WIDOWED

SPOUSE:_____

EDUCATION: (check highest level)　　ELEMENTARY_____　HIGH SCHOOL_____　COLLEGE_____

GRADUATE_____

ETHNICITY:_____　PERSONAL PHYSICIAN_____

LOCATION_____

Reason for last doctor visit?_____　Date of last physician exam_____

Have you previously been tested for an exercise Program?　　YES _____　　　NO _____　　　YEAR(s) _____

LOCATION OF TEST_____

Person to contact in case of an emergency_____　Phone #_____

(relationship)_____

### PLEASE CHECK YES or NO

| PAST (Have you ever had?) | YES | NO |
|---|---|---|
| High blood pressure | ☐ | ☐ |
| Heart problems | ☐ | ☐ |
| Disease of the arteries | ☐ | ☐ |
| Varicose veins | ☐ | ☐ |
| Lung disease | ☐ | ☐ |
| Asthma | ☐ | ☐ |
| Kidney disease | ☐ | ☐ |
| Hepatitis | ☐ | ☐ |
| Diabetes | ☐ | ☐ |
| Orthopedic problems | ☐ | ☐ |
| Arthritis | ☐ | ☐ |

| FAMILY (Have any immediate family or grandparents had?) | YES | NO |
|---|---|---|
| Heart attacks | ☐ | ☐ |
| High blood pressure | ☐ | ☐ |
| High cholesterol | ☐ | ☐ |
| Stroke | ☐ | ☐ |
| Diabetes | ☐ | ☐ |
| Congenital heart defect | ☐ | ☐ |
| Heart operations | ☐ | ☐ |
| Early death | ☐ | ☐ |
| Other family illness _____ | | |
| _____ | | |
| _____ | | |

| PRESENT SYMPTOMS (Have you recently had?) | YES | NO |
|---|---|---|
| Chest pain/discomfort | ☐ | ☐ |
| Shortness of breath | ☐ | ☐ |
| Dizzy spells | ☐ | ☐ |
| Skipped heart beats | ☐ | ☐ |
| Trouble sleeping | ☐ | ☐ |
| Ankle swelling | ☐ | ☐ |
| Leg pain/cramping | ☐ | ☐ |
| Frequent headaches | ☐ | ☐ |
| Frequent colds | ☐ | ☐ |
| Back pain | ☐ | ☐ |
| Orthopedic problems | ☐ | ☐ |

**(FOR STAFF COMMENTS)**

_____
_____
_____

**FIGURE 11.3.** Health History Questionnaire used at East Stroudsburg University. (*continued*)

---

**HEALTH HISTORY QUESTIONNAIRE**

**HOSPITALIZATIONS:** Please list recent hospitalizations (Women: do not list normal pregnancies)

Year                              Location                              Reason

_____

_____

---

**Any other medical problems/concerns not already identified?** Yes_____ No_____ (Please list below)

_____

---

**Have you ever had your cholesterol measures?** Yes_____ No_____; If yes, (value)_____ (Date)_____

---

**Are you taking any Prescription or Non-Prescription medications?** Yes_____ No_____ (include birth control pills)

Medication                    Reason for Taking                    For How Long?

_____

_____

---

**Do you currently smoke?** Yes_____ No_____ If so, what? Cigarettes_____ Cigars_____ Pipe_____

How much per day:     < .5 pack_____     0.5 to 1pack_____     1.5 to 2 packs_____     > 2 packs_____

**Have you ever quit smoking?** Yes_____ No_____ When?_____ How many years and how

much did you smoke?_____

---

**Do you drink any alcoholic beverages?** Yes_____ No_____ If Yes, how much in 1 week?

Beer_____(cans)          Wine_____(glasses)          Hard liquor_____(drinks)

---

**Do you drink any caffeinated beverages?** Yes_____ No_____ If Yes, how much in 1 week?

Coffee_____(cups)          Tea_____(glasses)          Soft drinks_____(cans)

---

**ACTIVITY LEVEL EVALUATION**

**What is your occupational activity level?**     sedentary_____; light_____; moderate_____; heavy_____

**Do you currently engage in vigorous physical activity on a regular basis?** Yes_____ No_____

If so, what type?_____ How many days per week?_____

How much time per day? (check one)     < 15 min_____     15–30 min_____     30–45 min_____     > 60 min_____

Do you ever have an uncomfortable shortness of breath during exercise? Yes_____ No_____

Do you ever have chest discomfort during exercise? Yes_____ No_____ If so, does it go away with rest?_____

**Do you engage in any recreational or leisure-time physical activities on a regular basis?** Yes_____ No_____

If so, what activities?_____

On average:   How often?_____times/week;   For how long?_____time/session

**FIGURE 11.3.** (*continued*)

**HEALTH HISTORY QUESTIONNAIRE**

**Are you currently following a weight reduction diet plan?**  Yes_____  No_____  Name:_____

If so, how long have you been dieting? _____months        Is the plan prescribed by your doctor?  Yes_____  No_____

**Have you used weight reduction diets in the past?**  Yes_____  No_____;        If yes, how often and which type(s)?

_____

_____

**Please indicate the reasons why you want to join the exercise program.**

To lose weight _____  Doctor's recommendation_____  For good health _____  Enjoyment_____

Release of tension_____  Improve physical appearance _____  Other _____

**FOR STAFF USE:**

_____

_____

**FIGURE 11.3.** (*continued*)

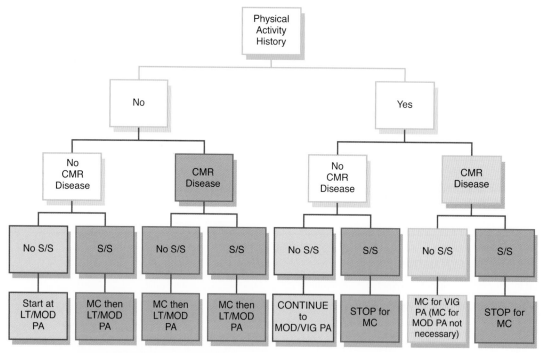

CMR: Cardiovascular, metabolic, and/or renal disease
S/S: Signs and symptoms suggestive of CMR disease
MC: Medical clearance
LT/MOD PA: Light to moderate physical activity
VIG PA: Vigorous physical activity

**FIGURE 11.4.** Decision tree for preparticipation screening; simplified algorithm.

**Exercise Preparticipation Health Screening Questionnaire for Exercise Professionals**

**Assess your client's health needs by marking all *true* statements.**

## Step 1

**SYMPTOMS**
**Does your client experience:**
____ chest discomfort with exertion
____ unreasonable breathlessness
____ dizziness, fainting, blackouts
____ ankle swelling
____ unpleasant awareness of a forceful, rapid or irregular heart rate
____ burning or cramping sensations in your lower legs when walking short distance

If you **did** mark any of these statements under the symptoms, **STOP**, your client should should seek medical clearance before engaging in or resuming exercise. Your client may need to use a facility with a **medically qualified staff**.

If you **did not** mark any symptoms, continue to steps 2 and 3.

## Step 2

**CURRENT ACTIVITY**
Has your client performed planned, structured physical activity for at least 30 min at moderate intensity on at least 3 days per week for at least the last 3 months?

Yes ☐  No ☐

Continue to Step 3.

## Step 3

**MEDICAL CONDITIONS**
**Has your client had or do they currently have:**
____ a heart attack
____ heart surgery, cardiac catheterization, or coronary angioplasty
____ pacemaker/implantable cardiac defibrillator/rhythm disturbance
____ heart valve disease
____ heart failure
____ heart transplantation
____ congenital heart disease
____ diabetes
____ renal disease

Evaluating Steps 2 and 3:

- If you **did not mark any of the statements in Step 3**, medical clearance is not necessary.
- If you marked Step 2 "**yes**" and **marked any of the statements in Step 3**, your client may continue to exercise at light to moderate intensity without medical clearance. Medical clearance is recommended before engaging in vigorous exercise.
- If you marked Step 2 "**no**" and **marked any of the statements in Step 3**, medical clearance is recommended. Your client may need to use a facility with a **medically qualified staff**.

**FIGURE 11.5.** Preparticipation physical activity screening questionnaire for exercise professionals.

It is important to note that the process of ACSM preparticipation physical activity screening has been divorced from the concept of the need for and supervisory qualifications of a graded exercise test and other health-related physical fitness assessments. Recent professional society opinions and research have devalued the use of graded exercise testing for many adults as part of the diagnostic workup for cardiovascular disease (3). Thus, preparticipation physical activity screening is about participating in a physical activity program not about exercise testing. We will discuss all three components of the preparticipation physical activity screening process in the following section.

### PHYSICAL ACTIVITY (OR EXERCISE) HISTORY

An individual who currently engages in physical activity is considered to be at lower risk for a cardiovascular event during exercise than one who is sedentary. Current physical activity is considered to be within the last 3 months. The threshold dose of physical activity that is necessary to lower one's risk, according to the ACSM, is 30 minutes or more of at least moderate physical activity on at least $3 \text{ d} \cdot \text{wk}^{-1}$. Moderate physical activity has several descriptors associated with it including exercise at a level that is between 40% and 60% of the individual's heart rate reserve or maximal oxygen uptake reserve. Moderate-intensity physical activity or exercise is further described as between 3 and 6 metabolic equivalents (METs) and at a rating of perceived exertion (RPE) of around 12–13 on the traditional 6–20 scale. Also, moderate-intensity causes noticeable increases in heart rate and breathing.

### KNOWN CARDIOVASCULAR, METABOLIC, AND/OR RENAL DISEASE

Clients with any of the CMR diseases are at a higher risk for an untoward event during exercise. Thus, the presence of a CMR disease will influence the level of preparticipation physical activity screening. A listing of the specific diseases and/or conditions covered are as follows:

- Heart attack
- Heart surgery, cardiac catheterization, or coronary angioplasty
- Pacemaker/implantable cardiac defibrillator/rhythm disturbance
- Heart valve disease
- Heart failure
- Heart transplantation
- Congenital heart disease (*congenital* refers to birth)
- Diabetes, type 1 and 2
- Renal disease such as renal failure

Those of you familiar with "older" systems of risk classification will note the absence of pulmonary diseases from this list of diseases and/or conditions. Pulmonary disease has been shown to be less likely to cause untoward events during exercise than CMR disease and thus has been removed from the list (3).

### ACSM MAJOR SIGNS OR SYMPTOMS SUGGESTIVE OF CARDIOVASCULAR DISEASE

There are several outward signs or symptoms that may indicate a client has current CMR disease. These signs and symptoms can be found in the following sections along with further discussion of these signs or symptoms. If a client has any of these signs or symptoms, then he or she is considered at a higher risk, and it is recommended that you seek medical clearance before they participate in a physical activity program. It is important to remember that these signs or symptoms must be interpreted within the clinical context in which they appear because they are not all specific for CMR disease.

### Discussion of ACSM Signs or Symptoms

There are eight signs and symptoms suggestive of CMR disease which include:

- Pain or discomfort in the chest, neck, jaw, arms, or other areas that may be due to ischemia or lack of oxygenated blood flow to the tissue, such as the heart (27). Remember that chest pain or angina is not always located in the chest area of a client. Women in particular may experience low back pain or feelings of indigestion as opposed to chest pain. Some key features of this pain that *favors an ischemic origin* include the following:

- *Character*: The pain is felt as constricting, squeezing, burning, "heaviness," or "heavy feeling."
- *Location*: The pain is substernal, across the midthorax, anteriorly; in one or both arms or shoulders; in neck, cheeks, or teeth; or in forearms, fingers, and/or in the interscapular region.
- *Provoking factors*: The pain comes on with exercise or exertion, excitement, other forms of stress, cold weather, or after meals (3).

- *Dyspnea* is the medical term for shortness of breath (27). Dyspnea is expected in most individuals during moderate to severe exertion such as stair climbing. However, shortness of breath at rest or with mild exertion may indicate cardiac and/or pulmonary disease and should be examined by a physician. Dyspnea (defined as an abnormally uncomfortable awareness of breathing) is one of the principal symptoms of cardiac and pulmonary disease. It commonly occurs during strenuous exertion in healthy, well-trained individuals and during moderate exertion in healthy, untrained individuals. However, it should be regarded as abnormal when it occurs at a level of exertion that is not expected to evoke this symptom in a given individual. Abnormal exertional dyspnea suggests the presence of cardiopulmonary disorders, in particular, left ventricular dysfunction or chronic obstructive pulmonary disease (3).

- Syncope, or fainting, and dizziness during exercise may indicate poor blood flow to the brain due to inadequate cardiac output from a number of cardiac disorders (27). However, syncope and dizziness upon sudden cessation of exercise is relatively common even among healthy individuals due to a sudden decrease in venous return and consequent reduction in blood flow to the brain. Cardiac disorders that are associated with syncope and dizziness are potentially life-threatening and include severe coronary artery disease, hypertrophic cardiomyopathy, aortic stenosis, and malignant ventricular dysrhythmias. Although dizziness or syncope shortly *after* cessation of exercise should not be ignored, these symptoms may occur even in healthy individuals as a result of a reduction in venous return to the heart (3).

- Orthopnea refers to trouble breathing while lying down. Paroxysmal nocturnal dyspnea refers to difficulty breathing while asleep, beginning usually 2–5 hours after the onset of sleep, which may be relieved by sitting on the side of the bed or getting out of bed (27). Both are indicative of poor left ventricular function. Patients with these conditions often report sleeping in recliners to lessen the symptoms of this disorder. Orthopnea is relieved promptly by sitting upright or standing. Although nocturnal dyspnea may occur in individuals with chronic obstructive pulmonary disease, it differs in that it is usually relieved following a bowel movement rather than specifically by sitting up (3).

- Ankle edema, or swelling, that is not due to injury is suggestive of heart failure, a blood clot, insufficiency of the veins, or a lymph system blockage (27). Generalized edema (known as anasarca) occurs in individuals with the nephrotic (from the kidneys) syndrome, severe heart failure, or hepatic (from the liver) cirrhosis. Bilateral ankle edema that is most evident at night is a characteristic sign of heart failure or bilateral chronic venous insufficiency. Unilateral edema of a limb often results from venous thrombosis or lymphatic blockage in the limb (3).

- Palpitations and tachycardia both refer to rapid beating or fluttering of the heart (27). The client may report a feeling of unpleasantness associated with the unusual heart rhythm. Palpitations (defined as an unpleasant awareness of the forceful or rapid beating of the heart) may be induced by various disorders of cardiac rhythm. These include tachycardia, bradycardia of sudden onset, ectopic beats, compensatory pauses, and accentuated stroke volume resulting from valvular regurgitation. Palpitations also often result from anxiety states and high cardiac output (or hyperkinetic) states, such as anemia, fever, thyrotoxicosis, arteriovenous fistula, and the so-called idiopathic hyperkinetic heart syndrome (3).

- Intermittent claudication refers to severe calf pain when walking (27). This pain indicates a lack of oxygenated blood flow to the working muscles similar in origin to chest pain. The pain does not occur with standing or sitting, is reproducible from day to day, is more severe when walking upstairs or up a hill, and is often described as a cramp, which disappears within 1–2 minutes after stopping exercise. Coronary artery disease is more prevalent in individuals with intermittent claudication. Patients with diabetes are at increased risk for this condition (3).

- Heart murmurs are unusual sounds caused by blood flowing through the heart (27). Although some murmurs may be innocent, heart murmurs may indicate valvular or other cardiovascular disease. From an exercise safety standpoint, it is especially important to exclude hypertrophic cardiomyopathy and aortic stenosis as underlying causes because these are among the more common causes of exertion-related sudden cardiac death. Unless previously diagnosed and determined to be safe, all murmurs should be evaluated by a physician (3).

- Unusual fatigue or shortness of breath that occurs during light exertion or normal activity and not during strenuous activity (27). Although there may be benign origins for these symptoms, they also may signal the onset of or change in the status of cardiovascular and/or metabolic disease (3).

### WHAT TO DO ONCE RISK IS ESTABLISHED?

Figure 11.4 is our attempt to clarify some of the decisions aided by the ACSM preparticipation physical activity screening process. The EP-C or CPT should always keep in mind that the ACSM preparticipation physical activity screening process is a guideline and may need to be modified based on several issues such as local medical practice or custom.

Essentially, Figure 11.4 represents a paradigm shift in preparticipation screening from previous ACSM screening paradigms, and we have chosen to colorize the figure to aid the EP-C or CPT with this decision tree. Medical clearance, which may include a medical examination by a health care professional including a physician, is suggested and recommended to be a part of the preparticipation physical activity screening workup if your client has signs and symptoms suggestive of CMR disease. We have denoted this outcome using the color blue in Figure 11.4. In fact, individuals who meet these criteria (signs and symptoms suggestive of CMR disease) should only participate after getting medical clearance to do so. Individuals who may be free of signs and symptoms but have the presence of CMR disease may benefit from medical clearance, and thus, we have used the color yellow for caution in Figure 11.4. This is very true in your clients who currently do not participate in a physical activity program. However, in most "apparently healthy" clients (free of CMR disease and signs and symptoms suggestive of CMR disease), it is acceptable to get them started in a moderate-intensity physical activity program without the need for previous medical clearance. We have used the color green for this outcome in Figure 11.4.

As you can see in Figure 11.4, the current physical activity history of a client does influence these decisions. For instance, if your client has not been physically active in the recent past (last 3 mo), then you are more likely to recommend medical clearance to start a low to moderate physical activity program, whereas the previously physically active client may be able to proceed to a more moderate to vigorous physical activity program.

The prudent EP-C or CPT would always err on the side of caution when there are uncertainties and request full medical clearance. The ePARmed-X+Physician Clearance Follow-Up Questionnaire may be used for medical clearance.

Vigorous exercise is often defined as greater than or equal to 60% of your client's functional capacity ($\geq$6 METs, $\geq$14 on a 6–20 RPE scale, and cause substantial increases in heart rate and breathing), whereas low to moderate exercise programs would be less than 60% of functional capacity (5,12,15,23).

Two previous features of the ACSM Risk Stratification/Classification process were the use and supervision of graded exercise testing. Nondiagnostic exercise testing is generally performed for exercise prescriptive and/or functional capacity purposes, whereas diagnostic exercise testing may be performed to assess the presence or impact of cardiovascular disease (34). Submaximal exercise testing may also be useful in individualizing your client's exercise prescription as well as gaining functional capacity information as is discussed in other chapters of this textbook. Research and expert opinion has recently questioned the value of the diagnostic exercise test (12,19).

The supervision criterion of exercise testing has also undergone much revision in recent years. Training in exercise testing administration is required and includes certification in emergency care (*i.e.*, AHA Advanced Cardiac Life Support Certification) as well as experience in exercise testing interpretation and emergency plan practice (12,18,19).

Thus, a competent EP-C or CPT may oversee the judicious use of the preparticipation physical activity screening and graded exercise test for exercise prescription purposes in their lower risk clients. However, other personnel may need to become involved if the preparticipation physical activity screening suggests the need for medical clearance (3,25).

## American Association of Cardiovascular and Pulmonary Rehabilitation (AACVPR) Risk Stratification

Other professional organizations have also published guidelines that address risk stratification and preparticipation physical activity screening (1–3,10,15,34). Most prominently among these are AHA and AACVPR. Similar to the recent changes in ACSM preparticipation exercise screening, other guidelines have been modified to reduce impediments to begin or continue safe and effective exercise programming.

The AACVPR has contributed to the field of preparticipation physical activity screening and risk stratification with guidelines revised most recently in 2013 (1–3,34). The AACVPR risk stratification scheme continues to utilize Low, Moderate, and High risk categories to identify level of risk of physical activity triggering an untoward event.

The AACVPR risk stratification scheme may serve as a nice bridge toward offering services and programming to more "risky" or diseased clients as might be found in clinical exercise programs such as cardiac rehabilitation or medical fitness facilities, perhaps supervised by a CEP or ACSM Registered Clinical Exercise Physiologist® (RCEP). The AACVPR risk stratification guidelines are listed in Figure 11.6 (3,34).

## Pitfalls of ACSM Preparticipation Physical Activity Screening

Perhaps the greatest pitfall of ACSM preparticipation physical activity screening is overlooking a sign or symptom of ongoing cardiovascular disease and then the client has a cardiac event while under your direction. Although the incidence of such events are rare (see "Exercise is Medicine" box), the prudent EP-C or CPT should exercise caution in minimizing such risk (14,29–31). To reduce the risk of such an event, the EP-C or CPT should obtain as much medical history information as possible through the HHQ and client interviews. When in doubt, particularly in a moderately risky client who may, in actuality, be of a higher risk client, the ACSM recommends consulting with a health care professional for advice on how to proceed. Remember, it is better to be conservative and prudent than to endanger your client's health (12).

Of course, this conservatism in preparticipation physical activity screening must be balanced by the public health argument of putting up too many obstacles or barriers to participation in the way of your client that you drive your client away from adopting a physically active, and healthy, lifestyle. Thus, your client might be encouraged to begin a low- to moderate-intensity program, where the overall risks of untoward events are minimal, before they undergo further medical evaluation (3). It is perhaps important for all individuals beginning a physical activity program that the initial intensity be low to moderate and increase gradually in a progressive overload fashion as discussed in other chapters in this text and the ACSM GETP (3,25).

## Recommendations versus Requirements

It is important to remember that the goal of GETP is to provide direction on how to screen participants and proceed with physical activity programming. In all cases, the EP-C or CPT should exercise caution and use their best judgment when handling an individual client. When in doubt, referring a client for a medical evaluation and clearance is always in good judgment.

**LOWEST RISK**

**Characteristics of patients at lowest risk for exercise participation (all characteristics listed must be present for patients to remain at lowest risk)**

- Absence of complex ventricular dysrhythmias during exercise testing and recovery
- Absence of angina or other significant symptoms (*e.g.*, unusual shortness of breath, light-headedness, or dizziness, during exercise testing and recovery)
- Presence of normal hemodynamics during exercise testing and recovery (*i.e.*, appropriate increases and decreases in heart rate and systolic blood pressure with increasing workloads and recovery)
- Functional capacity ≥7 metabolic equivalents (METs)

**Nonexercise Testing Findings**

- Resting ejection fraction ≥50%
- Uncomplicated myocardial infarction or revascularization procedure
- Absence of complicated ventricular dysrhythmias at rest
- Absence of congestive heart failure
- Absence of signs or symptoms of postevent/postprocedure myocardial ischemia
- Absence of clinical depression

**MODERATE RISK**

**Characteristics of patients at moderate risk for exercise participation (any one or combination of these findings places a patient at moderate risk)**

- Presence of angina or other significant symptoms (*e.g.*, unusual shortness of breath, light-headedness, or dizziness occurring only at high levels of exertion [≥7 METs])
- Mild-to-moderate level of silent ischemia during exercise testing or recovery (ST-segment depression <2 mm from baseline)
- Functional capacity <5 METs

**Nonexercise Testing Findings**

- Rest ejection fraction 40%–49%

**HIGHEST RISK**

**Characteristics of patients at high risk for exercise participation (any one or combination of these findings places a patient at high risk)**

- Presence of complex ventricular dysrhythmias during exercise testing or recovery
- Presence of angina or other significant symptoms (*e.g.*, unusual shortness of breath, light-headedness, dizziness at low levels of exertion [<5 METs] or during recovery)
- High level of silent ischemia (ST-segment depression ≥2 mm from baseline) during exercise testing or recovery
- Presence of abnormal hemodynamics with exercise testing (*i.e.*, chronotropic incompetence or flat or decreasing systolic blood pressure with increasing workloads) or recovery (*i.e.*, severe postexercise hypotension)

**Nonexercise Testing Findings**

- Rest ejection fraction <40%
- History of cardiac arrest or sudden death
- Complex dysrhythmias at rest
- Complicated myocardial infarction or revascularization procedure
- Presence of congestive heart failure
- Presence of signs or symptoms of postevent/postprocedure myocardial ischemia
- Presence of clinical depression

**FIGURE 11.6.** American Heart Association risk stratification. (Reprinted from Williams MA. Exercise testing in cardiac rehabilitation. Exercise prescription and beyond. *Cardiol Clin.* 2001;19[3]:415–31, with permission from Elsevier.)

It is important to note that to date, there are no published reports on the effectiveness of the ACSM preparticipation physical activity screening or the AACVPR risk classification schemes. Thus, although it is prudent to recommend that the EP-C or CPT follow or adopt such a preparticipation screening scheme, it is difficult to suggest this as a requirement to follow for a quality exercise program because it is lacking an evidence base (16).

 ## Contraindications to Exercise Testing

The process of evaluating risk (through a medical exam/health history and the ACSM preparticipation physical activity screening) may identify clinical characteristics of an individual that make physical activity risky and, thus, contraindicated. There are a host of clinical characteristics that have been identified and published by ACSM (as well as other organizations, such as the AHA) that are termed *contraindications*. These contraindications generally refer to exercise testing. This list can be found in Figure 11.7 (3). As you can see, many of these contraindications are cardiovascular disease–related only to be known by consultation with a physician and likely sophisticated medical testing. However, the resting blood pressure relative contraindication criterion (>200 mm Hg systolic blood pressure or 110 mm Hg diastolic blood pressure) is likely to be known by the EP-C or CPT during basic health-related physical fitness testing.

---

**Absolute Contraindications**

- Acute myocardial infarction within 2 days
- Ongoing unstable angina
- Uncontrolled cardiac arrhythmia with hemodynamic compromise
- Active endocarditis
- Symptomatic severe aortic stenosis
- Decompensated heart failure
- Acute pulmonary embolism, pulmonary infarction, or deep venous thrombosis
- Acute myocarditis or pericarditis
- Acute aortic dissection
- Physical disability that precludes safe and adequate testing

**Relative Contraindications**

- Known obstructive left main coronary artery stenosis
- Moderate to severe aortic stenosis with uncertain relationship to symptoms
- Tachyarrhythmias with uncontrolled ventricular rates
- Acquired advanced or complete heart block
- Recent stroke or transient ischemia attack
- Mental impairment with limited ability to cooperate
- Resting hypertension with systolic >200 mm Hg or diastolic >110 mm Hg
- Uncorrected medical conditions, such as significant anemia, important electrolyte imbalance, and hyperthyroidism

Fletcher GF, Ades PA, Kligfield P, et al. Exercise standards for testing and training: a scientific statement from the American Heart Association. *Circulation.* 2013;128(8):873–934.

---

**FIGURE 11.7.** Contraindications to exercise testing.

## What Does Contraindication Really Mean?

Just like ACSM preparticipation physical activity screening, these are guidelines that may be followed. A contraindication is a clinical characteristic that individuals may have that may make physical activity and thus, exercise testing, more risky than if the individual did not have that clinical characteristic. For instance, if an individual has unstable angina, or chest pain (unstable angina refers to chest pain that is not well controlled or predictable), then if they exercise their heart may become ischemic which could lead to a myocardial infarction, or heart attack. Although it is important to note that the incidence of cardiovascular complications is rare during exercise, a prudent EP-C or CPT would be advised to follow the contraindications listed to minimize this incidence (3,25,31). As previously discussed, many of the contraindications listed are not common, but the EP-C or CPT should protect the individual from all known and likely risks.

## Absolute versus Relative

The list of contraindications is often divided between those that are *absolute* and those that are *relative*. Essentially, absolute refers to those criteria that are absolute contraindications; individuals with those biomarkers should not be allowed to participate in any form of physical activity program and/or exercise test. However, those individuals with clinical contraindications that are listed as relative may be accepted or allowed into a physical activity assessment and/or program if it is deemed that the benefits for the individual outweigh the risks to the individual (24,25). For instance, if your client has a resting blood pressure of 210/105 mm Hg, it may be decided to allow your client (medical director decision, likely) into the physical activity program because the benefits to the individual may outweigh the risks of exercising with such as high blood pressure because the individual is controlled and stable in terms of their blood pressure.

## Repurposing Risk Factor Assessment and Management

As mentioned previously, the ACSM CVD Risk Assessment is no longer a mandatory component for determining if medical clearance is warranted before individuals begin an exercise program. However, identifying and controlling CVD risk factors remains an important objective of disease prevention and management. Therefore, under the new recommendations, the EP-C or CPT is encouraged to complete a CVD risk factor analysis with their patients and clients. The goal has simply shifted from using the ACSM CVD risk factor assessment as a tool for preparticipation health screening and risk stratification to identifying and managing CVD risk in patients and clients. As will be addressed later in this textbook, CVD risk factors may significantly impact exercise prescription.

Another important reason to provide CVD Risk Assessment is to help educate and inform the client about his or her need to make lifestyle modifications such as increasing physical activity and incorporating more healthful food choices in his or her diets.

## Review of ACSM Atherosclerotic Cardiovascular Disease (CVD) Risk Factors and Defining Criteria

Using the client's health history (and basic health evaluation data such as resting blood pressure), simply total the number of positive ACSM Coronary Artery Disease Risk Factor Thresholds the person meets. Having one or none of these indicates a low risk of future cardiovascular disease, whereas two or more risk factors indicate an increased risk of disease. Note that only one positive factor is assigned per ACSM Risk Factor Thresholds. For instance, in obesity, a body mass index (BMI) greater than $30 \text{ kg} \cdot \text{m}^{-2}$ and a waist circumference of 105 cm (for men) would count as only one positive factor. Likewise, having both high systolic and high diastolic resting blood pressure readings would result in only one positive factor. If a client is taking a medication for hypertension or high cholesterol, he or she is considered positive for the associated risk factor regardless of his or her actual resting blood pressure or blood cholesterol measurements. There is also one negative factor (having high high-density lipoprotein [HDL-C]) that would offset one positive risk factor. The following is a detailed list of the ACSM Atherosclerotic Cardiovascular Disease (CVD) Risk Factors and Defining Criteria (3, Table 3.1):

- Client's age of 45 years or older for males and 55 years or older for females (24)
- Family history of specific cardiovascular events including myocardial infarction (heart attack), coronary revascularization (bypass surgery or angioplasty), or sudden cardiac death. This applies to first-degree relatives only. First-degree relatives are biological parents, siblings, and children. The risk factor threshold is met when at least one male relative has had one of the three specific events prior to age 55 years or before age 65 years in a female relative (33).
- If the client currently smokes cigarettes, quit smoking within the last 6 months, or if he or she is exposed to secondhand smoke on a regular basis. Secondhand smoke exposure can be assessed by the presence of cotinine in your client's urine (11,20).
- A sedentary lifestyle is defined as not participating in a regular exercise program nor meeting the minimal recommendations of 30 minutes or more of moderate physical activity on 3 d $\cdot$ wk$^{-1}$ for a least 3 months (22).
- Obesity is defined as a BMI greater than or equal 30 kg $\cdot$ m$^{-2}$ or a waist circumference of greater than 102 cm ($\sim$40 in) for men and greater than 88 cm ($\sim$35 in) for women. If available, body fat percentage values could also be used with appropriate judgment of the EP-C or CPT (11).
- Hypertension refers to having a resting blood pressure equal to or above 140 mm Hg systolic or equal to or above 90 mm Hg diastolic or if the client is currently taking any of the numerous antihypertensive medications. Very importantly, these resting blood pressures must have been assessed on at least two separate occasions (7,8).
- Dyslipidemia refers to having a low-density lipoprotein cholesterol (LDL-C) equal or above 130 mg $\cdot$ dL$^{-1}$, an HDL-C of less than 40 mg $\cdot$ dL$^{-1}$, or if the client is taking a lipid-lowering medication. Use equal or greater than 200 mg $\cdot$ dL$^{-1}$ if only the total blood cholesterol measurement is available (21). Although not explicitly stated in the ACSM guidelines, the cholesterol risk factor is similar to the measurement of blood pressure in that it should be abnormal on at least two separate occasions to be counted as a risk factor. Also, LDL-C is typically not measured but rather estimated from HDL-C, total cholesterol (TC), and triglycerides (3).
- Diabetes is defined as having a fasting plasma glucose $\geq$126 mg $\cdot$ dL$^{-1}$ (7.0 mmol $\cdot$ L$^{-1}$) or 2 h plasma glucose values in oral glucose tolerance test (OGTT) $\geq$200 mg $\cdot$ dL$^{-1}$ (11.1 mmol $\cdot$ L$^{-1}$) or HbA1C $\geq$6.5%. There must be at least two separate abnormal results for the risk factor to be counted. Remember, FBG of 126 mg $\cdot$ dL$^{-1}$ or greater would indicate the individual has diabetes which would automatically place him or her in the high-risk level (4).
- High-serum HDL-C equal or greater than 60 mg $\cdot$ dL$^{-1}$ (this is a negative risk factor that would offset one positive risk factor). HDL-C participates in reverse cholesterol transport and thus may lower the risk of cardiovascular disease. Although it is not stated in the ACSM guidelines, it is suggested that a client have had his or her HDL-C measured on at least two separate occasions (3).

Comparing the clients personal data to the ACSM Atherosclerotic Cardiovascular Disease (CVD) Risk Factors and Defining Criteria outlined above will help the EP-C or CPT to educate the client about his or her current health risk and evaluate the effectiveness of the exercise protocol at managing and/or attenuating this risk.

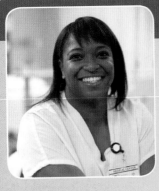

## Case Studies

Below are listed three case studies using one individual (Sam J.) for the purposes of exploring further the processes of ACSM preparticipation physical activity screening, contraindications to exercise, and ACSM Risk Factor Thresholds.

## ACSM Preparticipation Physical Activity Screening Case Study

The following case study is presented as an example of how to perform ACSM preparticipation physical activity screening:

Sam J., your client, decides he wants to exercise in your program. You take him through your routine preactivity screening. He presents to you with the following information: His father died of a heart attack at the age of 52 years. His mother was put on medication for hypertension 2 years ago at the age of 69 years. He presents no signs or symptoms of CMR disease and is a nonsmoker. His personal data shows that he is 38 years old. He weighs 170 lb and is 5 ft 8 in tall. His body fat percentage was measured at 22% via skinfolds. His cholesterol is 270 mg $\cdot$ dL$^{-1}$, HDL is 46 mg $\cdot$ dL$^{-1}$, and his resting blood glucose is 84 mg $\cdot$ dL$^{-1}$. His resting heart rate is 74 bpm, and his resting blood pressure measured 132/82 and 130/84 mm Hg on two separate occasions. He has a sedentary job in a factory and stands on his feet all day. He complains that as a supervisor on the job, he never gets a rest throughout his shift and often is required to work overtime. He routinely plays basketball once each week with his work buddies and then goes out for a few beers.

### Physical Activity History

He plays some basketball once a week and thus is not physically active by the ACSM definition.

### Presence of Cardiovascular, Metabolic, and/or Renal Disease

None noted.

### Major Symptoms or Signs suggestive of Cardiovascular, Metabolic, and/or Renal Disease

None noted.

### ACSM Preparticipation Physical Activity Screening Status

Medical clearance is not necessary before starting a physical activity program of a light to moderate intensity. He may progress to more vigorous-intensity exercise following ACSM GETP (3,25).

## Contraindications Case Study

Sam J. has a medical evaluation with his personal physician prior to joining your vigorous exercise program. His physician performs a medical evaluation (physical exam) and reports the following: Sam J. has no signs and symptoms of CMR disease and has the known risk factors you already uncovered (dyslipidemia and sedentary lifestyle as well as a family history). His physical exams results are unremarkable except for the relative contraindications listed below.

### Absolute Contraindications

None.

### Relative Contraindications

Sam suffers some from rheumatoid arthritis that is not usually made worse by exercise. In addition, Sam suffered a musculoskeletal injury to his low back last year that forced him to miss 1 week of work. However, his low back area has been problem free as of the last 6 months.

## Contraindication Analysis

Sam may not suffer from any technical contraindications that would prevent him from performing an exercise test for exercise prescription purposes as well as participating in an exercise program. Remember, relative contraindications are considered in terms of cost and benefit to your client. Certainly, as a prudent EP-C or CPT, you will want to conduct the exercise test for prescriptive purposes being careful not to exacerbate Sam's previous back injury. In addition, Sam having rheumatoid arthritis should signal you to take it easy with your client. A cautious physical activity program should be recommended for him that limits his use of his core and lower back muscles.

## ACSM CVD Risk Factors History

| | ACSM Coronary Artery Disease Risk Factor Thresholds | Comment |
|---|---|---|
| − | Age | |
| + | Family History | Father had heart attack (myocardial infarction) at age 52 yr old; mother with hypertension does not count |
| − | Cigarette Smoking | Okay, nonsmoker (not sure about passive smoke) |
| − | Hypertension | Okay, blood pressures measured are "fine" (132/84 mm Hg) |
| + | Dyslipidemia | TC = 270 mg · dL$^{-1}$ (LDL-C unknown) |
| − | Diabetes | Okay (FBG = 82 mg · dL$^{-1}$) |
| − | Obesity | Okay (BMI = 25.8 kg · m$^{-2}$) |
| + | Sedentary Lifestyle | Sedentary |
| | *High* HDL-C | Not positive (HDL = 46 mg · dL$^{-1}$) |
| 3 | (+) Risk Factors | |

## ACSM Risk Factor Analysis

Sam has a risk factor profile that is hyperlipidemic or dyslipidemic (his total cholesterol is 270 mg · dL$^{-1}$ or mg%). In addition, he is currently sedentary. Thus, a prudent EP-C or CPT would stress to this client the importance of adopting a physically active lifestyle with moderate physical activity to start. In addition a health care provider may wish to explore further Sam's dyslipidemia and treatment.

## Exercise is Medicine

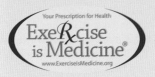

"Don't exercise too much; you may have a heart attack." How often have you heard that before? Dr. Paul Thompson and his colleagues from around the world have conducted many studies over the years to help refute that claim. In one particular study published back in 1996 in the *Archives of Internal Medicine*, Dr. Thompson studied the complications that may occur from participation in exercise (29). That study found that only 6 per 100,000 men die of exertion each year. In this article, Dr. Thompson suggested that the routine use of cardiovascular exercise tests has little diagnostic value for cardiovascular disease because of the rarity of sudden cardiac death in the population. In a scientific statement from the American Heart Association published in *Circulation* in 2007, the writing team (Dr. Thompson and his colleagues) further suggested that the risk of sudden death from exercise is greatest in those least accustomed to physical activity (31). This lends further support to the concepts of performing diagnostic exercise tests only on those at high risk for cardiovascular disease as well as using the principle of progressive overload in exercise training by starting those who are unaccustomed to exercise at a lower exercise load (intensity and duration) and gradually increasing the exercise load as they become more accustomed to exercise. Thus, the incidence of sudden cardiac death is lessened in your client. From this study and others, you can see the influence on the current ACSM preparticipation physical activity screening guidelines (3,25).

## SUMMARY

Preparticipation physical activity screening is a process that may include health/medical history and informed consent of an individual client. The process is one where the client is prepared for the upcoming physical activity program. Although there are several examples or models that can be followed for the preparticipation physical activity screening process, the bottom line is the need to evaluate a client's medical readiness to undertake the physical activity program planned for them. Thus, the preparticipation physical activity screening gives the relative assurance that the client is ready and able (based on national guidelines, such as from ACSM) to participate in the rigors of the physical activity training process. It is thus important that the EP-C or CPT perform the preparticipation physical activity screening on their client.

## STUDY QUESTIONS

1. Discuss each individual ACSM Risk Factor Threshold. Specifically, how do the individual ACSM Risk Factor Thresholds match up with the modifiable and nonmodifiable risk factors for coronary heart disease listed by the AHA?

2. Given the 2013 scientific statement from the AHA as well as the *2008 Physical Activity Guidelines for Americans*, does the ACSM preparticipation physical activity screening guidelines aid or hinder the concept of increasing physical activity behavior of all Americans?

3. Diabetes is relatively stressed in the ACSM preparticipation physical activity screening guidelines. (Diabetes is a CMR disease.) What are some of the complications of diabetes that justifies its inclusion in the preparticipation guidelines?

## REFERENCES

1. American Association of Cardiovascular and Pulmonary Rehabilitation. *Guidelines for Cardiac Rehabilitation and Secondary Prevention Programs.* 4th ed. Champaign (IL): Human Kinetics; 2004. 288 p.

2. American Association of Cardiovascular and Pulmonary Rehabilitation. *Guidelines for Pulmonary Rehabilitation Programs.* 3rd ed. Champaign (IL): Human Kinetics; 2004. 200 p.

3. American College of Sports Medicine. *ACSM's Guidelines for Exercise Testing and Prescription.* 10th ed. Philadelphia (PA): Wolters Kluwer; 2018.

4. American Diabetes Association. Diagnosis and classification of diabetes mellitus. *Diabetes Care.* 2007;30(Suppl 1):S42–7.

5. Brawner CA, Vanzant MA, Ehrman JK, et al. Guiding exercise using the talk test among patients with coronary artery disease. *J Cardiopulm Rehabil.* 2006;26(2):72–7.

6. Buchner DM. Physical activity to prevent or reverse disability in sedentary older adults. *Am J Prev Med.* 2003;25(3 Suppl 2):214–5.

7. Cardiovascular Risk Reduction Guidelines in Adults: Cholesterol Guideline Update (ATP IV) Hypertension Guideline Update (JNC 8) Obesity Guideline Update (Obesity 2) Integrated Cardiovascular Risk Reduction Guideline: timeline for release of updated guidelines [Internet]. Bethesda (MD): National Heart, Lung and Blood Institute, National Institutes of Health; [cited 2011 Jul 7]. Available from: http://www.nhlbi.nih.gov/guidelines/cvd_adult/background.htm

8. Chobanian AV, Bakris GL, Black HR, et al. The Seventh Report of the Joint National Committee on Prevention, Detection, Evaluation, and Treatment of High Blood Pressure: the JNC 7 report. *JAMA.* 2003;289(19):2560–72.

9. de Oliveira Luz LG, de Albuquerque Maranhao Neto G, de Tarso Veras Farinatti P. Validity of the Physical Activity Readiness Questionnaire (PAR-Q) in elder subjects. *Rer Brasileira de Cine Desempenho Hun.* 2007;9(4):366–71.

10. Executive summary of the clinical guidelines on the identification, evaluation, and treatment of overweight and obesity in adults. *Arch Intern Med.* 1998;158(17):1855–67.

11. Fletcher GF, Ades PA, Kligfield P, et al. Exercise standards for testing and training: a scientific statement from the American Heart Association. *Circulation.* 2013;128(8):873–934.

12. Garber CE, Blissmer B, Deschenes MR, et al. American College of Sports Medicine stand. Quantity and quality of exercise for developing and maintaining cardiorespiratory, musculoskeletal, and neuromotor fitness in apparently healthy adults: guidance for prescribing exercise. *Med Sci Sports Exer.* 2011;43(7):1334–59.

13. Gibbons RJ, Balady GJ, Bricker JT, et al. ACC/AHA 2002 guideline update for exercise testing: summary article. A report of the American College of Cardiology/American Heart Association Task Force on Practice Guidelines (Committee to Update the 1997 Exercise Testing Guidelines). *J Am Coll Cardiol.* 2002;40(8):1531–40.

14. Giri S, Thompson PD, Kiernan FJ, et al. Clinical and angiographic characteristics of exertion-related acute myocardial infarction. *JAMA.* 1999;282(18):1731–6.

15. Haskell WL, Lee IM, Pate RR, et al. Physical activity and public health: updated recommendation for adults from the American College of Sports Medicine and the American Heart Association. *Circulation.* 2007;116(9):1081–93.

16. Jamnik VK, Gledhill N, Shephard RJ. Revised clearance for participation in physical activity: greater screening responsibility for qualified university-educated fitness professionals. *Appl Physiol Nutr Metab.* 2007;32(6):1191–7.

17. Kaminsky LA, editor. *ACSM's Health-Related Physical Fitness Assessment Manual.* 4th ed. Philadelphia (PA): Lippincott Williams & Wilkins; 2013. 192 p.

18. Kern KB, Halperin HR, Field J. New guidelines for cardiopulmonary resuscitation and emergency cardiac care: changes in the management of cardiac arrest. *JAMA.* 2001;285(10): 1267–9.

19. Lahav D, Leshno M, Brezis M. Is an exercise tolerance test indicated before beginning regular exercise? A decision analysis. *J Gen Intern Med.* 2009;24(8):934–8.

20. Maron BJ, Araújo CG, Thompson PD, et al. Recommendations for prepartication screening and the assessment of cardiovascular disease in masters athletes: an advisory for healthcare professionals from the working groups of the World Heart Federation, the International Federation of Sports Medicine, and the American Heart Association Committee on Exercise, Cardiac Rehabilitation, and Prevention. *Circulation.* 2001;103(2):327–34.

21. National Cholesterol Education Program (NCEP) Expert Panel on Detection, Evaluation, and Treatment of High Blood Cholesterol in Adults (Adult Treatment Panel III). Third Report of the National Cholesterol Education Program (NCEP) Expert Panel on Detection, Evaluation, and Treatment of High Blood Cholesterol in Adults (Adult Treatment Panel III) final report. *Circulation.* 2002;106(25):3143–421.

22. Pate RR, Pratt M, Blair SN, et al. Physical activity and public health. A recommendation from the Centers for Disease Control and Prevention and the American College of Sports Medicine. *JAMA.* 1995;273(5):402–7.

23. Persinger R, Foster C, Gibson M, Fater DC, Porcari JP. Consistency of the talk test for exercise prescription. *Med Sci Sports Exerc.* 2004;36(9):1632–6.

24. *Physical Activity and Health: A Report of the Surgeon General.* Atlanta (GA): U.S. Department of Health and Human Services, Centers for Disease Control and Prevention, National Center for Chronic Disease Prevention and Health Promotion; 1996. 278 p.

25. Riebe D, Franklin BA, Thompson PD, et al. Updating ACSM's recommendations for exercise prepartication health screening. *Med Sci Sports Exerc.* 2015;47(11):2473–79.

26. Shephard RJ, Thomas S, Weller I. The Canadian Home Fitness Test. 1991 update. *Sports Med.* 1991;11(6):358–66.

27. Stedman, editor. *Stedman's Medical Dictionary for the Health Professions and Nursing.* 5th ed. Baltimore (MD): Lippincott Williams & Wilkins; 2005. 2154 p.

28. Swain DP. *ACSM's Resource Manual for Guidelines for Exercise Testing and Prescription.* 7th ed. Philadelphia (PA): Lippincott Williams & Wilkins; 2013. 896 p.

29. Thompson PD. The cardiovascular complications of vigorous physical activity. *Arch Intern Med.* 1996;156(20):2297–302.

30. Thompson PD, Buchner D, Pina IL, et al. Exercise and physical activity in the prevention and treatment of atherosclerotic cardiovascular disease: a statement from the Council on Clinical Cardiology (Subcommittee on Exercise, Rehabilitation, and Prevention) and the Council on Nutrition, Physical Activity, and Metabolism (Subcommittee on Physical Activity). *Circulation.* 2003;107(24):3109–16.

31. Thompson PD, Franklin BA, Balady GJ, et al. Exercise and acute cardiovascular events placing the risks into perspective: a scientific statement from the American Heart Association Council on Nutrition, Physical Activity, and Metabolism and the Council on Clinical Cardiology. *Circulation.* 2007;115(17):2358–68.

32. U.S. Department of Health and Human Services. *2008 Physical Activity Guidelines for Americans.* Washington (DC): U.S. Department of Health and Human Services; 2008 [cited 2015 Oct 30]. Available from: http://health.gov /paguidelines/guidelines

33. U.S. Preventive Services Task Force. Screening for coronary heart disease: recommendation statement. *Ann Intern Med.* 2004;140(7):569–72.

34. Williams MA. Exercise testing in cardiac rehabilitation. Exercise prescription and beyond. *Cardiol Clin.* 2001;19(3): 415–31.

# 12

# Client Fitness Assessments

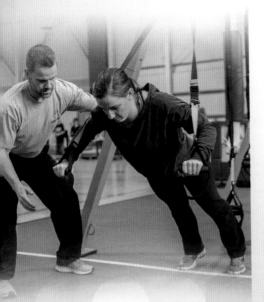

# INTRODUCTION

The assessment process can be extremely intimidating to clients, especially to those who are self-conscious about their appearance and intimidated by the idea of joining a fitness facility. As their Personal Trainer, it is important that you make your clients feel as comfortable as possible in the assessment process. During this process, share with your clients what you will be doing and how this will be accomplished. Clients may feel uncomfortable during certain parts of the assessment, such as during the weight assessment, measurement of waist circumference, and/or skinfold assessment. For example, if a client is overweight and a skinfold measurement at the abdomen site would be unsuccessful, do not attempt to take the abdomen site measurement. If the client is apprehensive about any part of the assessment process, let him or her know he or she can terminate the assessment at any time. Explain to the client the importance of accurately recording the measurements. If this explanation does not alleviate the client's anxiety, record any modifications to the measurement/assessment process for future reference. The success of the Personal Trainer–client relationship is built on a foundation of respect for the client. Respect can be established by providing information about the assessment process, listening to and addressing the client's concerns, and demonstrating competence in the assessment procedures. The Personal Trainer should guide the selection of the assessments (in consultation with the client) and the sequence of these assessments.

> The success of the Personal Trainer–client relationship is built on a foundation of respect for the client.

## Selection and Sequence of Assessments

A Personal Trainer has many options available to assess a client's health-related physical fitness. Among the considerations are the client's needs/desires, the situation or setting, and the Personal Trainer's training and experience. The exact sequence of assessments is dictated most by the setting and equipment available; however, a few generalizations regarding sequencing can be made. Resting measures (*i.e.*, resting heart rate [HR], resting blood pressure [BP], and body composition) typically should be taken prior to any exertional assessments, such as cardiorespiratory fitness (CRF) and flexibility. The Personal Trainer should perform assessments after the client has completed a health and physical activity questionnaire. One recommended order for performing assessments is the following (1):

1. HR: resting
2. BP: resting
3. Body composition: height and weight, body mass index (BMI), waist-to-hip ratio (WHR), and/or skinfolds
4. CRF assessment: Rockport 1-mile walk test procedures, 1.5-mile run test procedures, Queens College Step Test, and/or the Åstrand–Rhyming Submaximal Cycle Ergometer test
5. Muscular fitness: muscle strength and muscular endurance
6. Flexibility: sit-and-reach

# Heart Rate: Resting, Exercise, and Recovery

HR is the number of times the heart beats or contracts, usually reported in beats per minute (bpm). Although there are no known or accepted standards for resting HR, resting HR has often been thought of as an indicator of CRF because it tends to decrease as the client becomes more physically fit. There are also no standards for exercise HR, but the HR response to a standard amount of exercise is an important fitness variable and the foundation for many cardiorespiratory endurance tests. Recovery HR is often thought of as an excellent index of CRF and is used as a variable in some CRF tests (*e.g.*, Queens College Step Test). It is important to note that there are certain medications that may affect resting HR and HR response to exercise, so these statements may not always hold true in these cases. For example, β-blockers, often prescribed for hypertension, will significantly decrease resting HR and therefore may affect exercise responses to HR (1). This supports the importance of having the client complete the preparticipation screening questionnaire (refer to Chapter 11).

## Measurement of Heart Rate

There are many ways to assess or measure HR, including manual palpation at various anatomical sites and use of an HR monitor/watch or electrocardiogram.

### Palpation of Pulse

There are three common anatomical sites for the measurement of HR (3):

- *Radial*: Lightly press the index and middle fingers against the radial artery in the groove on the anterior surface of the lateral wrist (bordered by the abductor pollicis longus and extensor pollicis longus muscles). The radial palpation site is shown in Figure 12.1.
- *Brachial*: located in a groove between the triceps and biceps muscles on the medial side of the arm, anterior to the elbow, and palpated with the first two fingers in the medial part of this groove (see Fig. 12.1). This pulse location is also used for the auscultation of BP.
- *Carotid*: may be more visible or easily found than the radial pulse; press fingers lightly along the medial border of the sternocleidomastoid muscle in the lower neck region (on either side). Avoid the carotid sinus area (stay below the thyroid cartilage) to avoid the reflexive slowing of HR or drop in BP by the baroreceptor reflex. The carotid palpation site is shown in Figure 12.1 and should be used only if you or the client fails to feel the pulse in the radial or brachial sites.

The procedure for taking a pulse for HR determination is as follows (3):

1. Locate anatomic site.
2. Gently press down with the two fingers over palpation site.
3. Count the number of pulsations for a specific time period (*e.g.*, 10, 15, or 30 s).
4. Begin counting the first pulsation as 0 when timing is initiated simultaneously or, if a lag time occurs after the start time and the first pulsation, begin with the number 1.
5. Determine HR based on the number of pulsations in a given time period. Accuracy of HR increases with longer palpation times.
   - 10 seconds = multiply number of pulsations by 6
   - 15 seconds = multiply number of pulsations by 4
   - 30 seconds = multiply number of pulsations by 2

When clients experience difficulty in palpating the pulse, the use of an HR monitor as a learning tool to check the accuracy of the palpated HR with the monitor's HR may be desirable. The electrocardiogram is not often used by Personal Trainers to assess HR.

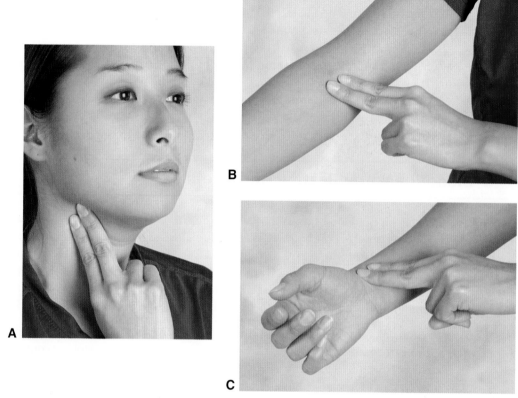

**FIGURE 12.1.** Locations for pulse determination.

All the given methods, when applied correctly, should yield similar results. The method for HR measurement by palpation of the pulse can be mastered through practice and should be taught to your clients. However, some clients, as a result of anatomical aberrations, are more difficult to palpate (3).

The measurement of HR by palpation of the carotid artery may lead to an underestimation of the true HR because the baroreceptors in the carotid sinus region often become stimulated when touched. This may reflexively reduce the client's HR as the baroreceptors sense a false increase in BP. Therefore, the radial or brachial arteries are the locations of choice for palpation.

The radial or brachial arteries are the locations of choice for palpation.

The baroreceptor reflex becomes a more important issue with HR counts longer than 15 seconds. It is recommended that a full 60-second count be performed for accuracy in resting HR. However, a 30-second time period may be sufficient for the count. "Resting" conditions must be present; for example, the client should be seated for at least 5 minutes with the back supported. Clients should be free of stimulants such as tobacco and caffeine for at least 30 minutes before taking the measurements (similar to resting BP). A resting HR may alternatively be assessed by having clients take their own pulse at home in bed upon waking in the morning. This resting HR may prove to be useful for the calculation of the exercise target HR zone.

## Measurement of Exercise Heart Rate

By the palpation method, measure the number of beats felt in a 15- or 30-second period and multiply by 4 (for 15 s) or 2 (for 30 s) to convert to a 1-minute value (bpm). Although the 30-second count may be more accurate and less prone to error than a 15-second count, the latter is typically used immediately postexercise because HR may decrease rapidly during recovery. When counting the exercise HR for a period less than 1 minute, you should start the time period and the count at zero (reference) at the first beat felt (3).

The use of HR monitors has increased in popularity as these monitors have become more available and affordable. Some monitors are prone to error (*i.e.*, not always consistent in measuring HR); however, newer technology has resolved the reliability problem previously associated with many of these monitors. HR monitors that rely on the opacity of blood at the earlobe or fingertip to measure/count flow are generally not as accurate as the monitors that use a chest electrode strap.

# Blood Pressure: Resting and Exercise

BP is the force of blood against the walls of the arteries and veins created by the heart as it pumps blood to every part of the body. BP is typically expressed in millimeters of mercury (mm Hg). BP is a dynamic variable with regard to location (*i.e.*, artery vs. vein and the level in an artery). Personal Trainers are most concerned with arterial BP at the level of the heart. This arterial, heart-level BP is the one typically measured at rest and during exercise (2). Definitions of BP are listed as follows, and more discussion concerning the regulation of BP can be found in Chapter 5.

- Systolic blood pressure (SBP) is the maximum pressure in the arteries when the ventricles of the heart contract during a heartbeat. The term derives from systole or contraction of the heart. The SBP occurs late in ventricular systole. SBP is thought to represent the overall functioning of the left ventricle and is thus an important indicator of cardiovascular function during exercise. SBP is typically measured from the brachial artery at the heart level and is expressed in units of mm Hg.
- Diastolic blood pressure (DBP) is the minimum pressure in the arteries when the ventricles relax. The term is derived from diastole or relaxation of the heart. The DBP occurs late in ventricular diastole and reflects the peripheral resistance to blood flow in the arterial vessels. DBP is typically measured from the brachial artery at the heart level and is expressed in units of mm Hg.

"Hypertension," or high BP, is a condition in which the resting BP, either SBP or DBP or both, is chronically elevated above the optimal or desired level. The standards for classifying resting hypertension are presented in Table 12.1. "Hypotension" is the term for low BP, and there are no accepted

| Table 12.1 | Classification of Resting Blood Pressure for Adults | |
|---|---|---|
| **Classification** | **Systolic (mm Hg)** | **Diastolic (mm Hg) (5th Phase)** |
| Normal | <120 | <80 |
| Prehypertension | 120–139 | 80–89 |
| Hypertension | | |
|    Stage 1 | 140–159 | 90–99 |
|    Stage 2 | >160 | >100 |

Reprinted with permission from the National High Blood Pressure Education Program. *The Seventh Report of the Joint National Committee on the Prevention, Detection and Treatment of High Blood Pressure.* Washington (DC): National High Blood Pressure Education Program; 2003.

standards for a value that classifies an individual with hypotension. Hypotension exists medically if the individual has symptoms related to low BP such as light-headedness, dizziness, or fainting (2). However, while there are classifications for hypertension, the Personal Trainer is not making a clinical diagnosis, instead they may refer the client to a health care professional for follow up. BP is typically assessed using the principle of indirect auscultation. Auscultation involves the use of a BP cuff, a manometer, and a stethoscope. Measurement of BP is a fundamental skill and is covered in detail in this chapter (11).

## Measurement of Blood Pressure

The measurement of BP is an integral component of a resting health-related physical fitness assessment. BP measurement is a relatively simple technique and may be used in risk stratification, as discussed in Chapter 11. Hypertension cannot be diagnosed from a single measurement; serial measurements must be obtained on separate days. The BP of a client should be based on the average of two or more resting BP recordings during each of two or more visits (1).

> Hypertension cannot be diagnosed from a single measurement; serial measurements must be obtained on separate days.

For accurate resting BP readings, it is important that the client be made as comfortable as possible. To accomplish this, take a few minutes to talk to the client after having him or her sit on a chair. Make sure the client does not have his or her legs crossed. Also, be sure to use the correct size of BP cuff. Choosing the correct cuff size is addressed later in this chapter. As with many other physiological and psychological measures, clients may experience "white coat syndrome" during the measurement of BP. White coat syndrome refers to an elevation of BP resulting from the anxiety or nervousness associated with being in a doctor's office or in a clinical setting (*i.e.*, clinician wearing a white lab coat). Thus, having a client in a relaxed state is important when taking a resting BP measurement.

### Korotkoff Sounds

To measure BP by auscultation, the Personal Trainer must be able to hear and distinguish between the sounds of the blood as it makes its way from an area of high pressure to that of lower pressure as the air is let out of the pumped-up cuff. These sounds are known as Korotkoff sounds. The sounds can be divided into five phases (3):

1. Phase 1 (SBP)
   - The first, initial sound or the onset of sound
   - Sounds like clear, repetitive tapping
   - Sound approximates the SBP, the maximum pressure that occurs near the end of systole of the left ventricle
2. Phase 2
   - Sounds like a soft tapping or murmur; sounds are often longer than those in the first phase; these sounds have also been described as having a swishing component.
   - Phase 2 sounds are typically 10–15 mm Hg after the onset or just below Phase 1 sounds.
3. Phase 3
   - Sounds like loud tapping; high in both pitch and intensity
   - Sounds are crisper and louder than Phase 2 sounds.
4. Phase 4 (also known as the true DBP)
   - Sounds like muffling of the sound; sounds become less distinct and less audible; another way of describing this sound is as soft or blowing.
   - This is often considered the true DBP and is typically recorded as the DBP.
5. Phase 5 (also known as the clinical DBP)
   - Sounds like the complete disappearance of sound

The true disappearance of sound usually occurs within 8–10 mm Hg of the muffling of sound, also known as Phase 4. Phase 5 is considered by some to be the clinical DBP. Phase 5 is the reading most often used for resting DBP in adults, whereas Phase 4 is considered the true DBP and should be recorded, if discerned.

### Instruments Used for Blood Pressure Measurement

A sphygmomanometer consists of a manometer and a BP cuff. The prefix *sphygmo* refers to the occlusion of the artery by a cuff. A manometer is simply a device used to measure pressure. Two common types of manometers are available for BP measurement: mercury (Fig. 12.2) and aneroid (Fig. 12.3). Mercury is the standard type used for accuracy; however, because of the toxic nature of mercury, aneroid sphygmomanometers are becoming more common in the workplace.

Position the manometer at your eye level to eliminate the potential for any reflex errors when reading either the mercury level or the needle if using the aneroid manometer. This is very important. Aneroid manometers are usually of a dial type (round), whereas mercury manometers are usually of a straight tube/column type. The cuff typically consists of a rubber bladder and two tubes, one to the manometer and one to a hand bulb with a valve that is used for inflation. The bladder must be of appropriate size for accurate readings. The sizing of a BP cuff should as follows:

- Width of bladder = 40%–50% of upper arm circumference
- Length of bladder = almost long enough (~80%) to circle upper arm

Three BP cuff sizes are commonly used in the health and fitness field: a pediatric or child cuff for small arm sizes (13–20 cm; 5–8 in), a normal adult cuff for arm size between 24 and 32 cm (9–11 in), and a large adult cuff for larger arm sizes (32–42 cm; 12–16 in). There are index lines on many of the newer sphygmomanometers cuffs to help "fit" the cuff for a client's arm circumference. In general,

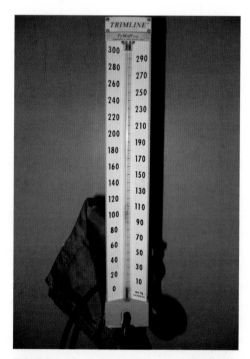

**FIGURE 12.2.** Sphygmomanometer, gravity mercury. Freestanding pressure manometer of the gravity mercury type, which uses the height of a mercury column in a glass tube to indicate cuff pressure.

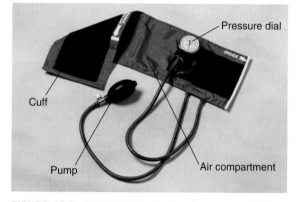

**FIGURE 12.3.** Aneroid sphygmomanometer and blood pressure cuff.

the appropriate BP bladder should encircle at least 80% of the arm's circumference. A cuff that is too small in length or width will generally result in a BP measurement that will be falsely high.

The cuff should be positioned at the level of the heart; if below the level of the heart, the BP reading will be falsely high. The cuff must be applied snugly or tightly. If the cuff is too loose, the BP measurement will typically be falsely high.

Equipment used in the measurement of BP is widely available commercially and varies greatly in quality. BP sphygmomanometer units can be purchased in most drug stores, from various health and fitness commercial catalogs, and at medical supply stores. Stethoscopes are also widely available and vary in quality. A high-quality stethoscope is worth the investment to help in hearing clear Korotkoff sounds (2). Electronic BP machines are increasingly available, with industrial models becoming commonplace in clinical settings. Commercial models have become widely available and relatively inexpensive to perform self-monitoring of BP. Many of these models have been shown to provide reasonably accurate readings (2).

### Resting Blood Pressure Measurement Procedures

**Visit thePoint to watch video 12.1 about blood pressure measurement.**

1. Position yourself to have the best opportunity to hear the BP and see the manometer scale. Take control of the client's arm while having it supported by some piece of furniture when listening to the sounds. Make sure that your stethoscope is flat and placed completely over the client's brachial artery. The room noise should be at a minimum and the temperature should be comfortable (21° C to 23° C [70° F to 74° F]). If you have some form of sinus congestion, your ability to hear the BP sounds may be diminished. Clearing your throat before attempting a BP measurement may be helpful. Of course, practice in the skill of resting BP measurement is important for its mastery.

2. The client should be seated, with the feet flat, the legs uncrossed, and the arm free of any clothing and relaxed. The arm you are using for the BP measurement should be well supported by you or resting on a piece of furniture. Your client's back should also be well supported.

3. Measurement should begin after at least 5 full minutes of quiet, seated rest. The client should be free of stimulants (nicotine products, caffeine products, recent alcohol use, or other cardiovascular stimulants) for at least 30 minutes prior to the resting measurement. In addition, your client should not have exercised strenuously for at least the prior 60 minutes.

4. There is no practical difference between a seated and supine resting BP; however, statistically, SBP tends to be higher by about 6–7 mm Hg and DBP by 1 mm Hg in the supine position.

5. It matters little which arm is chosen for the resting BP measurement; however, it is important to use the same arm for both resting and exercise measurements. The American Heart Association recommends that you measure both right and left arm BPs on your client on the initial evaluation and the arm with the higher pressure be chosen. However, if BP is normal in the right arm, it tends to be normal in the left arm. Conventionally, the left arm is typically used.

6. Center the rubber bladder of the BP cuff over the client's brachial artery; the lower border of the cuff should be 2.5 cm (1 in) above the antecubital fossa or crease of the elbow. Be sure to use the appropriate-size BP cuff, as discussed previously. Make sure to palpate the client's brachial artery to determine its location.

7. Secure the BP cuff snugly around the arm. Again, be sure to use the appropriate-size cuff. The client should have no clothing on the upper arm to secure the cuff properly. Clothing on the arm where you place the stethoscope will also muffle the intensity of the sound.

8. Position the client's arm so it is slightly flexed at the elbow; support the arm or rest it on some piece of furniture. If the client supports his or her own arm, the constant isometric contraction by the client may elevate the DBP. By having the client support the arm on a table, the "noise" heard during the procedure is reduced, which may increase measurement accuracy. Figure 12.4 depicts how the client's arm should be positioned with the BP cuff and stethoscope.

**FIGURE 12.4.** Position of the stethoscope head and blood pressure cuff.

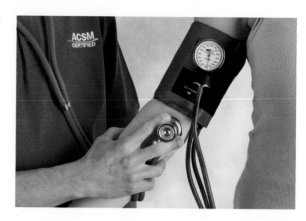

9. Position the BP cuff on the upper arm with the cuff at heart level. For every centimeter, the cuff is below heart level, the BP tends to be higher by 1 mm Hg. The reverse is true for a BP cuff that is above heart level.

10. Find the client's brachial artery. This artery, and thus pulse, is just medial to the biceps tendon. Mark the artery with an appropriate marker (water color) to "locate" the artery for the stethoscope bell placement. To best find the client's brachial artery, have the client face the palm upward and rotate the arm outward on the thumb side with the arm hyperextended.

11. Firmly place the bell of the stethoscope over the artery located in the antecubital fossa. Do not place the bell of the stethoscope under the lip of the BP cuff. There should be no air space or clothing between the bell of the stethoscope and the arm. The stethoscope earpieces should be directed facing slightly forward, toward your nose and in the same direction as your ear canal. Do not press too hard with the stethoscope bell on the arm. The earpieces of a stethoscope should be cleaned with rubbing alcohol before use each time.

12. Be sure to position the manometer (either mercury or aneroid) so that the dial or tube is clearly visible and at eye level to avoid any parallax (distortion from looking up or down) error.

13. Choose between any one of the following three accepted methods for BP cuff inflation. Quickly inflate the BP cuff to approximately:
    - 20 mm Hg above the SBP, if known
    - Up to 140–180 mm Hg for a resting BP
    - Up to 30 mm Hg above disappearance of the radial pulse if you palpate for radial pulse first. This is called the palpation method. Many educators favor the palpation method when the technician is first learning BP measurement to "feel" for and then listen to the SBP.

14. Deflate the pressure slowly; 2–3 mm Hg per heart beat (or 2–5 mm Hg per second) by opening the air exhaust valve on the hand bulb. Rapid deflation leads to underestimation of SBP and overestimation of DBP. Slow the deflation rate to 2 mm Hg per pulse beat when in the anticipated range of the systolic to diastolic BP; this will compensate for slow HRs. A falsely low BP tends to result from too rapid deflation of the cuff.

15. Record measures of SBP and DBP in even numbers. Always round off upward to the nearest 2 mm Hg. Always continue to listen to any BP sounds for at least 10 mm Hg below the fifth phase (to be sure you have correctly identified the fifth phase).

16. Rapidly deflate the cuff to zero after the DBP is obtained.

Wait for 1 full minute before repeating the BP measurement. Average at least two BP readings to get a "true sense" of an individual's BP. It is suggested that BP readings on clients be taken on at least two separate occasions to screen for hypertension. Also, the two readings on your client in any given session should be within 5 mm Hg of each other. If they are not, you should take another BP reading.

The norms (12) presented in Table 12.1 for resting BP are for those older than 18 years. To use these norms, individuals should not be taking any antihypertensive medications and should not be acutely ill during the measurement. When SBP and DBP fall into two different classifications, the higher classification should be selected. This classification is based on two or more readings taken at each of two or more visits after an initial BP screening. Generally, these norms are revised periodically. It is generally recommended that all persons older than 30 years have their BP checked annually (10).

 ## Body Composition

Body composition can be defined as the relative proportion of fat and fat-free tissue in the body (percent body fat).

Body composition can be defined as the relative proportion of fat and fat-free tissue in the body (percent body fat). The assessment of body composition is necessary for numerous reasons. There is a strong correlation (5) between obesity and increased risk of chronic diseases including coronary artery disease, diabetes, hypertension, certain cancers, and hyperlipidemia. There is a frequent need to evaluate body weight and body composition in the health and fitness field. Most often, this evaluation is done to establish a target, desirable, or optimal weight for an individual. There are several ways to evaluate the composition of the human body. Body composition can be estimated with both laboratory and field techniques that vary in terms of complexity, cost, and accuracy. For the purposes of this text, the following techniques are reviewed:

- Height and weight
- BMI
- WHR (waist and hip circumference measures)
- Skinfolds
- Bioelectrical impedance analysis (BIA)

### Height and Weight

Measure the client's height. Instruct the client with shoes removed to stand straight up, the client's heels should be together and their head should be level, they should take a deep breath and hold it, and look straight ahead. Record the height in centimeters or inches.

- 1 in = 2.54 cm
- 1 m = 100 cm
- For example: 6 ft = 72 in = 183 cm = 1.83 m

Measure the client's weight with his or her shoes removed and as much other clothing removed as is practical and possible. Convert weight from pounds to kilograms when necessary.

- 1 kg = 2.2 lb
- For example: 187 lb = 85 kg

Previously, one would compare the client's height and weight with one of the several height–weight tables that are available. With the many criticisms of the validity of the height–weight tables (including using a select group of individuals for development and the imprecise concept of "frame size"), there has been a strong trend recently to discontinue their use. Thus, this chapter discusses more advanced methods of anthropometry and body composition analysis.

### Body Mass Index

BMI, also called the Quetelet's index, is used to assess weight relative to height. BMI has a similar association with body fat as the height–weight tables previously discussed. This technique compares an individual's weight (in kilograms) with his or her height (in square meters), much like a height–weight table would. The BMI gives a single number for comparison, as opposed to the weight-to-height ranges located in the tables.

- BMI (kg · m$^{-2}$) = weight (kg) / height (m$^2$)
- For example, an individual who weighs 150 lb and is 5 ft, 8 in tall has a BMI of:

$$5 \text{ ft } 8 \text{ in} = 173 \text{ cm} = 1.73 \text{ m} = 2.99 \text{ m}^2 \text{ and } 150 \text{ lb} = 68.18 \text{ kg}$$

- BMI = 68.18 / 2.99 = 22.8 kg · m$^{-2}$

The major shortcoming with using BMI for body composition is that it is difficult for a client to relate to and/or interpret needed weight loss or weight gain. Also, the BMI does not differentiate fat weight from fat-free weight and has only a modest correlation with body fat percentage predicted from hydrostatic weighing (2). Standards and norms for BMI are presented in Table 12.2 and Figure 12.5.

## Waist-to-Hip Ratio

The WHR is a comparison between the circumference of the waist and the circumference of the hip. This ratio best represents the distribution of body weight, and perhaps body fat, in an individual. The pattern of body weight distribution is recognized as an important predictor of health risks of obesity. Individuals with more weight or circumference on the trunk are at higher risk of hypertension, type 2 diabetes, hyperlipidemia, and coronary artery disease than individuals who are of equal weight but have more of their weight distributed on

| Table 12.2 | Classification of Disease Risk Based on Body Mass Index (BMI) and Waist Circumference | | |
|---|---|---|---|
| | | Disease Risk[a] Relative to Normal Weight and Waist Circumference | |
| | BMI (kg · m$^{-2}$) | Men, ≤102 cm<br>Women, ≤88 cm | Men, >102 cm<br>Women, >88 cm |
| Underweight | <18.5 | — | — |
| Normal | 18.5–24.9 | — | — |
| Overweight | 25.0–29.9 | Increased | High |
| Obesity, class | | | |
| I | 30.0–34.9 | High | Very high |
| II | 35.0–39.9 | Very high | Very high |
| III | ≥40.0 | Extremely high | Extremely high |

Dashes (—) indicate that no additional risk at these levels of BMI was assigned. Increased waist circumference can also be a marker for increased risk, even in persons of normal weight.

[a]Disease risk for Type 2 diabetes, hypertension, and cardiovascular disease.

Reprinted from American College of Sports Medicine. *ACSM's Guidelines for Exercise Testing and Prescription.* 10th ed. Philadelphia (PA): Wolters Kluwer; 2018.

Adapted from National Institutes of Health. *Clinical Guidelines on the Identification, Evaluation, and Treatment of Overweight and Obesity in Adults* [Internet]. Bethesda (MD): National Institutes of Health. Available from: https://www.ncbi.nlm.nih.gov/books/NBK2003/pdf/Bookshelf_NBK2003.pdf.

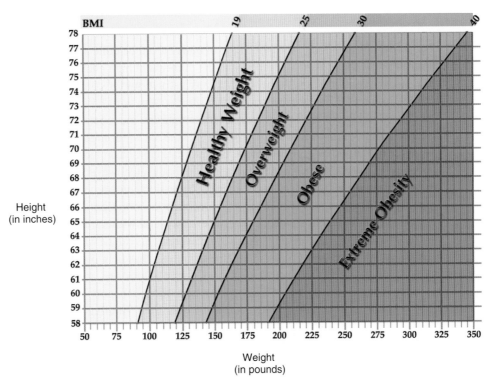

**FIGURE 12.5.** The risks of obesity. How is body fat measured? Body mass index (BMI) is a measure of weight in relation to a person's height. For most people, BMI has a strong relationship to weight. For adults, BMI can also be found by using this table. To use the BMI table, first find the client's weight at the bottom of the graph. Go straight up from that point until the line matches the client's height. Then, identify the client's weight group. (Anatomical Chart Company. *Risks of Obesity Anatomical Chart.* Baltimore [MD]: Lippincott Williams & Wilkins; 2004.)

the extremities. Some experts suggest that the waist circumference alone can be used as an indicator of health risk (1).

- Waist: The waist circumference has been frequently defined as the smallest circumference above the umbilicus or navel and below the xiphoid process (2).
- Hip: The hip circumference has been defined as the largest circumference around the buttocks, above the gluteal fold (posterior extension).
- WHR is a ratio (thus, there are no units).

**Visit thePoint to watch video 12.2 about using tape to measure waist circumference.** Measure the waist and hip circumferences in either inches or centimeters (1 in = 2.54 cm). A quality tape with a spring-loaded handle (*i.e.*, Gulick) should be used to measure circumferences. The technician should stand on the right side of the client, and the measurement should be made on bare skin. In addition, the measurement should be taken at the end of a normal exhalation by the client (2). Take multiple measurements until each is within 5 mm (¼ in) of each other. For example, if a male client has a waist circumference of 32 in (81.3 cm) and a hip circumference of 35 in (88.9 cm), his WHR is 32 / 35 = 0.91. Health risk is very high for young men when the WHR is more than 0.95 and for young women when the WHR is more than 0.86.

## Waist Circumference Alone

Some experts suggest that the waist circumference alone may be used as an indicator of health risk (1). For example, the health risk is high when the waist circumference is greater than or equal to 35 in (88 cm) for women and 40 in (102 cm) for men. A very low risk is associated with a waist circumference less than 27.5 in (70 cm) for women and 31.5 in (80 cm) for men.

# Skinfolds

Skinfold determination of the percentage of body fat can be quite accurate if the technician is properly trained in the use of skinfold calipers and the caliper is of high quality. If the technician is not properly trained, or does not adhere to the standardized instructions for skinfold measurement, significant error can be introduced into the assessment. Utilizing quality skinfold calipers is worth the investment, as poor quality skinfold calipers will provide inaccurate and inconsistent values. It should be remembered, however, that skinfold determination of percent body fat is still an estimate or a prediction of percentage body fat, not an absolute measurement. This estimate is based on the principle that the amount of subcutaneous fat is proportional to the total amount of body fat; however, the proportion of subcutaneous fat to total fat varies with sex, age, and ethnicity. Regression equations considering these factors have been developed to predict body density and percent body fat from skinfold measurements (6).

Use of skinfold measurement can also be very useful without determination of a body fat percent estimation. Use of the sum of the skinfold measurements can be a useful tool to track changes in body fat distribution that may occur with training. Calculating the sum of skinfolds prior to, and after training, or during routine follow-up testing, can provide the client with useful information on how their training program is impacting change in body composition.

> Use of skinfold measurement can also be very useful without determination of a body fat percent estimation.

Standardized descriptions as well as pictorial descriptions of skinfold sites are provided in Box 12.1 and Figure 12.6.

---

## Box 12.1 — Standardized Description of Skinfold Sites and Procedures

**Skinfold Site**

| | |
|---|---|
| Abdominal | Vertical fold; 2 cm to the right side of the umbilicus |
| Triceps | Vertical fold; on the posterior midline of the upper arm, halfway between the acromion and olecranon processes, with the arm held freely to the side of the body |
| Biceps | Vertical fold; on the anterior aspect of the arm over the belly of the biceps muscle, 1 cm above the level used to mark the triceps site |
| Chest/Pectoral | Diagonal fold; one-half the distance between the anterior axillary line and the nipple (men), or one-third of the distance between the anterior axillary line and the nipple (women) |
| Medial calf | Vertical fold; at the maximum circumference of the calf on the midline of its medial border |
| Midaxillary | Vertical fold; on the midaxillary line at the level of the xiphoid process of the sternum. An alternate method is a horizontal fold taken at the level of the xiphoid/sternal border on the midaxillary line. |
| Subscapular | Diagonal fold (45-degree angle); 1–2 cm below the inferior angle of the scapula |
| Suprailiac | Diagonal fold; in line with the natural angle of the iliac crest taken in the anterior axillary line immediately superior to the iliac crest |
| Thigh | Vertical fold; on the anterior midline of the thigh, midway between the proximal border of the patella and the inguinal crease (hip) |

**Procedures**

- All measurements should be made on the right side of the body with the subject standing upright.
- Caliper should be placed directly on the skin surface, 1 cm away from the thumb and finger, perpendicular to the skinfold, and halfway between the crest and the base of the fold.
- Pinch should be maintained while reading the caliper.
- Wait 1–2 s before reading caliper.
- Take duplicate measures at each site and retest if duplicate measurements are not within 1–2 mm.
- Rotate through measurement sites or allow time for skin to regain normal texture and thickness.

From American College of Sports Medicine. *ACSM's Guidelines for Exercise Testing and Prescription.* 10th ed. Philadelphia (PA): Lippincott Williams & Wilkins; 2018.

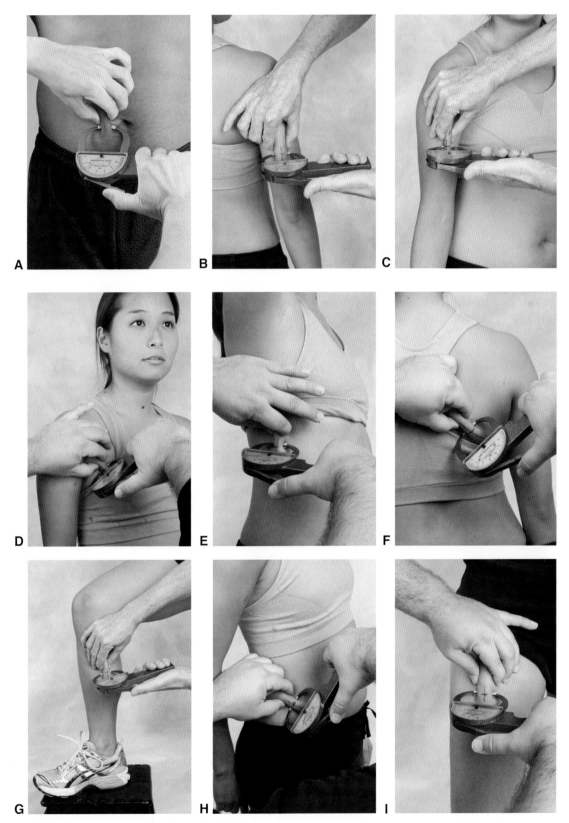

**FIGURE 12.6.** Anatomical sites for skinfold measurement.

### Skinfold Measurement Procedures

The following procedures help standardize the skinfold measurement (3).

Visit thePoint to watch videos 12.3 and 12.4 about using skinfolds to measure body fat in men and women.

1. Firmly grasp a double fold of skin (a skinfold) and the subcutaneous fat between the thumb and index finger of your left hand and lift up and away from the body. Be certain that you have not grasped any muscle in this procedure and that you have taken up all the fat. You can also have the subject first flex the muscle below the site to help distinguish muscle from fat before you measure. Be sure, however, to have the subject relax the area prior to measurement.

2. You should grasp the skinfold site with your two fingers about 8 cm (3 in) apart on a line that is perpendicular to the long axis of the skinfold site. You should be able to form a fold that has roughly parallel sides. Larger skinfolds (obese individuals) will require separating your fingers farther than 8 cm. All skinfolds should be taken on the right side of the body.

3. Hold the calipers in your right hand with the scale facing up to ease your viewing. Place the contact surfaces of the calipers 1 cm (0.5 in) below your fingers. The calipers should be placed on the exact skinfold site, whereas your fingers should be above the site by 1 cm. Place the tips of the calipers on the double fold of skin and fat. By marking the skin on the specific sites (see Fig. 12.6), you will be able to accurately place the caliper head at the correct location. This will allow for measurement at the same site during duplicate measures.

4. Release the scissor-like grip of the calipers claws while continuing to support the weight of the calipers with that hand. Be sure to maintain a firm hold on the skinfold throughout the entire measurement process.

5. Record the reading on the calipers scale 1–2 seconds (not longer) after releasing the scissor grip lever to allow the jaws of the calipers to measure the skinfold site. Measure the skinfold to the nearest 0.5 mm (if using the Lange brand calipers). Be careful to avoid jaw slippage of the calipers.

6. Measure each skinfold site at least twice. Rotate through the measurement sites to allow time for the skin to regain its normal texture and thickness. If duplicate measurements are not within 1 or 2 mm (or 10%), retest this site.

7. Sum the mean, or average, of each skinfold site to determine percent body fat. You can use specific skinfold equations to determine body density and percent body fat and these equations can be found in other sources (1,3,5). For the purpose of this text, we suggest using the Jackson–Pollock 3-Site Skinfold Formula as discussed below. Percentile rankings for percent body fat for men and women can be found in Table 12.3.

### Jackson–Pollock 3-Site Skinfold Formula for Percent Body Fat

Jackson and Pollock (7) have developed several skinfold formulas for the prediction of percent body fat or body composition (often referred to as the Jackson–Pollock formulas). Jackson and Pollock developed two three-site skinfold formulas in 1980 and 1985, as well as a seven-site skinfold formula (1). The 1980 formula provides percent body fat averages for the skinfold measurement for the chest, abdomen, and thigh for men and triceps, suprailiac, and thigh for women. Sum the means of the three skinfold site measures and use the nomogram provided in this text (Fig. 12.7) for percent body fat estimation or tables published in other resources (2). Using the Jackson–Pollock nomogram provided in Figure 12.7 involves plotting your client's age along the "Age in years" section and connecting that point with a straight line to a point plotted along the "Sum of three skinfolds" section. Where the line dissects, the "Percent body fat" section of the nomogram represents the client's percent body fat.

## Bioelectrical Impedance

BIA is a noninvasive and easy-to-administer method for assessing body composition. The basic premise behind the procedure is that the volume of fat-free tissue in the body will be proportional to the electrical conductivity of the body. Thus, the bioelectrical impedance analyzer passes a small

| Table 12.3 | | Fitness Categories for Body Composition (% Body Fat) for Men and Women by Age | | | | | |
|---|---|---|---|---|---|---|---|
| | | Age, yr (Men) | | | | | |
| % | | 20–29 | 30–39 | 40–49 | 50–59 | 60–69 | 70–79 |
| 99 | Very lean[a] | 4.2 | 7.3 | 9.5 | 11.1 | 12.0 | 13.6 |
| 95 | | 6.4 | 10.3 | 13.0 | 14.9 | 16.1 | 15.5 |
| 90 | Excellent | 7.9 | 12.5 | 15.0 | 17.0 | 18.1 | 17.5 |
| 85 | | 9.1 | 13.8 | 16.4 | 18.3 | 19.2 | 19.0 |
| 80 | | 10.5 | 14.9 | 17.5 | 19.4 | 20.2 | 20.2 |
| 75 | Good | 11.5 | 15.9 | 18.5 | 20.2 | 21.0 | 21.1 |
| 70 | | 12.6 | 16.8 | 19.3 | 21.0 | 21.7 | 21.6 |
| 65 | | 13.8 | 17.7 | 20.1 | 21.7 | 22.4 | 22.3 |
| 60 | | 14.8 | 18.4 | 20.8 | 22.3 | 23.0 | 22.9 |
| 55 | Fair | 15.8 | 19.2 | 21.4 | 23.0 | 23.6 | 23.6 |
| 50 | | 16.7 | 20.0 | 22.1 | 23.6 | 24.2 | 24.1 |
| 45 | | 17.5 | 20.7 | 22.8 | 24.2 | 24.9 | 24.5 |
| 40 | | 18.6 | 21.6 | 23.5 | 24.9 | 25.6 | 25.2 |
| 35 | Poor | 19.8 | 22.4 | 24.2 | 25.6 | 26.4 | 25.7 |
| 30 | | 20.7 | 23.2 | 24.9 | 26.3 | 27.0 | 26.3 |
| 25 | | 22.1 | 24.1 | 25.7 | 27.1 | 27.9 | 27.1 |
| 20 | | 23.3 | 25.1 | 26.6 | 28.1 | 28.8 | 28.0 |
| 15 | Very poor | 25.1 | 26.4 | 27.7 | 29.2 | 29.8 | 29.3 |
| 10 | | 26.6 | 27.8 | 29.1 | 30.6 | 31.2 | 30.6 |
| 5 | | 29.3 | 30.2 | 31.2 | 32.7 | 33.5 | 32.9 |
| 1 | | 33.7 | 34.4 | 35.2 | 36.4 | 37.2 | 37.3 |
| *n* = | | 1,938 | 10,457 | 16,032 | 9,976 | 3,097 | 571 |

Total *n* = 42,071

| | | Age, yr (Women) | | | | | |
|---|---|---|---|---|---|---|---|
| % | | 20–29 | 30–39 | 40–49 | 50–59 | 60–69 | 70–79 |
| 99 | Very lean[b] | 11.4 | 11.0 | 11.7 | 13.5 | 13.8 | 13.7 |
| 95 | | 14.1 | 13.8 | 15.2 | 16.9 | 17.7 | 16.4 |
| 90 | Excellent | 15.2 | 15.5 | 16.8 | 19.1 | 20.1 | 18.8 |
| 85 | | 16.1 | 16.5 | 18.2 | 20.8 | 22.0 | 21.2 |
| 80 | | 16.8 | 17.5 | 19.5 | 22.3 | 23.2 | 22.6 |

*(continued)*

| Table 12.3 | Fitness Categories for Body Composition (% Body Fat) for Men and Women by Age (continued) | | | | | | |
|---|---|---|---|---|---|---|---|
| | | Age, yr (Women) | | | | | |
| **%** | | **20–29** | **30–39** | **40–49** | **50–59** | **60–69** | **70–79** |
| **75** | Good | 17.7 | 18.3 | 20.5 | 23.5 | 24.5 | 23.7 |
| **70** | | 18.6 | 19.2 | 21.6 | 24.7 | 25.5 | 24.5 |
| **65** | | 19.2 | 20.1 | 22.6 | 25.7 | 26.6 | 25.4 |
| **60** | | 20.0 | 21.0 | 23.6 | 26.6 | 27.5 | 26.3 |
| **55** | Fair | 20.7 | 22.0 | 24.6 | 27.4 | 28.3 | 27.1 |
| **50** | | 21.8 | 22.9 | 25.5 | 28.3 | 29.2 | 27.8 |
| **45** | | 22.6 | 23.7 | 26.4 | 29.2 | 30.1 | 28.6 |
| **40** | | 23.5 | 24.8 | 27.4 | 30.0 | 30.8 | 30.0 |
| **35** | Poor | 24.4 | 25.8 | 28.3 | 30.7 | 31.5 | 30.9 |
| **30** | | 25.7 | 26.9 | 29.5 | 31.7 | 32.5 | 31.6 |
| **25** | | 26.9 | 28.1 | 30.7 | 32.8 | 33.3 | 32.6 |
| **20** | | 28.6 | 29.6 | 31.9 | 33.8 | 34.4 | 33.6 |
| **15** | Very poor | 30.9 | 31.4 | 33.4 | 34.9 | 35.4 | 35.0 |
| **10** | | 33.8 | 33.6 | 35.0 | 36.0 | 36.6 | 36.1 |
| **5** | | 36.6 | 36.2 | 37.0 | 37.4 | 38.1 | 37.5 |
| **1** | | 38.4 | 39.0 | 39.0 | 39.8 | 40.3 | 40.0 |
| *n* = | | 1,342 | 4,376 | 6,392 | 4,496 | 1,576 | 325 |

Total *n* = 18,507

Norms are based on Cooper Clinic Patients.
[a]Very lean, no less than 3% body fat is recommended for men.
[b]Very lean, no less than 10%–13% body fat is recommended for women.
Adapted with permission from *Physical Fitness Assessments and Norms for Adults and Law Enforcement*. The Cooper Institute, Dallas, Texas. 2013. For more information: www.cooperinstitute.org

electrical current into the body and then measures the resistance to that current. The theory behind BIA is that fat is a poor electrical conductor containing little water (14%–22%), whereas lean tissue contains mostly water (more than 90%) and electrolytes and is a good electrical conductor. Thus, fat tissue provides impedance to electrical current. In actuality, BIA measures total body water and uses calculations for percent body fat using some assumptions about hydration levels of individuals and the exact water content of various tissues. The following conditions must be controlled to ensure that the subject has a normal hydration level so the BIA measurement is valid.

- No eating or drinking within 4 hours of the test
- No exercise within 12 hours of the test
- Urinate (or void) completely within 30 minutes of the test
- No alcohol consumption in the previous 48 hours before test

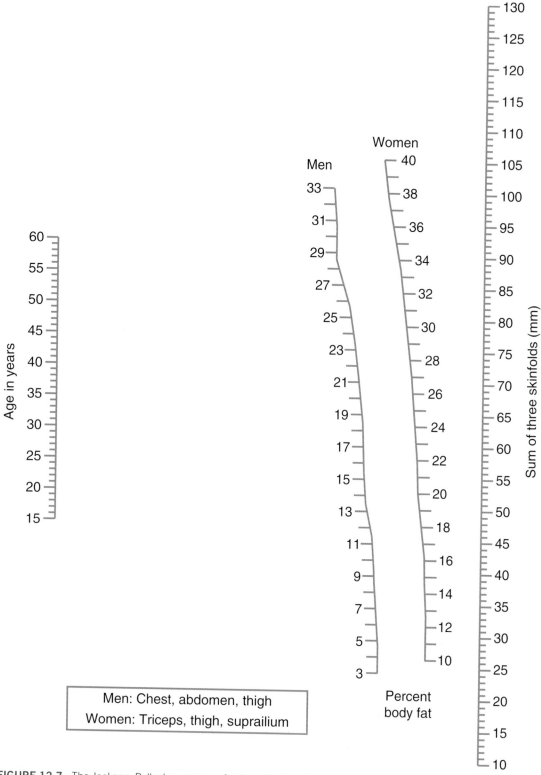

**FIGURE 12.7.** The Jackson–Pollock nomogram for the estimate of percent body fat. (Reprinted with permission from Baun WB, Baun MR. A nomogram for the estimate of percent body fat from generalized equations. *Res Q Exerc Sport.* 1981;52[3]:382. Reprinted by permission of the Society of Health and Physical Educators, www.shapeamerica.org)

| Box 12.2 | Summary of Body Composition Techniques |
|---|---|

| Procedure | Comments |
|---|---|
| Skinfold analysis | Highly regarded, many sites and formulas, technician training important, small prediction error (SEE about ±3.5%) |
| Bioelectrical impedance | Numerous pretest conditions need to be met (hydration of client), technician training minimal, under ideal conditions similar prediction error to skinfolds (SEE about ±3.5%–5.0%) |

SEE, standard error of estimate.
Adapted and modified from American College of Sports Medicine. *ACSM's Resource Manual for Guidelines for Exercise Testing and Prescription.* 7th ed. Philadelphia (PA): Lippincott Williams & Wilkins; 2014. p. 302.

BIA measurement offers an advantage over skinfold measurement in that there is no physical discomfort associated with the procedure. In addition, clients will feel less self-conscious with BIA measurement, as minimal skin exposure is required, relative to that needed for skinfold measurement. Cost of BIA devices, however, can be a disadvantage relative to skinfold measurement. A summary of the various body composition techniques discussed in this chapter is provided in Box 12.2 (2).

## Calculation of Ideal or Desired Body Weight

Along with the determination of percent body fat, it is often desirable to determine an ideal or desired body weight based on a desired percent of fat for the individual (Box 12.3). Obviously, this process can be problematic in that a desirable percent body fat for an individual must be determined. The determination of a desirable body weight is useful in weight loss and weight maintenance (7).

| Box 12.3 | Ideal Body Weight Calculations |
|---|---|

$$\text{Ideal body weight (IBW)} = \frac{\text{LBM (lean body mass)}}{1.00 - (\text{desired \% body fat} / 100)}$$

For example, if a man weighs 190 lb (86.4 kg) and is determined to have 22.3% body fat, then fat weight = body weight × (% body fat / 100)

$$= 190 \times (22.3 / 100)$$
$$= 42.37 \text{ lb (19.25 kg)}$$

LBM = body weight − fat weight = 190 − 42.37 = 147.63 lb (67.1 kg)

$$\text{IBW} = \frac{147.63}{1.00 - (15 / 100)} \quad (15\% \text{ used for a man; as a guideline})$$

$$= 173.68 \text{ (78.9 kg) at 15\% body fat}$$

Weight loss = body weight − IBW

In this example, 190 − 173.68 = 16.3 lb (7.4 kg) to lose to achieve ideal body weight.

# Cardiorespiratory Fitness Assessment

CRF is related to the ability to perform large muscle, dynamic, moderate- to high-intensity exercise for prolonged periods of time and reflects the functional capabilities of the heart, blood vessels, blood, lungs, and relevant muscles during various types of exercise demands. CRF is a synonym for many terms that may be used for the same thing (2). The following is a list of the terms that all mean essentially the same thing:

- Maximal aerobic capacity
- Functional capacity
- Physical work capacity
- Maximal oxygen uptake ($\dot{V}O_{2max}$) or maximal oxygen consumption or maximal oxygen intake
- Cardiovascular endurance, fitness, or capacity
- Cardiopulmonary endurance, fitness, or capacity

CRF can be measured or predicted by many methods. This chapter discusses the prediction of CRF using field tests such as the 1.5-mile run test and step tests as well as laboratory tests such as the submaximal cycle ergometer protocols. The Personal Trainer needs to decide which test is the most appropriate to determine CRF for a client. The measurement of CRF can be used in the following:

- Exercise prescription and programming
- Progress in, and motivation of, an individual in an exercise program (providing both feedback and motivation to keep a client interested in exercise)
- Prediction of medical conditions such as coronary artery disease (to further identify or diagnose health problems)

> CRF is related to the ability to perform large muscle, dynamic, moderate- to high-intensity exercise for prolonged periods of time and reflects the functional capabilities of the heart, blood vessels, blood, lungs, and relevant muscles during various types of exercise demands.

The true measurement of CRF involves maximal exertion as a result of graded exercise testing along with the collection of expired gases during this exercise test. The measurement of expired gases is not always applicable, nor desirable, in many settings such as corporate fitness and wellness programs that wish to measure or quantify CRF; also, this procedure is likely beyond the scope of practice of many Personal Trainers (2).

## Pretest Considerations

It is important to standardize pretesting conditions for all clients who undergo these various tests for CRF. Standardization can also increase the accuracy of prediction of CRF as well as aid in client safety. Instructions to clients prior to the test can increase their comfort as well. These general instructions are as follows (1):

- Abstain from prior eating (4 h).
- Abstain from prior strenuous exercise (>24 h).
- Abstain from prior caffeine ingestion (>12–24 h).
- Abstain from prior nicotine use (>3 h).
- Abstain from prior alcohol use (>24 h).
- Medication considerations (if the client's medications affect resting or exercise HR, it will invalidate the test)

# Various Field Tests for Prediction of Cardiorespiratory Fitness

A field test generally requires the client to perform a task in a nonlaboratory or field setting, such as running 1.5 miles (2.4 km) at near-maximal exertion. Thus, field tests, perhaps considered by some to be submaximal, may be inappropriate for safety reasons for sedentary individuals at moderate to high risk for cardiovascular or musculoskeletal complications.

> Field tests, perhaps considered by some to be submaximal, may be inappropriate for safety reasons for sedentary individuals at moderate to high risk for cardiovascular or musculoskeletal complications.

Two types of field tests are commonly used for the prediction of aerobic capacity: a timed completion of a set distance (*e.g.*, 1.5-mile run) or a maximal distance for a set time (*e.g.*, 12-min walk/run). Field tests are relatively easy and inexpensive to administer and thus are ideal for testing large groups of clients (2,4). Although the particular CRF assessment to select can be a difficult choice, there are criteria you may use to help select the best test for your client:

- What the data will be used for (*e.g.*, exercise programming)
- Need for data accuracy
- Client's age and health status
- Available resources

In general, both walk/run performance tests and step tests are appropriate for a wide range of clients, as long as the appropriate health risk screening has occurred first. One note of importance is that in the performance of a field test (both walk/run and step tests), the client can approach a level of near-maximal exertion, and this clearly may not be desirable for all clients.

## Walk/Run Performance Tests

There are two common field test protocols that use a walk or run performance to predict CRF. These walk or run tests tend to be more accurate (*i.e.*, less error in prediction) than the step tests discussed next. The performance tests can be classified into two groups: walk/run tests or pure walk tests. In the walk/run test, the client can walk, run, or use a combination of both to complete the test. In the pure walking test, clients are strictly limited to walking (always having one foot on the ground at any given time) the entire test. Another classification for these tests is whether the test is performed over a set distance (*e.g.*, 1 mile or 1.6 km) or over a set time period (*e.g.*, 12 min). The first test discussed uses a 1.5-mile (2.4 km) distance and requires the client to complete the distance in the shortest time possible, either by running the whole distance, if possible, or by combining periods of running and walking to offset the fatigue of continuous running in a less fit individual. The second test uses a set 1-mile course and requires the subject to walk the entire distance.

### The 1.5-Mile Test Procedures

1. This test is contraindicated for unconditioned beginners, individuals with symptoms of heart disease, and those with known heart disease or risk factors for heart disease. Clients should be able to jog for 15 minutes continuously to complete this test and obtain a reasonable prediction of their aerobic capacity.
2. Ensure that the area for performing the test measures 1.5 miles in distance. A standard ¼-mile track would be ideal (6 laps in lane 1 = 1.5 miles). For a metric 400-m track, this would be 6 laps (1.49 miles) plus approximately 46 ft to equal 1.5 miles.
3. Inform clients of the purpose of the test and the need to pace themselves over the 1.5-mile distance. Effective pacing and the clients' motivation are key variables in the outcome of the test.

4. Have clients start the test and start a stopwatch to coincide with the start. Give your clients feedback on time throughout the assessment to help them with pacing.
5. Record the total time to complete the test and use the formula below to predict CRF as measured by $\dot{V}O_{2max}$ and recorded in $mL \cdot kg^{-1} \cdot min^{-1}$:
   - For men and women: $\dot{V}O_{2max}$ $(mL \cdot kg^{-1} \cdot min^{-1}) = 3.5 + 483\,/\,time$, where time = time to complete 1.5 miles in nearest hundredth of a minute
   - For example, if the time to complete 1.5 miles was 14:20 (14 min and 20 s), then time used in the formula would be 14.33 min (20 / 60 = 0.33).
     - $\dot{V}O_{2max}$ $(mL \cdot kg^{-1} \cdot min^{-1}) = 3.5 + 483\,/\,14.33 = 37.2\ mL \cdot kg^{-1} \cdot min^{-1}$

### Rockport 1-Mile Walk Test Procedures

This test may be useful for those who are unable to run because of a low fitness level and/or injury. The client should be able to walk briskly (and should get the exercise HR above 120 bpm) for 1 mile to complete this test.

The 1-mile walk test requires that clients walk as fast as they can around a measured 1-mile course. The clients must not break into a run! Walking can be defined as having one foot in contact with the ground at all times, whereas running involves an airborne phase. The time it takes to walk this 1 mile is measured and recorded (8,9).

Immediately at the end of the 1-mile walk, the client counts the recovery HR (or pulse) for 10 seconds and multiplies by 4 to determine a 1-minute recovery HR (bpm). In another version of the test, HR is measured in the final minute of the 1-mile walk (during the last quarter mile). It has been shown that using an HR monitor may give the client more accurate results than manual palpation of HR.

The formula to determine $\dot{V}O_{2max}$ $(mL \cdot kg^{-1} \cdot min^{-1})$ is sex-specific (the constant 6.315 is added to the formula for men only). This formula was derived on apparently healthy individuals ranging in age from 30 to 69 years (6).

$$\dot{V}O_{2max}\ (mL \cdot kg^{-1} \cdot min^{-1}) = 132.853 - (0.1692 \cdot WT) - (0.3877 \cdot AGE) + (6.315,\ for\ men) - (3.2649 \cdot TIME) - (0.1565 \cdot HR)$$

where WT = weight in kilograms, AGE = age in years, TIME = time for 1 mile in nearest hundredth of a minute (e.g., 14:42 = 14.7 [42 / 60 = 0.7]), and HR = recovery HR in bpm.

For example, a male, 30 years of age, with a weight of 180 lb (81 kg) completed the 1-mile run in 14:42 minutes and had a recovery HR of 140 bpm; then, his estimated $\dot{V}O_{2max}$ would be

$$\dot{V}O_{2max}\ (mL \cdot kg^{-1} \cdot min^{-1}) = 132.853 - (0.1692 \times 81) - (0.3877 \times 30) + (6.315) - (3.2649 \times 14.7) - (0.1565 \times 140) = 43.9\ mL \cdot kg^{-1} \cdot min^{-1}$$

## Step Tests

Step tests have been around for more than 50 years in fitness testing. We will discuss the use of the Queens College Step Test (2) for the prediction of CRF (there are several popular step test protocols). This test relies on having the client step up and down on a standardized step or bench (standardized for step height) for a set period of time at a set stepping cadence. After the test time period is complete, a recovery HR is obtained and used in the prediction of CRF. The lower the recovery HR, the more fit the individual. Most step tests use the client's HR response to a standard amount of exertion (2).

In general, step tests require little equipment to conduct (a watch, a metronome, and a standardized height step bench). Special precautions for safety are needed for those clients who may have balance problems or difficulty with stepping. It should also be remembered that while step tests may be considered submaximal for many clients, they might be at or near maximal exertion for other clients.

| Table 12.4 | Calculation of Maximal Oxygen Consumption as Determined from the Recovery Heart Rate | |
|---|---|---|
| **For Men** | | **For Women** |
| $\dot{V}O_{2max}$ (mL · kg$^{-1}$ · min$^{-1}$) = 111.33 − (0.42 × HR) | | $\dot{V}O_{2max}$ (mL · kg$^{-1}$ · min$^{-1}$) = 65.81 − (0.1847 × HR) |

HR, recovery heart rate (bpm).

### Queens College Step Test Procedures

1. The Queens College Step Test requires that the individual step up and down on a standardized step height of 16.25 in (41.25 cm) for 3 minutes. Many gym bleachers have a riser height of 16.25 in.

2. The men step at a rate (cadence) of 24 steps per minute, whereas women step at a rate of 22 per minute for a total of 3 minutes of exercise. This cadence should be closely monitored and set with the use of an electronic metronome. A 24-steps-per-minute cadence means that the complete cycle of step-up with one leg, step-up with the other, step-down with the first leg, and finally step-down with the last leg is performed 24 times in a minute (up one leg — up the other leg — down the first leg — down the second leg). Set the metronome at a cadence of four times the step rate, in this case 96 bpm for men, to coordinate each leg's movement with a beat of the metronome. The women's step rate would be 88 bpm. Thus, although it may be possible to test more than one client at a time, depending on equipment, it is problematic to test men and women together.

3. After 3 minutes of stepping are completed, the client stops and has his or her pulse taken (preferably at the radial site) while standing and within the first 5 seconds. A 15-second pulse count is then taken. Multiply this pulse count by 4 to determine HR in bpm. Thus, the recovery HR should occur between 5 and 20 seconds of immediate recovery from the end of the step test.

4. The client's $\dot{V}O_{2max}$ (in mL · kg$^{-1}$ · min$^{-1}$) is determined from the recovery HR using the sex-specific formulas as given in Table 12.4.

## Submaximal Cycle Ergometer Tests

CRF may be predicted using several testing methodologies that can vary from submaximal to maximal in nature. We will next discuss the approach of laboratory submaximal exercise testing for the prediction of CRF. Maximal testing is not always a feasible or desirable approach in some settings; thus, the Personal Trainer may need to be able to perform a submaximal exercise test on a client in a laboratory setting. Per Olaf Åstrand (a famous exercise physiologist from Sweden) along with his wife, Irma Rhyming, developed a simple protocol in the 1950s to be used for the prediction of CRF from laboratory submaximal cycle exercise results known as the Åstrand–Rhyming protocol (Fig. 12.8). This protocol uses a single-stage approach for the prediction of CRF, which may be a simpler, and more preferable protocol for use by a Personal Trainer. Another protocol, developed by the YMCA (4), is commonly used and a brief overview is included here, more details on this more complicated test can be found in *ACSM's Health-Related Physical Fitness Assessment Manual*, 4th edition (2).

Maximal testing is not always a feasible or desirable approach in some settings; thus, the Personal Trainer may need to be able to perform a submaximal exercise test on a client in a laboratory setting. Two common tests include the Åstrand–Rhyming Test and YMCA Submaximal Cycle Test.

### Åstrand–Rhyming Test Procedures

In summary, the client performs a 6-minute submaximal exercise bout on the cycle ergometer. Thus, this is typically a single-stage test. The client's HR response to this bout will determine his

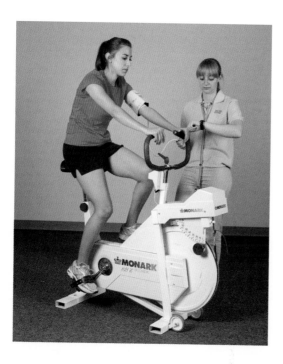

**FIGURE 12.8.** Submaximal exercise testing on a cycle ergometer.

or her maximal aerobic capacity or CRF by plotting his or her HR response to this one stage on a test-specific nomogram (Fig. 12.9).

1. *Explain the test to the client*: Adequately screen the client via a Health History Questionnaire and/or a Physical Activity Readiness Questionnaire (PAR-Q) and perform American College of Sports Medicine (ACSM) Pre-participation screening. Note: Physician supervision is not necessary with submaximal testing in low- and moderate-risk adults. More information on this can be found in Chapter 11 as well as the *ACSM's Guidelines for Exercise Testing and Prescription* (*ACSM GETP*) (1).

2. *Explain and obtain informed consent*: The safety of this test is reported as >300,000 tests performed without a major complication (1). Informed consent is further discussed in Chapter 11 and *ACSM GETP* (1). It is very important that the clients understand that they are free to stop the tests anytime, but they are also responsible for informing you of any and all symptoms they might develop.

3. Discuss with the client the general procedures to handle any emergencies.

4. Take the baseline or resting measures of HR and BP with the client seated.

5. *Adjust seat height*: The knee should be flexed at approximately 5°–10° in the pedal down position with the toes on the pedals. (Another way to check seat height is to have the client place his or her heels on the pedals; with the heels on the pedals, the leg should be straight in the pedal down position. Another option is to align the seat height with the client's greater trochanter, or hip, with the client standing next to the cycle.) Most important is for the client to be comfortable with the seat height. Have the client turn the pedals to test for the seat height appropriateness. While pedaling, the client should be comfortable and there should be no rocking of their hips (you can check on hip rocking by viewing your client from behind). Also, be sure that your client maintains an upright posture (by adjusting the handlebars, if necessary) and does not grip the handlebars too tight. Be sure to record the seat height for any follow-up testing.

6. Start the test.

7. Have the client freewheel, without any resistance (0 kg), at the pedaling cadence of 50 rpm (set the metronome at 100).

8. Remind the client that maintaining 50 rpm throughout the test is essential. The test results will not be valid if there is a large variance in pedaling cadence.

9. Set the first stage's work output according to protocol table (Table 12.5).

**Visit thePoint to watch video 12.5 about determining the correct seat height on a cycle ergometer.**

| Age | Correction Factor |
|-----|-------------------|
| 15 | 1.10 |
| 25 | 1.00 |
| 35 | 0.87 |
| 40 | 0.83 |
| 45 | 0.78 |
| 50 | 0.75 |
| 55 | 0.71 |
| 60 | 0.68 |
| 65 | 0.65 |

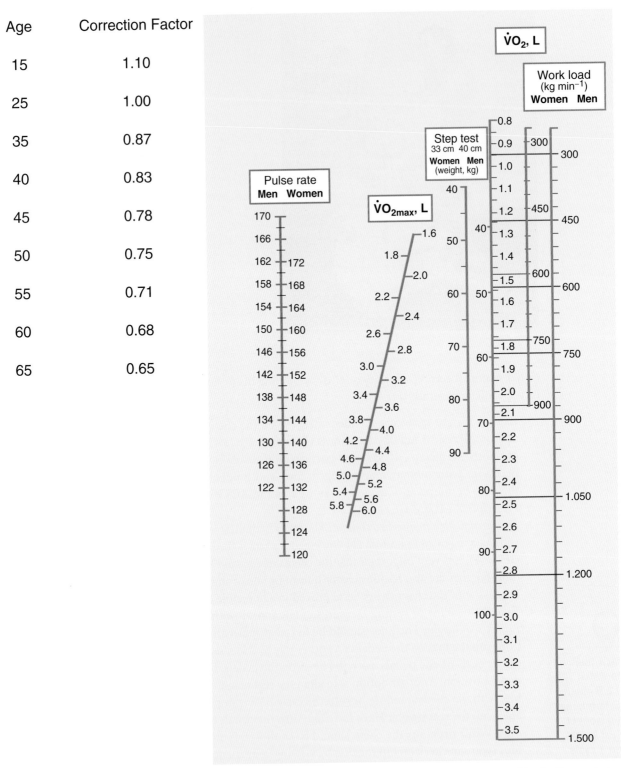

**FIGURE 12.9.** Åstrand–Rhyming submaximal cycle ergometer test nomogram and age-correction factors. (Used with permission from Åstrand PO, Rhyming I. A nomogram for calculation of aerobic capacity from pulse rate during submaximal work. *J Appl Physiol.* 1954;7:218–21.)

| Table 12.5 | Åstrand Cycle Submaximal Ergometer Test Initial Workloads |
|---|---|
| **Men** | |
| Unconditioned | 300 or 600 kg · m · min$^{-1}$ (50 or 100 W) |
| Conditioned | 600 or 900 kg · m · min$^{-1}$ (100 or 140 W) |
| **Women** | |
| Unconditioned | 300 or 450 kg · m · min$^{-1}$ (50 or 75 W) |
| Conditioned | 450 or 600 kg · m · min$^{-1}$ (75 or 100 W) |

10. Start the clock/timer.
11. Measure HR after each minute starting at minute 2. Count the HR for 10–15 seconds. An HR monitor may be used. Record the HR on the data collection sheet.
12. Measure and record the BP after the third-minute HR; ACSM guidelines for test termination and BP are applicable (1).
13. The fifth- and sixth-minute HR will be used in the test determination of $\dot{V}O_{2max}$ as long as there is not more than a five-beat difference between the two HRs.
14. The following applies for HRs.
    - If there is a difference of less than or equal to 5 bpm, consider the test finished.
    - If there is a difference of greater than 5 bpm, continue on for another minute and check HR again.
15. Regularly check the work output of the cycle ergometer with the pendulum resistance scale on the side of the ergometer and the rpm of client. For the resistance, do not use the scale on the top front panel for measurement. Adjust the work output if necessary.
16. Regularly check the client's rpm and correct if necessary. The Åstrand–Rhyming protocol requires the following for test completion:
    - Obtain fifth- and sixth-minute HR (within 5 bpm).
    - For the most accurate prediction of $\dot{V}O_{2max}$, the protocol requires the HR be between 125 and 170 bpm.
    - If the HR response to the initial work rate is not above 125 bpm after 6 minutes, the test is continued for another 6-minute interval by increasing the work rate by 300 kg · m · min$^{-1}$ (1 kg).
    - The HRs at the fifth and sixth minutes, if acceptable to the aforementioned criteria, are averaged for the nomogram method (Fig. 12.9).
17. Allow the client to cool down after the protocol is complete. Have the client continue to pedal at 50 rpm and decrease the resistance to 0.5–1 kg for 3 minutes of cool-down or recovery. Take the client's HR and BP at the end of the 3-minute active recovery period. Next, allow the client to sit quietly in a chair for 2–3 minutes to continue the recovery process. Be sure to check the client's HR and BP before allowing the client to leave the laboratory. HR and BP should be near resting measures before departing.

## Prediction of Cardiorespiratory Fitness or $\dot{V}O_{2max}$ from Åstrand–Rhyming Results

There are two methods available:

1. A popular nomogram technique described in this text (see Fig. 12.9)
2. A calculation-based formula not described in this chapter (this method can be found in the *ACSM's Health-Related Physical Fitness Assessment Manual* [2])

To use Figure 12.9, plot the HR (average for fifth and sixth minutes) on the appropriate gender scale and plot the corresponding work rate in $kg \cdot m \cdot min^{-1}$ on sex-specific workload scale. Connect the two points with a straight line and read off the $\dot{V}O_{2max}$ in $L \cdot min^{-1}$. Use the correction factor table (see Fig. 12.9) to correct the $\dot{V}O_{2max}$ by the person's age (nearest 5 years). Convert absolute $\dot{V}O_{2max}$ in $L \cdot min^{-1}$ to relative $\dot{V}O_{2max}$ ($mL \cdot kg^{-1} \cdot min^{-1}$) using the client's body weight. For example:

- If the estimated $\dot{V}O_{2max}$ (in $L \cdot min^{-1}$) was 3.65 for a 40-year-old man, the age-corrected $\dot{V}O_{2max}$ would be 3.03 $L \cdot min^{-1}$ (3.65 × 0.83).
- If the person weighs 147 lb (66.8 kg), his or her relative $\dot{V}O_{2max}$ ($mL \cdot kg^{-1} \cdot min^{-1}$) would be 3.03 $L \cdot min^{-1}$ × 1,000 = 3,030 $mL \cdot min^{-1}$ / 66.8 kg = 45.4 $mL \cdot kg^{-1} \cdot min^{-1}$.

### YMCA Submaximal Cycle Test Procedures

The YMCA Submaximal Cycle Test involves a branching, multistage format to establish a relationship between HR and work rate to estimate CRF (2). The test requires a minimum of two stages, with the possibility of four stages. Each stage is 3 minutes in duration. The goal of the protocol is to complete two separate stages that result in HR values between 110 and 150 bpm (2). All clients begin with a workload of 150 $kg \cdot m \cdot min^{-1}$. The second stage is dependent on the HR response from stage one. Detailed steps for the YMCA protocol are included as follows.

1–6. Steps 1–6 for performing the YMCA Submaximal Cycle Test are the same as described in steps 1–6 for the Åstrand–Rhyming protocol.
7. The exercise test should start with a 2- to 3-minute warm-up phase. Once the test protocol begins, the client is to be instructed to maintain a 50 rpm pedaling rate.
8. HR should be monitored near the end of minutes 2 and 3 of each stage.
9. The initial stage, Stage 1, is set for a workload of 150 $kg \cdot m \cdot min^{-1}$. This requires a resistance of 0.5 kg and pedal rate of 50 RPM.
10. The workload for the Stage 2, is dependent on the HR from Stage 1 taken during the last minute of the initial stage and use the following:
    - HR <80 bpm – change the resistance to 2.5 kg (125 W; 750 kgm/min)
    - HR 80–89 bpm – change the resistance to 2.0 kg (100 W; 600 kgm/min)
    - HR 90–100 bpm – change the resistance to 1.5 kg (75 W; 450 kgm/min)
    - HR >100 bpm – change the resistance to 1.0 kg (50 W; 300 kgm/min)
11. Use additional stages in order to obtain two consecutive steady state HRs between 110 bpm and 70% HR reserve (calculation: $[(HR_{max} - HR_{rest}) \times .70] + HR_{rest}$) or 85% of age-predicted maximal HR (calculation: $HR_{max} \times 0.85$).
12. If additional stages are necessary, increase the resistance from stage 2 by 0.5 kg or 25 W per stage.
13. Test should be terminated when subject reaches calculated HR zone, fails to conform to the test protocol, experiences adverse signs or symptoms, requests to stop, or experiences an emergency situation.
14. A cool-down period should be conducted, equivalent to the workload of stage one.
15. Normative tables can be found elsewhere (4).

## Norms for Cardiorespiratory Fitness ($\dot{V}O_{2max}$)

CRF is commonly expressed as $\dot{V}O_{2max}$. $\dot{V}O_{2max}$ is expressed as milliliters of oxygen consumed per kilogram of body weight per minute ($mL \cdot kg^{-1} \cdot min^{-1}$). Table 12.6 shows the norms for $\dot{V}O_{2max}$ for men and women.

| Table 12.6 | Percentile Values for Maximal Aerobic Power (mL · kg⁻¹ · min⁻¹) |

$\dot{V}O_{2max}$ (mL $O_2$ · kg⁻¹ · min⁻¹)

| | | MEN | | | | |
|---|---|---|---|---|---|---|
| | | Age Group (yr) | | | | |
| Percentile | | 20–29 (*n* = 513) | 30–39 (*n* = 963) | 40–49 (*n* = 1,327) | 50–59 (*n* = 1,078) | 60–69 (*n* = 593) |
| 95 | Superior | 66.3 | 59.8 | 55.6 | 50.7 | 43.0 |
| 90 | Excellent | 61.8 | 56.5 | 52.1 | 45.6 | 40.3 |
| 85 | | 59.3 | 54.2 | 49.3 | 43.2 | 38.2 |
| 80 | | 57.1 | 51.6 | 46.7 | 41.2 | 36.1 |
| 75 | Good | 55.2 | 49.2 | 45.0 | 39.7 | 34.5 |
| 70 | | 53.7 | 48.0 | 43.9 | 38.2 | 32.9 |
| 65 | | 52.1 | 46.6 | 42.1 | 36.3 | 31.6 |
| 60 | | 50.2 | 45.2 | 40.3 | 35.1 | 30.5 |
| 55 | Fair | 49.0 | 43.8 | 38.9 | 33.8 | 29.1 |
| 50 | | 48.0 | 42.4 | 37.8 | 32.6 | 28.2 |
| 45 | | 46.5 | 41.3 | 36.7 | 31.6 | 27.2 |
| 40 | | 44.9 | 39.6 | 35.7 | 30.7 | 26.6 |
| 35 | Poor | 43.5 | 38.5 | 34.6 | 29.5 | 25.7 |
| 30 | | 41.9 | 37.4 | 33.3 | 28.4 | 24.6 |
| 25 | | 40.1 | 35.9 | 31.9 | 27.1 | 23.7 |
| 20 | | 38.1 | 34.1 | 30.5 | 26.1 | 22.4 |
| 15 | Very Poor | 35.4 | 32.7 | 29.0 | 24.4 | 21.2 |
| 10 | | 32.1 | 30.2 | 26.8 | 22.8 | 19.8 |
| 5 | | 29.0 | 27.2 | 24.2 | 20.9 | 17.4 |

| | | WOMEN | | | | |
|---|---|---|---|---|---|---|
| | | Age Group (yr) | | | | |
| Percentile | | 20–29 (*n* = 410) | 30–39 (*n* = 608) | 40–49 (*n* = 843) | 50–59 (*n* = 805) | 60–69 (*n* = 408) |
| 95 | Superior | 56.0 | 45.8 | 41.7 | 35.9 | 29.4 |
| 90 | Excellent | 51.3 | 41.4 | 38.4 | 32.0 | 27.0 |
| 85 | | 48.3 | 39.3 | 36.0 | 30.2 | 25.6 |
| 80 | | 46.5 | 37.5 | 34.0 | 28.6 | 24.6 |

*(continued)*

| Table 12.6 | Percentile Values for Maximal Aerobic Power (mL · kg$^{-1}$ · min$^{-1}$) (continued) |
|---|---|

$\dot{V}O_{2max}$ (mL O$_2$ · kg$^{-1}$ · min$^{-1}$)

| | | WOMEN | | | | |
|---|---|---|---|---|---|---|
| | | **Age Group (yr)** | | | | |
| **Percentile** | | **20–29** (*n* = 410) | **30–39** (*n* = 608) | **40–49** (*n* = 843) | **50–59** (*n* = 805) | **60–69** (*n* = 408) |
| 75 | Good | 44.7 | 36.1 | 32.4 | 27.6 | 23.8 |
| 70 | | 43.2 | 34.6 | 31.1 | 26.8 | 23.1 |
| 65 | | 41.6 | 33.5 | 30.0 | 26.0 | 22.0 |
| 60 | | 40.6 | 32.2 | 28.7 | 25.2 | 21.2 |
| 55 | Fair | 38.9 | 31.2 | 27.7 | 24.4 | 20.5 |
| 50 | | 37.6 | 30.2 | 26.7 | 23.4 | 20.0 |
| 45 | | 35.9 | 29.3 | 25.9 | 22.7 | 19.6 |
| 40 | | 34.6 | 28.2 | 24.9 | 21.8 | 18.9 |
| 35 | Poor | 33.6 | 27.4 | 24.1 | 21.2 | 18.4 |
| 30 | | 32.0 | 26.4 | 23.3 | 20.6 | 17.9 |
| 25 | | 30.5 | 25.3 | 22.1 | 19.9 | 17.2 |
| 20 | | 28.6 | 24.1 | 21.3 | 19.1 | 16.5 |
| 15 | Very Poor | 26.2 | 22.5 | 20.0 | 18.3 | 15.6 |
| 10 | | 23.9 | 20.9 | 18.8 | 17.3 | 14.6 |
| 5 | | 21.7 | 19.0 | 17.0 | 16.0 | 13.4 |

Percentiles from cardiopulmonary exercise testing on a treadmill with measured $\dot{V}O_{2max}$ (mL O$_2$ · kg$^{-1}$ · min$^{-1}$). Data obtained from the Fitness Registry and the Importance of Exercise National Database (FRIEND) Registry for men and women who were considered free from known CVD.
Adapted with permission from Kaminsky LA, Arena R, Myers J. Reference standards for cardiorespiratory fitness measured with cardiopulmonary exercise testing: data from the Fitness Registry and the Importance of Exercise National Database. *Mayo Clin Proc.* 2015;90(11):1515–23. Reprinted from American College of Sports Medicine. *ACSM's Guidelines for Exercise Testing and Prescription.* 10th ed. Philadelphia (PA): Wolters Kluwer; 2018.

 ## Muscular Strength Assessment: One Repetition Maximum

Muscular strength is defined as a one-time maximal force that may be exerted and is localized to a joint or muscle group. There are many assessment tests for muscular strength, but only one test will be focused on this chapter. A good way of expressing muscular strength is as a ratio to total body weight.

A good way of expressing muscular strength is as a ratio to total body weight.

The one repetition maximum (1-RM) stands for a one-time maximum amount of weight lifted. Research has shown that the single best weightlifting test for predicting total dynamic strength is the 1-RM bench press. This test measures the strength of the muscles involved in arm extension: the triceps, pectoralis major, and anterior deltoid. It is important to note that the 1-RM involves vigorous exertion on the part of the client to complete this test. As a result, explanation of proper technique is crucial in an attempt to prevent injury. Although this test provides useful information concerning the total dynamic strength of the client, this test may not be appropriate for everyone (*e.g.*, elderly, those with significant ortho-pedic limitations). An assessment of the risk versus benefit of performing the 1-RM test needs to be performed by the Personal Trainer prior to conducting the test. Other assessments of muscular strength can be found in Chapter 4 of the *ACSM GETP*, 10th edition (1). The Personal Trainer may choose an assessment that best fits not only their client but also the facility in which they are performing the assessment.

Although determining a 1-RM can be time-consuming and somewhat complicated to perform, the procedures for the 1-RM bench press test are as follows:

1. Allow the client to become comfortable with the bench press and its operation by practicing a light warm-up of 5–10 repetitions at 40%–60% of perceived maximum.
2. For the test, the client is to keep his or her back on the bench, both feet on the floor, and the hands should be shoulder width apart with palms up on the bar. It is necessary for the Personal Trainer to ensure that the client is using a closed grip with the thumbs on one side of the bar and the other fingers on the other side encircling the bar. Free weight equipment is preferred over equipment like Universal or Nautilus. A spotter must be present for all lifts. The spotter hands the bar to the subject. The client starts the lift with the bar in the up position and arms fully extended. The bar is lowered to the chest and then pushed back up until the arms are locked. Be mindful of breathing; avoid a Valsalva maneuver (holding breath).
3. Following a 1-minute rest with light stretching, the subject does three to five repetitions at 60%–80% of perceived maximum.
4. The client should be close to the perceived maximum. Add a small amount of weight and a 1-RM lift is attempted. If the lift is successful, a rest period of 3–5 minutes is provided. The goal is to find the 1-RM in three to five maximal efforts. The process continues until a failed attempt occurs. The greatest amount of weight lifted is considered 1-RM.
5. An interesting way of expressing muscular strength is as a ratio to total body weight. For a ratio determination of the amount of weight lifted compared to the individual's body weight (for normative comparison purposes), divide the maximum weight lifted in pounds by the sub-ject's weight in pounds. Compare the calculated value to the norms (upper body) presented in Table 12.7.

The given procedure can also be utilized for the 1-RM leg press (lower body). The norms for this test are presented in Table 12.8 (1).

## Muscular Endurance Assessment: Push-up Tests

Muscular endurance is also joint and muscle group specific, and there are many tests available for this component of health-related physical fitness. Muscular endurance denotes the ability to apply a force repeatedly over time. Two common assessments for muscular endurance are the partial curl-up and push-up tests. However, recent evidence has suggested the partial curl-up test may not provide sufficient information re-garding muscular fitness and therefore has been removed from the most recent ACSM-related assessments (1).

A common assessment for muscular endurance is the push-up test.

Box 12.4 presents the procedures for the push-up test. The normative data for comparison pur-poses can be found in Table 12.9 for the push-up test (1).

| Table 12.7 | Fitness Categories for Upper Body Strength[a] for Men and Women by Age |
| --- | --- |

**Bench Press Weight Ratio = weight pushed in lb ÷ body weight in lb**

| | | MEN | | | | | |
| --- | --- | --- | --- | --- | --- | --- | --- |
| | | Age | | | | | |
| % | | <20 | 20–29 | 30–39 | 40–49 | 50–59 | 60+ |
| 99 | Superior | >1.76 | >1.63 | >1.35 | >1.20 | >1.05 | >0.94 |
| 95 | | 1.76 | 1.63 | 1.35 | 1.20 | 1.05 | 0.94 |
| 90 | Excellent | 1.46 | 1.48 | 1.24 | 1.10 | 0.97 | 0.89 |
| 85 | | 1.38 | 1.37 | 1.17 | 1.04 | 0.93 | 0.84 |
| 80 | | 1.34 | 1.32 | 1.12 | 1.00 | 0.90 | 0.82 |
| 75 | Good | 1.29 | 1.26 | 1.08 | 0.96 | 0.87 | 0.79 |
| 70 | | 1.24 | 1.22 | 1.04 | 0.93 | 0.84 | 0.77 |
| 65 | | 1.23 | 1.18 | 1.01 | 0.90 | 0.81 | 0.74 |
| 60 | | 1.19 | 1.14 | 0.98 | 0.88 | 0.79 | 0.72 |
| 55 | Fair | 1.16 | 1.10 | 0.96 | 0.86 | 0.77 | 0.70 |
| 50 | | 1.13 | 1.06 | 0.93 | 0.84 | 0.75 | 0.68 |
| 45 | | 1.10 | 1.03 | 0.90 | 0.82 | 0.73 | 0.67 |
| 40 | | 1.06 | 0.99 | 0.88 | 0.80 | 0.71 | 0.66 |
| 35 | Poor | 1.01 | 0.96 | 0.86 | 0.78 | 0.70 | 0.65 |
| 30 | | 0.96 | 0.93 | 0.83 | 0.76 | 0.68 | 0.63 |
| 25 | | 0.93 | 0.90 | 0.81 | 0.74 | 0.66 | 0.60 |
| 20 | | 0.89 | 0.88 | 0.78 | 0.72 | 0.63 | 0.57 |
| 15 | Very poor | 0.86 | 0.84 | 0.75 | 0.69 | 0.60 | 0.56 |
| 10 | | 0.81 | 0.80 | 0.71 | 0.65 | 0.57 | 0.53 |
| 5 | | 0.76 | 0.72 | 0.65 | 0.59 | 0.53 | 0.49 |
| 1 | | <0.76 | <0.72 | <0.65 | <0.59 | <0.53 | <0.49 |
| n | | 60 | 425 | 1,909 | 2,090 | 1,279 | 343 |

Total n = 6,106

| Table 12.7 | Fitness Categories for Upper Body Strength[a] for Men and Women by Age (continued) |
|---|---|

**Bench Press Weight Ratio = weight pushed in lb ÷ body weight in lb**

| | | WOMEN | | | | | |
|---|---|---|---|---|---|---|---|
| | | **Age** | | | | | |
| **%** | | **<20** | **20–29** | **30–39** | **40–49** | **50–59** | **60+** |
| 99 | Superior | >0.88 | >1.01 | >0.82 | >0.77 | >0.68 | >0.72 |
| 95 | | 0.88 | 1.01 | 0.82 | 0.77 | 0.68 | 0.72 |
| 90 | Excellent | 0.83 | 0.90 | 0.76 | 0.71 | 0.61 | 0.64 |
| 85 | | 0.81 | 0.83 | 0.72 | 0.66 | 0.57 | 0.59 |
| 80 | | 0.77 | 0.80 | 0.70 | 0.62 | 0.55 | 0.54 |
| 75 | Good | 0.76 | 0.77 | 0.65 | 0.60 | 0.53 | 0.53 |
| 70 | | 0.74 | 0.74 | 0.63 | 0.57 | 0.52 | 0.51 |
| 65 | | 0.70 | 0.72 | 0.62 | 0.55 | 0.50 | 0.48 |
| 60 | | 0.65 | 0.70 | 0.60 | 0.54 | 0.48 | 0.47 |
| 55 | Fair | 0.64 | 0.68 | 0.58 | 0.53 | 0.47 | 0.46 |
| 50 | | 0.63 | 0.65 | 0.57 | 0.52 | 0.46 | 0.45 |
| 45 | | 0.60 | 0.63 | 0.55 | 0.51 | 0.45 | 0.44 |
| 40 | | 0.58 | 0.59 | 0.53 | 0.50 | 0.44 | 0.43 |
| 35 | Poor | 0.57 | 0.58 | 0.52 | 0.48 | 0.43 | 0.41 |
| 30 | | 0.56 | 0.56 | 0.51 | 0.47 | 0.42 | 0.40 |
| 25 | | 0.55 | 0.53 | 0.49 | 0.45 | 0.41 | 0.39 |
| 20 | | 0.53 | 0.51 | 0.47 | 0.43 | 0.39 | 0.38 |
| 15 | Very poor | 0.52 | 0.50 | 0.45 | 0.42 | 0.38 | 0.36 |
| 10 | | 0.50 | 0.48 | 0.42 | 0.38 | 0.37 | 0.33 |
| 5 | | 0.41 | 0.44 | 0.39 | 0.35 | 0.31 | 0.26 |
| 1 | | <0.41 | <0.44 | <0.39 | <0.35 | <0.31 | <0.26 |
| *n* | | 20 | 191 | 379 | 333 | 189 | 42 |

Total *n* = 1,154

[a]One repetition maximum (1-RM) bench press, with bench press weight ratio = weight pushed in pounds per body weight in pounds. 1-RM was measured using a Universal Dynamic Variable Resistance (DVR) machine.
Adapted with permission from *Physical Fitness Assessments and Norms for Adults and Law Enforcement*. The Cooper Institute, Dallas, Texas. 2013. For more information: www.cooperinstitute.org

| Table 12.8 | Fitness Categories for Leg Strength By Age and Sex[a] |
|---|---|

**Leg Press Weight Ratio = weight pushed in lb ÷ body weight in lb**

**MEN**

| Percentile | | Age (Yr) | | | | |
|---|---|---|---|---|---|---|
| | | 20–29 | 30–39 | 40–49 | 50–59 | 60+ |
| 90 | Well above average | 2.27 | 2.07 | 1.92 | 1.80 | 1.73 |
| 80 | Above average | 2.13 | 1.93 | 1.82 | 1.71 | 1.62 |
| 70 | | 2.05 | 1.85 | 1.74 | 1.64 | 1.56 |
| 60 | Average | 1.97 | 1.77 | 1.68 | 1.58 | 1.49 |
| 50 | | 1.91 | 1.71 | 1.62 | 1.52 | 1.43 |
| 40 | Below average | 1.83 | 1.65 | 1.57 | 1.46 | 1.38 |
| 30 | | 1.74 | 1.59 | 1.51 | 1.39 | 1.30 |
| 20 | Well below average | 1.63 | 1.52 | 1.44 | 1.32 | 1.25 |
| 10 | | 1.51 | 1.43 | 1.35 | 1.22 | 1.16 |

**WOMEN**

| Percentile | | Age (Yr) | | | | |
|---|---|---|---|---|---|---|
| | | 20–29 | 30–39 | 40–49 | 50–59 | 60+ |
| 90 | Well above average | 1.82 | 1.61 | 1.48 | 1.37 | 1.32 |
| 80 | Above average | 1.68 | 1.47 | 1.37 | 1.25 | 1.18 |
| 70 | | 1.58 | 1.39 | 1.29 | 1.17 | 1.13 |
| 60 | Average | 1.50 | 1.33 | 1.23 | 1.10 | 1.04 |
| 50 | | 1.44 | 1.27 | 1.18 | 1.05 | 0.99 |
| 40 | Below average | 1.37 | 1.21 | 1.13 | 0.99 | 0.93 |
| 30 | | 1.27 | 1.15 | 1.08 | 0.95 | 0.88 |
| 20 | Well below average | 1.22 | 1.09 | 1.02 | 0.88 | 0.85 |
| 10 | | 1.14 | 1.00 | 0.94 | 0.78 | 0.72 |

[a]One repetition maximum (1-RM) leg press with leg press weight ratio = weight pushed per body weight. 1-RM was measured using a Universal Dynamic Variable Resistance (DVR) machine.
Study population for the data set was predominantly white and college educated.
Adapted from Institute for Aerobics Research, Dallas, 1994. Study population for the data set was predominantly white and college educated. A Universal Dynamic Variable Resistance (DVR) machine was used to measure the 1-repetition maximum (RM).

| Box 12.4 | Push-up Test Procedures for Measurement of Muscular Endurance |
|---|---|

**Visit thePoint to watch video 12.6, which demonstrates the push-up test for men and women.**

1. The push-up test is administered with male subjects starting in the standard "down" position (hands pointing forward and under the shoulder, back straight, head up, using the toes as the pivotal point) and female subjects in the modified "knee push-up" position (legs together, lower leg in contact with mat with ankles plantarflexed, back straight, hands shoulder width apart, head up, using the knees as the pivotal point) (Fig. 12.10).

2. The subject must raise the body by straightening the elbows and return to the "down" position, until the chin touches the mat. The stomach should not touch the mat.

3. For both men and women, the subject's back must be straight at all times, and the subject must push up to a straight arm position.

4. The maximal number of push-ups performed consecutively without rest is counted as the score.

5. The test is stopped when the client strains forcibly or is unable to maintain the appropriate technique within two repetitions.

Adapted with permission from the Canadian Society for Exercise Physiology. *Canadian Physical Activity, Fitness & Lifestyle Approach: CSEP-Health & Fitness Program's Health-Related Appraisal & Counselling Strategy.* 3rd ed. Ottawa (Canada): Canadian Society for Exercise Physiology; 2003. © 2003 Canadian Society for Exercise Physiology.

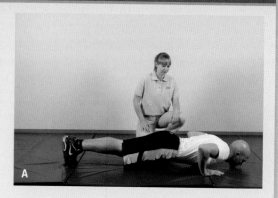

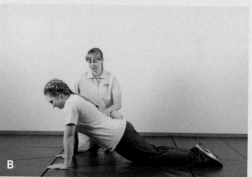

**FIGURE 12.10.** Client performing a pushup: **(A)** male and **(B)** female. (From American College of Sports Medicine. *ACSM's Health-Related Physical Fitness Assessment Manual.* 3rd ed. Baltimore [MD]: Lippincott Williams & Wilkins; 2010.)

| Table 12.9 | Fitness Categories by Age Groups and Sex for Push-ups |
|---|---|

| | Age (yr) | | | | | | | | | |
|---|---|---|---|---|---|---|---|---|---|---|
| Category | 20–29 | | 30–39 | | 40–49 | | 50–59 | | 60–69 | |
| Sex | M | W | M | W | M | W | M | W | M | W |
| Excellent | ≥36 | ≥30 | ≥30 | ≥27 | ≥25 | ≥24 | ≥21 | ≥21 | ≥18 | ≥17 |
| Very good | 29–35 | 21–29 | 22–29 | 20–26 | 17–24 | 15–23 | 13–20 | 11–20 | 11–17 | 12–16 |
| Good | 22–28 | 15–20 | 17–21 | 13–19 | 13–16 | 11–14 | 10–12 | 7–10 | 8–10 | 5–11 |
| Fair | 17–21 | 10–14 | 12–16 | 8–12 | 10–12 | 5–10 | 7–9 | 2–6 | 5–7 | 2–4 |
| Poor | ≤16 | ≤9 | ≤11 | ≤7 | ≤9 | ≤4 | ≤6 | ≤1 | ≤4 | ≤1 |

M, men; W, women.
Reprinted with permission from the Canadian Society for Exercise Physiology. *Canadian Physical Activity, Fitness & Lifestyle Approach: CSEP-Health & Fitness Program's Health-Related Appraisal & Counselling Strategy.* 3rd ed. Ottawa (Canada): Canadian Society for Exercise Physiology; 2003. © 2003 Canadian Society for Exercise Physiology.

# Flexibility Assessment: Sit-and-Reach Test

Although there is no single best test of overall flexibility, the sit-and-reach test is the most common and most practical to use. Preceded by a proper warm-up, the sit-and-reach test can be easy to administer and interpret. The Personal Trainer should be made aware that this test measures only flexibility of the hamstrings, hip, and lower back. The practical significance of using the sit-and-reach test to measure of flexibility is the significant number of people who complain of low back pain. It is likely that this pain is caused by decreased flexibility, primarily of the hamstrings (which have their anatomical origin in the posterior hip region). For a detailed description of the procedure, see Box 12.5. Percentile rankings for men and women can be found in Table 12.10 (6).

> Preceded by a proper warm-up, the sit-and-reach test can be easy to administer and interpret.

---

## Box 12.5    Trunk Flexion (Sit-and-Reach) Test Procedures

*Pretest*: Participant should perform a short warm-up prior to this test and include some stretches for the targeted muscle groups (*e.g.*, modified hurdler's stretch). It is also recommended that the participant refrain from fast, jerky movements, which may increase the possibility of an injury. The participant's shoes should be removed for the assessment.

1. For the Canadian Trunk Forward Flexion test, the client sits without shoes and the soles of the feet flat against the flexometer (sit-and-reach box) at the 26-cm mark. Inner edges of the soles are placed within 6 in (15.2 cm) of the measuring scale (Fig. 12.11). Note that specific norms are available for each of these tests.

2. The participant should slowly reach forward (no bouncing) with both hands as far as possible (to the point of mild discomfort), holding this position approximately 2 seconds. Be sure that the participant keeps the hands parallel and does not lead with one hand. Fingertips can be overlapped and should be in contact with the measuring portion of the sit-and-reach box or the yardstick. To assist with the best attempt, the participant should exhale and drop the head between the arms when reaching. Testers should ensure that the knees of the participant stay extended; however, the participant's knees should not be pressed down. The participant should breathe normally during the test and should not hold his or her breath anytime.

3. The score is the most distant point (in centimeters or inches depending on the test used) reached with the fingertips. The better of two trials should be recorded. Norms for the Canadian test are presented in Table 12.10. Note that these norms use a sit-and-reach box in which the "zero" point is set at the 26-cm mark. If you are using a box in which the zero point is set at 23 cm (*e.g.*, Fitnessgram), subtract 3 cm from each value in this table.

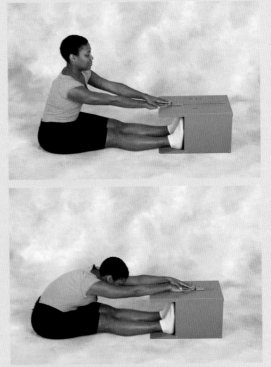

**FIGURE 12.11.** Client performing a sit-and-reach test using a sit-and-reach box. (From American College of Sports Medicine. *ACSM's Health-Related Physical Fitness Assessment Manual*. 3rd ed. Baltimore [MD]: Lippincott Williams & Wilkins; 2010.)

Diagrams of these procedures are available from Canadian Society for Exercise Physiology. *Canadian Physical Activity, Fitness & Lifestyle Approach: CSEP-Health & Fitness Program's Health-Related Appraisal & Counselling Strategy*. 3rd ed. Ottawa (Canada): Canadian Society for Exercise Physiology; 2003. © 2003 Canadian Society for Exercise Physiology.

| Table 12.10 | Fitness Categories for Canadian Trunk Forward Flexion Test Using a Sit-and-Reach Box (cm)[a] by Age and Sex | | | | | | | | |
| --- | --- | --- | --- | --- | --- | --- | --- | --- | --- |
| | Age (yr) | | | | | | | | |
| Category | 20–29 | | 30–39 | | 40–49 | | 50–59 | | 60–69 | |
| Sex | M | W | M | W | M | W | M | W | M | W |
| Excellent | ≥40 | ≥41 | ≥38 | ≥41 | ≥35 | ≥38 | ≥35 | ≥39 | ≥33 | ≥35 |
| Very good | 34–39 | 37–40 | 33–37 | 36–40 | 29–34 | 34–37 | 28–34 | 33–38 | 25–32 | 31–34 |
| Good | 30–33 | 33–36 | 28–32 | 32–35 | 24–28 | 30–33 | 24–27 | 30–32 | 20–24 | 27–30 |
| Fair | 25–29 | 28–32 | 23–27 | 27–31 | 18–23 | 25–29 | 16–23 | 25–29 | 15–19 | 23–26 |
| Poor | ≤24 | ≤27 | ≤22 | ≤26 | ≤17 | ≤24 | ≤15 | ≤24 | ≤14 | ≤22 |

[a]These norms are based on a sit-and-reach box in which the "zero" point is set at 26 cm. When using a box in which the zero point is set at 23 cm, subtract 3 cm from each value in this table.
M, men; W, women.
From the Canadian Society for Exercise Physiology. *Canadian Physical Activity, Fitness & Lifestyle Approach: CSEP-Health & Fitness Program's Health-Related Appraisal & Counselling Strategy.* 3rd ed., © 2003, Canadian Society for Exercise Physiology.

## Assessments as a Motivational Device

Health-related physical fitness assessments can serve not only for exercise programming but also for motivational purposes when the results of the various assessments are explained and used in the goal-setting approach. It is important to note that a particular physical fitness assessment that is not used in programming decisions and instilling motivation should be questioned as to its use. In other words, simply testing all clients for all available assessments should be avoided.

Physical fitness assessment should be performed on a regular basis to determine whether established goals have been met. As goals are set, often a time frame for the attainment of those goals is included (*e.g.*, lose 2% body fat in 3 mo). For instance, if the individual has a goal to improve his or her overall flexibility in 3 months, then the sit-and-reach test should be performed every 4–6 weeks to measure progress toward that goal. A word of caution about follow-up assessments is that frequent assessments may fail to demonstrate desired changes as some components of physical fitness may take time and effort to change (*e.g.*, significant and lasting body composition changes are not likely to occur in short time intervals). A standard for follow-up may be 4 weeks to 3 months, depending on what is being assessed.

Frequent assessments may fail to demonstrate desired changes as some components of physical fitness may take time and effort to change.

## SUMMARY

The results of a health-related physical fitness assessment represent a potential time of change. If a client scores *poorly* or has failed to demonstrate progress in certain areas (such as CRF with the submaximal cycle ergometer test), then answers should be sought as to why the changes were not evident and how the exercise program should be adjusted to produce the desired changes in the future. The results of the health-related physical fitness assessments should be used with an outcome in mind. It is important to realize that not all individuals are going to adapt to programming suggestions in the same way. Thus, each round of health-related physical fitness assessments calls for a reexamination of the client's goals and objectives. Perhaps, new measurable goals may be identified for that individual at some distant time interval.

# REFERENCES

1. American College of Sports Medicine. *ACSM's Guidelines for Exercise Testing and Prescription.* 10th ed. Philadelphia (PA): Wolters Kluwer; 2018.

2. American College of Sports Medicine. *ACSM's Health-Related Physical Fitness Assessment Manual.* 4th ed. Baltimore (MD): Lippincott Williams & Wilkins; 2013. 192 p.

3. American College of Sports Medicine. *ACSM's Resource Manual for Guidelines for Exercise Testing and Prescription.* 7th ed. Baltimore (MD): Lippincott Williams & Wilkins; 2014. 896 p.

4. Golding LA, Myers CR, Sinning WE, editors. *Y's Way to Physical Fitness.* 3rd ed. Champaign (IL): Human Kinetics; 1989. 192 p.

5. Heyward V, Gibson A. *Advanced Fitness Assessment and Exercise Prescription.* 7th ed. Champaign (IL): Human Kinetics; 2014. 552 p.

6. Howley E, Thompson D. *Fitness Professional's Handbook.* 7th ed. Champaign (IL): Human Kinetics; 2017. 592 p.

7. Jackson AS, Pollock ML. Practical assessment of body composition. *Physician Sports Med.* 1985;13(5):76–90.

8. Kline GM, Porcari JP, Hintermeister R, et al. Estimation of $\dot{V}O_{2max}$ from a one-mile track walk, gender, age, and body weight. *Med Sci Sports Exerc.* 1987;19(3):253–9.

9. Nieman D. *Fitness and Sports Medicine: A Health-Related Approach.* 4th ed. Mountain View (CA): Mayfield; 1999.

10. Perloff D, Grim C, Flack J, et al. Human blood pressure determination by sphygmomanometry. *Circulation.* 1993;88(5 pt 1):2460–70.

11. Prisant LM, Alpert BS, Robbins CB, et al. American national standard for nonautomated sphygmomanometers. Summary report. *Am J Hypertens.* 1995;8:210–3.

12. U.S. Department of Health and Human Services, National Institutes of Health, National Heart, Lung and Blood Institute. *Seventh Report of the Joint National Committee on Prevention, Detection, Evaluation, and Treatment of High Blood Pressure (JNC7)* (NIH Publication No. 03-5233) [Internet]. Bethesda (MD): National Institutes of Health; [cited 2008 Aug 27]. Available from: http://www.nhlbi.nih.gov /guidelines/hypertension/

# PART V

# Developing the Exercise Program

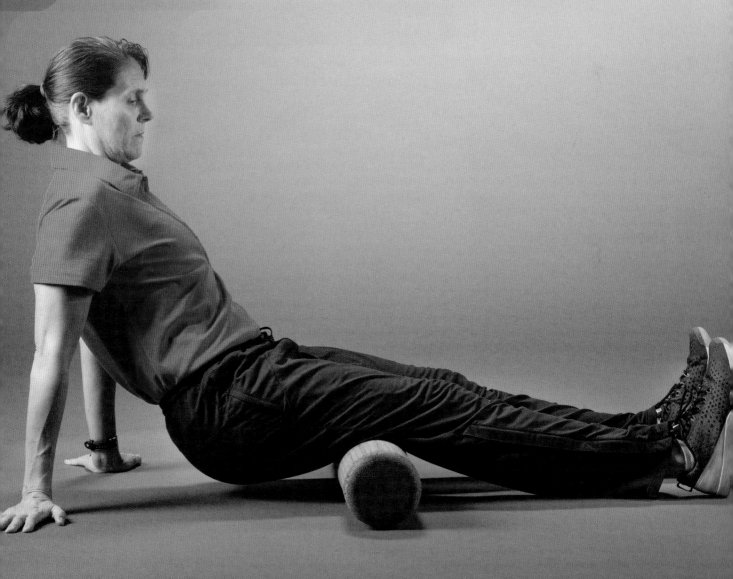

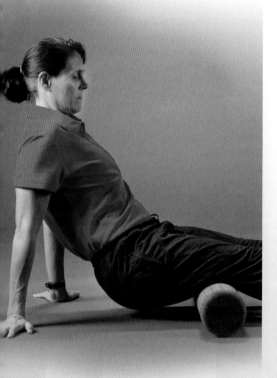

# 13 Comprehensive Program Design

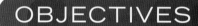

## OBJECTIVES

**Personal Trainers should be able to:**

- Describe the physiological and psychological benefits of a comprehensive exercise program.
- Describe the components of a comprehensive exercise program.
- Consider advanced training options.
- Understand the anatomy of an exercise session.

# INTRODUCTION

Personal Trainers have the opportunity to assist clients in creating exercise programs that not only help to prevent a number of hypokinetic diseases (*e.g.*, coronary heart disease, diabetes, low back pain) but also improve fitness and quality of life. As highlighted in this chapter, a comprehensive exercise program provides many physiological and psychological benefits. A well-rounded fitness plan follows a general format including a warm-up, the conditioning phase, such as cardiorespiratory exercise and/or resistance exercise, a cool-down, and flexibility exercise, and, when indicated, neuromotor exercise training (Box 13.1) (5). For some clients, more advanced options with a greater focus on skill-related components of physical fitness may also be appropriate.

In addition to health benefits of a fitness program, Personal Trainers should also be concerned with clients' sedentary behavior (*e.g.*, computer use, smartphone use, watching television). Sedentary behavior is associated with elevated risk of mortality due to heart disease and depression, increased waist circumference, and elevated blood pressure, among other concerns associated with chronic disease (5). Detrimental effects of sedentary activities are possible even among individuals who meet physical activity recommendations within their fitness program and thus including short bouts of physical activity to break up sedentary activities is recommended (5).

Detrimental effects of sedentary activities are possible even among individuals who meet physical activity recommendations within their fitness program and thus including short bouts of physical activity to break up sedentary activities is recommended (5).

 ## Benefits of a Comprehensive Exercise Program

A comprehensive exercise program has many potential physiological as well as psychological benefits. This section provides Personal Trainers with insight into the range of physical and mental health benefits possible with a regular exercise program.

---

**Box 13.1**   **Components of the Exercise Training Session (2,11)**

- **Warm-up:** At least 5–10 minutes of low- to moderate-intensity cardiorespiratory and muscular endurance activities
- **Conditioning:** At least 20–60 minutes of aerobic, resistance, neuromotor, and/or sports activities (Exercise bouts of 10 min are acceptable if the individual accumulates at least 20–60 min · d$^{-1}$ of daily aerobic exercise.)
- **Cool-down:** At least 5–10 minutes of low- to moderate-intensity cardiorespiratory and muscular endurance activities
- **Flexibility:** At least 10 minutes of stretching exercises performed after the warm-up or cool-down phase

Reprinted from American College of Sports Medicine. ACSM position stand. Exercise and physical activity for older adults. *Med Sci Sports Exerc.* 2009;41(7):1510–30. Data from American College of Sports Medicine. ACSM position stand. Quantity and quality of exercise for developing and maintaining cardiorespiratory, musculoskeletal, and neuromuscular fitness in apparently healthy adults: guidance for prescribing exercise. *Med Sci Sports Exerc.* 2011;43(7):1334–59, and U.S. Department of Health and Human Services. *Physical Activity Guidelines Advisory Committee Report, 2008* [Internet]. Washington (DC): U.S. Department of Health and Human Services; [cited 2017 Mar 1]. Available from: http://www.health.gov/paguidelines/Report/pdf/CommitteeReport.pdf.

# Physiological Benefits

Physiological changes as a result of a comprehensive exercise program provide many fitness and health benefits.

## Improvement in Cardiovascular and Respiratory Function

Aerobic activities in which large muscle groups are used dynamically for extended periods of time place demands on the cardiovascular and respiratory systems in addition to the skeletal-muscle system (6). By placing a stress on these systems, cardiorespiratory fitness can be improved. Increases in cardiorespiratory fitness are associated with a reduction in death from all causes. Conversely, low cardiorespiratory fitness is associated with increased risk of premature death, in particular death from cardiovascular disease (6).

## Reduction in Coronary Artery Disease Risk Factors

Prevention of risk factors (primordial prevention) and treatment of risk factors (primary prevention) are both important considerations considering the high prevalence of heart disease. Some primordial risk factors cannot be changed or prevented (*e.g.*, age, sex, or genetics), but others including physical inactivity can be addressed. Risk factors such as dyslipidemia, prediabetes, hypertension, and obesity are positively impacted with regular physical activity (7). Greater cardiorespiratory fitness in individuals with preexisting disease is associated with decreased risk of clinical events (5).

## Decreased Morbidity and Mortality

Physical activity and exercise are known to prevent the development of several life-threatening diseases as well as premature death (10). Morbidity and mortality rates in a population can be directly affected by the quality and quantity of physical activity and exercise. Morbidity refers to the amount of disease in a given population, whereas mortality refers to the amount of death in a population. All-cause mortality is delayed with regular physical activity. Mortality is also delayed when individuals who were previously sedentary or insufficiently active increase their physical activity to meet the recommended levels of physical activity (5). The Centers for Disease Control and Prevention publishes a weekly report providing information on these rates in the United States, called the Morbidity/Mortality Weekly Report.

> Physical activity and exercise are known to prevent the development of several life-threatening diseases as well as premature death (10).

## Decreased Risk of Falls

According to the Centers for Disease Control and Prevention, each year about 1 in 4 adults older than 65 years will experience a fall that leads to moderate or severe injury (9). Severe falls can cause injuries affecting mobility as well as brain trauma, and can lead to other health conditions or disease. Falls may be linked to lack of muscular strength and endurance, balance, and coordination. Regular physical activity, muscular fitness, cardiovascular fitness, flexibility training, and balance exercises can improve daily functioning and decrease the risk of falling (2). Neuromotor exercise training (also called functional fitness training), which includes balance, coordination, gait, agility, and proprioceptive training, is a beneficial component of a comprehensive exercise program for older persons to reduce the risk of falls (5).

> Participation in a comprehensive exercise program (including cardiovascular and resistance training) will attenuate muscle loss or promote lean muscle gains, which can potentially maintain metabolic rate.

## Increased Metabolic Rate

Metabolism is the rate at which bodily tissues break down and utilize energy consumed (calories). Unfortunately, metabolic rate declines steadily as a part of the aging process (2). If energy is not utilized, it is most often stored in fat cells. Typically, as individuals age, they become less and less physically active, losing muscle mass, thus contributing to this steady decline in metabolic rate (2). Participation in a comprehensive exercise program (including cardiovascular and resistance training) will attenuate muscle loss or promote lean muscle gains, which can potentially maintain metabolic rate.

### Improvement in Bone Health

As with heart disease, bone health is affected by factors that cannot be modified (*e.g.*, age, sex, race, genetics) as well as those that can be changed (*e.g.*, diet, physical activity). Exercises to increase bone mass or to slow/prevent age-related bone loss require loading of the bone in a site-specific manner (7). Impact and weight-bearing activities (*e.g.*, plyometrics, jumping, resistance training) provide for a stress on the bone to promote positive adaptations in the bone (3).

### Weight Loss and Reduced Obesity

Obesity is related to many chronic diseases (*e.g.*, coronary heart disease, hypertension, stroke, Type 2 diabetes, dyslipidemia, some cancers) (7). Physical activity is recommended as part of a complete weight management plan for prevention of excessive fat gain, for weight maintenance, and to enhance weight loss strategies. In fact, evidence suggests a dose response with exercise meaning there may be greater weight loss with greater amounts of physical activity. Although American College of Sports Medicine (ACSM) recommends participation in at least 150 minutes per week of moderate-intensity activity for weight maintenance and reduction in chronic disease risk; 250–300 minutes per week of moderate-intensity activity may lead to greater weight loss (1).

## Psychological

In addition to the many physiological benefits, regular exercisers may also experience a number of potential psychological benefits.

### Decreased Anxiety and Depression

Depression is marked by feelings of sadness and unhappiness along with being self-critical and having low self-esteem (7). In addition to impairing daily function and potentially creating difficulties in work and home life, depression is also associated with health risks, such as heart disease (7). Exercise (both aerobic exercise and resistance training) has been found to be helpful in treating mild-to-moderate depressive symptoms (18), to lessen depressive symptoms (11), to potentially reduce the risk of developing depression (11), and to work in conjunction with medication-based antidepressive therapy for those with diagnosed major depression (20).

Anxiety is an emotional state marked by excessive anticipatory worry and tension (7). Unlike fear which is a reaction to a present danger, anxiety is future-oriented; anxiety-related worry is related to upcoming events, real or imagined, over which the person has little control (7). Symptoms of anxiety disorders include both acute, short-lived psychological responses that are linked to a particular situation (called state anxiety) as well as chronic, long-term tendencies to become anxious (called trait anxiety) (18). Exercise has been linked to reductions in both state and trait anxiety (16).

### Enhanced Feelings of Well-Being

Exercise provides enhancement of self-esteem, more restful sleep, and faster recovery from psychosocial stressors (14). Exercise also has the potential to enhance emotional well-being and to improve mood (19) and to enhance feelings of "energy" and quality of life (5).

### Positive Effect on Stress

High stress is when the perceived demands appear to exceed the resources available to handle those demands (7). Stress is associated with a number of health risks, including weakening of the immune system, overeating, and adverse shifts in blood lipid levels (7). People with depression, those suffering from stress and hostility, have the same risk of heart attack as those who smoke or have high blood pressure. However, exercise and physical activity have potentially positive effects on stress. For example, exercise training has been shown to reduce depression, overall stress, as well as hostility by 50%–70% (17).

### Better Cognitive Function (Older Adults)

Regular physical activity (both aerobic exercise and resistance training) is associated with reduced risk for dementia or cognitive decline in older adults (2). For example, individualized aerobic training at the ventilatory threshold was found to improve cognitive functioning to the same level as a mental training program (13). Exercise and fitness effects are the greatest for tasks that require complex mental processing (2), in particular, executive-control tasks such as coordination, inhibition, scheduling, planning, and working memory (12).

##  Components of a Comprehensive Exercise Program

The optimal exercise program should address the health-related physical fitness components of cardiorespiratory fitness, muscular strength and endurance, flexibility, body composition, and neuromotor fitness (6). In addition, skill-related physical fitness components can also be added, and they include agility, coordination, balance, power, reaction time, and speed (6). Including activities to improve aerobic fitness, muscular fitness, and flexibility are recommended for everyone. Neuromotor exercise, which includes skill-related physical fitness components, is advocated for those at higher risk for falling, in particular, older individuals, although there are likely benefits for younger adults as well (6). Additionally, some clients have goals related to sport or competitive activities in which the skill-related components need to be addressed.

> The optimal exercise program should address the health-related physical fitness components of cardiorespiratory fitness, muscular strength and endurance, flexibility, body composition, and neuromotor fitness (6).

The FITT-VP principles of exercise prescription allow for complete design of the frequency (F), intensity (I), time (T) (or duration), and type (T) (or mode) of exercise plus the overall volume (V) or amount and progression (P) of the exercise (6). Within the FITT-VP framework, the Personal Trainer can develop individual exercise prescriptions (as discussed in more detail in the upcoming chapters in this section), which include cardiorespiratory and muscular fitness exercises as well as flexibility-promoting activities.

## Cardiorespiratory Fitness

Cardiorespiratory endurance refers to the ability of the heart and blood vessels (circulatory system) and the lungs (respiratory system) to provide oxygen to the body during sustained physical activity (6). Another term commonly used is "aerobic" fitness, as these activities require sufficient oxygen in order to be continued. Maximal oxygen consumption ($\dot{V}O_{2max}$) can be measured directly by analyzing expired gases or may be estimated from submaximal effort (see Chapter 12 for examples of submaximal exercise tests) or maximal effort. The higher the $\dot{V}O_{2max}$, the greater is the individual's aerobic capacity.

## Frequency

Although some activity is better than none, the recommended frequency for aerobic exercise is 3–5 days per week (6). When determining optimal frequency, intensity should be considered. More frequent exercise sessions (*e.g.*, 5 d · wk$^{-1}$) are typically used in conjunction with moderate-intensity exercise programs. As intensity levels increase, the number of days per week needed for health benefits decreases; the incidence of injury may also increase with vigorous intensity exercise done more than 5 days per week (6).

> Although some activity is better than none, the recommended frequency for aerobic exercise is 3–5 days per week (6).

## Intensity

Exercise intensity can be quantified using various methods, including heart rate reserve (HRR), percentage of age-predicted maximal heart rate (%HR$_{max}$), oxygen uptake reserve ($\dot{V}O_2R$), and perceived exertion. The intensity recommended for a given individual depends on the person's habitual activity and fitness level (6). For individuals who are sedentary and very deconditioned, the recommended intensity is very low (*i.e.*, 30%–39% HRR or $\dot{V}O_2R$) but progressively increases with higher activity and fitness levels (*i.e.*, for habitually active individuals with high fitness, 60%–89% HRR or $\dot{V}O_2R$) (6). See Table 15.2 in Chapter 15 for specific ranges for various intensity levels.

## Time (or Duration)

Exercise duration is the amount of time the exercise is performed, typically expressed as minutes per day or minutes per week. General baseline targets for time spent exercising depend on the intensity of the exercise. Thus, the recommendations link duration and intensity (6):

- Moderate-intensity exercise is recommended at least 30 minutes per day on at least 5 days per week for a total of at least 150 minutes per week, *or*
- Vigorous-intensity exercise is recommended at least 20–25 minutes per day on at least 3 days per week for a total of at least 75 minutes, *or*
- A combination of moderate- and vigorous-intensity exercise at least 20–30 minutes on 3–4 days per week.

> General baseline targets for time spent exercising depend on the fitness level of the individual and the intensity of the exercise.

A dose-response relationship exists between physical activity and health outcomes. Thus, benefits may begin at low levels for sedentary individuals (*e.g.*, <20 min · d$^{-1}$), whereas extending the time or intensity may provide additional health benefits for those who are already regular exercisers (6). For example, one may gain even greater benefits with the following:

- Moderate-intensity exercise of 300 minutes per week, *or*
- Vigorous-intensity exercise of 150 minutes per week, *or*
- A combination of moderate- and vigorous-intensity exercise

Going above the baseline of 150 minutes per week of moderately intense exercise also is important to assist with weight loss, or to help maintain weight loss. In these situations, the recommended duration of exercise is 50–60 minutes per day, or 250–300 minutes per week (6). These recommendations provide a framework in which the Personal Trainer can develop a health-enhancing exercise program.

## Type (or Mode)

Examples of aerobic activities include walking, jogging, running, cycling, swimming, and using aerobic-based machines (*e.g.*, stair climber, elliptical machines). Although most of these activities require low to moderate skills and can be used even by those with low fitness levels, others require considerable skill, fitness, and practice to master. Table 15.11 in Chapter 15 provides a classification system which acknowledges the fitness and skill level required for optimal use of various aerobic exercises. Activities appropriate for everyone have minimal skill or fitness prerequisites (*e.g.*, walking). As fitness increases, more intense activities can be included (*e.g.*, jogging). Still, other activities have a major skill component (*e.g.*, swimming) that must be acquired before including in aerobic training or have a competitive nature (*e.g.*, team sports) that requires at least average physical fitness.

### Volume (Amount)

Exercise volume plays an important role for realizing health/fitness outcomes, particularly with respect to body composition and weight management. Exercise volume should be used to estimate the overall energy expenditure for an exercise prescription. Exercise volume is typically measured in metabolic equivalent (MET) $\cdot$ min $\cdot$ wk$^{-1}$ and/or kcal $\cdot$ wk$^{-1}$ (note that volume can also be tracked on a daily basis). Box 13.2 reflects the standard measures of exercise intensity (METs, MET-min, and kcal $\cdot$ min$^{-1}$) for different physical activities. These values can then be used to calculate volume of activity per week that is accumulated as part of the exercise program. The recommended volume that is consistently associated with lower rates of cardiovascular disease and premature mortality is greater than 500–1,000 MET $\cdot$ min $\cdot$ wk$^{-1}$ (11). This is approximately equal to 1,000 kcal $\cdot$ wk$^{-1}$ of moderate-intensity physical activity, ~150 min $\cdot$ wk$^{-1}$ of moderate-intensity exercise, an intensity of 3–5.9

---

### Box 13.2    Calculation of METs, MET-min, and kcal $\cdot$ min$^{-1}$ (2,11,21)

**Metabolic equivalents (METs):**

An index of energy expenditure. "[A MET is] the ratio of the rate of energy expended during an activity to the rate of energy expended at rest. . . . [One] MET is the rate of energy expenditure while sitting at rest . . . by convention, [1 MET is equal to] an oxygen uptake of 3.5 [mL $\cdot$ kg$^{-1}$ $\cdot$ min$^{-1}$]" (21).

**MET-min:**

An index of energy expenditure that quantifies the total amount of physical activity performed in a standardized manner across individuals and types of activities (21). Calculated as the product of the number of METs associated with one or more physical activities and the number of minutes the activities were performed (*i.e.*, METs × min). It is usually standardized per week or per day as a measure of exercise volume.

**Kilocalorie (kcal):**

The energy needed to increase the temperature of 1 kg of water by 1° C. To convert METs to kcal $\cdot$ min$^{-1}$, it is necessary to know an individual's body weight. It is usually standardized as kilocalories per week or per day as a measure of exercise volume.

$$\text{kcal} \cdot \text{min}^{-1} = (\text{METs} \times 3.5 \text{ mL} \cdot \text{kg}^{-1} \cdot \text{min}^{-1} \times \text{body weight in kg}) \div 200$$

**Example**

Calculate weekly volume for a 70-kg male jogging (at ~7 METs) 3 days per week for 30 minutes.

$$7 \text{ METs} \times 30 \text{ min} \times 3 \text{ times per week} = 630 \text{ MET-min} \cdot \text{wk}^{-1}$$

or

$$(7 \text{ METs} \times 3.5 \text{ mL} \cdot \text{kg}^{-1} \cdot \text{min}^{-1} \times 70 \text{ kg}) \div 200 = 8.6 \text{ kcal} \cdot \text{min}^{-1}$$

$$8.6 \text{ kcal} \cdot \text{min}^{-1} \times 30 \text{ min} \times 3 \text{ times per week} = 774 \text{ kcal} \cdot \text{wk}^{-1}$$

Reprinted from American College of Sports Medicine. ACSM position stand. Exercise and physical activity for older adults. *Med Sci Sports Exerc.* 2009;41(7):1510–30. Data from American College of Sports Medicine. ACSM position stand. Quantity and quality of exercise for developing and maintaining cardiorespiratory, musculoskeletal, and neuromuscular fitness in apparently healthy adults: guidance for prescribing exercise. *Med Sci Sports Exerc.* 2011;43(7):1334–59, and U.S. Department of Health and Human Services. *Physical Activity Guidelines Advisory Committee Report, 2008* [Internet]. Washington (DC): U.S. Department of Health and Human Services; [cited 2017 Mar 1]. Available from: http://www.health.gov/paguidelines/Report/pdf/CommitteeReport.pdf.

| Table 13.1 | Activity Status and Aerobic Training Focus |
|---|---|
| **Activity Status** | **Aerobic Training Focus** |
| Beginner: those who are inactive with no or minimal physical activity and thus are deconditioned | *No prior activity*: Focus is on light- to moderate-level activity for 20–30 min over the course of the day. Accumulating time in 10-min bouts is an option. Overall, the target is 60–150 min · wk$^{-1}$. <br><br> *Minimal prior activity* (*i.e.*, once the previous target level is met): Focus is on light- to moderate-level activity for 30–60 min · d$^{-1}$. Accumulating time in 10-min bouts is an option. Overall, the target is 150–200 min · wk$^{-1}$. |
| Intermediate: those who are sporadically active but do not have an optimal exercise plan and thus are moderately deconditioned | *Fair to average fitness*: Focus is on moderate activity for 30–90 min · d$^{-1}$. Overall, the target is 200–300 min · wk$^{-1}$. |
| Established: those who are regularly engaging in moderate to vigorous exercise | *Regular exerciser* (moderate to vigorous): Focus is on moderate to vigorous activity for 30–90 min · d$^{-1}$. Overall, the target is 200–300 min · wk$^{-1}$ of moderate-intensity activity or 100–150 min of vigorous-intensity activity or a combination of moderate- and vigorous-intensity activity. |

Adapted with permission from Bushman B, editor. *ACSM's Complete Guide to Fitness & Health*. Champaign (IL): Human Kinetics; 2011.

METs (for people weighing 68–91 kg or 150–200 lb). In deconditioned people, lower exercise volumes can have significant benefits, but even greater volumes may be needed for weight management.

### Progression Rate

Progression depends on an individual's health status, training response, fitness, and the exercise program goals. Progression allows for improvements in cardiorespiratory fitness while avoiding stagnation in training. The Personal Trainer may need to increase any or all of the FITT components to provide progression to the exercise program. Typically, only one variable is increased at a time. Initially, an increase in time (minutes per session) is recommended. After about 1 month, the frequency, intensity, and time should be gradually increased over the next 4–8 months to meet the recommendations presented in *ACSM's Guidelines for Exercise Testing and Prescription* (6). A longer trajectory is recommended for those who are very deconditioned. Any progression should avoid making large increases in the FITT components to minimize risks of injury, muscular soreness, or overtraining.

> Progression depends on an individual's health status, training response, fitness, and the exercise program goals. Progression allows for improvements in cardiorespiratory fitness while avoiding stagnation in training.

Chapter 15 provides more detail on cardiorespiratory fitness training programs and incorporating the FITT-VP principle into a usable program for a client. A sample progression, including activity status and training focus, is provided in Table 13.1.

## Muscular Fitness

Muscular fitness includes both muscular strength and muscular endurance. Muscular strength refers to the ability of a muscle or muscle group to exert force (*e.g.*, one repetition maximum [1-RM]). Muscular endurance refers to the ability of a muscle or muscle group to continue to perform without fatigue (*i.e.*, repeated contractions or to sustain a contraction).

To improve muscular fitness, the muscles must be exposed to an overload (stress beyond the typical activity). This is done via resistance training. Over time, as the muscles adapt to a given overload, the training stimulus must be increased to continue to have gains. This is referred to as progressive overload. Details on resistance training programs are found in Chapter 14 and a sample progression is found in Table 13.2. As with cardiorespiratory training programs, the FITT-VP principle can be applied to resistance training.

### Frequency

The frequency of resistance training varies depending on the goals of the client. For general muscular fitness, resistance training the major muscle groups (chest, shoulders, back, abdomen, hips, and legs) 2–3 days per week is recommended (6). At least 48 hours should separate workouts targeting any given muscle group to allow time for adaptations to occur (4,6). Depending on client schedules, Personal Trainers may incorporate whole-body sessions in which all the major muscle groups are exercised in one session (repeating this sequence a couple times per week) or may train a few

| Table 13.2 | Sample Resistance Training Progression | | | |
|---|---|---|---|---|
| Stage[a] | Exercises[b] | No. of Sets | No. of Repetitions | No. Days Per Week[c] |
| Beginner: Moving through this level typically takes about 2–3 mo, although remaining at this level until the client feels comfortable enough to advance is appropriate. | Do a total of six exercises. Select *one* exercise from each of the following areas: hips and legs, chest, back, shoulders, low back, and abdominals. | 1–2 | 8–12 (10–15 for older adults) | 2–3 |
| Intermediate to established: Moving through the intermediate to established level typically takes 3–12 mo depending on the client's level of consistency. | Do a total of 10 exercises. Select *one* exercise from each of the following areas: hips and legs, quadriceps, hamstrings, chest, back, shoulders, biceps, triceps, low back, and abdominals. | 2 | 8–12 (10–15 for older adults) | 2–3 |
| More advanced: Some clients may have higher level goals in the area of muscular fitness and thus will include an expanded training program. | Do a total of 10 exercises. Select *two* exercises from each of these larger muscle group areas: hips and legs, quadriceps, hamstrings, chest, and back. | 2–3 | 8–12 | 2–3 |
| | Do a total of five exercises. Select *one* exercise from each of these smaller muscle group and trunk areas: shoulders, biceps, triceps, low back, and abdominals. | 2 | 8–12 | 2–3 |

[a]The time spent at each stage will depend on the client's muscular fitness level. Transition slowly between the stages (*e.g.*, over time, a beginner can add additional exercises or increase the number of sets to move toward the intermediate level of resistance training).
[b]Different exercises can be performed on different days.
[c]Schedule training days so that at least 48 hours separate training sessions that target the same muscle group.
Source: Adapted with permission from Bushman B, editor. *ACSM's Complete Guide to Fitness & Health*. Champaign (IL): Human Kinetics; 2011.

selected muscle groups each session (multiple sessions) (6). In the latter scenario, more frequent resistance training will occur but individual muscle groups will still only be targeted two to three times per week.

### Intensity

Intensity of resistance training is inversely related to the number of repetitions; with higher resistance, the number of repetitions will be fewer. To improve muscular fitness, typically 8–12 repetitions per set are completed, at an intensity of between 60% and 80% of the client's 1-RM (*i.e.*, the greatest amount of resistance overcome in a single repetition) (6). For older and very deconditioned individuals, a lower intensity (40%–50% of 1-RM) with 10–20 repetitions is recommended initially (5). To lower the chance of injury or extreme muscle soreness after exercise, the number of repetitions selected should allow for muscle fatigue at the end of the set but not failure (6).

> Intensity of resistance training is inversely related to the number of repetitions; with higher resistance, the number of repetitions will be fewer.

### Time (or Duration)

The total time spent will vary with the program, in particular if a whole-body approach is used or if a split program targeting different muscles groups on separate days is applied. For adults, each muscle group should be trained with two to four sets with rest intervals of 2–3 minutes between sets (6). Four sets are more effective than two sets, but also realize that for novices, even a single set per exercise will improve muscular strength (6). When determining the number of sets, attention should be made to adherence and thus may be influenced by the individuals schedule, time availability, and level of commitment (6).

### Type (or Mode)

Resistance training can be done using free weights, machines (stacked weights or pneumatic resistance), rubber bands/cords, and even body weight. For examples of different activities that can be used for the major body areas, see Table 13.3. In addition, Personal Trainers should include multijoint (*e.g.*, bench press, leg press) as well as potentially single-joint (*e.g.*, biceps curl, quadriceps extension) exercises (6). When selecting exercises, the Personal Trainer should ensure opposing muscle groups, agonists and antagonists, are included in order to prevent muscle imbalances. For example, including lower back extensions and abdominal crunches to strengthen both the lower back and the abdomen will provide for muscle balance.

### Volume

Muscular groups should be trained for a minimum of two to four sets. These may be the same exercise or from a combination of exercises affecting the same muscle group (5,6). For example, either four sets of bench presses or a combination of two sets of bench presses and two sets of dips may be used to train the pectoral muscles (6).

### Progression

Progressive overload in resistance training can be done in many ways. One can increase the amount of resistance lifted, increase the number of repetitions, increase the number of sets done per muscle group, or increase the number of days per week the muscle groups are trained. However, if individuals seek to maintain a given level of muscular fitness, it is not necessary to continue to progressively increase the training stimulus. Muscular strength may be maintained by training muscle groups as little as 1 day per week as long as the training intensity or the resistance lifted is held constant (5,6).

| Table 13.3 | Examples of Resistance Training Exercises for Major Body Areas | |
|---|---|---|
| **Body Area** | **Exercises** | |
| Hips and legs (gluteals, quadriceps, hamstrings) | Machine leg press<br>Dumbbell squat | Ankle weight hip flexion and extension<br>Band leg lunge |
| Legs (quadriceps) | Machine leg extension | Ankle weight knee extension |
| Legs (hamstrings) | Machine leg curl | Ankle weight knee flexion |
| Chest (pectoralis) | Machine chest press<br>Band seated chest press | Dumbbell chest press<br>Push-up and modified push-up |
| Back (latissimus dorsi) | Machine lat pull-down<br>Dumbbell one-arm row | Machine seated row<br>Band seated row |
| Shoulders (deltoid) | Machine overhead press<br>Dumbbell or band upright row | Dumbbell lateral raise |
| Arms (biceps) | Machine biceps curl | Dumbbell or band biceps curl |
| Arms (triceps) | Machine biceps press<br>Band triceps extension | Dumbbell lying triceps extension |
| Low back (erector spinae) | Machine back extension<br>Prone plank | Kneeling hip extension |
| Abdominals | Curl-up<br>Diagonal curl-up | Machine abdominal curl |

Adapted with permission from Bushman B, editor. *ACSM's Complete Guide to Fitness & Health.* Champaign (IL): Human Kinetics; 2011.

# Flexibility

Flexibility exercises have the potential to improve joint range of motion (ROM) and physical function (5). Although the Personal Trainer may not be able to point to benefits such as a reduction in cardiovascular disease risk, stretching is recommended as part of a comprehensive training program for adults (6).

## Frequency

Stretching activities should be included a minimum of 2–3 days each week for most adults, although daily flexibility exercise is most effective (6).

A stretch should not create discomfort; if so, the client should release slightly. A stretch should never be painful.

## Intensity

Describing the intensity of stretching to a client can be difficult as it is not a measurable entity like a treadmill speed. The Personal Trainer can use cues to help guide clients, such as moving within the ROM to point of mild tightness without discomfort (6). A stretch should not create discomfort; if so, the client should release slightly. A stretch should never be painful.

### Time (or Duration)

At least 10 minutes is recommended per session in order to allow all the major muscle–tendon groups to be targeted with at least four repetitions of each stretch (6).

### Type (or Mode)

Flexibility can be improved using a wide variety of activities, including static stretching (active and passive), dynamic or slow movement stretching, and proprioceptive neuromuscular facilitation (6). Interestingly, when properly performed, even ballistic or "bouncing" stretches can be as effective as static stretches for increasing joint ROM in individuals engaging in activities that involve ballistic movements such as tennis or basketball (6).

### Volume

Each flexibility exercise per joint should be held at the point of tightness for 10–30 seconds. Time/duration and repetitions of the flexibility exercises should be adjusted to accumulate a total of 60 seconds of stretching at each joint. Recommendations for using proprioceptive neuromuscular facilitation (PNF) are to hold a 20%–75% maximum voluntary contraction for 3–6 seconds, followed by 10–30 seconds of assisted stretch. Performing flexibility exercises at least 2–3 days per week is recommended with daily flexibility exercise being most effective (5,6). Details on flexibility and various stretching program options are presented in Chapter 16.

## Neuromotor Exercise

Neuromotor exercise involves motor skills including balance, coordination, agility, and proprioceptive training (5). These activities have recently been termed *functional fitness or movement,* and additional information regarding this type of training can be found in Chapter 17. Neuromotor-enhancing activities focus on the communication between feedback from the periphery (*e.g.,* arms and legs) and the interpretation by the central nervous system (*e.g.,* brain and spinal cord). As with any training, providing a challenge, or overload, will allow for improvements. This training is of particular importance for older adults who are at a higher fall risk or who have mobility impairments (6). In addition, all adults may gain benefits, especially if participation in recreation or occupational pursuits requires agility and balance (6).

### Frequency

Neuromuscular exercise is recommended at least 2–3 days per week for 20–30 minutes of duration the previously mentioned populations (6). This recommendation is based on conventional use rather than evidence-based documentation of benefit as programs range from 1 to 7 days per week (7).

### Intensity

The intensity of balance-related training can be manipulated by the Personal Training through three aspects:

1. Base of support (narrowing the base of support will increase the challenge)
2. Center of mass (displacing the center of mass increases difficulty)
3. Peripheral cues (visual, vestibular, and proprioceptive pathways)

Some examples of how these three domains can be manipulated are included in Table 13.4 (7).

| Table 13.4 | Factors Affecting Intensity of Balance Training (4) | | |
|---|---|---|---|
| Domain | Less Difficult | Moderate | More Difficult |
| Base of support | Feet apart (with or without assistive device) | Feet together Semitandem stand | Heel-to-toe stand One-legged stand |
| Center of mass | Leaning forward and backward Leaning side to side | Turning in a circle Shifting weight from side to side Stepping over an obstacle | Crossover walking Balancing on a large ball or rocker platform |
| Peripheral feedback | These are more difficult and are recommended only after particular activity was done successfully with peripheral feedback. | Closing the eyes (seated position) while leaning forward, backward, and side to side Standing on a foam pad while shifting weight or bringing feet close together | Closing eyes (standing position) while leaning in various directions or reducing base of support Standing on a foam pad in a heel-to-toe stance or one-legged stance |

Data from American College of Sports Medicine. ACSM position stand. Progression models in resistance training for healthy adults. *Med Sci Sports Exerc.* 2009;41(3):687–708.

### Time (or Duration)

The minimum effective dose of balance training has yet to be defined (5). Improvements have been noted with 20–30 minutes or more per day for a total of 60 minutes per week (6). When activities like tai chi are incorporated, typically durations are 45–60 minutes, but the minimum effective time for neuromotor exercise training is not known (7).

### Type (or Mode)

Various activities (see Table 13.5 for example of a progressive balance program), as well as tai chi, Pilates, and yoga, can be used (6).

## Advanced Training Options

Personal Trainers may want to consider advanced training options for new clients with an extensive background in fitness training (such as athletes) or for long-term clients who have made great progress since starting their beginner comprehensive fitness programs. Advanced training options can increase the challenge of an exercise program by manipulating current exercises through the FITT-VP principle (frequency, intensity, time, type, volume, and progression) (see Tables 13.6, 13.7, and 13.8 for examples of how the FITT components can be manipulated for beginner, intermediate, and established exercisers) or through prescribing new or additional exercises that focus on the skill-related components of physical fitness.

> Advanced training options can increase the challenge of an exercise program by manipulating current exercises through the FITT-VP principle (frequency, intensity, time, type, volume, and progression) or through prescribing new or additional exercises that focus on the skill-related components of physical fitness.

For some clients, development of the skill-related components of physical fitness is a training goal. The skill-related components of physical fitness include the following (6):

- Speed refers to the ability to perform a movement within a short about of time (*e.g.*, a 100-m sprinter moving quickly toward the finish line).
- Agility refers to the ability to change the position of the body in space with speed and accuracy (*e.g.*, cutting in a new direction to successfully execute a play in basketball).

| Table 13.5 | Sample Progressive Balance Program | | | |
|---|---|---|---|---|
| | **Level 1** | **Level 2** | **Level 3** | **Challenge** |
| Seated balance activities | Seated chair lean | Add arm movements:<br>■ Raise one arm at a time to the front and then to the sides.<br>■ Raise both arms to the front and then to the sides.<br>Add leg movements:<br>■ Raise one knee at a time.<br>■ Raise one leg (straightened) at a time. | Combine arm and leg movements. | ■ Sit on a pillow.<br>■ Sit on a stability ball.<br>■ Close one eye.<br>■ Close both eyes.<br>■ Turn head to the right and then to the left. |
| Standing balance activities | Upright stance (variations including wide stance, narrow stance, semitandem, and tandem) | In all four variations, add:<br>■ Forward and backward sway<br>■ Lateral sway (side to side) | Add arm movements to sway:<br>■ Raise one arm at a time to the front and then to the sides.<br>■ Raise both arms to the front and then to the sides. | ■ Close one eye.<br>■ Close both eyes.<br>■ Turn head to the right and then to the left.<br>■ Hold an item, such as a book. |
| Movement balance activities | Walk forward and backward. | ■ Wide-stance walk<br>■ Narrow-stance walk<br>■ Walk on heels<br>■ Walk on toes | ■ Tandem walk forward and backward<br>■ Walk while carrying an item<br>■ Walk with head turns | ■ Barefoot<br>■ One eye closed<br>■ Surface change (mat, sand, etc.)<br>■ Obstacles |
| | Walk side to side. | ■ Sidestep on heels<br>■ Sidestep on toes<br>■ Turn in a circle | ■ Sidestep while carrying an item<br>■ Sidestep with head turns<br>■ Crossover walk: cross one foot over the other foot | |

Adapted with permission from Bushman B, editor. *ACSM's Complete Guide to Fitness & Health.* Champaign (IL): Human Kinetics; 2011.

| Table 13.6 | Sample Beginner Adult Exercise Program[a] | | | |
|---|---|---|---|---|
| **Week** | **Aerobic** | **Resistance** | **Stretching**[b] | **Comments** |
| 1–2 | 3 d · wk$^{-1}$; 10–20 min · d$^{-1}$; light intensity (level 3 or 4) | 2 d · wk$^{-1}$; one set, 8–12 reps of six exercises[c] | 2 d · wk$^{-1}$; 10 min of stretching activities | An easy beginning aerobic activity is walking at a comfortable pace. For inactive clients, target 10 min at a time for aerobic activity. Include some stretching activities (see Chapter 16) after the walk. For resistance training, see Table 13.3, for details on what activities to include. |
| 3–4 | 3 d · wk$^{-1}$; 20–30 min · d$^{-1}$; light to moderate intensity (level 4 or 5) | 2 d · wk$^{-1}$; one or two sets, 8–12 reps of six exercises[c] | 2 d · wk$^{-1}$; 10 min of stretching activities | The focus for the client over the next couple of weeks will be getting comfortable with at least 20 min of aerobic exercise at least 3 d · wk$^{-1}$. Continue with the resistance training program. |
| 5–7 | 3 or 4 d · wk$^{-1}$; 30–40 min · d$^{-1}$; moderate intensity (level 5) | 2 d · wk$^{-1}$; two sets, 8–12 reps of six exercises[c] | 2 d · wk$^{-1}$; 10 min of stretching activities | For the next 3 wk, the client's focus is on getting comfortable with up to 40 min of aerobic exercise at least 3 d · wk$^{-1}$ (for each week, add 5–10 min per session). Continue with the resistance training program, completing two sets per exercise and adding more weight if the 12 reps for a given exercise now feel easy. |
| 8–10 | 3 or 4 d · wk$^{-1}$; 35–50 min · d$^{-1}$; moderate intensity (level 5 or 6) | 2 d · wk$^{-1}$; two sets, 8–12 reps of six exercises[c] | 2 d · wk$^{-1}$; 10 min of stretching activities | Over the past couple of months, the client will develop a good aerobic fitness base. For some variety, other activities such as biking or swimming can be included (for more ideas, see Chapter 15). If the client likes walking, that is also an option. For your resistance training program, consider adding some variety and trying some other exercises (see Table 13.3 for ideas). |

[a]All activity sessions should be preceded and followed by a 5- to 10-minute warm-up and cool-down.
[b]Include stretching activities after aerobic exercise to improve flexibility. For specific stretches to target the major muscle groups, see Chapter 16.
[c]Resistance training is more fully outlined in Chapter 14. Beginners should select one exercise for each of the following body areas (see Table 13.3): hips and legs, chest, back, shoulders, low back, and abdominals.
*Source:* Adapted with permission from Bushman B, editor. *ACSM's Complete Guide to Fitness & Health.* Champaign (IL): Human Kinetics; 2011.

| Table 13.7 | Sample Intermediate-Level Adult Exercise Program[a] | | | |
|---|---|---|---|---|
| **Week** | **Aerobic** | **Resistance** | **Stretching[b]** | **Comments** |
| 1–2 | 3 or 4 d · wk$^{-1}$; 35–50 min · d$^{-1}$; moderate intensity (level 5 or 6) | 2 d · wk$^{-1}$; one or two sets, 8–12 reps of 8–10 different exercises[c] | 2 or 3 d · wk$^{-1}$; 10 min of stretching activities | Aerobic activity is included for a total of 150–200 min · wk$^{-1}$ (moderate-intensity activity). For resistance training, include exercises for biceps and triceps (in addition to the body areas previously targeted) and add exercises for the quadriceps and hamstrings in the second week, so by the end of this stage, the client will include a total of 10 exercises (see Table 13.3). |
| 3–5 | 3–5 d · wk$^{-1}$; 30–60 min · d$^{-1}$; moderate intensity (level 5–7) | 2 d · wk$^{-1}$; one or two sets, 8–12 reps of 10 different exercises[c] | 2 or 3 d · wk$^{-1}$, 10 min of stretching activities | The focus for the next 3 wk is to increase the time spent in aerobic exercise or to increase the intensity (don't do both at the same time). If the client feels more comfortable with moderate-intensity activity, 200 min · wk$^{-1}$ is appropriate. If the client is ready to increase intensity (*e.g.*, jogging rather than walking), cut back on the time to 20–30 min · d$^{-1}$ (note that the target for vigorous-intensity activity is 75–100 min · wk$^{-1}$). A mix of moderate- and vigorous-intensity activity is also an option (see Chapter 15 for more details). Continue with the resistance training program. |
| 6–10 | 3–5 d · wk$^{-1}$; 30–50 min · d$^{-1}$; moderate intensity (level 6) | 2 d · wk$^{-1}$; two sets, 8–12 reps of 10 exercises[c] | 2 or 3 d · wk$^{-1}$, 10 min of stretching activities | For the client's aerobic activity, either increase the time spent per day or increase the number of days per week. Ultimately, the weekly total should be 200–300 min of moderate-intensity activity or 100–150 min of vigorous-intensity activity (recall that 2 min of moderate activity equals 1 min of vigorous activity) or a combination of moderate and vigorous activity. For resistance training, consider trying some different exercises this week while still targeting the same muscle groups (see Table 13.3 for details). |

[a]All activity sessions should be preceded and followed by a 5- to 10-minute warm-up and cool-down.
[b]Include stretching activities after aerobic exercise to improve flexibility. Target all the muscle groups, holding each for 15–60 seconds. For specific stretches to target the major muscle groups, see Chapter 16.
[c]Resistance training is more fully outlined in Chapter 14. Select one exercise for each of the following body areas: hips and legs, chest, back, shoulders, low back, and abdominals. In the progression the number of body areas targeted is increased by adding quadriceps and hamstrings as well as biceps and triceps. This provides 10 body areas to target. Examples of exercises for each body area are found in Table 13.3.
Adapted with permission from Bushman B, editor. *ACSM's Complete Guide to Fitness & Health.* Champaign (IL): Human Kinetics; 2011.

| Table 13.8 | | Sample Established Adult Exercise Program[a] | | |
| --- | --- | --- | --- | --- |
| **Week** | **Aerobic** | **Resistance** | **Stretching**[b] | **Comments** |
| 1–2 | ■ 5 d · wk$^{-1}$ for moderate exercise, or<br>■ 3 d · wk$^{-1}$ for vigorous exercise, or<br>■ 3–5 d · wk$^{-1}$ for a mix of moderate and vigorous exercise | 2 d · wk$^{-1}$; two sets, 8–12 reps of 10 different exercises[c] | 2 or 3 d · wk$^{-1}$, minimum; 10 min of stretching activities | Target for aerobic activity is 200–300 min of moderate-intensity activity or 100–150 min of vigorous-intensity activity (recall that 2 min of moderate activity equals 1 min of vigorous activity) or a combination of moderate and vigorous activity. Resistance training exercise examples are found in Table 13.3. |
| 3–4 | 2 or 3 d · wk$^{-1}$ of moderate activity and 1 or 2 d of vigorous activity | 2 d · wk$^{-1}$; two sets, 8–12 reps of 10 different exercises[c] | 3 d · wk$^{-1}$, minimum; 10 min of stretching activities | For the next couple of weeks, try mixing up the activities. Suggest a new aerobic activity or change the intensity of an activity already part of the client's exercise program. Continue with the resistance training program. |
| 5–6 | ■ 5 d · wk$^{-1}$ for moderate exercise, or<br>■ 3 d · wk$^{-1}$ for vigorous exercise, or<br>■ 3–5 d · wk$^{-1}$ for moderate and vigorous exercise | 2 d · wk$^{-1}$; two sets 8–12 reps of 10 exercises[c] | 3 d · wk$^{-1}$, minimum; 10 min of stretching activities | Continue with the aerobic training program. For resistance training, consider trying some different exercises (see Table 13.3 and Chapter 14). If the client typically uses machines, suggest a couple of new exercises using dumbbells to provide the muscles with a new challenge. Be sure to watch for good form when the client tries new activities. |
| 7–8 | ■ 5 d · wk$^{-1}$ for moderate exercise, or<br>■ 3 d · wk$^{-1}$ for vigorous exercise, or<br>■ 3–5 d · wk$^{-1}$ for moderate and vigorous exercise | 2 d · wk$^{-1}$; three sets, 8–10 reps of 10 exercises[c] | 3 d · wk$^{-1}$, minimum; 10 min of stretching activities | Continue with the aerobic training program. For resistance training, consider doing three sets rather than two (this may require the client to cut back on reps to add the additional set). |

[a]All activity sessions should be preceded and followed by a 5- to 10-minute warm-up and cool-down.
[b]Include stretching activities after aerobic exercise to improve flexibility. For specific stretches to target the major muscle groups, see Chapter 16.
[c]Resistance training is more fully outlined in Chapter 14. Select one exercise for each of the following body areas: hips and legs, chest, back, shoulders, low back, abdominals, quadriceps, hamstrings, biceps, and triceps.
Source: Adapted with permission from Bushman B, editor. *ACSM's Complete Guide to Fitness & Health*. Champaign (IL): Human Kinetics; 2011.

- Coordination refers to the ability to use the senses, such as sight and hearing, together with body parts in performing tasks smoothly and accurately (*e.g.*, returning a serve in racquet sports).
- Balance refers to the maintenance of equilibrium while stationary or moving (*e.g.*, performing gymnastic moves on top of a balance beam).
- Power refers to the rate at which one can perform work (*e.g.*, a defensive back runs through the offensive line to sack the quarterback before the ball is thrown).
- Reaction time refers to the time elapsed between stimulation and the beginning of the response (*e.g.*, a soccer ball kicked toward a goal and the goalie's reaction to block it).

These skill-related components can be achieved simultaneously through several types of advanced training options such as high-intensity interval training, high-velocity weight training, Olympic weight lifting, plyometric training, balance training, sport-specific and nonsport-specific agility, and coordination drills (see Table 13.9 for examples of activities involving the skill-related components of fitness).

### Power, Agility, and Speed

Personal Trainers can use several advanced training methods, such as plyometric exercises, to train their clients to improve power, agility, and speed. Plyometrics refer to exercises that link strength with speed of movement to produce power and were first known simply as "jump training."

| Table 13.9 | Activities/Exercises Involving Skill-Related Components of Physical Fitness |
|---|---|
| **Skill Component** | **Activity/Exercise Examples** |
| Speed | Sprint drills<br>Plyometric exercises (high-intensity jumps, bounds, and sprints)<br>High-velocity resistance training<br>Mixed martial arts (speed bag punching, sparring) |
| Power | Olympic weight lifting (clean and jerk, snatch)<br>High-velocity resistance training<br>Plyometric exercises (box jumps, push-up claps)<br>Medicine ball exercises (ball slams, passing exercises) |
| Agility | Plyometric exercises (multidirectional jumps, bounds, and sprints)<br>Sport-specific agility drills (shuttle drills, lateral shuffle drills) |
| Reaction time | Stimulus-response exercises (sprints initiated by whistle/start gun, quick response sport-specific ball handling)<br>Mixed martial arts (blocking exercises, sparring) |
| Coordination | Multisensory integration exercises (sport-specific ball handling drills, racquet sports drills, batting exercises)<br>Multimovement weight lifting (clean and snatch)<br>Mixed martial arts (sparring)<br>Yoga/Pilates |
| Balance | Stability exercises (traditional exercises performed on an uneven surface such as a foam pad or BOSU ball)<br>Yoga/Pilates<br>Static stretching |

Plyometric exercises begin with a quick stretch of the muscle fibers (the eccentric phase) and then followed by a fast shortening of the same muscle fibers (the concentric phase) (15). This mode of training may improve a client's ability to increase speed of movement and power production as well as increase agility levels because plyometric exercises often change directions rapidly.

Another training method Personal Trainers can use to improve their clients' fitness levels is power resistance training. Muscular power production is used in various movements in sports, work, and daily living. Power can be increased through resistance training and by performing repetitions of lower loads at a high velocity (4). Some resistance training options Personal Trainers can use to develop more power in their clients are high-velocity resistance training and Olympic weight training. Both modes of resistance training yield increases in power production.

### Reaction Time, Coordination, and Balance

Balance, coordination, and reaction time are not only needed for recreational purposes but also used in daily routines. There are many exercises and drills that Personal Trainers can use to condition their clients that require them to jump, run, slide, and bound in nontraditional movement patterns that will develop their coordination, reaction time, and balance skills. All three of these skills involve muscle activation along with sensory integration to perform exercise-related tasks in a more highly skilled way. Flexibility exercises have been shown to increase balance and reaction time (5,8).

##  Anatomy of an Exercise Session

The components of an exercise training session include the following: warm-up, conditioning exercise, cool-down, and stretching. Although the focus of exercise sessions can vary widely, this framework is appropriate for various conditioning stimuli.

## Warm-Up

The warm-up is, at a minimum, 5–10 minutes of low to moderate activity intended to literally warm up the muscles in preparation for the conditioning phase. This transitional phase provides opportunity for the body to adjust from resting status to the higher physiologic, biomechanical, and bioenergetic demands of the conditioning phase (6). Warm-up activities include cardiovascular and muscular endurance activities.

## Conditioning Phase

The conditioning phase is the main focus of the exercise session and may include one or more of the following: cardiorespiratory (aerobic) exercise, resistance training, neuromotor activities, and sport-specific activities. The conditioning phase will follow the FITT principles described previously in this chapter and as will be covered in greater detail in the upcoming chapters in this section.

## Cool-Down

The cool-down involves similar cardiovascular and muscular endurance activities as found in the warm-up but now the transition is from the higher intensity of the conditioning phase back toward resting status. During this time of low- to moderate-intensity activity, the body will experience a decrease in heart rate and systolic blood pressure, and metabolic end products (*e.g.*, lactate) produced during more intense activity will be removed. Allowing for a gradual return toward baseline will help the client avoid postexercise hypotension (low blood pressure) and potential dizziness (due to blood pooling in the legs rather than flowing back to the heart and brain). The cool-down should be at least 5–10 minutes, longer for higher intensity conditioning phase sessions (6).

## Stretching

The stretching phase is considered distinct from the warm-up and cool-down phases (6). For adults in a general fitness program and for athletes in sports in which flexibility is important, stretching after the warm-up is typically recommended (6). Stretching can also be included after the cool-down. For some sports (*e.g.*, those focused on muscular strength, power, and endurance), some research suggests stretching following the activity rather than following the warm-up (6). When properly performed, even ballistic or "bouncing" stretches can be as effective as static stretches for increasing joint ROM in individuals engaging in activities that involve ballistic movements such as tennis or basketball (6).

## SUMMARY

A complete fitness program provides many physiological and psychological benefits. With an understanding of these benefits, a Personal Trainer can provide clients with the appropriate guidance regarding cardiorespiratory exercise, resistance training, and flexibility exercises as well as balance training or skill-related activities as needed to achieve individual client goals.

## REFERENCES

1. American College of Sports Medicine. ACSM position stand. Appropriate physical activity interventions strategies for weight loss and prevention of weight regain for adults. *Med Sci Sports Exerc.* 2009;41(2):459–71.

2. American College of Sports Medicine. ACSM position stand. Exercise and physical activity for older adults. *Med Sci Sports Exerc.* 2009;41(7):1510–30.

3. American College of Sports Medicine. ACSM position stand. Physical activity and bone health. *Med Sci Sports Exerc.* 2004;36(11):1985–96.

4. American College of Sports Medicine. ACSM position stand. Progression models in resistance training for healthy adults. *Med Sci Sports Exerc.* 2009;41(3):687–708.

5. American College of Sports Medicine. ACSM position stand. Quantity and quality of exercise for developing and maintaining cardiorespiratory, musculoskeletal, and neuromuscular fitness in apparently healthy adults: guidance for prescribing exercise. *Med Sci Sports Exerc.* 2011;43(7):1334–59.

6. American College of Sports Medicine. *ACSM's Guidelines for Exercise Testing and Prescription.* 10th ed. Philadelphia (PA): Wolters Kluwer; 2018.

7. American College of Sports Medicine. *ACSM's Resource Manual for Guidelines for Exercise Testing and Prescription.* 6th ed. Philadelphia (PA): Wolters Kluwer/Lippincott Williams & Wilkins; 2010. 868 p.

8. Behm D, Bambury A, Cahill F, Power K. Effect of acute static stretching on force, balance, reaction time, and movement time. *Med Sci Sports Exerc.* 2004;36(8):1397–402.

9. Centers for Disease Control and Prevention. *Important Facts About Falls* [Internet]. Atlanta (GA): Centers for Disease Control and Prevention; [cited 2017 Feb 27]. Available from: http://www.cdc.gov/HomeandRecreationalSafety/Falls/adultfalls.html

10. Centers for Disease Control and Prevention. *Physical Activity and Health* [Internet]. Atlanta (GA): Centers for Disease Control and Prevention; [cited 2017 Feb 27]. Available from: https://www.cdc.gov/physicalactivity/basics/pa-health/index.htm

11. Christmas C, Andersen RA. Exercise and older patients: guidelines for the clinician. *J Am Geriatric Soc.* 2000;48(3):318–24.

12. Colcombe S, Kramer AF. Fitness effects on the cognitive function of older adults: a meta-analytic study. *Psychol Sci.* 2003;14(2):125–30.

13. Fabre C, Chamari K, Mucci P, Massé-Biron J, Préfaut C. Improvement of cognitive function by mental and/or individualized aerobic training in healthy elderly subjects. *Int J Sports Med.* 2002;23:415–21.

14. Landers DM. The influence of exercise on mental health. Washington (DC): President's Council on Physical Fitness and Sports Research; [cited 2017 Feb 27]. Available from: http://fitness.foundation/research-digest

15. Lloyd RS, Meyers RW, Oliver JL. The natural development and trainability of plyometric ability during childhood. *Strength Cond J.* 2011;33(2):23–32.

16. Long BC, Van Stavel R. Effects of exercise training on anxiety: a meta-analysis. *J Appl Sport Psychol.* 1995;7:167–89.

17. Milani RV, Lavie CJ. Reducing psychosocial stress: a novel mechanism of improving survival from exercise training. *Am J Med.* 2009;122(10):931–8.

18. Paluska SA, Schwenk TL. Physical activity and mental health: current concepts. *Sports Med.* 2000;29(3):167–80.

19. Penedo FJ, Dahn JR. Exercise and well-being: a review of mental and physical health benefits associated with physical activity. *Curr Opin Psych.* 2005;18(2):189–93.

20. Trivedi MH, Greer RL, Grannemann BD, Chambliss HO, Jordan AN. Exercise as an augmentation strategy for treatment of major depression. *J Psychiatr Pract.* 2006;12(4):205–13.

21. U.S. Department of Health and Human Services. *Physical Activity Guidelines Advisory Committee Report*, 2008 [Internet]. Washington (DC): U.S. Department of Health and Human Services; [cited 2017 Mar 1]. Available from: http://www.health.gov/paguidelines/Report/pdf/CommitteeReport.pdf

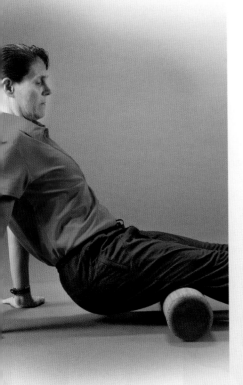

CHAPTER **14**

# Resistance Training Programs

## OBJECTIVES

**Personal Trainers should be able to:**

- Define resistance training principles.
- Review how and why resistance training should be performed.
- Design, evaluate, and implement resistance training programs.
- Evaluate clients' resistance training needs and progress.

# INTRODUCTION

Resistance training, also known as strength training or weight training, is a standard part of a comprehensive personal training program. A resistance training program can affect almost every system in the body and is used in a wide variety of populations. The benefits of resistance training are numerous and include increases in strength, muscle mass, and bone density. Almost every population can benefit from resistance training, from children preparing for youth sports to individuals trying to counteract the effects of the aging process.

A resistance training program can affect almost every system in the body and is used in a wide variety of populations, from children preparing for youth sports to individuals trying to counteract the effects of the aging process.

## The History and Science behind Resistance Training

At the end of the Second World War, Captain Thomas Delorme, MD, experimented with the use of progressive resistance exercise as a rehabilitation modality for injured soldiers (5). A few years later, Delorme and A. L. Watkins published the first paper in a scientific journal on the topic of long-term resistance training (6). After the initial work by Delorme and Watkins, the most influential personalities in resistance training were Mr. Bob Hoffman of York Barbell Club, who pioneered the interest in Olympic-style weightlifting and weight training with free weights through his publications and sales of barbells and dumbbells, and Mr. Joe Weider and his brother Ben, who promoted the bodybuilding industry.

The science of resistance training did not pick up again until two notable former weightlifters and future scientists, Dr. Patrick O'Shea from Oregon State University and Dr. Richard Berger from Temple University, fueled an explosion of scientific work in the 1960s and 1970s (49,50). Since then, published research on resistance training has grown exponentially with a gradual widening in research focus from enhancing athletic performance to also improving health and fitness (8). Although resistance training programs are critical for athletic and sports performance, they have now become a foundation of a variety of rehabilitation disciplines from orthopedic to cardiac to obesity management programs. Research on resistance training now appears in many medical and scientific journals such as the American College of Sports Medicine (ACSM's) *Medicine & Science in Sports & Exercise* and the National Strength and Conditioning Association's *Journal of Strength and Conditioning Research*. Thousands of scientific articles examining various aspects of resistance training with regard to designing optimal exercise prescriptions across the population spectrum are in print. However, in addition to these legitimate research articles, an abundance of resistance training mythology continues to be touted in popular books, magazines, and on the Internet. A demanding challenge has been placed on the Personal Trainer to sift through and carefully evaluate the scientific evidence from the marketing ploys. Resistance training programs and protocols should be guided by scientific evidence and not by dubious testimonials. Personal Trainers are advised to follow evidence-based practices to promote safety and effectiveness for clients.

## General Resistance Training Principles

The terms *resistance exercise* and *resistance training* are often used interchangeably; however, there is an important distinction between the two terms. Resistance exercise refers to a single exercise session, whereas resistance training refers to the combination of many consecutive resistance exercise sessions over time. Thus, a resistance exercise protocol is an exercise prescription for a single

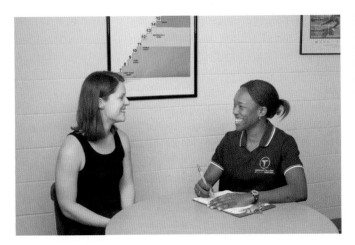

**FIGURE 14.1.** Exercise prescription in resistance training is an individualized process that requires a series of steps from a needs analysis and goal setting to evaluations and making changes in the workouts over time.

Resistance exercise refers to a single exercise session, whereas resistance training refers to the combination of many consecutive resistance exercise sessions over time.

session (most commonly called a "workout") and a resistance training program is an overall plan guiding the specific exercise parameters chosen for each exercise protocol.

Designing a resistance training program is a very individualized process, and the needs and goals of the client are paramount to the selection of program characteristics (Fig. 14.1). However, be aware that although a client may be training to maximize muscle hypertrophy, the client will also develop some muscular strength and endurance. Thus, the program will be at the same time both specific and general. The general principles of any effective resistance training program are as follows:

- Specificity of training: Only the muscles that are trained will adapt and change in response to a given program. For this reason, resistance programs must target all muscles for which a training effect is desired.
- Specific Adaptations to Imposed Demands (SAID) principle: SAID indicates that the adaptation will be specific to the demands that the exercise places on the individual. For example, if a high number of repetitions are used, the muscles will increase their ability to perform a high number of repetitions (muscular endurance).
- Progressive overload: As the body adapts to a given stimulus, an increase in the stimulus is required for further adaptations and improvements. Thus, if the load or volume is not increased over time, progress will be limited.
- Variation in training: No one program should be used without changing the exercise stimulus over time. An example of increasing variety in training is periodized training.
- Periodization: The phasic manipulation of the training variables (volume, intensity, frequency, and rest intervals) as a means of optimizing desired physiological outcomes while concurrently reducing the incidence of overtraining. Periodization allows for optimal training and recovery time in a resistance training program.
- Prioritization of training: It is difficult to train for all aspects of muscular fitness. Thus, within a periodized training program, one needs to focus or prioritize the training goals for each training cycle. This technique is often used in athletics paralleling competitive season schedules.

 **Program Design Process**

The key to a great program design is to identify the specific variables that need to be controlled to best predict and/or ensure the desired training outcomes. The most challenging aspect of resistance training exercise prescription is deciding which changes in program design will best meet an individual's training goals. Appropriate changes in the resistance training program are required over time. This means that sound decisions must take into consideration the needs of the sport or activity, the individual training response, and available testing data. Therefore, the resistance training exercise prescription is a continual process of planning, assessing, and changing.

Planning a resistance training exercise prescription allows one to quantify the exercise stimulus. Planning ranges from the initial development of a single exercise session to the variation of the training program over time. A successful Personal Trainer needs the ability to quantify a client's workout and evaluate progress made to ensure the program is safe and effective and will lead to optimal physical development of the client.

## Training Potential

The gains made in any variable related to muscular performance will ultimately be linked to an individual's genetic potential. A deconditioned individual will likely achieve large initial gains because of the great adaptive potential available. As training proceeds, the rate of adaptation slows, as an individual approaches genetic limits. Over time, the physiological adaptation as measured from baseline will continue to increase albeit at a much slower rate. At this point in the training process, because gains are less noticeable, other goals for the resistance training program must be targeted to prevent the client from losing interest because of a lack of progress. Appreciation of the process by which adaptations occur over time is critical in developing an optimal program.

## Initial Assessments

When working with a new client, Personal Trainers should always devote adequate time to evaluate the clients' prior resistance exercise experience and discuss their training goals carefully before beginning any exercise sessions. The initial assessment should include the following:

- A needs analysis focusing on learning about the client's personal goals and needs
- The intended time frame for achieving these goals
- Targeted areas or muscle groups
- Health issues (*e.g.*, cardiovascular disease, asthma, diabetes, osteoporosis, osteoarthritis, immune system disorders, neurologic disorders), musculoskeletal limitations, recent surgeries, chronic injuries, sites of pain, and so on

Personal Trainers should try to understand the motivation underlying their clients' goals. In addition, Personal Trainers should assess the level of support their clients feel they have, available from family or friends (see Chapter 8 for additional discussion of social support). Finally, Personal Trainers should discuss any prior resistance training experience their clients have had in order to uncover potential challenges or barriers to training and develop appropriate strategies for motivation. Personal Trainers work with clients to develop strategies to overcome potential barriers to resistance training. These initial assessments will help Personal Trainers determine which muscle groups, energy systems, and muscle actions need to be trained and how these and the other acute program variables should be manipulated to meet the specific needs of the training program.

Before developing a resistance training program, Personal Trainers should take the time to conduct a baseline fitness assessment, consisting of anthropometric measurements (height, weight, circumferences, skinfolds, etc.), resting hemodynamics (heart rate, blood pressure), body composition, and tests of muscular strength and endurance (see Chapter 12 for more information on assessment). Determination of initial fitness is necessary to the development of an effective training program.

Muscular strength assessments include the one repetition maximum (1-RM) testing on a variety of exercises, especially those exercises that involve the major muscle groups such as bench press and squat, but only if tolerable to the client (22). The 1-RM test allows the Personal Trainer to determine loading values for a particular exercise. There are specific procedures that should be followed when conducting a 1-RM test to help ensure safety, reliability, and validity of the test (1). Although 1-RM is a measure of maximal strength, muscular power can be tested by using the medicine ball "put" for the upper body power assessment and the vertical jump test or standing long jump for the lower body muscular power assessment (1,32,33,35). Muscular endurance testing might include curl-ups, push-ups, or maximal amount of repetitions that can be performed at a given percentage of the 1-RM load (32,35).

## Follow-up Assessments

It is exciting and motivating for clients to see improvements toward reaching their goals. To see these improvements, it is important that Personal Trainers keep records of their clients' progress. Individualized training logs are a useful tool for monitoring progress. These logs should record specific exercises, resistance or load, number of sets, and number of repetitions (consider discussing using a rating of perceived exertion [RPE] scale or a 0–10 scale rating effort as well) (30,43). The training log provides a record of the resistance and knowledge of performance of previous exercise sessions, which is necessary for assigning the appropriate resistance for successive sessions. Kept over time, these logs provide the Personal Trainer with a means to examine and evaluate program effectiveness or to identify areas of weakness.

Formal reassessment of a client's progress should occur periodically for encouragement but not so often that there has not been adequate time for noticeable changes to develop. These follow-up assessments should include the same measures as administered at the baseline assessment, including anthropometrics and tests of muscular strength, power, and endurance.

Based on these assessments, the concepts of progression, variation, and overload can be applied to the resistance training program to achieve optimal physiological adaptations and to accommodate changing fitness levels and goals of clients. These assessments give Personal Trainers a basis for modifying the short term acute program variables, including choice of exercise, order of exercises, intensity, number of sets, set structure, rest periods, load or resistance, and repetition speed. Variation can be incorporated by altering joint angles and positioning, primary exercises versus assistance exercises, or multijoint exercises versus single-joint exercises to stress the muscles and joints specified by the client's needs analysis. Progressive overload can be accomplished by increasing the intensity and/or volume by increasing the resistance, number of sets, number of repetitions, or number of exercises or by decreasing or increasing the rest intervals.

## Individualization

Clients are not replicas of each other. Similar training programs provided to different clients will result in varied training responses. Therefore, skilled and effective Personal Trainers do not give standard programs to multiple clients. Exercises need to be modified to best suit the anatomical characteristics, needs, and abilities of each client. Additionally, the Personal Trainer must make modifications in the progression of the program based on the training response of the specific client. Adjustments to programs should focus on optimizing the individual's physiological adaptations.

## Client Feedback

To design an effective resistance training program, the Personal Trainer needs to pay special attention to feedback from the client. Clients may request favorite exercises or muscle groups, or they may complain of pain or fatigue requiring program modifications. Personal Trainer must be alert to this feedback and encourage further feedback to ensure that the program and strategy meet the expectations of the client. This can be accomplished by asking the client for feedback, for example, "How do you think the workout went?" "Did you feel that you worked out hard enough? Too hard? Just right?" "What did you find went especially well or easier? What was particularly challenging?" Always pay attention to physical signs of overuse or exhaustion, such as dizziness, light-headedness, complexion changes, profuse sweating, facial expressions, and muscular exhaustion. Clearly, working a client to the point of vomiting or passing out is not safe and will not leave a good impression with clients or any spectators who are present when medical attention arrives.

Of special concern for Personal Trainers is the careful and proper progression in the resistance training program, especially for beginners or those coming back from an injury lay off. Too much exercise, too heavy of exercise, and/or accentuated eccentric exercise can lead to an excessive amount of muscle tissue damage and breakdown. This can result in delayed onset muscle soreness (DOMS) or in extreme cases rhabdomyolysis. Rhabdomyolysis is a clinical pathology that is characterized by the rapid breakdown of muscle tissue resulting in high amounts of intramuscular proteins (*e.g.*, myoglobin, myosin protein) entering into the blood stream that are potentially harmful to kidneys and can cause kidney failure and sometimes death (16).

> *Rhabdomyolysis* is a clinical pathology that is characterized by the rapid breakdown of muscle tissue resulting in high amounts of intramuscular proteins (*e.g.*, myoglobin, myosin protein) entering into the blood stream that are potentially harmful to kidneys and can cause kidney failure and sometimes death.

The most common manifestation of muscle injury is DOMS. DOMS symptoms are a first sign that the individual has done too much too soon. DOMS is a condition of heightened postexercise soreness that presents in the initial 24–48 hours after the exercise session and may last upwards of 5–7 days. Although some swelling, pain, and soreness are common and classical signs of muscle tissue adaptation following a workout, DOMS should *not* be considered a goal of the training program (*i.e.*, no pain no gain). If these symptoms are extreme, tissue damage may be more serious and DOMS is likely to reduce training potential as well as having a deleterious effect on performance (3).

To avoid overshooting a client's tolerance, Personal Trainers carefully progress the client to heavier loads with prudent volume changes, thus allowing for adequate recovery from each workout. A simple Likert-type (Box 14.1) scale can be used to gauge the level of soreness for the client. Individuals having a score of 3 or more should have the resistance intensity and/or volume reduced dramatically and should increase the amount of rest allowed in a periodized training program. Although some muscle soreness is a normal result of muscular adaptation, extreme soreness is a sign of physiological overshoot.

---

### Box 14.1   Likert-Type Chart to Determine Muscle Soreness

| | |
|---|---|
| 0 | |
| 1 | **Minor soreness** |
| 2 | |
| 3 | **Moderate soreness** |
| 4 | |
| 5 | **Extreme soreness** |
| 6 | |

Pay attention to the client's hydration levels and medications to help minimize potential muscle damage from a workout. Dehydration can cause muscle damage, limit one's force production, and decrease the training potential of the workout. Monitor water intake and provide scheduled fluid consumption throughout the workout. Be aware that medications such as statins or diuretics could also influence muscle tissue damage. For example, rhabdomyolysis may develop from disease, infections, metabolic disorders, or even statins used for the control of cholesterol levels which are unrelated to resistance training. Symptoms of rhabdomyolysis include severe muscle aches, weakness, and extremely dark reddish-brown urine. Kidney shock and acute renal failure can develop in up to 2 days after major tissue trauma. If rhabdomyolysis is suspected, seek medical help immediately.

Personal Trainers should always explain the muscle group(s) that the exercise is intended to target, and clients should be taught how to differentiate between muscle fatigue and soreness, and extreme soreness, pain, or injury. Clients must be told that new exercises often feel uncomfortable or awkward but that if pain is felt in any joint or nonsynergistic or stabilizer muscle, that exercise should be discontinued. The exercises should be stopped immediately if the client complains of pain or the Personal Trainer suspects that the client is in pain. The last thing a Personal Trainer wants to do is induce or aggravate an injury.

Feedback from the client can also come from paying close attention to the technique of the client during an exercise. Deterioration in technique often results from fatigue or insufficient flexibility in the range of motion (ROM) involved in the exercise. Proper technique should always be a priority. When technique is compromised during an exercise, the exercise should be either stopped or modified to reestablish correct technique to avoid injury.

In summary, it is important to properly assess workouts and prevent extreme muscle injury from occurring. The resistance load and volume of training need to be carefully progressed and monitored to limit muscle tissue damage and develop a physiological toleration to heavier resistance and volumes of exercise stress. Emphasizing proper technique and paying attention to the basic principle of progression are important to an effective and safe exercise prescription.

## Setting and Evaluating Goals

Optimal program design needs to be individualized for each client's goals. Personal Trainers encounter an assortment of clients with a plethora of goals, including weight loss; weight gain; building strength; building muscle; shaping/toning; improving overall health; improving speed, agility, power, balance, and coordination; decreasing blood pressure or cholesterol level; managing diabetes and other chronic diseases; injury rehabilitation; or sport-specific training. Often, the desired goals of clients are unrealistic. When improvements do not meet expectations, motivation can be lost, frustration may set in, and nonadherence to the program can occur. Therefore, it is crucial that the Personal Trainer help the client understand what realistic and obtainable goals are, considering the time course, the individual's training history and status, fitness level, and genetic potential. The expectations of the client must be realistic and measurable (see Chapter 8), considering the physiological time course of neural and cellular adaptations. Goal setting and time frame, as well as the individual's age, physical maturity, training history, and psychological and physical tolerance, should also be considered. Progression toward the goals must be gradual to minimize the risk of injury.

Common program goals in resistance training are related to improvements in function, such as increased muscular strength, power, and local muscular endurance, or decreased body fat (Fig. 14.2). Other functional gains such as increased coordination, agility, balance, and speed are also common goals of a program. Factors such as balance may have implications for injury prevention by limiting falls in older individuals. Other goals may relate to physiological changes related to increased body mass through muscle hypertrophy, improved blood pressure, decreased body fat, and increased metabolic rate for caloric expenditure.

**FIGURE 14.2.** Setting goals and evaluating progress in a resistance training program are vital to realistic progress and gains.

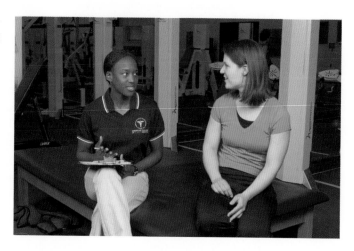

For the most part, training goals or objectives should be measurable variables (*e.g.*, 1-RM strength, vertical jump height, and fat mass loss) so that one can objectively judge whether or not gains were made or goals were achieved. Examination and evaluation of a workout log is invaluable in assessing the effects of various resistance training programs. Formal strength tests to determine functional changes in strength can be done on a variety of equipment, including isokinetic dynamometers, free weights, and machines. Using the results of these objective tests can help in modifying the exercise program to reach previous training goals or to develop new goals.

Athletic performance and good health are not always the same thing. A person being a competitive athlete does not mean that he or she makes healthy choices or has a healthy lifestyle. Many elite athletes train in ways that far exceed what is recommended for good health (*e.g.*, lifting $7 \text{ d} \cdot \text{wk}^{-1}$ or running 140 miles in a week or training $4–6 \text{ h} \cdot \text{d}^{-1}$). In fact, they may actually do exercises that would be considered contraindicated for the average healthy person. Thus, goals in resistance training have to be put in the context of the desired outcome for each individual but also within what is healthy.

> Athletic performance and good health are not always the same thing.

## Maintenance of Training Goals

A concept called "capping" may need to be applied to various training situations in which small gains will require very large amounts of time to achieve, and yet in the long run, these small gains are not necessary for success. Capping a training goal is a tough decision that comes only after an adequate period of training time and observation of what the realistic potential for further change is for a particular variable. This may be related to a performance goal (*e.g.*, bench press 1-RM strength) or some form of physical development (*e.g.*, calf size). At some point, one must make a value judgment on how to best spend training time. By not adding any further training time to develop a particular muscle characteristic (*e.g.*, strength, size, and power), one decides that the current gains are "good enough," and it is time to go into a maintenance training program. Thus, more training time is available to address other training goals. Ultimately, this decision may result in greater total development of the individual.

Decisions such as capping are part of the many types of clinical decisions that must be made when monitoring the progress of resistance training programs. Are the training goals realistic in relation to the sport or health enhancement for which the client is being trained? Is the attainment of a particular training goal vital to the program's success? These difficult questions need to be continually asked in the goal development phase of each training cycle for any program.

## Unrealistic Goals

Too often, goals are open-ended and unrealistic. Careful attention must be paid to the magnitude of the performance goal and the amount of training time needed to achieve it. Although scientific studies may last up to 6 months, most real-life training programs are developed as a part of a lifestyle for an individual's sports career or whole life. Over time, clients' goals change, and thus, resistance training programs must also change to reflect these changing needs.

Goals may at times exceed the reality of genetic limitations. For example, some men desire near impossible and extreme muscle size (*e.g.*, 23-in biceps, 36-in thighs, 20-in neck, and 50-in chest) or strength (*e.g.*, 400-lb bench press), or in contrast, some women desire drastic decreases in body weight and limb size and/or shape. Genetic limits in anatomical structure or somatotype may make these changes unattainable. Ultimately, for both men and women, goals must be carefully and honestly examined to determine if the resistance training program can actually stimulate the changes desired.

> Ultimately, for both men and women, goals must be carefully and honestly examined to determine if the resistance training program can actually stimulate the changes desired.

Big marketing of the newest high-tech fitness equipment and training programs can also create unrealistic training expectations in clients. Airbrushed pictures of movie actors and models advertising a specific program or product project body images that are desired but totally unobtainable. Most people make mistakes in goal development by wanting too much too soon, with too little effort expended. Making progress in a resistance training program requires a long-term commitment to a total training program. Thus, resistance training is one aspect of an overall healthy lifestyle that includes cardiovascular conditioning and proper nutrition.

## Resistance Training Modalities

Many different training tools (*e.g.*, free weights, machines, and medicine balls) can be used in resistance training programs. Each tool fits into a category of training, which has certain inherent strengths and weaknesses. The modality chosen should depend on the accessibility of equipment, needs, goals, experiences, and limitations of the client.

### Variable-Resistance Devices

Variable-resistance equipment operates through a lever arm, cam, or pulley arrangement. Its purpose is to alter the resistance throughout the exercise's ROM in an attempt to match the increases and decreases in strength (*i.e.*, strength curve). Proponents of variable-resistance machines believe that by increasing and decreasing the resistance to match the exercise's strength curve, the muscle is forced to contract maximally throughout the ROM, resulting in maximal gains in strength.

There are three major types of strength curves: ascending, descending, and bell-shaped (Fig. 14.3). In an exercise with an ascending strength curve, it is possible to lift more weight if only the top ½ or ¼ of a repetition is performed rather than if the complete ROM of a repetition is performed. For example, an exercise with an ascending strength curve is the squat exercise. If an exercise has a descending strength curve, it is possible to lift more weight if only the bottom half of a repetition is performed. Such an exercise is upright rowing. A bell-shaped curve is an exercise in which it is possible to lift more resistance, if only the middle portion of the ROM is performed and not the beginning or end portions of the range of the motion. Elbow flexion has a bell-shaped strength curve. Because there are three major types of strength curves, variable-resistance machines have to be able to vary the resistance in three major patterns to match the strength curves of all exercises. To date, this has not been accomplished. Additionally, because of variations in limb length (point of

**FIGURE 14.3.** Three basic strength curves exist for every exercise, with hybrids of them for certain movements.

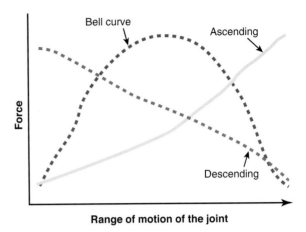

attachment of a muscle's tendon to the bones) and body size, it is hard to conceive of one mechanical arrangement that would match the strength curve of all individuals for a particular exercise.

Biomechanical research indicates that certain types of cam-operated variable-resistance equipment do not match the strength curves of specific exercises such as the elbow curl, fly, knee extension, knee flexion, and pullover exercises (10,37). In women, one type of cam equipment was shown to match the strength curves of females fairly well (14), although not for all aspects of each exercise. For example, in women, the cam resulted in too much resistance near the end of the knee extension exercise and provided too much resistance during the first half and too little during the second half of elbow flexion and extension. The knee flexion machine matched the female's strength curve well throughout the ROM. This research indicates that not all machines are appropriate for all populations or for all exercises.

Elastic resistance bands have become popular within the fitness world because they are relatively easy to work with and less intimidating to clients. Although very effective as a training modality if the resistance can be heavy enough (23), care must be taken when using elastic bands with certain types of exercises that do not match the ascending strength curve. A possible drawback to elastic bands is that the constantly increasing resistance offered as the band is stretched. In other words, elastic bands have a resistance pattern that only matches an ascending strength curve. At the beginning of a muscle flexion, the resistance is low, and at the end of the flexion, the resistance is very high. If the setup is not correct, only part of the muscle involved in the latter part of the flexion may be optimally stimulated. Thus, proper starting angle, band fit, and stretch are essential for optimal training outcome. Also, because of the physics of elastic bands, the resistance during the extension phase will be lower than that during the flexion phase, again reducing the training stimulus. In addition, elastic bands give minimal feedback to clients or trainers in that the resistance cannot be quantified.

## Dynamic Constant External Resistance Devices

Isotonic is traditionally defined as a muscular contraction in which the muscle exerts a constant tension. The execution of free-weight exercises and exercises on various weight training machines, although usually considered isotonic, is not by nature isotonic. The force exerted by a muscle in the performance of such exercises is not constant but varies with the mechanical advantage of the joint involved in the movement and the length of the muscle at a particular point in the movement. A more workable definition of isotonic is a resistance training exercise in which the external resistance or weight does not change and both a lifting (concentric) phase and a lowering (eccentric) phase occur during each repetition. Thus, free-weight exercises and exercise machines that do not vary the resistance are isotonic in nature. Because there is confusion concerning the term *isotonic*, the term *dynamic constant external resistance training* has been adopted.

The types of devices used for dynamic constant external resistance include dumbbells, barbells, kettle bells, weight machines, and medicine balls. These are generally devices that do not use pulleys or levers. The major disadvantage to this type of device is that it does not stimulate the neuromuscular systems involved maximally throughout the entire ROM. The changes in the musculoskeletal leverage occurring during a movement also change the force requirement and thus the exercise stimulus. However, these types of devices require recruitment of muscles, other than the primary movers of an exercise, to act as stabilizers. This increases the total amount of physiological work the body must do to perform the exercise as well as providing exercise stimuli to the stabilizing muscles that are very important in a real-world setting or for athletic performance. These types of modalities are referred to as "free form" exercises, as they operate in multiple dimensions of space (frontal, sagittal, and transverse planes). Other benefits to most constant external resistance devices include little or no limitation in the ROM allowed and easy adaptation of the exercise to accommodate individual differences such as the clients' body size or physical capabilities. Equipment fit is also not a limiting factor for large and small body sizes and limb lengths.

## Static Resistance Devices

Specialized static or isometric contraction devices, in which a person pulls or pushes against an immovable resistance, are rarely used. Pushing an overloaded barbell against the safety racks, or using a wall or partner for an isometric contraction, is occasionally used for an individual to overcome a sticking point, and this form of resistance exercise is called "functional isometrics." Isometrics or static resistance training refers to a muscular action in which no change in the length of the muscle takes place. This type of resistance training is normally performed against an immovable object such as a wall, barbell, or weight machine loaded beyond the maximal concentric strength of an individual.

Isometrics can also be performed by having a weak muscle group contract against a strong muscle group (*e.g.*, trying to bend the left elbow by contracting the left elbow flexors maximally while resisting the movement by pushing down on the left hand with the right hand with just enough force to prevent any movement at the left elbow). If the left elbow flexors are weaker than the right elbow extensors, the left elbow flexors would be performing an isometric action at 100% of a maximal voluntary contraction.

Isometric training leads to static strength gains, but the gains are substantially less than 5% per week (9). Increases in strength resulting from isometric training are related to the number of muscle actions performed, the duration of the muscle actions, whether the muscle action is maximal or submaximal, the angle at which the exercise is performed, and the frequency of training. Most studies involving isometric training manipulate several of these factors simultaneously. It is difficult, therefore, to evaluate the importance of any one factor. Enough research has been conducted, however, to allow some recommendations concerning isometric training. Isometric exercises are thought to strengthen muscle fibers within 15° of the position being held isometrically, and therefore, clients should perform multiple positions with isometric contraction to ensure full ROM strengthening. Also, isometric training is good for individuals with joint disorders in which pain is elicited by motion (*i.e.*, rheumatoid arthritis).

## Other Resistance Devices

Isokinetic devices allow one to maintain a maximum resistance throughout the whole ROM by controlling the speed of the movement. These devices use friction, compressed air, or pneumatics, which often allow for both the concentric and the eccentric component of a repetition, or hydraulics for the concentric component of a repetition. Isokinetic exercises, although popular in the rehabilitation setting, have never caught on as a typical modality used in a weight room.

The initial excitement for this training modality was related to the ability to train at fast velocities similar to the high-speed movements seen in sport and real life. Isokinetic refers to a muscular action performed at constant angular limb velocity. Unlike other types of resistance training, there is no set resistance to meet; rather, the velocity of movement is controlled. The resistance offered by the isokinetic machine cannot be accelerated; any force applied against the equipment results in an equal reaction force. The reaction force mirrors the force applied to the equipment by the user throughout the range of movement of an exercise, making it theoretically possible for the muscle(s) to exert a continual, maximal force through the movement's full ROM.

Pneumatic resistance (compressed air) exercise has become relatively popular as it allows both the concentric and eccentric portions of a repetition and can be adjusted during a repetition or a set of exercises with handheld buttons. This type of device has been popular for working with older populations. In addition, with no deceleration, it can be used effectively to train power with joint exercises not possible with conventional machines. Power is as important for older adults to maintain function as it is for athletes' performance. Because of the fixed nature of the configuration for most pneumatic machines, they are unable to address key factors such as balance and control in a multidimensional environment.

Hydraulics equipment has also become more popular with many fitness clubs promoting it as a safe and nonintimidating form of resistance exercise. Although this modality has no deceleration in its repetition range and has been used as a type of power training modality, it also has no eccentric component, which limits its efficiency as twice the number of repetitions may be required to get the same effect as a typical concentric–eccentric repetition (7). Training the eccentric phase is important to protect the body from injury and also to enhance the ability to recover from injury. Furthermore, concentric-only training appears to be less resistant to detraining.

## Machines versus Free-Weight Exercises

> A topic of great debate, especially in the health and fitness world, is the use of free weights versus machine resistance exercises.

A topic of great debate, especially in the health and fitness world, is the use of free weights versus machine resistance exercises. These different exercise modalities were discussed previously in the sections on constant external resistance and variable-resistance devices. The following is a comparison of the two modalities.

1. Machines are not always designed to fit the proportions of all individuals. Clients who are obese; who have special physical considerations or disabilities; and who are shorter, taller, or wider than the norm may not be able to fit comfortably in the machines. In contrast, free-weight exercises can easily be adapted to fit most clients' physical size or special requirements.

2. Machines use a fixed ROM; thus, the individual must conform to the movement limitations of the machine. Often, these movements do not mimic functional or athletic movements. Free weights allow full ROM, and the transfer to the real-world movements is greater than that for machines.

3. Most machines isolate a muscle or muscle group, thus negating the need for other muscles to act as assistant movers and stabilizers. Free-weight exercises almost always involve assisting and stabilizing muscles. On the other hand, if the goal is to isolate a specific muscle or muscle group, as in some rehabilitation settings or because of physical disabilities, machine exercises may be preferred.

4. Although it is never advisable to perform resistance exercise alone, machines do allow greater independence, as the need for a spotter or helper is usually diminished once the client has learned the technique of the exercise. However, there is a misconception of extra safety that may lead to a lack of attention being paid to the exercise. Injuries are still possible when using machines, specifically when there is a breakdown in lifting form or improper seat height, lifting form, and/or joint alignment.

5. Machine exercises may be more useful than free-weight exercises in some special populations. One reason for this is that machines are often perceived to be less intimidating to a beginner. As the resistance training skill and experience level increases, free-weight exercise can gradually be introduced, if desired. However, it is important to inform clients of the benefits that free weights have compared with machines (*e.g.*, increased musculoskeletal loading that reduces the risk of developing osteoporosis, improved balance).

6. Certain free-weight exercises (*e.g.*, Olympic-style lifts) and hydraulic and pneumatic machines allow training of power, as no joint deceleration occurs.

7. Rotational resistance accommodates certain body movements (*e.g.*, shoulder adduction) that would be difficult to work through a full ROM with free weights.

From the comparison earlier, it seems that variable resistive devices (machines) in general are at a comparative disadvantage to constant resistance devices (free weights). However, machine exercises are still recommended for certain populations and can be very useful when used appropriately. In fact, a safe and optimally effective resistance training program involves a combination of both free-weight and machine exercises, taking into consideration many aspects of the client's needs and the advantages of the different modalities. Both modalities can be used to add variation to the training program and are effective "tools" in a Personal Trainer's "tool box." To summarize, for the general population, a combination of free weights and variable-resistance machines are generally most effective. Machines and other variable-resistance devices are recommended as an adjunct to a free-weight training program in mid-level and advanced clients.

> For the general population, a combination of free weights and variable-resistance machines are generally most effective.

## The Needs Analysis

Before designing a training program, a needs analysis of the client should be performed to design the most effective program (8). Once the needs and goals of the client have been established, the Personal Trainer can address questions that will come up when designing the workout using the acute program variables.

A needs analysis for strength training involves answering some important initial questions that affect the program design components (18). The needs analysis requires that the following questions be considered:

1. What is the main goal of the resistance training program?
2. What muscle groups need to be trained?
3. What are the basic energy sources (*e.g.*, anaerobic, aerobic) that need to be trained?
4. What type of muscle action (*e.g.*, isometric, eccentric actions) should be used?
5. What are the primary sites of injury for the particular sport or prior injury history of the individual?

### Resistance Training Goals

The first question to be asked of the client concerns the main goal for the resistance training program. A discussion with the client of what type of outcome (*i.e.*, general health, muscular strength, muscular endurance, muscular hypertrophy, and/or muscular power) they desire will help the Personal Trainer develop an appropriate program. Each of the aforementioned program goals will require a different program design to optimize the stated goals. Reviewing these with the client allows for discussion of realistic expectations and time commitments before continuing with more extensive program evaluation procedures.

## Biomechanical Analysis to Determine Which Muscles Need to Be Trained

In determining the client's needs and goals, an examination of the muscles and the specific joint angles to be trained needs to be conducted. For any activity, including a sport, this involves a basic analysis of the movements performed and the most common sites of injury. With the proper equipment and a background in basic biomechanics, a more definitive approach to this question is possible. With the use of a slow motion videotape, a Personal Trainer can better evaluate specific aspects of movements and can conduct a qualitative analysis of the muscles, angles, velocities, and forces involved. The decisions made at this stage help define one of the acute program variables — choice of exercise.

Specificity is a major tenet of resistance training and is based on the concept that the exercises and resistances used should result in training adaptations that will transfer to better performance in sport or daily activity. Resistance training is used because it is often difficult, if not impossible, to overload a sport skill or other physical movement without risk of injury or dramatically altering skill technique. Specificity assumes that muscles must be trained similarly to the sport or activity in terms of the following:

- The joint around which movement occurs
- The joint ROM
- The pattern of resistance throughout the ROM (ascending, descending, or bell-shaped)
- The pattern of limb velocity throughout the ROM
- The types of muscle contraction (*e.g.*, concentric, eccentric, or isometric)

Resistance training for any sport or activity of daily living should include full ROM exercises around all the major body joints. For example, for general fitness and muscular development, the major muscle groups of the hips and legs, chest, back, shoulders, low back, and abdominals should be the training focus. For those who are interested in enhancing sport performance, specific sport activity movements should be included in the workout to maximize the contribution of strength training to those movements. The best way to select appropriate exercises is to biomechanically analyze, in quantitative terms, the sport or physical activity. Unfortunately, such analyses of each sport or activity are not readily available to the Personal Trainer. Thus, the Personal Trainer must use biomechanical principles in a qualitative manner to intelligently select exercises. Ideally, this analysis should be followed up with appropriate resistance exercises in the weight room that train the specific muscles and joint angles involved.

> Biomechanical principles can be used in a qualitative manner to intelligently select exercises.

## Transfer Specificity

Each resistance exercise used in a program will have various amounts of transfer to another activity, referred to as "transfer specificity." When training for improved health and well-being, transfer is related to its effects on specific clinical outcomes (*e.g.*, bone mineral density). However, training for enhancing sport performance requires equally specific exercises. Every training activity has a percentage of carryover to other activities, but no conditioning activity has perfect carryover. Although some activities have a higher percentage of carryover than others, because of similarities in neuromuscular recruitment patterns, energy systems, and biomechanical characteristics, only by practicing the exact task (*e.g.*, lifting groceries or shoveling snow) or sport (*e.g.*, running or basketball) itself, is the training 100% transferred.

Unfortunately, most of the time, one cannot use the specific sport or activity as the training stimulus because it is not possible or safe to gain the needed "overload" on the neuromuscular system. Thus, this is why resistance training is used in the conditioning process. The optimal training program needs to maximize carryover to the sport or activity.

## Determining the Energy Sources Used in the Activity

Performance of every sport or activity uses a percentage of all three energy sources. The energy sources (see Chapter 5) to be trained have a major impact on the program design. Resistance training usually stresses the anaerobic energy sources (adenosine triphosphate–creatine phosphate [ATP–CP] energy source and glycolytic energy source) more than aerobic metabolism (11). Individuals who have gained initial cardiovascular fitness will have difficulty improving maximal oxygen consumption values using conventional resistance training alone (26). However, resistance training can be used to improve endurance performance by improving running efficiency and economy (15). In addition, systematic reviews of the literature have reported that concurrent resistance and endurance training has a positive effect on endurance performance among well-trained runners and cyclists (52,53).

## Selecting a Resistance Modality

Decisions regarding the use of isometric, dynamic concentric, dynamic eccentric, and isokinetic modalities of exercise are important in planning *any type* of resistance training program. Not all equipment uses concentric and eccentric muscle actions, and this can impact training effectiveness (*e.g.*, hydraulics) (7). Whether for sport, fitness, or rehabilitation, basic biomechanical analysis is used to decide which muscles to train and to identify the type of muscle action is involved in the activity. Most resistance training programs use several types of muscle actions.

## Injury Prevention Exercises

Personal Trainers need to know the prior injury profile of their client and the common sites of potential injury from the sport or recreational activity performed or other daily activities. The prescription of resistance training exercises will be directed at enhancing the strength and function of tissue to better resist injury, enhance recovery if injured, and minimizes the extent of damage related to an injury. The term *prehabilitation* (the opposite of rehabilitation) has become popular. Prehabilitation refers to preventing initial injury by training the joints and muscles that are most susceptible to injury in an activity (such as a rotator cuff program for throwing athletes). The prevention of reinjury is also an important goal of a resistance training program. Thus, understanding the sport's or activity's typical injury profile (*e.g.*, knees in downhill skiing, elbows and shoulders in baseball pitching, extended hours sitting or standing for work) and the individual's prior history of injury can help in properly designing a resistance training program.

## Acute Program Variables

Developed more than 20 years ago, the paradigm of acute program variables allows one to define every workout (19). Every resistance exercise protocol or workout is derived from five acute program variables. The classical acute program variables are (a) choice of exercises, (b) order of exercises, (c) amount of resistance and number of repetitions, (d) number of sets, and (e) duration of rest periods between sets and exercises. In turn, the choices made for each of these variables define the exercise stimuli and ultimately, with repeated exposure, the training adaptations. Essentially, the choices made for the specific combination of acute program variables create an exercise stimulus "fingerprint" that is specific and unique to that workout protocol. Thus, by making specific choices for the acute program variables that are related to the needs and goals of the client, the Personal Trainer is able to create many different types of workouts (8).

The classical acute program variables are choice of exercises, order of exercises, amount of resistance and number of repetitions, number of sets, and duration of rest periods between sets and exercises.

## Choice of Exercises

The choice of exercise will be related to the biomechanical characteristics of the goals targeted for improvement. The number of possible joint angles and exercises is almost as limitless as the body's functional movements. As muscle tissue that is not activated will not benefit from resistance training, the exercises should be selected so they stress the muscles, joints, and joint angles specified by the client's needs analysis. To aid the Personal Trainer in making the correct choices, exercises can be divided into several different categories based on their function and/or muscle involvement.

Exercises can be designated as primary exercises or assistance exercises. Primary exercises train the prime movers in a particular movement and are typically major muscle group exercises (e.g., leg press, bench press, hang pulls). Assistance exercises are exercises that train predominantly a single muscle group (e.g., triceps press, biceps curls) that aids (synergists or stabilizers) in the movement produced by the prime movers.

Exercises can be classified as multijoint or single-joint exercises. Multijoint exercises require the coordinated action of two or more muscle groups and joints. Power cleans, power snatches, dead lifts, and squats are good examples of whole-body multijoint exercises. The bench press, which involves movement of both the elbow and shoulder joints, is also a multijoint, multi-muscle group exercise, although it involves only movement in the upper body. Some examples of other multijoint exercises are the lat pull-down, military press, and squat. Exercises that attempt to isolate a particular muscle group's movement of a single joint are known as single-joint and/or single-muscle group exercises. Biceps curls, knee extensions, and knee curls are examples of isolated single-joint, single-muscle group exercises. Many assistance exercises may be classified as single-muscle group or single-joint exercises.

The inclusion of both bilateral (both limbs) and unilateral (single limb) exercises in a program will ensure proper balance in the development of the body. Bilateral differences in muscle force production can be developed with one limb working harder on every repetition than the other, leading to an obvious force production deficit and imbalances between limbs. Unilateral exercises (e.g., dumbbell biceps curl) play an important role in helping maintain equal strength in both limbs.

Multijoint exercises require neural coordination among muscles and thus promote coordinated multijoint and multi-muscle group movements. Although multijoint exercises require a longer initial learning or neural phase than single-joint exercises (4), including multijoint exercises in a resistance training program is crucial, especially when whole-body strength movements are required for a particular activity. Multijoint exercises activate several different muscle groups at the same time and thus are time-efficient. Therefore, they can be especially useful for an individual or a team with a limited amount of time for each training session. Other benefits of multijoint exercises include enhanced hormonal response and greater metabolic demands. Be aware that many multijoint exercises, especially those with an explosive component, require advanced lifting techniques (e.g., power cleans, power snatches). These exercises need additional coaching, practice, and skill development beyond the basic movement patterns. Almost all sports and functional activities in everyday life (e.g., climbing stairs) depend on structural multijoint movements. Whole-body strength/power movements are the basis for success in most sports. Clearly, all running, jumping, or striking activities, as well sport-specific movements such as tackling in American football, a takedown in wrestling, or hitting a baseball, depend on whole-body strength/power movements. Thus, incorporating multijoint exercises in a resistance training program is important for all competitive or recreational athletes.

## Order of Exercises

The order in which exercises are performed is an important acute program variable that affects the quality and focus of the workout. ACSM recommends that by exercising the larger muscle groups first, a superior training stimulus is presented to all of the muscles involved (2).

Exercising the larger muscles first is thought to stimulate optimal neural, metabolic, endocrine, and circulatory responses, which may augment the training response to subsequent exercises later in the workout. This concept also applies to the sequencing of multijoint and single-joint exercises. The more complex multijoint technique-intensive exercises (*e.g.*, power cleans, squats) should be performed initially followed by the less complex single-joint exercises (*e.g.*, leg extension, biceps curls).

The rationale for this exercise sequencing recommendation is that the exercises performed in the beginning of the workout require the greatest amount of muscle mass and energy for optimal performance. This has been observed by Simão et al. (45,46), who found that performing exercises of both the large and the small muscle groups at the end of an exercise sequence resulted in significantly fewer repetitions in the three sets of an exercise in both men and women. This decrease in the number of repetitions performed was especially apparent in the third set when an exercise was performed last in an exercise sequence (45,46). These sequencing strategies focus on attaining a greater training effect for the large muscle group exercises. If multijoint exercises are performed early in the workout, more resistance can be used because of less fatigue in the smaller muscle groups that assist the prime movers during the multijoint exercises. Also, alternating upper and lower body exercises and/or pushing and pulling exercises allows more time for the assisting muscles to recover between exercises.

> If multijoint exercises are performed early in the workout, more resistance can be used because of less fatigue in the smaller muscle groups that assist the prime movers during the multijoint exercises.

Because the order of exercise affects the outcome of a training program, it is important to have the exercise order correspond to the specific training goals. In general, the sequence of exercises for both multiple and single muscle group exercise sessions should be as follows:

1. Large muscle group before small muscle group exercises
2. Multijoint before single-joint exercises
3. Alternate push/pull exercises for total body sessions
4. Alternate upper/lower body exercises for total body sessions
5. Explosive/power type lifts (*e.g.*, Olympic lifts) and plyometric exercises before basic strength and single-joint exercises
6. Exercises for priority weak areas before exercises for strong areas
7. Most intense to least intense (particularly when performing several exercises consecutively for the same muscle group)

## Resistance and Repetitions

The amount of resistance used for a specific exercise is one of the key variables in any resistance training program. The resistance is the major stimulus related to changes observed in measures of strength, hypertrophy, and local muscular endurance. When designing a resistance training program, the resistance for each exercise must be chosen carefully. The use of either repetition maximums (RMs) (the maximal load that can be lifted the specified number of repetitions) or the absolute resistance, which allows only a specific number of repetitions to be performed, is the easiest method for determining resistance. Typically, a single training RM target (*e.g.*, 10 RM) or an RM target range (*e.g.*, 3–5 RM) is used. The absolute resistance is then adjusted to match the changes in strength over the training program. Every set is done until failure (*e.g.*, momentary muscular fatigue) to ensure that the resistance used corresponds to the prescribed number of repetitions. This is because performing 3–5 repetitions with a resistance that allows for only 3–5 repetitions produces very different results than performing 13–15 repetitions using a resistance that would allow for only 13–15 repetitions.

> When designing a resistance training program, the resistance for each exercise must be chosen carefully.

Another method of determining resistances for an exercise involves using a percentage of the 1-RM (*e.g.*, 70% or 85% of the 1-RM). If the client's 1-RM for an exercise is 200 lb (90.9 kg), a 70% resistance would be 140 lb (63.6 kg). This method requires that the maximal strength in all exercises used in the training program must be evaluated regularly. In some exercises, percentage of 1-RM needs to be used, as going to failure or near-failure is not practical (*e.g.*, power cleans, Olympic-style lifts). Without regular 1-RM testing (*e.g.*, each week), the percentage of 1-RM actually used during training, especially at the beginning of a program, will decrease, and the training intensity will be reduced. From a practical perspective, the use of percentages of 1-RM as the resistance for many exercises may not be administratively effective because of the amount of testing time required. In addition, for beginners, the reliability of a 1-RM test can be poor. Instead, by using the RM target or RM target range, the Personal Trainer has the ability to alter the resistance in response to changes in the number of repetitions that can be performed at a given absolute resistance.

As is the case for any of the acute program variables, the loading intensity should depend on the goal and training status of the client. The intensity of the loading (as a percentage of 1-RM) has an effect on the number of repetitions that can be performed, and vice versa. The number of repetitions that can be performed at a given intensity ultimately determines the effects of training on strength development (12,13). If a given absolute resistance allows a specific number of repetitions (defined as the RM), then any reductions in the number of repetitions without an increase in the resistance will cause a change in the training stimulus. In this case, the change in the stimulus will lead to a change in the motor units recruited to perform the exercise and thus the neuromuscular adaptations. Differences exist between free weights and machines for percentage of RM used. For example, in a squat exercise, one may be able to perform only 8–10 repetitions, whereas in the leg press, 15–20 repetitions are possible. Differences exist related to the amount of balance and control that is needed in the exercise and the size of the muscle groups. For example, free-weight exercises require more neural control and activation of assistance muscles; also as the muscle group gets smaller, the magnitude of the response to a given percentage of the 1-RM is reduced.

The neuromuscular adaptations to resistance training depend on the amount and modality of resistance used. These adaptations follow the SAID principle presented earlier in this chapter. Compared with lower resistances, heavier resistances will allow lower numbers of repetitions (1–6) but will lead to greater improvements in maximal strength (2,47). Thus, if maximal strength development is desired, heavier loads should be used. Alternately, if muscular endurance is the goal, a lower load should be used, which will in turn allow a greater number of repetitions (12–15 RM) to be conveyed (2,45). Alternately, adaptations specific to muscular hypertrophy necessitate a differential training style. A recent review of the literature recommends a range of approximately 6–12 repetitions to optimize metabolic stress leading to hypertrophic adaptations (44) (see Tables 14.1, 14.2, and 14.3 for more information relative to the guidelines set for by ACSM with regard to intensity of training.)

## Number of Days per Week of Training (Frequency)

Frequency of training (*i.e.*, number of days per week) is another program variable that needs to be determined when developing an optimal resistance exercise program. Factors such as desired outcome, training status, competition season (for athletes), and type of training session (full-body or split routine) are a few of the variables that should be considered when developing the frequency recommendations of a resistance training program.

When health-related benefits are the desired outcome for the program, ACSM has proposed that 2–3 days per week using a full-body resistance training program are sufficient. However, additional training days may be necessary for intermediate (4–5 d $\cdot$ wk$^{-1}$) and advanced trained individuals (4–6 d $\cdot$ wk$^{-1}$) for continued strength related gains. There are additional recommendations for frequency of training when hypertrophic, muscular endurance, power, or motor adaptations are

## Table 14.1 ACSM Recommendations for Muscular Strength (1,2)

### Novice and Intermediate Individuals

| | |
|---|---|
| Volume | 1–3 sets per exercise |
| Intensity | 60%–70% 1-RM<br>8–12 reps |
| Rest period | 2–3 min between sets for core lifts<br>1–2 min for assistance exercises |
| Frequency | Novice: 2–3 d · wk$^{-1}$<br>Intermediate: 3–4 d · wk$^{-1}$ |

### Advanced Individuals

| | |
|---|---|
| Volume | Multiple set programs with systematic variations in volume and intensity |
| Intensity | Cycling load of 80%–100% 1-RM<br>Progressing to heavy loads 1–6 reps |
| Rest period | 2–3 min between sets for core lifts<br>1–2 min for assistance exercises<br>Extended rest periods may be necessary |
| Frequency | 4–6 d · wk$^{-1}$ |

Data from American College of Sports Medicine. *ACSM's Guidelines for Exercise Testing and Prescription.* 10th ed. Philadelphia (PA): Wolters Kluwer; 2018, and American College of Sports Medicine. American College of Sports Medicine position stand. Progression models in resistance training for healthy adults. *Med Sci Sports Exerc.* 2009;41(3):687–708.

## Table 14.2 ACSM Recommendations for Muscular Hypertrophy (1,2)

### Novice and Intermediate Individuals

| | |
|---|---|
| Volume | 1–3 sets per exercise |
| Intensity | 70%–85% 1-RM<br>8–12 reps |
| Rest period | 1–2 min |
| Frequency | Novice: 2–3 d · wk$^{-1}$<br>Intermediate: up to 4 d · wk$^{-1}$ for split routines |

### Advanced Individuals

| | |
|---|---|
| Volume | 3–6 sets per exercise in a periodized manner |
| Intensity | 70%–100% 1-RM be used<br>1–12 reps per set<br>6–12 reps for the majority |
| Rest period | 2–3 min for heavy loading<br>1–2 min moderate to moderate–high intensity |
| Frequency | 4–6 d · wk$^{-1}$ |

Data from American College of Sports Medicine. *ACSM's Guidelines for Exercise Testing and Prescription.* 10th ed. Philadelphia (PA): Wolters Kluwer; 2018, and American College of Sports Medicine. American College of Sports Medicine position stand. Progression models in resistance training for healthy adults. *Med Sci Sports Exerc.* 2009;41(3):687–708.

| Table 14.3 | ACSM Recommendations for Muscular Power (1,2) |
|---|---|
| **Novice and Intermediate Individuals** | |
| Volume | 1–3 sets per exercise |
| Intensity | Light to moderate load<br>30%–60% of 1-RM for upper body exercises<br>0%–60% of 1-RM for lower body exercises<br>3–6 repetitions not to failure |
| Rest period | 2–3 min between sets for primary exercises when intensity is high<br>1–2 min for assistance exercises or lower intensity exercises |
| Frequency | Novice: 2–3 d · wk$^{-1}$<br>Intermediate: 3–4 d · wk$^{-1}$ |
| **Advanced Individuals** | |
| Volume | 3–6 sets per exercise |
| Intensity | Heavy loading<br>85%–100% of 1-RM (necessary for increasing force)<br>Light to moderate loading<br>30%–60% of 1-RM for upper body exercises<br>0%–60% of 1-RM for lower body exercises<br>Performed at an explosive velocity<br>1–6 reps in a periodized manner |
| Rest period | 2–3 min between sets for primary exercises when intensity is high<br>1–2 min for assistance exercises or lower intensity exercises |
| Frequency | 4–5 d · wk$^{-1}$ |

Data from American College of Sports Medicine. *ACSM's Guidelines for Exercise Testing and Prescription.* 10th ed. Philadelphia (PA): Wolters Kluwer; 2018, and American College of Sports Medicine. American College of Sports Medicine position stand. Progression models in resistance training for healthy adults. *Med Sci Sports Exerc.* 2009;41(3):687–708.

the desired outcome (2). Tables 14.1, 14.2, and 14.3 provide more information on the training frequency recommendations for differential program variables.

## Number of Sets for Each Exercise

The number of sets does not have to be the same for all exercises in a workout program. For resistance-trained individuals, multiple-set programs have been found to be superior for strength, power, hypertrophy, and high-intensity endurance improvements (27,31). Additionally, recent meta-analytic research has shown a dose-response relationship between set number and muscular strength and hypertrophy (28,29,36). These findings have prompted support from ACSM for periodized multiple-set programs when long-term progression (not maintenance) is the goal (2). Both single- and multiset programs appear to be effective for increasing strength in untrained clients during short-term training periods (*i.e.*, 6–12 wk). However, multiple-set programs are superior for long-term progression. Single-set programs are effective for developing and maintaining a certain level of muscular strength and endurance. For some fitness enthusiasts, this level of muscular fitness may be adequate. Also, one-set programs sometimes result in greater compliance by those who are limited in their time for exercise and also need to perform cardiovascular exercise, flexibility exercise, and so on. Having a client do one set is better than no sets at all. However, no study has shown single-set training to be superior to multiple-set training in either trained or untrained individuals.

The number of sets is one of the critical variables in the exercise volume equation (*e.g.*, volume = sets × reps × resistance). The principle of variation in training or, more specifically, "periodized training" involves the number of sets and volume performed. Exercise volume is a vital concept in resistance training progression, especially for those who have already achieved a basic level of training or strength fitness. Some short-term studies (2,47) and most long-term studies (2,47) support the contention that the greater training stimulus associated with the higher volume from multiple sets is needed to create further improvement and progression in physical adaptation and performance. Meta-analytic research has shown that as experience in training increases, the need for greater volumes of training also increases (28,29,36). Use of a constant-volume program can lead to staleness and lack of adherence to training. Making variations in training volume (*i.e.*, both low- and high-volume exercise protocols) are critical during a long-term training program to continue to provide appropriate overload stimulus, yet also to provide adequate rest and recovery periods. This concept is addressed later in this chapter under "periodization of exercise." Please see Tables 14.1, 14.2, and 14.3 for more information on training recommendations from ACSM.

> The number of sets performed for each exercise is one variable in what is referred to as the volume of exercise equation (*e.g.*, sets × reps × resistance) calculation.

## Duration of Rest Period between Sets and Exercises

The rest periods play an important role in dictating the metabolic stress of the workout and influence the amount of resistance that can be used during each set or exercise. A major reason for this is that the primary energy system used during resistance exercise, the ATP–CP system, needs to be replenished, and this process takes time (see Chapter 5). Therefore, the duration of the rest period significantly influences the metabolic, hormonal, and cardiovascular responses to a short-term bout of resistance exercise as well as the performance of subsequent sets (24,25). For advanced training emphasizing absolute strength, rest periods of at least 2–3 minutes (with the possibility of extended rest periods as long as 3–5 min) are recommended for primary, large muscle mass multijoint exercises (such as squat or dead lift), whereas shorter rest may be sufficient for assistant, smaller muscle mass single-joint exercises (2). For novice-to-intermediate resistance exercise protocols, rest periods of 2–3 minutes may suffice for large muscle mass multijoint exercises because the lower absolute resistance used at this training level seems to be less stressful to the neuromuscular system. Performance of maximal resistance exercises requires maximal energy substrate availability at the onset of the exercise and thus requires relatively long rest periods between sets and exercises.

> The duration of the rest period significantly influences the metabolic, hormonal, and cardiovascular responses to a short-term bout of resistance exercise as well as the performance of subsequent sets (24,25).

Based on a recent review, a minimum of 3 minutes rest is recommended when training for muscular power (*e.g.*, plyometric jumps) due to the need to perform maximal effort movements (51). Alternately, when training for muscular hypertrophy, shorter rest intervals of 30–60 seconds between sets is advocated. The shorter rest interval stimulates greater hormonal activity associated with a hypertrophic effect (51).

Resistance training that stresses both the glycolytic and ATP–CP energy systems appears to be superior in enhancing muscle hypertrophy (*e.g.*, bodybuilding); thus, less rest between sets appears to be more effective in high levels of muscular definition. If the goal is to optimize both strength and muscle mass, both long rest with heavy loading and short rest with moderate loading types of workout protocols should be included. However, it should be kept in mind that short-rest resistance training programs can potentially cause greater psychological anxiety and fatigue because of the greater discomfort, muscle fatigue, and high metabolic demands of the program (48). Therefore, psychological ramifications of using short-rest workouts must be carefully considered and discussed with the client before the training program is designed. The increase in anxiety appears to be associated with the high metabolic demands found with short-rest exercise protocols (*i.e.*, 1 min or less). Despite the high psychological demands, the changes in mood states do not constitute abnormal psychological changes and may be a part of the normal arousal process before a demanding workout.

The key to determining optimal rest-period lengths is to observe the client. Symptoms of loss of force production in the beginning of the workout and clinical symptoms of nausea, dizziness, and fainting are clear signs of the inability to tolerate the workout. When such symptoms occur, the workout should be stopped and longer rest periods used in subsequent workouts. With aging, rest periods need to be carefully heeded. Aging decreases the ability to tolerate changes in muscle and blood pH and underscores the need for gradual progression of cutting rest period lengths between sets and exercises (24). Typical rest periods are characterized as

- Very short rest periods: 1 minute or shorter
- Short rest periods: 1–2 minutes
- Moderate rest periods: 2–3 minutes
- Long rest periods: 3–4 minutes
- Very long rest periods: 5 minutes or longer

The heavier the resistance, the more rest that should be allowed between sets and exercises. Also, more rest allows for a greater number of repetitions to be performed at a specific RM load (17,25,51). The gradual use of shorter rest periods stimulates improvements in the body's blood bicarbonate and intramuscular buffering systems (17,25) (see Tables 14.1, 14.2, and 14.3 for the recommended rest period intervals set forth by ACSM).

# Variation of Acute Program Variables

As long as the demands placed on the neuromuscular system are similar, the acute program variables can be manipulated in various ways to develop different workouts for the single-exercise sessions used over time. The number of sets, number of repetitions, relative resistance used, and rest periods do not have to be the same for each exercise in a session. They can be varied either within an exercise or, more frequently, between different exercises in an exercise protocol. The use of light exercise levels can be used when it is necessary to rest higher threshold motor units (*i.e.*, motor neuron and associated muscle fibers). Motor recruitment follows a "size principle." Because not all motor units are recruited with each resistance loading or contraction of a muscle, different loadings can result in varying amounts and types of muscle tissue being used. Heavier loads with adequate volume recruit more muscle tissue than high repetitions of lower load levels (8). Understanding and using the size principle is vital for developing variation in resistance training and ultimately periodized training.

## Muscle Actions

Muscles produce force while performing one of three different actions:

1. When sufficient force is produced to overcome the external load and shorten the muscle, the muscle action is termed a *concentric muscular action* or *contraction*.
2. When the muscle produces force but there is no change in the length of the muscle, the muscular action is termed an *isometric muscular action*.
3. When the production of force occurs while the muscle is lengthening (*i.e.*, resisting the movement), the muscular action is termed an *eccentric muscular action*.

In the past, the term *contraction* was used for each of the three muscle actions; however, only concentric muscle actions actually involve a classic muscle shortening or true contraction. Any exercise can include any combination of the three muscle actions; however, most exercises are performed using either isometric muscle action or both concentric and eccentric muscle actions. However, the most effective training programs appear to use concentric–eccentric repetitions (7). The skeletal muscle force–velocity relationship patterns encompass high- to low-speed eccentric muscle actions, maximal isometric muscle actions, and slow- to high-velocity concentric muscle actions, creating a descending hierarchy of force productions.

> The most effective training programs appear to use concentric–eccentric repetitions (7).

## True Repetition and Range of Movement

Muscle actions involving movement of a joint are termed *dynamic*, and thus, exercises involving joint movements are called dynamic exercises. A full-range dynamic exercise usually contains both a concentric phase and an eccentric phase. The order of the phases depends on the choice of exercise. A squat, for example, starts with the eccentric phase, whereas a pull-up normally starts with the concentric phase. It is important to perform the exercise so that the joints involved move through a full ROM. This is especially true for single-joint exercises. For example, in the arm curl, a full repetition should start with the elbow almost completely extended, progress until the elbow is maximally flexed, and finish with the elbow almost completely extended again. By using the whole ROM, the whole length of the muscle is stimulated, leading to adaptations throughout the whole muscle. However, ROM may need to be carefully monitored and perhaps restricted when working with clients who have orthopedic injuries or limitations or anatomical joint laxity such as in the knee, elbow, or shoulder.

# Periodization of Exercise

Periodization is a concept that is applied in the design of workouts used in an exercise program (33). Periodization refers to systematic variation in acute program variables such as the prescribed volume and intensity during different phases of a resistance training program. A traditional linear periodization program contains four phases:

1. Hypertrophy phase, consisting of high volume and short rest periods
2. Strength/power phase, consisting of reduced volume but increased load and rest periods
3. Peaking phase, consisting of low volume but high load and longer rest periods
4. Recovery phase, consisting of low volume and load

> Periodization refers to systematic variation in the prescribed volume and intensity during different phases of a resistance training program.

There is no set formula for how a program should be periodized because it depends on the specific goals and needs of the client (38). Table 14.4 presents an example of a traditional four-phase periodized training program aimed at producing maximal strength.

Periodization acts as a way to systematically vary the workout over time. Incorporating periodization into the training program systematically varies the acute program variables, which exposes muscles to different stimuli, leading to greater muscular adaptation and performance. In addition, rest is encouraged at different points in the training program, which allows for appropriate recovery and the prevention of both short- and long-term overtraining. Another important benefit to periodization is that it can reduce the potential boredom found with repeating the same resistance exercise program over and over again which may improve program adherence. Many different models for periodization have been developed. Thus, the model to be used should be selected on the basis of the needs and desires of the client.

| Table 14.4 | Traditional American-Style Periodization Schedule | | | |
| --- | --- | --- | --- | --- |
| Goal | Hypertrophy | Maximal Strength/Power | Peak | Recovery |
| Repetitions | High | Moderate–low | Low | Moderate |
| Sets | High | Moderate | Low | Moderate |
| Rest | Short | Moderate | Long | Moderate |
| Load | Low | Moderate | Very high | Low |
| Volume | High–moderate | Moderate | Low | Low |

The terms *micro-*, *meso-*, and *macrocycle* refer to the time course of the different phases of periodization. The macrocycle is the largest training cycle time frame. A common example of a macrocycle is a calendar year, and all phases are included in this cycle. A mesocycle refers to the next smaller group of training cycles that make up the macrocycle, usually four to six in a year. Finally, the microcycle is the smallest component, which usually ranges in time from 1 to 4 weeks and is typically dedicated to one type of workout variable in that phase (*e.g.*, high-volume, low-intensity power).

The use of periodized resistance training has been shown to be superior to constant training methods (27). Periodized training involves the planned variation in the intensity of exercises and in the volume of a workout. Typically, one periodizes large muscle group exercises. However, periodization schemes can be created for smaller muscle groups as well. Although opinions among trainers differ regarding the number and time course of the cycles that are most effective, a primary theory suggests that a greater variation in the training stimulus will produce greater overall adaptations in the body. This idea has led to different variations in the classic periodization model. In general, there are two basic types that have been developed for maximal strength development: linear and nonlinear periodized protocols.

## Linear Periodization

Classic periodization methods use a progressive increase in the intensity with small variations in each 1- to 4-week microcycle. An example of a classic 16-week, four-cycle linear periodized program is presented in Table 14.5.

Although there are some variations within each microcycle, the general trend for the 16-week program is a steady linear increase in the intensity of the training program. Microcycle 5 is a 2-week active rest period in which no lifting is done or only a very light, low-volume training is used prior to the next mesocycle. Because of the straight-line increase in the intensity of the program, it has been termed "linear" periodized training. Linear periodization originally evolved from training

> Classic periodization methods use a progressive increase in the intensity with small variations in each 1- to 4-week microcycle.

| Table 14.5 | An Example of a Classic Linear Periodized Program Using 4-Week Microcycles | | | |
| --- | --- | --- | --- | --- |
| Microcycle 1 (4 wk) | Microcycle 2 (4 wk) | Microcycle 3 (4 wk) | Microcycle 4 (4 wk) | Microcycle 5 (2 wk) |
| 3–5 sets of 12–15 RM | 4–5 sets of 8–10 RM | 3–4 sets of 4–6 RM | 3–5 sets of 1–3 RM | Active rest/recovery |

for single-peak performance events (*e.g.*, track and field, weightlifting). Thus, consecutive or linear buildup in the training intensity to the peak was used.

The volume of the training program in the classic periodization program will gradually decrease in concert with an increase in intensity. The volume–intensity trade-off can be lessened as an individual improves training status. In other words, advanced athletes can tolerate higher volumes of exercise during heavy and very heavy microcycles. A meta-analysis of the research has shown that progressing to an average of eight sets per muscle group is the optimal dose needed to stimulate muscular strength adaptations in muscular strength in advanced lifters as compared to an average of three sets per muscle group for beginners and four sets for intermediate lifters (36).

One must be very careful not to train with high volumes and heavy weights too quickly; monitor the stress of the workouts and the total conditioning program. Pushing too hard has the potential for creating a serious overtraining syndrome. Overtraining can compromise progress for weeks or even months. Although it takes a great deal of excessive work to produce this type of overtraining effect, highly motivated individuals can easily make these mistakes out of sheer desire to make gains and see rapid progress in their training.

The idea of high-volume exercise in the early microcycles is that it may promote the muscle hypertrophy needed to eventually enhance strength in the later phases of training. Thus, the later cycles of training are dependent on the early cycles of training. Programs that attempt to gain strength without developing the needed hypertrophy of muscle tissue are limited in their potential.

The increases in the intensity of the periodized program allows for development of the needed nervous system adaptations for enhanced motor unit recruitment. As the program progresses, the heavier weights require that higher threshold motor units become involved in the force production process. The subsequent increase in muscle protein from the early cycle training enhances force production from the motor units. Thus, it is clear to see how the different parts of the 16-week training program are integrated.

One mesocycle is the completion of all of the cycles in this 16-week program. A year training program (macrocycle) is made up of several mesocycles. Multiple and short mesocycles allow for delineating different trainable features of muscle. In theory, each mesocycle can progress the body's musculature upward toward one's genetic limitations. Thus, the theoretical basis for a linear method of periodization consists of developing the body with a sequential loading from light to heavy and from high volume to low volume, thereby addressing the goals of the program for that training cycle while providing active rest at the completion of the mesocycle. This is repeated again and again with each mesocycle, and progress is made in the training program over an entire macrocycle.

## Reverse Linear Programs

A twist on traditional linear periodization is termed *reverse linear periodization*. As the name states, it is a technique that follows the tenants of linear periodization for volume and strength; however, it is in the reverse order. One study has shown that this type of periodization is beneficial when muscular endurance is the primary program outcome (42).

## Nonlinear Periodized Programs

More recently, the concept of nonlinear periodized training programs (also called daily undulating periodization or DUP) has been developed to maintain variation in the training stimulus (39,41). Nonlinear periodized training enhances program implementation because it is flexible and can accommodate schedule, business, or competitive demands placed on the individual. The nonlinear program allows variation in the intensity and volume within each week over the course of the training program (*e.g.*, 12 wk). Active rest is then taken after the 12-week mesocycle.

The nonlinear program allows variation in the intensity and volume within each week over the course of the training program (*e.g.*, 12 wk).

| Table 14.6 | An Example of a Nonlinear Periodized Training Protocol[a] | | |
|---|---|---|---|
| **Monday** | **Wednesday** | **Friday** | **Monday** |
| 1 set 12–15 RM | 3 sets of 8–10 RM | 4 sets of 4–6 RM | Power day 6 sets of 3 at 30%–45% of 1-RM using power exercises (*e.g.*, hang pulls) or plyometrics |

[a]This protocol uses a 4-day rotation with 1-day rest between workouts.

The change in the intensity and volume of training will vary within the cycle, which could be 7–14 days. An example of a nonlinear periodized training program over a 12-week mesocycle is shown in Table 14.6.

Recent research has shown that nonlinear periodized training can have similar or greater beneficial effects on resistance training outcomes when compared with traditional linear periodization. Rhea and colleagues (41) showed the nonlinear periodization training elicited a greater percentage of strength gains as compared with linear training. Additionally, Prestes and colleagues (40) found that undulating periodization induces greater increases in maximal strength as compared with linear periodization. These studies suggest that daily variations in the undulation training had a superior effect on maximizing strength as compared with weekly or monthly variation.

One of the theorized reasons for the success of nonlinear periodization is that unlike linear programs, the different components of muscle size, strength, and power are trained with the goal of attempting to train different features of muscle within the same time frame (*e.g.*, hypertrophy and power and strength). Thus, an individual stimulates multiple physiological adaptations within the same 7- to 10-day period of the 12-week mesocycle.

Often, busy travel, school, or competition schedules conflict with time requirements of traditional training program. A DUP program is highly adaptable to variations in a client's schedule. This type of training model may enhance adherence as it may "fit" the client's schedule better than the traditional linear method. Additionally, constantly altering program variables keeps the program interesting and challenging for clients, thereby reducing the boredom of repeating the same program. Theoretically, a DUP program can be different with each and every training session. Because the workouts are not linear, the different workouts change with different training sessions. If the Monday workout is missed, the rotation is just changed. For example, if a client misses a workout scheduled for Monday, with DUP, that workout is performed on the next training day and the sequence is continued. In this way, no workout stimulus is missed in the training program. With a DUP type program, any mesocycle will be completed when a certain number of workouts are completed (*e.g.*, 48) rather than counting the completion of a set number of weeks.

> With a nonlinear periodization or DUP type program, any mesocycle will be completed when a certain number of workouts are completed (*e.g.*, 48) rather than counting the completion of a set number of weeks.

## Unplanned/Flexible Nonlinear Periodized Programs

One of the new advances in periodization is called "unplanned nonlinear periodization." The name is somewhat of a misnomer, as an overall plan is developed for a 12-week mesocycle, but the actual day that a given workout will be performed is based on the readiness to train. Thus, it is also termed "flexible nonlinear periodization." In unplanned or flexible nonlinear periodization, a workout plan is set for the mesocycle but deciding what workout is to be done on what day is left to the Personal Trainer, who will base it on the client's fatigue level, psychological state, or fitness, to use only the most optimal workout that can be performed on a given day. In this model, the training session category (*e.g.*, light, moderate, power, or heavy) is prescribed on the basis of the physiological ability or state of the client at the time of the session. Thus, if the client is very fatigued before a particular exercise session, some workouts would not be prescribed. For example, a power training or plyometrics training day or a high-volume, low-rest training day would not be a good choice because fatigue would reduce the workout quality. After a specific workout is completed, it is checked off in the major planning matrix for the 12-week mesocycle. Again, the goal for any mesocycle in this type of nonlinear periodization program is to complete each planned workout rather than "x" number of weeks.

In any periodization model, it is the primary exercises that are typically periodized, but one can also use a two-cycle periodization program to vary the small muscle group exercises. For example, in the "triceps pushdown" one could rotate between the moderate (8–10 RM) and the heavy (4–6 RM) cycle intensities. This would provide not only the hypertrophy needed for such isolated muscles of a joint but also the strength needed to support heavier workouts of the large muscle groups.

In summary, different approaches can be used to periodize a resistance training program. Programs can be linear, reverse linear, nonlinear "daily undulating," or unplanned/flexible nonlinear schedules. Periodized programs are more effective than constant-intensity training programs for increasing strength. Effective periodization is accomplished by melding specific program goals (strength, hypertrophy, muscular endurance, or some combination) with appropriate variations in volume–intensity and frequency of training. The key to workout success is variation, and different periodization approaches can be used to accomplish this training need.

> Effective periodization is accomplished by melding specific program goals (strength, hypertrophy, muscular endurance, or some combination) with appropriate variations in volume–intensity and frequency of training.

## Progression from Beginner to Advanced

The level of fitness and resistance training experience of the client is perhaps the most important factor to be considered when designing a resistance training program. Resistance exercise can place a large stress on the body, and certain exercises require high levels of skill to avoid injury. Thus, exercise technique is the most important aspect of resistance training for beginners. At the beginning of the training program, correct technique should be significantly emphasized, and the resistance and volume should be kept low.

> Resistance exercise can place a large stress on the body, and certain exercises require a high level of technique to avoid injury.

From a short-term performance-enhancement point of view, a single set per exercise may be enough for beginners to achieve the stimulus needed from an exercise. However, depending on the individual, multiple sets, even for beginners may be beneficial (2,28,31,41). Some studies have found that multiple sets even for beginners create larger improvements than single sets, whereas no study has found that single sets are superior (2,36,41). One reason for this is that more repetitions can lead to faster improvements in exercise technique, especially for multijoint exercises. The squat exercise is an example of an exercise that requires a great deal of technique to be performed correctly. Thus, only doing one set of a few squats does not allow the client many practice trials of this complex movement.

There is a dose-response relationship with progressive resistance training. As a person becomes accustomed to a given stimulus or dose of exercise, additional stress is needed to elicit the given response or increase in strength, muscular endurance, hypertrophy, power, or all four.

As the client progresses past the initial few months of training, multisets should be used for each exercise session. As the skill and experience level of the client improves, more technical exercises can be taught. Advanced resistance training can include highly technical exercises such as the clean or the snatch as well as advanced modalities such as plyometric exercises. The progression will differ among individuals, and the Personal Trainer must evaluate each client extensively and continuously before including more advanced exercises, to ensure that the exercises match the client's skill and experience level.

## Client Interactions

As a Personal Trainer working with clients, it is important to encourage and motivate them as well as to provide innovative, optimal, individualized resistance training programs. Clients hire Personal Trainers for a variety of reasons. Many clients hire Personal Trainers because they feel they need constant guidance. In addition, Personal Trainers provide them with a support system. Most importantly, clients desire to hire professionals with training and knowledge in conditioning science. They want a professional to help them perform exercises properly and who understands exercise prescription to allow them to achieve their personal goals and objectives. For some clients, it is an important part of their sports conditioning program. Ultimately, the Personal Trainer must form a special relationship with each and every client that is based on professionalism, trust, and openness (Fig. 14.4).

> Personal trainers should convey the specific benefits of resistance training, including increases in strength, muscle mass, and bone mass, particularly to clients who may be skeptical about why resistance training is important.

Clients should feel that their Personal Trainer genuinely cares about them and is personally vested in helping them achieve their goals. Clients expect their Personal Trainer to be a source of knowledge and an educator. Clients expect their Personal Trainer to be able to explain things or answer the question "why?" Thus, clients appreciate having their Personal Trainer explain the reason they are doing a particular exercise or combination of sets and reps in their program. Personal training has been found to be superior to unsupervised training, even for people who understand resistance training (34).

Personal Trainers should convey the specific benefits of resistance training, including increases in strength, muscle mass, and bone mass, particularly to clients who may be skeptical about why resistance training is important. Some uneducated clients may have false impressions of the outcomes from resistance training or on how to go about attaining optimal gains. Some men may do too much of one exercise (*e.g.*, biceps curls) trying to get huge, thereby creating muscular imbalance or women may hold back from performing any heavy loading because of the "fear of getting big muscles." These mistakes may at best diminish the gains that could be realized with resistance training and at worse result in serious overtraining or acute injury.

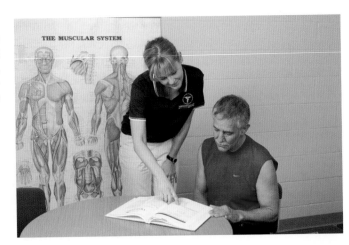

**FIGURE 14.4.** Having education and being a credible source of knowledge as a fitness expert is part of what Personal Trainers must provide to their clients. This takes continual study and preparation to stay current and up-to-date on basic topics and hot topics of the day.

Clients consider Personal Trainers experts and will often want to hear their opinion on fads facing the fitness industry. Often, clients' knowledge of resistance training comes from infomercials or magazine advertisements. Personal Trainers need to stay up to date with the scientific literature in order to provide accurate information and current research to their clients. Additionally, Personal Trainers should develop a network of experts who can act as resources for when clients ask questions that the Personal Trainer does not know the answer. It is always best to admit you do not know the answer than conveying potentially incorrect information. Furthermore, because Personal Trainers are required to obtain continuing education credits to maintain their certifications, staying current is critical to success.

## Demonstration of Proper Lifting Technique

A key aspect in personal training is the ability to demonstrate a given lift or technique. Providing the client with a good visual representation of the lift will allow the client to then replicate the movement pattern. The Personal Trainer should demonstrate each lift with proper form with a verbal explanation of the lift or technique and then actually physically demonstrate proper form of the given lift.

## Spotting in Resistance Exercise

Resistance training often requires that the Personal Trainer have physical contact with the client to ensure correct positioning, fit and setup of a machine, and proper technique in both machine and free-weight exercises. Personal Trainers should take time to explain to clients the spotting procedures in resistance training and the level of physical interaction required. Always ask your clients before physically touching them to ensure that they are comfortable with it. For example, when performing elbow extension exercises, it is sometimes helpful for the Personal Trainer to place his or her hands on the client's elbows as a reminder to keep the elbow from pointing outward. In these cases, explain to the client, "I am going to put my hands on your elbows to remind you to keep them from pointing outward. is this okay with you?" In most cases, clients will have no problem with this physical contact, but it is always better to ask than to assume.

> Ask your clients before physically touching them to ensure that they are comfortable with it.

## Know Proper Spotting Technique

Good spotting technique is vital for a safe resistance training program. Personal Trainers must understand the movement technique of every exercise and how to position clients to get the proper anatomical positioning throughout the exercises. In addition, Personal Trainers need to know where to position themselves to spot appropriately for each exercise. The goal of correct spotting is to prevent injury. A lifter should always have an exercise spotted, and the Personal Trainer must mediate this process, alone or with additional help. A checklist for the Personal Trainer is the following:

1. Know proper exercise technique.
2. Know proper spotting technique.
3. Be sure you are strong enough to assist the lifter with the resistance being used or get help.
4. Know how many repetitions the lifter intends to do.
5. Be attentive to the lifter at all times.
6. Stop lifters if exercise technique is incorrect or they break form.
7. Know the plan of action if a serious injury occurs.

## Resistance Exercises

A large number of resistance exercises can be used in a program. It is beyond the scope of this chapter to go through each and every exercise. The reader is referred to a comprehensive list of more than 125 exercise descriptions of both machine and free-weight exercises along with spotting techniques by Kraemer and Fleck (20). Each program should be designed on the basis of the principles outlined in this chapter. Periodization is very important, and many Personal Trainers are now using nonlinear methods to keep the clients interested and the programs effective (21). Free weights and machines can be used for each exercise as well as bilateral and unilateral exercises. See Figures 14.5A to 14.5O for examples of 15 basic exercises: (A) squat, (B) supine leg press, (C) 45° leg press, (D) lunge, (E) leg extensions, (F) leg curls, (G) machine vertical bench press, (H) smith supine bench press, (I) free-weight supine bench press, (J) dumbbell bench press, (K) machine seated rows, (L) front lat pull-down, (M) dumbbell arm curls, (N) barbell arm curls, and (O) triceps push-down.

Visit thePoint to watch video 14.1, which demonstrates a body weight squat.

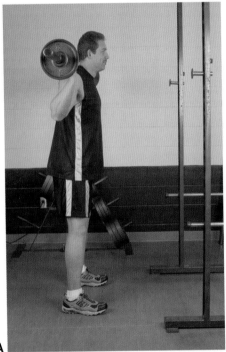
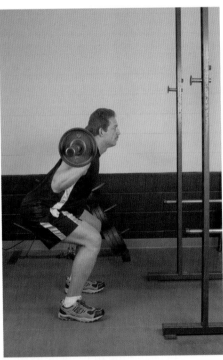

A

Start                          Finish

**FIGURE 14.5. A.** Back squat (thighs). Place the barbell on the back of the shoulders and grasp the barbell at the sides, with feet shoulder-width apart, toes slightly out. Dismount bar from rack. Descend until thighs are parallel to the floor and then extend the knees and hips until legs are straight, returning you to the starting position. Repeat for the appropriate number of repetitions. Keep the head forward with the chin level, back straight, and feet flat on the floor; keep equal distribution of weight throughout forefoot and heel and either squat within the power rack or have spotter(s).

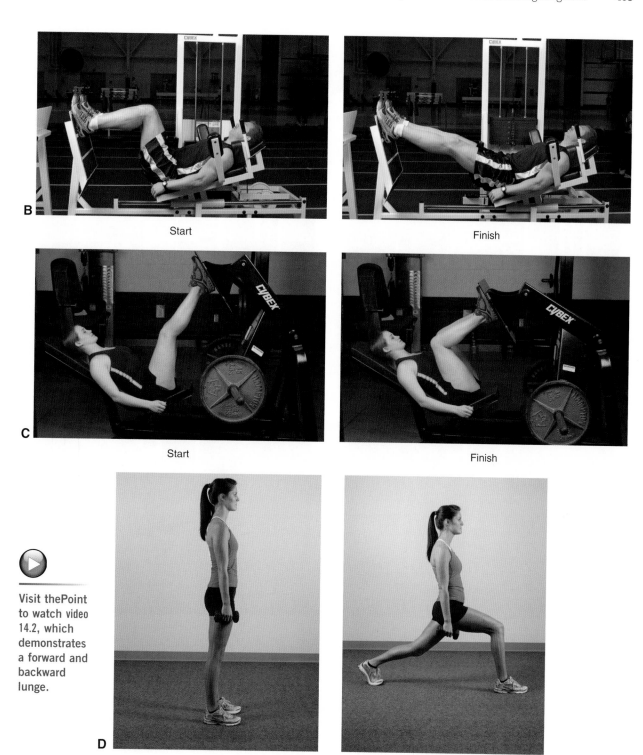

**Visit thePoint to watch video 14.2, which demonstrates a forward and backward lunge.**

**FIGURE 14.5.** (*Continued*) **B.** Supine leg press (thighs). Lie flat on the sled with shoulders against the pad. Place the feet on the platform, making sure that they are securely on the base plate. Extend the hips and knees. Flex the hips and knees until the knees are just short of complete flexion and return to the starting position to complete the repetition. Keep the feet flat on the platform and do not lock the knees. A full ROM should be used; keep the knees in the same direction as the feet. **C.** 45° leg press (thighs). Lie down on the machine with the back on the padded supports. Place the feet on the platform. Grasp the handles on the side and release the weight. Lower the weight by flexing the hips and knees until the hips are completely flexed and then extend the knees to complete the repetition. Make sure that the feet are flat on the platform and the knees track over the feet. **D.** Lunge (thighs, unilateral). Standing straight up with feet shoulder-width apart, stand holding the dumbbells at the sides. Lunge forward with one leg at a time, keeping the hips in the middle of the two legs, with the trailing knee just above the ground. Return to the standing position to complete the repetition and then repeat with the opposite leg. Keep the back straight and chin level with the ground.

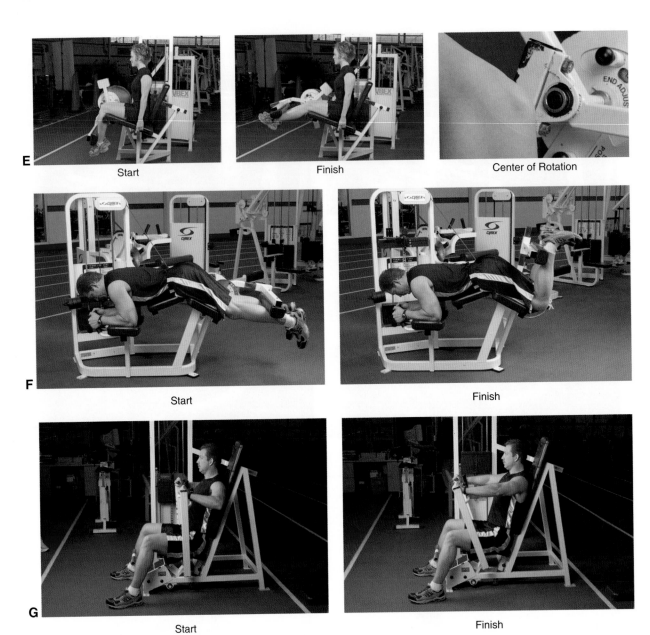

**FIGURE 14.5.** (*Continued*) **E.** Leg extensions (thighs, bilateral or unilateral). Sit on the machine with the back straight against the back pad or seat and grasp the handles on the side of the machine. Place the legs under the padded lever, making sure that they are positioned just above the ankles. Most machines will allow adjusting the length of the lever. Lift the lever until the legs are almost straight and return to the starting position to complete the repetition. It is important not to "rip" the plates off the stack, as this can add stress to the knees. This exercise can be done with a single leg (unilateral) or with both legs (bilateral). Make sure that the knees are aligned with the machine's center of rotation. **F.** Leg curls (hamstrings, bilateral or unilateral). Lying face down, grab the support handles in the front of the machine with the heels just beyond the edge of the lever pads. Lift the lever arm by flexing the knees until they are straight. Return to the starting position to complete the repetition. Keep the body on the bench and focus on moving only the legs. Many machines are angled so that the user is in a better position for the exercise movement to reduce stress on the lower back. Other forms of leg curls are standing and seated forms. This exercise can be done with a single leg (unilateral) or with both legs (bilateral). **G.** Vertical machine bench press (chest–triceps, bilateral). Sit on the seat, making sure that the line of the grips is just below the chest. The bar line should be an inch above the chest. Grasp the handles with an overhand grip and make sure that the feet are flat on the ground. Push the lever arm straight out until the elbows are straight. Return to the starting position to complete one repetition.

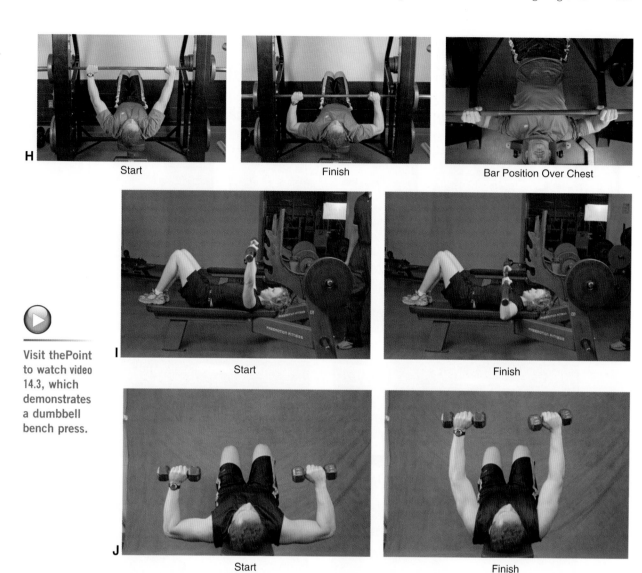

Visit thePoint to watch video 14.3, which demonstrates a dumbbell bench press.

**FIGURE 14.5.** (*Continued*) **H.** Smith supine bench press (chest–triceps, bilateral). Lie flat on the bench with the upper chest under the bar, as shown in the bar position figure above. Place the feet flat on the floor unless the bench is too high, in which case put them flat on the bench. Keep the shoulders and hips on the bench at all times during the lift. Grasp the bar with elbows at 45° angles. Disengage the bar hooks from the smith machine. Lower the weight to the chest and then press the bar up until arms are extended to complete the repetition. When completed, rehook the bar to the machine. **I.** Free-weight supine bench press (chest–triceps, bilateral). Lie flat on the bench with the upper chest under the bar, as shown in the bar position figure above. Place the feet flat on the floor unless the bench is too high, in which case put them flat on the bench. Keep the shoulders and hips on the bench at all times during the lift. Grasp the bar with elbows at 45° angles. Lower the weight to the chest and then press the bar up until the arms are extended to complete the repetition. When completed, rerack the bar with a spotter's help. **J.** Dumbbell bench press (chest–upper arms–triceps, unilateral). Start in a seated position on the bench with a dumbbell in each hand resting on the lower thigh. Lift the weights to the shoulder and lie back on the bench or have the spotter give you the dumbbells once you are in a position. Position the dumbbells to the side of the upper chest. Press the dumbbells up until the arms are extended and then return to complete a repetition. When completed, return to the seated position with the dumbbells on your thighs or have the spotter take the dumbbells. If heavy weights are used, two spotters may be necessary.

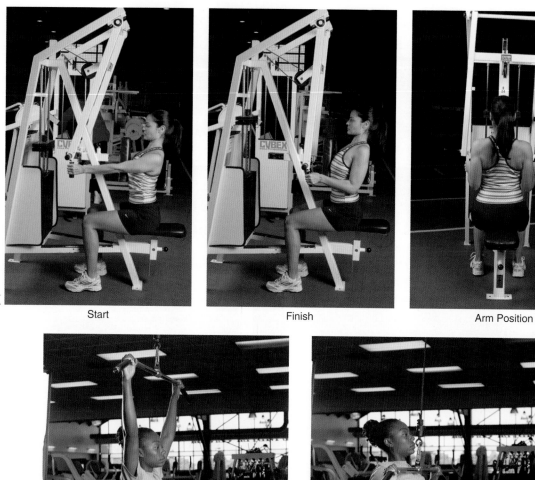

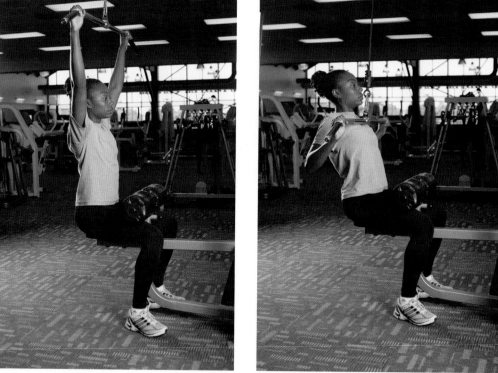

**FIGURE 14.5.** (*Continued*) **K.** Machine seated rows (upper back, bilateral). Take a seated position with the chest against the pad. Grasp the lever vertical handles with a vertical or horizontal overhand grip. Pull the lever back until the elbows are in line with the upper body and return to complete the repetition. Check the seat height so that the chest is directly in front of the lever handles and check whether the client is pulling in a straight line parallel to the ground. The client can use an overhand grip as a variation to the movement, using the other horizontal handles. **L.** Front lat pull-down (upper back, bilateral). Use a locked grip (thumb around the bar) and grasp the cable bar with a wide grip. Sit with thighs under machine support. Proceed to pull down the bar to the upper chest. Return to the starting position to complete the repetition.

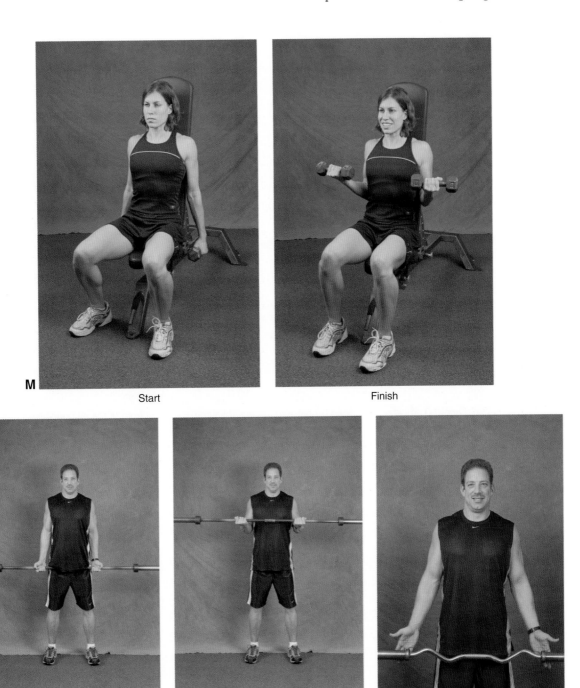

**FIGURE 14.5.** (*Continued*) **M.** Dumbbell arm curls (upper arm–biceps, unilateral). Take a seated position with two dumbbells held at the sides, with the palms facing in and the arms hanging straight down. Raise the dumbbells and rotate the forearm so that the palms face the shoulder. Lower to the original position to complete one repetition. One can also alternate one arm at a time. **N.** Barbell arm curls (upper arm–biceps, bilateral). In the standing position with the feet shoulder-width apart, grasp the straight barbell with an underhand grip and palms facing up. Raise the bar until the forearms are vertical and then lower the bar to the starting position to complete a repetition. One can also perform this exercise with an e-z bar with the palms facing inward.

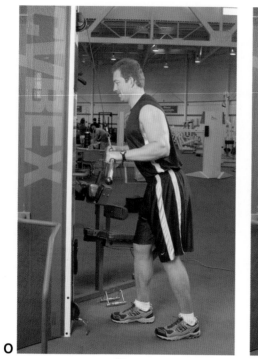
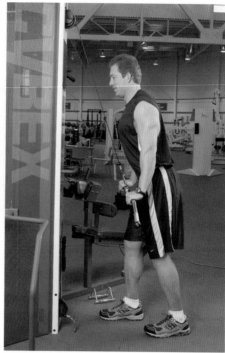

Start | Finish

**FIGURE 14.5.** (*Continued*) **O.** Triceps push-down (upper arm–triceps, bilateral). Stand in front of the lat pull station or high pulley station and take an overhand grasp on the bar with your elbows at the sides. Start at chest level and extend the arms down until straight and return to the starting position to complete the repetition. Position the hands above the bar prior to the push-down phase of the repetition. Other types of attachments also can be used (*e.g.*, rope, v-bar).

## SUMMARY

Development of a resistance training program is a systematic process in which science and art come together to allow the Personal Trainer to specifically address a client's needs for neuromuscular fitness. A sequence of events in the exercise prescription process consists of getting a client's medical clearance, personal training history, goal generation, a needs analysis, and a general preparation phase of initial training and testing before putting together workouts based on the acute program variables that will be used in a resistance training program. This program is then updated and revised with the same process over time. Education, client interactions, and motivation are vital components of successful resistance training programs that meet each client's goals and objectives.

## REFERENCES

1. American College of Sports Medicine. *ACSM's Guidelines for Exercise Testing and Prescription*. 10th ed. Philadelphia (PA): Wolters Kluwer; 2018.
2. American College of Sports Medicine. American College of Sports Medicine Position Stand. Progression models in resistance training for healthy adults. *Med Sci Sports Exerc.* 2009;41(3):687–708.
3. Cheung K, Hume P, Maxwell L. Delayed onset muscle soreness: treatment strategies and performance factors. *Sports Med.* 2003;33(2):145–64.
4. Chilibeck P, Calder A, Sale D, Webber C. A comparison of strength and muscle mass increases during resistance training in young women. *Eur J Appl Physiol Occup Physiol.* 1998;77(1–2):170–5.

5. Delorme TL. Restoration of muscle power by heavy resistance exercises. *J Bone Joint Surg*. 1945;27:645–667.

6. Delorme TL, Watkins AL. Techniques of progressive resistance exercise. *Arch Phys Med*. 1948;29:263–73.

7. Dudley GA, Tesch PA, Miller BJ, Buchanan P. Importance of eccentric actions in performance adaptations to resistance training. *Aviat Space Environ Med*. 1991;62(6):543–50.

8. Fleck SJ, Kraemer WJ. *Designing Resistance Training Programs*. 3rd ed. Champaign (IL): Human Kinetics; 2004. 392 p.

9. Fleck SJ, Schutt RC. Types of strength training. *Clin Sports Med*. 1985;4:159–69.

10. Harman E. Resistive torque analysis of 5 nautilus exercise machines. *Med Sci Sports Exerc*. 1983;15:113.

11. Hickson JF, Bruno MJ, Wilmore JH, Constable SH. Energy cost of weight training exercise. *Natl Strength Cond Assoc J*. 1984;6:522–3.

12. Hoeger WWK, Barette SL, Hale DF, Hopkins DR. Relationship between repetitions and selected percentages of one repetition maximum. *J Appl Sport Sci Res*. 1990;4(2): 47–54.

13. Hoeger WWK, Hopkins DR, Barette SL, Hale DF. Relationship between repetitions and selected percentages of one repetition maximum: a comparison between untrained and trained males and females. *J Appl Sport Sci Res*. 1987;1(1):1–13.

14. Johnson JH, Colodny S, Jackson D. Human torque capability versus machine resistive torque for four eagle resistance machines. *J Appl Sport Sci Res*. 1990;4:83–7.

15. Johnson RE, Quinn TJ, Kertzer R, Vroman NB. Strength training in female distance runners: impact on running economy. *J Strength Cond Res*. 1997;11(4):224–9.

16. Khan FY. Rhabdomyolysis: a review of the literature. *Neth J Med*. 2009;67(9):272–83.

17. Kraemer WJ. A series of studies — the physiological basis for strength training in American football: fact over philosophy. *J Strength Cond Res*. 1997;11(3):131–42.

18. Kraemer WJ. Exercise prescription in weight training: a needs analysis. *Natl Strength Cond Assoc J*. 1983;5(1):64–5.

19. Kraemer WJ. Exercise prescription in weight training: manipulating program variables. *Natl Strength Cond Assoc J*. 1983;5:58–9.

20. Kraemer WJ, Fleck SJ. *Optimizing Strength Training: Designing Nonlinear Periodization Workouts*. Champaign (IL): Human Kinetics; 2007. 256 p.

21. Kraemer WJ, Fleck SJ. *Strength Training for Young Athletes*. 2nd ed. Champaign (IL): Human Kinetics; 2005. 296 p.

22. Kraemer WJ, Fry AC. Strength testing: development and evaluation of methodology. In: Maud P, Foster C, editors. *Physiological Assessment of Human Fitness*. Champaign (IL): Human Kinetics; 1995. p. 115–38.

23. Kraemer WJ, Keuning M, Ratamess NA, et al. Resistance training combined with bench-step aerobics enhances women's health profile. *Med Sci Sports Exerc*. 2001;33(2):259–69.

24. Kraemer WJ, Marchitelli L, Gordon SE, et al. Hormonal and growth factor responses to heavy resistance exercise protocols. *J Appl Physiol*. 1990;69(4):1442–50.

25. Kraemer WJ, Noble BJ, Clark MJ, Culver BW. Physiologic responses to heavy-resistance exercise with very short rest periods. *Int J Sports Med*. 1987;8(4):247–52.

26. Kraemer WJ, Patton JF, Gordon SE, et al. Compatibility of high-intensity strength and endurance training on hormonal and skeletal muscle adaptations. *J Appl Physiol*. 1995;78(3):976–89.

27. Kraemer WJ, Ratamess N, Fry AC, et al. Influence of resistance training volume and periodization on physiological and performance adaptations in collegiate women tennis players. *Am J Sports Med*. 2000;28(5):626–33.

28. Krieger JW. Single versus multiple sets of resistance exercise: a meta-regression. *J Strength Cond Res*. 2009;23(6): 1890–901.

29. Krieger JW. Single vs. multiple sets of resistance exercise for muscle hypertrophy a meta-analysis. *J Strength Cond Res*. 2010;24(4):1150–9.

30. Lagally KM, Robertson RJ. Construct validity of the OMNI resistance exercise scale. *J Strength Cond Res*. 2006; 20(2):252–6.

31. Marx JO, Ratamess NA, Nindl BC, et al. Low-volume circuit versus high-volume periodized resistance training in women. *Med Sci Sports Exerc*. 2001;33(4):635–43.

32. Mathews DK. *Measurement in Physical Education*. 4th ed. Philadelphia (PA): W.B. Saunders; 1973. 484 p.

33. Matveyev L. *Fundamentals of Sports Training*. Moscow (Russia): Progress; 1982.

34. Mazzetti SA, Kraemer WJ, Volek JS, et al. The influence of direct supervision of resistance training on strength performance. *Med Sci Sports Exerc*. 2000;32(6):1175–84.

35. National Strength and Conditioning Association. In: Baechle TR, Earle RW, editors. *Essentials of Strength Training and Conditioning*. 3rd ed. Champaign (IL): Human Kinetics; 2008. 656 p.

36. Peterson MD, Rhea MR, Alvar BA. Applications of the dose-response for muscular strength development: a review of meta-analytic efficacy and reliability for designing training prescription. *J Strength Cond Res*. 2005;19(4): 950–8.

37. Pizzimenti MA. Mechanical analysis of the nautilus leg curl machine. *Can J Sport Sci*. 1992;17(1):41–8.

38. Plisk SS, Stone MH. Periodization strategies. *Strength Cond J*. 2003;25(6):19–37.

39. Poliquin C. Five steps to increasing the effectiveness of your strength training program. *NSCA J*. 1988;10(3):34–9.

40. Prestes J, Frollini AB, De Lima C, et al. Comparison between linear and daily undulating periodized resistance training to increase strength. *J Strength Cond Res*. 2009; 23(9):2437–42.

41. Rhea MR, Ball SD, Phillips WT, Burkett LN. A comparison of linear and daily undulating periodized programs with equated volume and intensity for strength. *J Strength Cond Res*. 2002;16(2):250–5.

42. Rhea MR, Phillips WT, Burkett LN, et al. A comparison of linear and daily undulating periodized programs with equated volume and intensity for local muscular endurance. *J Strength Cond Res*. 2003;17(1):82–7.

43. Robertson RJ, Goss FL, Rutkowski J, et al. Concurrent validation of the OMNI Perceived Exertion Scale for Resistance Exercise. *Med Sci Sports Exerc*. 2003;35(2):333–41.

44. Schoenfeld BJ. The mechanisms of muscle hypertrophy and their application to resistance training. *J Strength Cond Res*. 2010;24(10):2857–72.

45. Simão R, Farinatti PTV, Polito MD, Maior AS, Fleck SJ. Influence of exercise order on the number of repetitions performed and perceived exertion during resistance exercises. *J Strength Cond Res.* 2005;19(1):152–6.

46. Simão R, Farinatti PTV, Polito MD, Viveiros L, Fleck SJ. Influence of exercise order on the number of repetitions performed and perceived exertion during resistance exercises in women. *J Strength Cond Res.* 2007;21(1):23–8.

47. Tan B. Manipulating resistance training program variables to optimize maximum strength in men: a review. *J Strength Cond Res.* 1999;13(3):289–304.

48. Tharion WJ, Rausch TM, Harman EA, Kraemer WJ. Effects of different resistance exercise protocols on mood states. *J Appl Sport Sci Res.* 1991;5(2):60–5.

49. Todd T, Todd J. Dr. Patrick O'Shea: a man for all seasons. *J Strength Cond Res.* 2001;15(4):401–4.

50. Todd T, Todd J. Pioneers of strength research: the legacy of Dr. Richard A. Berger. *J Strength Cond Res.* 2001;15(3): 275–8.

51. Willardson JM. A brief review: factors affecting the length of the rest interval between resistance exercise sets. *J Strength Cond Res.* 2006;20(4):978–84.

52. Yamamoto LM, Klau JF, Casa DJ, Kraemer WJ, Armstrong LE, Maresh CM. The effects of resistance training on road cycling performance among highly trained cyclists: a systematic review. *J Strength Cond Res.* 2010;24(2): 560–6.

53. Yamamoto LM, Lopez RM, Klau JF, Casa DJ, Kraemer WJ, Maresh CM. The effects of resistance training on endurance distance running performance among highly trained runners: a systematic review. *J Strength Cond Res.* 2008;22(6):2036–44.

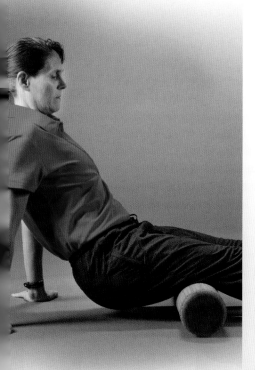

# 15 Cardiorespiratory Training Programs

## OBJECTIVES

**The Personal Trainer should be able to:**

- Understand the development of cardiovascular exercise guidelines over time.

- Apply the FITT-VP principles of exercise prescription to cardiovascular exercise training.

- Understand the physiological basis of the warm-up and cool-down.

- Use metabolic equations or MET values to determine desired workload.

# INTRODUCTION

According to the most recent American College of Sports Medicine (ACSM) Position Stand (3), "the scientific evidence demonstrating the beneficial effects of exercise is indisputable, and the benefits of exercise far outweigh the risks in most adults." Regular cardiorespiratory, resistance, flexibility, and neuromotor exercise training is considered "essential for most adults" (3). This chapter will focus on one of the primary components of a balanced exercise program: cardiorespiratory endurance training. The other major components, resistance and flexibility training, are described in Chapters 14 and 16, respectively.

## History of Physical Activity Recommendations

In 1953, more than 55% of U.S. children failed to meet a minimum standard of muscular fitness and health compared with about 8% for European children (10). These troubling findings became a primary impetus for policy makers to focus on developing and improving fitness standards and recommendations. Expert panel meetings were held in the 1960s and 1970s to summarize all the research that was conducted by that time. Most of the research at this point was primarily focused on describing and comparing the benefits of different exercise training regimens in order to improve cardiovascular fitness. In 1973, an article by Michael Pollock (14) served as the basis of the first ACSM Position Statement entitled "The Recommended Quantity and Quality of Exercise for Developing and Maintaining Fitness in Healthy Adults" (5). This statement provided the first guidelines for improving cardiorespiratory fitness, including performing moderate-to-vigorous cardiorespiratory exercise using large muscle groups 15–60 minutes for 3–5 days per week.

As time continued and research expanded, it became apparent that significant health-related benefits could be achieved at lower levels of physical activity. In 1990, a distinction was made between physical activity recommendations for *health* and physical activity recommendations for *fitness*. Later recommendations by the Centers for Disease Control and Prevention (CDC) and the ACSM (12) were combined with the 1996 Surgeon General's (16) guidelines that clearly highlighted the health benefits of physical activity. These documents were based on evidence that significant health benefits could be achieved with the accumulation of at least 30 minutes of moderate-intensity physical activity on most days of the week (12). A unique characteristic of these CDC/ACSM recommendations is the option for "accumulating" physical activity across the day. The concept of accumulating activity was a large deviation from previous guidelines, which had recommended continuous exercise of at least 20 minutes in duration. In 1998, ACSM updated its position stand and included a more balanced approach by adding muscular fitness and flexibility components to the cardiorespiratory recommendations (4). More recent documents continue to underscore the importance of cardiorespiratory endurance exercise to promote and maintain health. For example, in the 2007 report "Physical Activity and Public Health: Updated Recommendation for Adults from the American College of Sports Medicine and the American Heart Association" (9), regular participation in cardiorespiratory training was emphasized. This report highlighted that ". . . all healthy adults aged 18–65 yr need moderate-intensity aerobic physical activity for a minimum of 30 min on five days each week or vigorous-intensity aerobic activity for a minimum of 20 min on three days each week" (9, p. 1423).

All healthy adults aged 18–65 yr need moderate-intensity aerobic physical activity for a minimum of 30 min on five days each week or vigorous-intensity aerobic activity for a minimum of 20 min on three days each week (9, p. 1423).

| Table 15.1 | Evidence Statements and Summary of Recommendations for the Individualized Exercise Prescription of Cardiorespiratory Exercise | |
| --- | --- | --- |
| **Component** | **Evidence-Based Recommendation** | **Evidence Category[a]** |
| Frequency | $\geq$5 d $\cdot$ wk$^{-1}$ of moderate exercise, or $\geq$3 d $\cdot$ wk$^{-1}$ of vigorous exercise, or a combination of moderate and vigorous exercise on $\geq$3–5 d $\cdot$ wk$^{-1}$ | A |
| Intensity | Moderate- and/or vigorous-intensity exercise for most adults | A |
| | Light- to moderate-intensity exercise may be beneficial in deconditioned persons | B |
| Time | 30–60 min $\cdot$ d$^{-1}$ (150 min $\cdot$ wk$^{-1}$) of purposeful moderate exercise, or 20–60 min $\cdot$ d$^{-1}$ (75 min $\cdot$ wk$^{-1}$) of vigorous exercise, or a combination of moderate and vigorous exercise per day for most adults | A |
| | <20 min $\cdot$ d$^{-1}$ (<150 min $\cdot$ wk$^{-1}$) of exercise can be beneficial in previously sedentary persons | B |
| Type | Regular, purposeful exercise that involves major muscle groups and is continuous and rhythmic in nature | A |
| Volume | $\geq$500–1,000 MET $\cdot$ min $\cdot$ wk$^{-1}$ | C |
| Pattern | One continuous session per day or in multiple $\geq$10-min sessions to accumulate the desired duration and volume of exercise per day | A |
| | <10 min per session may yield favorable adaptation in very deconditioned individuals | B |
| Progression | Gradual progression of exercise volume by adjusting exercise duration, frequency, and/or intensity until desired exercise goal (maintenance) is attained | B |

[a]Table evidence categories: A, randomized controlled trials (rich body of data); B, randomized controlled trials (limited body of data); C, nonrandomized trials, observational studies; D, panel consensus judgment.
Adapted with permission from Garber CE, Blissmer B, Deschenes MR, et al. American College of Sports Medicine position stand. Quantity and quality of exercise for developing and maintaining cardiorespiratory, musculoskeletal, and neuromuscular fitness in apparently healthy adults: guidance for prescribing exercise. *Med Sci Sports Exerc*. 2011;43(7):1334–59.

The *Physical Activity Guidelines for Americans* published in 2008 (15) expanded these guidelines to include children, adolescents, adults, older adults, women during pregnancy and postpartum, adults with disabilities, and people with chronic medical conditions. This report emphasized that adults need to accumulate at least 150 minutes per week of moderate-intensity physical activity (with additional benefits noted for more physical activity) or 75 minutes per week of vigorous-intensity physical activity (15). The most recent ACSM Position Stand (3) supersedes all previous reports. This position stand includes over 400 references providing an extensive summary of the scientific evidence and most up-to-date recommendations for professionals concerning individualized exercise prescription (3). Table 15.1 provides an excerpt of the recommendations for cardiorespiratory exercise as presented in the 2011 ACSM Position Stand (3). This chapter will be based on these recent guidelines.

 ## General Training Principles

Cardiorespiratory endurance training refers to the ability of an individual to perform large muscle, repetitive, moderate- to high-intensity exercise for an extended period. The goal is to increase heart rate (HR) and respiration in order to place an appropriate physiological stress on the cardiorespiratory system. This required stress is often referred to as "overload." The term *overload* is commonly

Overload of the cardiovascular and respiratory systems is required to have beneficial adaptations in cardiorespiratory endurance.

used when referring to resistance or strength training (*i.e.*, lifting a weight heavier than typically done in daily activity to stress the muscle, resulting in increases in strength and potential hypertrophy) but also applies to cardiorespiratory training. Overload of the cardiovascular and respiratory systems is required to have beneficial adaptations in cardiorespiratory endurance. Cardiorespiratory fitness is a function of enhancing both the central oxygen delivery (*i.e.*, heart and circulatory) processes and the peripheral oxygen-uptake mechanisms of the working muscles. Enhancing the body's ability to deliver and utilize oxygen for metabolic processes allows one to do more work. Typical measurements used to determine improvements in cardiorespiratory fitness include increases in maximal oxygen consumption ($\dot{V}O_{2max}$) and decreases in HR or $\dot{V}O_2$ in response to a given submaximal workload.

The benefits of cardiorespiratory endurance include the following (7):

- Decreased risk of premature death from all causes and specifically from heart disease and Type 2 diabetes
- Reduction in death from all causes
- Increased likelihood of increased habitual activity levels that are also associated with health benefits

More benefits from regular physical activity and/or exercise are listed in Box 15.1 (7). Clearly, including cardiorespiratory endurance training in an exercise program has many benefits and is instrumental in designing a balanced health-related program.

The training methods used to bring about the appropriate overload for cardiorespiratory adaptations are quite varied. When the cardiorespiratory system is challenged (or overloaded) by endurance training (*i.e.*, exercise of a certain intensity for a certain period of time), then adaptation occurs. Over time, functional (*i.e.*, fitness or performance) changes or improvements follow. There is no single or best "one-size-fits-all" exercise program to apply universally. Determining how to stress the system appropriately for a given individual is one of the roles of a Personal Trainer. A Personal Trainer must understand that each client comes with unique characteristics (*i.e.*, health risk factors, fitness levels, and exercise goals) that must be considered when designing a client's optimal fitness program. Thus, prior to developing the program, the client's risk category, appropriate exercise level, and the need for physician oversight need to be determined.

To overload or challenge the cardiorespiratory system requires performing activities that increase HR and respiration. Altering the mode or type of exercise brings about specific adaptations as well as more generalized cardiorespiratory fitness gains. The minimal amount of overload needed to bring about the desired adaptation is referred to as the "threshold" for change. If the training level exceeds the threshold, then characteristic physiological adaptations occur. Although exceeding the threshold is required for physiological adaptations to occur, excessive overload can result in diminished performance. The term *retrogression* (8) is used to describe the decrease in physiological capacities resulting from excessive stress that is placed on the cardiorespiratory system. If a client is injured or has to decrease his or her exercise below the threshold level, then the body will regress toward pretraining status. Reducing the overload on the system results in a loss of physiological adaptation. This process of losing fitness gains is referred to as regression or de-adaptation (8). The Personal Trainer must carefully balance the FITT-VP principles of exercise prescription (*i.e.*,

The Personal Trainer must carefully balance frequency, intensity, duration, volume, and progression of the workouts to avoid over-challenging the client beyond an appropriate amount of overload.

frequency [F; number of days per week], intensity [I; how hard the workout is for the client], time [T; minutes per workout], type [T; mode of activity], volume [V; total amount of energy expenditure achieved per week], and progression [P; gradual increase in the overload]) to ensure that one properly overloads the cardiorespiratory system without overchallenging the client beyond an appropriate amount of overload (3).

| **Box 15.1** | **Benefits of Regular Physical Activity/Exercise** |
|---|---|

**Improvement in Cardiovascular and Respiratory Function**

- Increased maximal oxygen uptake resulting from both central and peripheral adaptations
- Decreased minute ventilation at a given absolute submaximal intensity
- Decreased myocardial oxygen cost for a given absolute submaximal intensity
- Decreased heart rate and blood pressure at a given submaximal intensity
- Increased capillary density in skeletal muscle
- Increased exercise threshold for the accumulation of lactate in the blood
- Increased exercise threshold for the onset of disease signs or symptoms (*e.g.*, angina pectoris, ischemic ST-segment depression, claudication)

**Reduction in Coronary Artery Disease Risk Factors**

- Reduced resting systolic/diastolic pressures
- Increased serum high-density lipoprotein cholesterol and decreased serum triglycerides
- Reduced total body fat and reduced intraabdominal fat
- Reduced insulin needs and improved glucose tolerance
- Reduced blood platelet adhesiveness and aggregation

**Decreased Morbidity and Mortality**

- Primary prevention (*i.e.*, interventions to prevent the initial occurrence)
- Higher activity and/or fitness levels are associated with lower death rates from coronary artery disease

- Higher activity and/or fitness levels are associated with lower incidence rates for combined cardiovascular diseases, coronary artery disease, stroke, Type 2 diabetes, osteoporotic fractures, cancer of the colon and breast, and gallbladder disease
- Regular physical activity/exercise interventions act as secondary prevention (*i.e.*, interventions after a cardiac event help prevent another)
- Based on meta-analyses (pooled data across studies), cardiovascular and all-cause mortality are reduced in postmyocardial infarction patients who participate in cardiac rehabilitation exercise training, especially as a component of multifactorial risk factor reduction
- Randomized controlled trials of cardiac rehabilitation exercise training involving postmyocardial infarction patients do not support a reduction in the rate of nonfatal reinfarction

**Other Benefits**

- Decreased anxiety and depression
- Enhanced physical function and independent living in older persons
- Enhanced feelings of well-being
- Enhanced performance of work, recreational, and sport activities
- Reduced risk of falls and injuries from falls in older persons
- Prevention or mitigation of functional limitations in older adults
- Effective therapy for many chronic diseases in older adults

Reprinted from American College of Sports Medicine. *ACSM's Guidelines for Exercise Testing and Prescription*. 10th ed. Philadelphia (PA): Wolters Kluwer, 2018. Data from American College of Sports Medicine. ACSM position stand. Exercise and physical activity for older adults. *Med Sci Sports Exerc*. 2009;41(7):1510–30. Data from U.S. Department of Health and Human Services. *Physical Activity and Health: A Report of the Surgeon General*. Atlanta (GA): U.S. Department of Health and Human Services, Public Health Service, Centers for Disease Control and Prevention, National Center for Chronic Disease Prevention and Health Promotion; 1996.

##  Design of a Cardiorespiratory Training Session

A cardiorespiratory exercise session includes a warm-up, an endurance phase, and a cool-down. The warm-up prepares the person for the endurance phase, where a target intensity is to be achieved allowing for appropriate overload. The cool-down allows the person to transition back toward resting levels. Development of the structure of the entire exercise program sequence is presented in Chapter 18.

A cardiorespiratory exercise session includes a warm-up, an endurance phase, and a cool-down.

## Warm-Up

A properly constructed exercise program will include a transition period from rest to the target exercise intensity. This transition period is called the warm-up. During the warm-up, the client should gradually increase body temperature by incorporating low-level activity similar to what will be done during the endurance phase. For example, an appropriate warm-up for a brisk walking exercise program would include slow walking. The muscle groups used are similar in the two activities — slow walking being a low-intensity activity, which naturally leads to the brisk walking of the exercise program. The warm-up may also include gentle dynamic stretching activities, although stretching should not be done with cold muscles. The specific activities included in a warm-up will vary depending on the target activity to be included in the endurance phase. In general, the warm-up should include 5–10 minutes of low-intensity large muscle activity that progresses to an intensity at the lower end of the target exercise range for the endurance phase (7).

The intent of a warm-up is to prepare the muscles and cardiorespiratory system for the upcoming workout. It is a time of transition and should provide a gradual (rather than an abrupt) increase in HR, respiration, and body temperature. Taking sufficient time to prepare the body for physical activity increases the safety and enjoyment of the target exercise during the endurance phase. The benefits of completing a warm-up include the following (7):

- May reduce the susceptibility of injury to muscles or joints by increasing the extensibility of connective tissue
- May improve joint range of motion and function
- May improve muscle performance
- May help prevent ischemia (lack of oxygen) of the heart muscle, which may occur in clients with sudden strenuous exertion

## Endurance Phase

The warm-up allows a transition from rest to the endurance phase, which is at a higher level of intensity. The object of the endurance phase is to provide the appropriate overload to promote beneficial cardiorespiratory adaptations. Thus, the Personal Trainer must consider and balance the exercise prescription principles (FITT-VP). Each of these factors, as they pertain to cardiorespiratory endurance, is discussed in more detail later in this chapter.

## Cool-Down

The cool-down is a transition from the higher intensity of the endurance phase back toward resting levels. The cool-down allows HR, blood pressure, and respiration rate to shift downward and back toward resting levels. By allowing a gradual progression toward resting rather than abruptly stopping exercise, the client will avoid an acute, excessive drop in blood pressure that could result in dizziness (this differs from the positive adaptation that exercise can provide to lower blood pressure chronically). A gradual decrease in intensity also helps remove metabolic end products (*e.g.*, lactate) from muscles used more intensely during the conditioning phase (7).

> The cool-down allows HR, blood pressure, and respiration rate to shift downward and back toward resting levels.

Approximately 10 minutes of diminishing intensity activities are appropriate for a typical cool-down (7). For exercise done at higher intensity during the endurance phase, a longer cool-down may be warranted. However, for the client who uses brisk walking as an exercise mode for the endurance phase, an appropriate cool-down could be a bit shorter and could include slow walking for 5 minutes followed by 5 minutes of dynamic body stretches.

# Exercise Prescription for Cardiovascular Endurance

## Frequency

According to the ACSM Guidelines (3,7), the optimal frequency of aerobic exercise appears to be 3–5 days per week (3,7) for most adults, with the frequency varying with the intensity. For sedentary individuals, incorporating even a couple of days per week can initiate improvements in cardiorespiratory fitness (8). Although additional benefits may be achieved beyond 5 days per week, improvements are attenuated as the frequency increases such that a plateau in benefits is often seen with exercise done greater than 5 days per week (3,7). Admittedly, individuals focused on competition or high-level performance will likely train 6 or more days per week in the hopes of getting additional gains. However, training at high intensity or vigorous activity for greater than 5 days per week might increase the incidence of injury and is not recommended for most adults (7). Clearly different goals will require altering the exercise program and thus involve different associated risks.

There is an inverse relationship between the recommendations for frequency and intensity such that if the exercise intensity is held at the lower end of the target range, then the frequency can be increased and vice versa (7). In some situations, for deconditioned individuals, multiple short daily exercise sessions may be more appropriate (7).

## Intensity

Initial fitness levels determine the appropriate exercise intensity needed to achieve the required overload. Intensity levels are necessarily higher in fit than in unfit individuals because the threshold for cardiorespiratory benefits is higher. Higher intensity exercise carries more cardiovascular and orthopedic risk. For individuals with lower fitness, intensity levels as low as 45% oxygen uptake reserve ($\dot{V}O_2R$) or below may provide sufficient challenge to increase $\dot{V}O_{2max}$ (7). In contrast, highly trained athletes may train at 95% $\dot{V}O_{2max}$ or higher (7). Moderately trained individuals may find that 70%–80% $\dot{V}O_{2max}$ provides a sufficient training stimulus (7). Intensity can be determined using various methods. Table 15.2 provides an overview of the intensity classifications for cardiorespiratory endurance (7). Details on these various methods will be outlined in this section.

### Methods of Estimating Intensity for Cardiorespiratory Endurance Exercise

Some methods of estimating intensity require knowledge of $\dot{V}O_{2max}$ or maximal heart rate ($HR_{max}$) and/or resting heart rate ($HR_{rest}$). Others rely on estimations of $HR_{max}$ based on age. Personal Trainers must use the information available to determine the most appropriate exercise prescription, realizing the shortcomings of the various methods. A good Personal Trainer has the willingness and ability to modify the exercise program to provide the appropriate overload and prescription to the client.

### Oxygen Uptake Reserve

Exercise intensity can be determined from $\dot{V}O_2R$, which is the difference between $\dot{V}O_{2max}$ and resting oxygen consumption ($\dot{V}O_{2\,rest}$). To use $\dot{V}O_2R$ to determine intensity, one must have access to $\dot{V}O_{2max}$ information and know that $\dot{V}O_{2\,rest}$ is estimated to be $3.5\ mL \cdot kg^{-1} \cdot min^{-1}$ (also referred to as one metabolic equivalent or 1 MET) and is used for all individuals. The following equations are to determine target intensity if $\dot{V}O_{2max}$ is known.

$$\text{Target } \dot{V}O_2 \text{ (lower end of range)} = [(0.40) \times (\dot{V}O_{2max} - \dot{V}O_{2\,rest})] + \dot{V}O_{2\,rest}$$

$$\text{Target } \dot{V}O_2 \text{ (upper end of range)} = [(0.89) \times (\dot{V}O_{2max} - \dot{V}O_{2\,rest})] + \dot{V}O_{2\,rest}$$

| Table 15.2 | **Methods of Estimating Intensity for Cardiorespiratory Endurance Exercise** | | | | | | | |
|---|---|---|---|---|---|---|---|---|
| | | | | | Intensity (%$\dot{V}O_{2max}$) Relative to Maximal Exercise Capacity in MET | | | Absolute Intensity (METs) |
| Intensity | Relative Intensity | | | | | | | |
| | %HRR ($\dot{V}O_2R$) | % HR$_{max}$ | % $\dot{V}O_{2max}$ | Perceived Exertion (Rating on 6–20 RPE Scale) | 20 MET | 10 MET | 5 MET | |
| Very low (light) | ≤30 | ≤57 | ≤37 | ≤9 | ≤34 | ≤37 | ≤44 | ≤2 |
| Low (light) | 30–39 | 57–63 | 37–45 | 9–11 | 34–42 | 37–45 | 44–51 | 2.0–2.9 |
| Moderate | 40–59 | 64–76 | 46–63 | 12–13 | 43–61 | 46–63 | 52–67 | 3.0–5.9 |
| Vigorous | 60–89 | 77–95 | 64–90 | 14–17 | 62–90 | 64–90 | 68–91 | 6.0–8.7 |
| Near maximal to maximal | ≥90 | ≥96 | ≥91 | ≥18 | ≥91 | ≥91 | ≥92 | ≥8.8 |

MET, metabolic energy equivalents; HRR, heart rate reserve; HR$_{max}$, maximal heart rate; $\dot{V}O_{2max}$, maximum oxygen consumption; $\dot{V}O_2R$, oxygen uptake reserve; RPE, rating of perceived exertion.
Adapted from American College of Sports Medicine. *ACSM's Guidelines for Exercise Testing and Prescription*. 9th ed. Philadelphia (PA): Lippincott Williams & Wilkins; 2013.

Although ACSM recommends a range of between 40% and 50% up to 89% of $\dot{V}O_2R$ (7), the actual percentages that the Personal Trainer uses to determine the appropriate $\dot{V}O_2$ range must be made with the client's fitness level and goals in mind. Low-fit clients will need to start on the lower end of the range (or even lower), whereas other clients will require intensities toward the upper end of the range to receive the appropriate overload.

Factors such as environmental conditions may make the relative intensity higher than prescribed.

Once the target oxygen consumption is calculated, the Personal Trainer must determine the correct workload for each activity using charts or metabolic calculations. A clear shortcoming of this technique is that the $\dot{V}O_2$ level determines intensity based on workload and not the individual's response. In other words, determining an outdoor running pace based on the percentage of $\dot{V}O_{2max}$ alone would be inaccurate when faced with a hot, humid environment. Certain environmental conditions may make the relative intensity higher than prescribed. Blindly using workloads without monitoring the physiological responses, such as HR, are not recommended.

To determine workload settings based on $\dot{V}O_2$ data, standard metabolic equations are used (8). These equations are found in Box 15.2. These equations are an estimate of the oxygen consumption required by the body during constant, submaximal activity (including walking, jogging/running, stationary cycling, arm cranking, and stepping). Box 15.3 provides a computational example of the various equations to determine a client's exercise prescription. Additionally, normative values for $\dot{V}O_{2max}$ are found in Table 15.3, which allows the Personal Trainer to see the percentile rank for males and females of various ages.

These metabolic equations should be used carefully because underestimating the workload may leave a client below the appropriate target intensity (and the accompanying health benefits) and

| Box 15.2 | **Metabolic Calculations for the Estimation of Energy Expenditure ($\dot{V}O_{2max}$ [mL $\cdot$ kg$^{-1}$ $\cdot$ min$^{-1}$]) during Common Physical Activities** |
|---|---|

| Activity | Resting Component | Horizontal Component | Vertical Component/ Resistance Component | Limitations |
|---|---|---|---|---|
| Walking | 3.5 | 0.1 $\times$ speed[a] | 1.8 $\times$ speed[a] $\times$ grade[b] | Most accurate for speeds of 1.9–3.7 mi $\cdot$ h$^{-1}$ (50–100 m $\cdot$ min$^{-1}$) |
| Running | 3.5 | 0.2 $\times$ speed[a] | 0.9 $\times$ speed[a] $\times$ grade[b] | Most accurate for speeds ≥5 mi $\cdot$ h$^{-1}$ (134 m $\cdot$ min$^{-1}$) |
| Stepping | 3.5 | 0.2 $\times$ steps $\cdot$ min$^{-1}$ | 1.33 $\times$ (1.8 $\times$ step height[c] $\times$ steps $\cdot$ min$^{-1}$) | Most accurate for stepping rates of 12–30 steps $\cdot$ min$^{-1}$ |
| Leg cycling | 3.5 | 3.5 | (1.8 $\times$ work rate[d])/ body mass[e] | Most accurate for work rates of 300–1,200 kg $\cdot$ m $\cdot$ min$^{-1}$ (50–200 W) |
| Arm cycling | 3.5 | | (3 $\times$ work rate[d])/body mass[e] | Most accurate for work rates between 150 and 750 kg $\cdot$ m $\cdot$ min$^{-1}$ (25–125 W) |

Header for the Vertical/Resistance columns: **Sum of Resting + Horizontal + Vertical/Resistance Components**

[a]Speed in m $\cdot$ min$^{-1}$.
[b]Grade is grade percentage expressed in decimal format (*e.g.,* 10% = 0.10).
[c]Step height in m.
*Multiply by the following conversion factors:*
  lb to kg: 0.454;
  mi to km: 1.609;
  W to kg $\cdot$ m $\cdot$ min$^{-1}$: 6.12;
  in to cm: 2.54;
  mi $\cdot$ h$^{-1}$ to m $\cdot$ min$^{-1}$: 26.8;
  $\dot{V}O_{2max}$ L $\cdot$ min$^{-1}$ to kcal $\cdot$ min$^{-1}$: 4.9;
  ft to m: 0.3048;
  kg $\cdot$ m $\cdot$ min$^{-1}$ to W: 0.164;
  $\dot{V}O_2$ MET to mL $\cdot$ kg$^{-1}$ $\cdot$ min$^{-1}$: 3.5.
[d]Work rate in kilogram meters per minute (kg $\cdot$ m $\cdot$ min$^{-1}$) is calculated as resistance (kg) $\times$ distance per revolution of flywheel $\times$ pedal frequency per minute. Note: Distance per revolution is 6 m for Monark leg ergometer, 3 m for the Tunturi and BodyGuard ergometers, and 2.4 m for Monark arm ergometer.
[e]Body mass in kg.
$\dot{V}O_{2max}$, maximal volume of oxygen consumed per unit of time.
American College of Sports Medicine. *ACSM's Guidelines for Exercise Testing and Prescription.* 7th ed. Baltimore (MD): Lippincott Williams & Wilkins; 2005.

overestimating the workload commonly results in frustration with exercise and poor adherence. These equations will give initial starting points, but intensity levels may still need to be adjusted on the basis of individual HR responses and perceived levels of exertion.

Another option that does not require extensive calculations is to take the oxygen consumption values (for the upper and lower end of the target range) and convert them to MET values. To determine METs, divide the $\dot{V}O_2$ values by 3.5 (1 MET = 3.5 mL $\cdot$ kg$^{-1}$ $\cdot$ min$^{-1}$). Once the target intensity is expressed as a MET level, then Tables 15.4–15.8 can be used to determine appropriate workloads for walking, jogging/running, leg and arm cycle ergometry, and stair stepping (7).

## Box 15.3    Example for Metabolic Equations

Client Name: Anne
Characteristics:

Age = 29 yr　　　　　　　Weight = 150 lb (68.2 kg)　　　　　　　Height = 69 in (1.75 m)

$\dot{V}O_{2max}$ = 45 mL · kg$^{-1}$ · min$^{-1}$ (12.9 MET)

To calculate $\dot{V}O_2R$, use the following formula:

$$\text{Target } \dot{V}O_2R = [(\text{percentage}) \times (\dot{V}O_{2max} - \dot{V}O_{2\,rest})] + \dot{V}O_{2\,rest}$$

Anne's $\dot{V}O_{2max}$ puts her just above the 80th percentile (see Table 15.3), in the excellent category. As a result, her Personal Trainer decides to prescribe a range of 60%–80% $\dot{V}O_2R$.

To determine the target $\dot{V}O_2$ range, the calculations for Anne are as follows:

$$\text{Target } \dot{V}O_2 \text{ (lower end)} = [(0.60) \times (45 - 3.5)] + 3.5 = 28.4 \text{ mL} \cdot \text{kg} \cdot \text{min}^{-1} \text{ (8.1 MET)}$$

$$\text{Target } \dot{V}O_2 \text{ (upper end)} = [(0.80) \times (45 - 3.5)] + 3.5 = 36.7 \text{ mL} \cdot \text{kg} \cdot \text{min}^{-1} \text{ (10.5 MET)}$$

Thus, the workouts will range between 28.4 and 36.7 mL · kg · min$^{-1}$ (8.1–10.5 MET). Anne indicates that using her club membership, she enjoys brisk walking and jogging on the treadmill as well as some stationary cycling and bench stepping. She needs help to determine the right intensity settings so that she gets sufficient stress but does not work too hard.

### Walking

When using the equation for walking (given below), the Personal Trainer selects walking on the treadmill as the lower end of the intensity range. The Personal Trainer must determine the grade necessary to reach 28.4 mL · kg$^{-1}$ · min$^{-1}$, as Anne has indicated that she feels comfortable walking at around 3.7 mph (5.9 kph).

The equation for walking is as follows:

$$\dot{V}O_2 \text{ (mL} \cdot \text{kg}^{-1} \cdot \text{min}^{-1}) = (0.1 \times \text{speed}) + (1.8 \times \text{speed} \times \text{grade}) + 3.5 \text{ mL} \cdot \text{kg}^{-1} \cdot \text{min}^{-1}$$

Because Anne enjoys walking at 3.7 mph (5.9 kph), the first thing the Personal Trainer must calculate is the speed in m · min$^{-1}$ (as required in the formula). This can be accomplished by multiplying speed in mph by 26.8 (26.8 m · min$^{-1}$ = 1 mph). Therefore, 3.7 mph (5.9 kph) is 99.2 m · min$^{-1}$. Then, grade must be determined.

$$28.4 \text{ mL} \cdot \text{kg}^{-1} \cdot \text{min}^{-1} = (0.1 \times 99.2) + (1.8 \times 99.2 \times \text{grade}) + 3.5 \text{ mL} \cdot \text{kg}^{-1} \cdot \text{min}^{-1}$$

Solving for determination of grade:

$$28.4 = (0.1 \times 99.2) + (1.8 \times 99.2 \times \text{grade}) + 3.5 \text{ mL} \cdot \text{kg}^{-1} \cdot \text{min}^{-1}$$

$$28.4 = (9.92 + 3.5) + (178.56 \times \text{grade})$$

$$28.4 - 14.22 = 178.56 \times \text{grade}$$

$$13.42 / 178.56 = \text{grade}$$

$$\text{Grade} = 0.08 = 8\%$$

For the lower end of the intensity range, Anne will walk on the treadmill at 3.7 mph with an 8% grade.

### Running

When working toward the upper end of the intensity range, Anne will be running on the treadmill. She prefers to have little grade, and thus, the formula for running will be used to determine the speed. The running equation (see Box 15.2) is as follows:

$$\dot{V}O_2 \text{ (mL} \cdot \text{kg}^{-1} \cdot \text{min}^{-1}) = (0.2 \times \text{speed}) + (0.9 \times \text{speed} \times \text{grade}) + 3.5 \text{ mL} \cdot \text{kg}^{-1} \cdot \text{min}^{-1}$$

| Box 15.3 | **Example for Metabolic Equations** (*continued*) |
|---|---|

Therefore, if Anne wants to run with a 1% grade (note: 1% = 0.01) on the treadmill, the running formula can be used to determine the speed.

$$36.7 \text{ mL} \cdot \text{kg}^{-1} \cdot \text{min}^{-1} = (0.2 \times \text{speed}) + (0.9 \times \text{speed} \times 0.01) + 3.5 \text{ mL} \cdot \text{kg}^{-1} \cdot \text{min}^{-1}$$

Solving for determination of speed:

$$36.7 - 3.5 = (0.2 \times \text{speed}) + (0.009 \times \text{speed})$$

$$33.2 = 0.209 \times \text{speed}$$

$$33.2 / 0.209 = \text{speed} = 158.9$$

$$\text{Speed} = 158.9 \text{ m} \cdot \text{min}^{-1} = 5.9 \text{ mph (9.4 kph)}$$

For the upper end of the intensity range, Anne will run on the treadmill at 5.9 mph with a 1% grade.

### Cycling

Anne will be cycling on a Monark cycle ergometer. Her Personal Trainer will determine the workload at the lower and upper ends of her target range (corresponding with 28.4 and 36.7 mL $\cdot$ kg$^{-1}$ $\cdot$ min$^{-1}$). The formula for cycling from Box 15.2 is as follows:

$$\dot{V}O_2 \text{ (mL} \cdot \text{kg}^{-1} \cdot \text{min}^{-1}) = \frac{1.8 \times \text{work rate in kg m} \cdot \text{min}^{-1}}{\text{Body mass}} + 7$$

The Personal Trainer discussed a preferred cycling cadence with Anne and found that she is most comfortable at 70 revolutions per minute (rpm). This will be used to determine the resistance level. Although resistance is often thought of as kilopounds (kp), note that 1 kp is equivalent to 1 kilogram (kg). In the formulas below, 1 kp = 1 kg, and these terms are used interchangeably. First, the overall work rate is calculated as follows:

$$28.4 \text{ mL} \cdot \text{kg}^{-1} \cdot \text{min}^{-1} = \frac{1.8 \times \text{work rate in kg m} \cdot \text{min}^{-1}}{68.2} + 7$$

Thus for the lower end of the range, the work rate is 811 kp $\cdot$ m $\cdot$ min$^{-1}$. To determine the resistance (in kilopounds) to place on the flywheel, the following calculation is used:

$$\text{Work rate (kp} \cdot \text{m} \cdot \text{min}^{-1}) = \text{revolutions per minute}$$

$$\times \text{length of flywheel in meters} \times \text{resistance in kilopounds}$$

Because Anne desires to pedal at a rate of 70 rpm on a Monark bike (whose distance per revolution is a constant of 6 m), the calculation of resistance is as follows:

$$811 \text{ kp m} \cdot \text{min}^{-1} = 70 \text{ rpm} \times 6 \text{ m} \times \text{resistance (kp)}$$

Solving for determination of resistance:

$$811 = 420 \times \text{resistance}$$

$$811 / 420 = \text{resistance} = 1.9 \text{ (round to 2.0 kp)}$$

$$\text{Resistance} = 1.9 \text{ or } 2.0 \text{ kp}$$

For the upper end of the target intensity, the work rate is determined using the following formula:

$$36.7 \text{ mL} \cdot \text{kg}^{-1} \cdot \text{min}^{-1} = \frac{1.8 \times \text{work rate in kg m} \cdot \text{min}^{-1}}{68.2} + 7$$

(*continued*)

## Box 15.3    Example for Metabolic Equations (continued)

Thus, the work rate is 1,125 kp · m · min$^{-1}$. Assuming 70 rpm, the resistance at this level would be approximately 3.0 kp.

$$1,125 \text{ kpm} \cdot \text{min}^{-1} = 70 \text{ rpm} \times 6 \text{ m} \times \text{resistance}$$

Solving for determination of resistance:

$$1,125 = 420 \times \text{resistance}$$

$$1,125 \, / \, 420 = \text{resistance} = 2.7$$

$$\text{Resistance} = 2.7 \text{ (round to 3.0 kp)}$$

### Stepping

Anne owns a 12-in step (12 in = 0.3048 m) and is interested in knowing the stepping rate (frequency in steps per minute) she would need to use to step up and down and stay within her target intensity range. A step is defined as an up–up–down–down, four-part movement (6): (a) step up, (b) pushing with this leg to raise the body and placing the other leg on the box, (c) stepping down with the first, and (d) stepping down with second leg in a repetitive fashion.

Once again, her Personal Trainer uses the formulas in Box 15.2 for stepping. The formula for stepping is as follows:

$$\dot{V}O_2 \, (\text{mL} \cdot \text{kg}^{-1} \cdot \text{min}^{-1}) = (0.2 \text{ frequency}) + (1.33 \times 1.8 \times \text{height} \times \text{frequency}) + 3.5$$

For the lower end of Anne's target range, the frequency would be 26 steps per minute:

$$28.4 \text{ mL} \cdot \text{kg}^{-1} \cdot \text{min}^{-1} = (0.2 \times \text{frequency}) + (1.33 \times 1.8 \times 0.3048 \times \text{frequency}) + 3.5$$

$$28.4 - 3.5 = (0.2 \times \text{frequency}) + (0.72 \times \text{frequency})$$

$$24.9 \, / \, 0.92 = 27 \text{ steps per minute}$$

For the upper end of Anne's target range, the frequency would be 36 steps per minute:

$$36.7 \text{ mL} \cdot \text{kg}^{-1} \cdot \text{min}^{-1} = (0.2 \times \text{frequency}) + (1.33 \times 1.8 \times 0.3048 \times \text{frequency}) + 3.5$$

$$36.7 - 3.5 = (0.2 \times \text{frequency}) + (0.72 \times \text{frequency})$$

$$33.2 \, / \, 0.92 = 36 \text{ steps per minute}$$

Anne now has some starting points for her exercise. Initially, she can begin toward the lower end of the range. Over time, she will progress toward the higher end of her intensity range. Heart rate and ratings of perceived exertion will be used to fine-tune this prescription.

For Personal Trainers interested in more details on the metabolic equations, please see Chapter 6 in the *ACSM's Guidelines for Exercise Testing and Prescription*, 10th edition (7).

## Table 15.3  Fitness Categories for Maximal Aerobic Power for Men and Women by Age

### MEN

| % | | Age 20–29 | | | | Age 30–39 | | | |
|---|---|---|---|---|---|---|---|---|---|
| | | Balke Treadmill (Time) | Max V̇O₂ (mL · kg⁻¹ · min⁻¹) | 12-min Run (Miles) | 1.5-Mile Run (Time) | Balke Treadmill (Time) | Max V̇O₂ (mL · kg⁻¹ · min⁻¹) | 12-min Run (Miles) | 1.5-Mile Run (Time) |
| 99 | Superior | 31:03 | 59.8 | 1.98 | 8:35 | 30:00 | 58.3 | 1.93 | 8:49 |
| 95 | | 28:01 | 55.4 | 1.86 | 9:18 | 27:02 | 54.0 | 1.82 | 9:34 |
| 90 | Excellent | 26:40 | 53.5 | 1.80 | 9:40 | 25:22 | 51.6 | 1.75 | 10:02 |
| 85 | | 25:30 | 51.8 | 1.75 | 10:00 | 24:12 | 49.9 | 1.70 | 10:24 |
| 80 | | 25:00 | 51.1 | 1.73 | 10:09 | 23:03 | 48.3 | 1.66 | 10:47 |
| 75 | Good | 23:09 | 48.4 | 1.66 | 10:45 | 22:10 | 47.0 | 1.62 | 11:06 |
| 70 | | 22:30 | 47.5 | 1.63 | 10:59 | 21:30 | 46.0 | 1.59 | 11:22 |
| 65 | | 22:00 | 46.8 | 1.61 | 11:10 | 21:00 | 45.3 | 1.57 | 11:33 |
| 60 | | 21:05 | 45.4 | 1.58 | 11:31 | 20:05 | 44.0 | 1.54 | 11:56 |
| 55 | Fair | 20:30 | 44.6 | 1.55 | 11:45 | 20:00 | 43.9 | 1.53 | 11:58 |
| 50 | | 20:00 | 43.9 | 1.53 | 11:58 | 19:00 | 42.4 | 1.49 | 12:25 |
| 45 | | 19:02 | 42.5 | 1.49 | 12:23 | 18:05 | 41.1 | 1.46 | 12:50 |
| 40 | | 18:30 | 41.7 | 1.47 | 12:38 | 17:39 | 40.5 | 1.44 | 13:04 |
| 35 | Poor | 18:00 | 41.0 | 1.45 | 12:53 | 17:00 | 39.5 | 1.41 | 13:24 |
| 30 | | 17:15 | 39.9 | 1.42 | 13:16 | 16:20 | 38.6 | 1.39 | 13:46 |
| 25 | | 16:31 | 38.8 | 1.39 | 13:40 | 15:41 | 37.6 | 1.36 | 14:09 |
| 20 | | 15:46 | 37.8 | 1.36 | 14:06 | 15:00 | 36.7 | 1.33 | 14:34 |
| 15 | Very poor | 15:00 | 36.7 | 1.33 | 14:34 | 14:01 | 35.2 | 1.29 | 15:13 |
| 10 | | 13:31 | 34.5 | 1.27 | 15:35 | 13:00 | 33.8 | 1.25 | 15:58 |
| 5 | | 11:18 | 31.3 | 1.18 | 17:22 | 11:11 | 31.1 | 1.18 | 17:29 |
| 1 | | 7:40 | 26.1 | 1.04 | 21:25 | 8:00 | 26.5 | 1.05 | 20:58 |
| | | | $n = 2,463$ | | | | $n = 13,308$ | | |

**Total $n$** = 15,771

(continued)

## Table 15.3 Fitness Categories for Maximal Aerobic Power for Men and Women by Age (continued)

### MEN

| % | | Age 40-49 | | | | Age 50-59 | | | |
|---|---|---|---|---|---|---|---|---|---|
| | | Balke Treadmill (Time) | Max $\dot{V}O_2$ (mL·kg⁻¹·min⁻¹) | 12-min Run (Miles) | 1.5-Mile Run (Time) | Balke Treadmill (Time) | Max $\dot{V}O_2$ (mL·kg⁻¹·min⁻¹) | 12-min Run (Miles) | 1.5-Mile Run (Time) |
| 99 | Superior | 28:30 | 56.1 | 1.87 | 9:10 | 27:00 | 54.0 | 1.81 | 9:34 |
| 95 | | 26:00 | 52.5 | 1.77 | 9:51 | 23:31 | 49.0 | 1.67 | 10:38 |
| 90 | Excellent | 24:00 | 49.7 | 1.69 | 10:28 | 24:56 | 46.7 | 1.61 | 11:11 |
| 85 | | 23:00 | 48.2 | 1.65 | 10:48 | 20:31 | 44.6 | 1.55 | 11:45 |
| 80 | | 21:44 | 46.4 | 1.60 | 11:16 | 19:39 | 43.4 | 1.52 | 12:07 |
| 75 | Good | 20:41 | 44.9 | 1.56 | 11:41 | 18:36 | 41.9 | 1.48 | 12:36 |
| 70 | | 20:01 | 43.9 | 1.53 | 11:58 | 18:00 | 41.0 | 1.45 | 12:53 |
| 65 | | 19:30 | 43.2 | 1.51 | 12:11 | 17:14 | 39.9 | 1.42 | 13:17 |
| 60 | | 19:00 | 42.4 | 1.49 | 12:25 | 16:45 | 39.2 | 1.40 | 13:32 |
| 55 | Fair | 18:00 | 41.0 | 1.45 | 12:53 | 16:01 | 38.1 | 1.37 | 13:57 |
| 50 | | 17:25 | 40.1 | 1.43 | 13:11 | 15:29 | 37.4 | 1.35 | 14:16 |
| 45 | | 17:00 | 39.5 | 1.41 | 13:24 | 15:00 | 36.7 | 1.33 | 14:34 |
| 40 | | 16:15 | 38.5 | 1.38 | 13:49 | 14:16 | 35.6 | 1.30 | 15:03 |
| 35 | Poor | 15:45 | 37.7 | 1.36 | 14:07 | 13:52 | 35.0 | 1.29 | 15:20 |
| 30 | | 15:01 | 36.7 | 1.33 | 14:34 | 13:00 | 33.8 | 1.25 | 15:58 |
| 25 | | 14:30 | 35.9 | 1.31 | 14:53 | 12:30 | 33.0 | 1.23 | 16:21 |
| 20 | | 13:48 | 34.9 | 1.28 | 15:22 | 12:00 | 32.3 | 1.21 | 16:46 |
| 15 | Very poor | 13:00 | 33.8 | 1.25 | 15:58 | 11:00 | 30.9 | 1.17 | 17:38 |
| 10 | | 12:00 | 32.3 | 1.21 | 16:46 | 10:00 | 29.4 | 1.13 | 18:38 |
| 5 | | 10:01 | 29.5 | 1.13 | 18:37 | 8:20 | 27.0 | 1.07 | 20:53 |
| 1 | | 7:01 | 25.1 | 1.01 | 22:20 | 5:25 | 22.8 | 0.95 | 25:01 |

$n = 19,566$          $n = 11,693$

**Total $n$** = 31,259

**MEN**

| % | | Age 60-69 | | | | Age 70-79 | | |
|---|---|---|---|---|---|---|---|---|
| | Balke Treadmill (Time) | Max $\dot{V}O_2$ (mL·kg⁻¹·min⁻¹) | 12-min Run (Miles) | 1.5-Mile Run (Time) | Balke Treadmill (Time) | Max $\dot{V}O_2$ (mL·kg⁻¹·min⁻¹) | 12-min Run (Miles) | 1.5-Mile Run (Time) |
| 99 Superior | 25:00 | 51.1 | 1.73 | 10:09 | 24:00 | 49.7 | 1.69 | 10:28 |
| 95 Excellent | 21:18 | 45.8 | 1.59 | 11:26 | 18:45 | 42.1 | 1.48 | 12:31 |
| 90 | 19:08 | 42.6 | 1.50 | 12:21 | 17:00 | 39.5 | 1.41 | 13:24 |
| 85 | 18:00 | 41.0 | 1.45 | 12:53 | 16:00 | 38.1 | 1.37 | 13:58 |
| 80 | 17:01 | 39.6 | 1.41 | 13:23 | 15:00 | 36.7 | 1.33 | 14:34 |
| 75 Good | 16:07 | 38.3 | 1.38 | 13:53 | 14:01 | 35.2 | 1.29 | 15:13 |
| 70 | 15:29 | 37.4 | 1.35 | 14:16 | 13:05 | 33.9 | 1.26 | 15:54 |
| 65 | 15:00 | 36.7 | 1.33 | 14:34 | 12:33 | 33.1 | 1.23 | 16:19 |
| 60 | 14:14 | 35.5 | 1.30 | 15:04 | 12:01 | 32.3 | 1.21 | 16:45 |
| 55 Fair | 13:45 | 34.9 | 1.28 | 15:25 | 11:26 | 31.5 | 1.19 | 17:15 |
| 50 | 13:02 | 33.8 | 1.25 | 15:56 | 10:51 | 30.7 | 1.17 | 17:47 |
| 45 | 12:30 | 33.0 | 1.23 | 16:21 | 10:21 | 29.9 | 1.15 | 18:16 |
| 40 | 12:00 | 32.3 | 1.21 | 16:46 | 10:00 | 29.4 | 1.13 | 18:38 |
| 35 Poor | 11:30 | 31.6 | 1.19 | 17:11 | 9:04 | 28.1 | 1.09 | 19:39 |
| 30 | 11:00 | 30.9 | 1.17 | 17:38 | 8:52 | 27.8 | 1.09 | 19:53 |
| 25 | 10:05 | 29.6 | 1.14 | 18:32 | 8:05 | 26.7 | 1.06 | 20:51 |
| 20 | 9:30 | 28.7 | 1.11 | 19:10 | 7:24 | 25.7 | 1.03 | 21:47 |
| 15 Very poor | 8:36 | 27.4 | 1.08 | 20:12 | 6:39 | 24.6 | 1.00 | 22:54 |
| 10 | 7:26 | 25.7 | 1.03 | 21:44 | 5:30 | 22.9 | 0.95 | 24:52 |
| 5 | 6:00 | 23.7 | 0.97 | 23:58 | 4:01 | 20.8 | 0.89 | 27:56 |
| 1 | 3:05 | 19.4 | 0.85 | 6:18 | 2:15 | 18.2 | 0.82 | 32:46 |

$n = 3,285$

$n = 467$

**Total $n$** = 3,752

(continued)

## Table 15.3    Fitness Categories for Maximal Aerobic Power for Men and Women by Age (continued)

WOMEN

| % | Category | Age 20–29 | | | | Age 30–39 | | | |
|---|---|---|---|---|---|---|---|---|---|
| | | Balke Treadmill (Time) | Max V̇O₂ (mL · kg⁻¹ · min⁻¹) | 12-min Run (Miles) | 1.5-Mile Run (Time) | Balke Treadmill (Time) | Max V̇O₂ (mL · kg⁻¹ · min⁻¹) | 12-min Run (Miles) | 1.5-Mile Run (Time) |
| 99 | Superior | 27:19 | 54.4 | 1.83 | 9:29 | 26:00 | 52.5 | 1.77 | 9:51 |
| 95 | | 24:00 | 49.7 | 1.69 | 10:28 | 22:27 | 47.4 | 1.63 | 11:00 |
| 90 | Excellent | 22:00 | 46.8 | 1.61 | 11:10 | 21:00 | 45.3 | 1.57 | 11:33 |
| 85 | | 21:00 | 45.3 | 1.57 | 11:33 | 20:00 | 43.9 | 1.53 | 11:58 |
| 80 | | 20:01 | 43.9 | 1.53 | 11:58 | 19:00 | 42.4 | 1.49 | 12:25 |
| 75 | Good | 19:00 | 42.4 | 1.49 | 12:25 | 18:00 | 41.0 | 1.45 | 12:53 |
| 70 | | 18:01 | 41.0 | 1.45 | 12:53 | 17:01 | 39.6 | 1.41 | 13:23 |
| 65 | | 18:00 | 41.0 | 1.45 | 12:53 | 16:19 | 38.6 | 1.39 | 13:47 |
| 60 | | 17:00 | 39.5 | 1.41 | 13:24 | 15:49 | 37.8 | 1.37 | 14:04 |
| 55 | Fair | 16:15 | 38.5 | 1.38 | 13:49 | 15:18 | 37.1 | 1.34 | 14:23 |
| 50 | | 15:45 | 37.7 | 1.36 | 14:07 | 15:00 | 36.7 | 1.33 | 14:34 |
| 45 | | 15:01 | 36.7 | 1.33 | 14:34 | 14:00 | 35.2 | 1.29 | 15:14 |
| 40 | | 14:36 | 36.0 | 1.32 | 14:50 | 13:26 | 34.4 | 1.27 | 15:38 |
| 35 | Poor | 14:00 | 35.2 | 1.29 | 15:14 | 13:00 | 33.8 | 1.25 | 15:58 |
| 30 | | 13:08 | 34.0 | 1.26 | 15:52 | 12:09 | 32.5 | 1.22 | 16:38 |
| 25 | | 12:24 | 32.9 | 1.23 | 16:26 | 12:00 | 32.3 | 1.21 | 16:46 |
| 20 | | 12:00 | 32.3 | 1.21 | 16:46 | 11:00 | 30.9 | 1.17 | 17:38 |
| 15 | Very poor | 11:00 | 30.9 | 1.17 | 17:49 | 10:01 | 29.5 | 1.13 | 18:37 |
| 10 | | 10:01 | 29.5 | 1.13 | 18:37 | 9:01 | 28.0 | 1.09 | 19:43 |
| 5 | | 8:21 | 27.1 | 1.07 | 20:31 | 7:35 | 25.9 | 1.30 | 21:31 |
| 1 | | 6:00 | 23.7 | 0.97 | 23:58 | 5:27 | 22.9 | 0.95 | 24:57 |
| | | *n* = 1,397 | | | | *n* = 4,642 | | | |

**Total *n* = 6,039**

| | | WOMEN | | | | | | | |
|---|---|---|---|---|---|---|---|---|---|
| | | Age 40–49 | | | | Age 50–59 | | | |
| % | | Balke Treadmill (Time) | Max $\dot{V}O_2$ (mL·kg⁻¹·min⁻¹) | 1.5-Mile Run (Time) | 12-min Run (Miles) | Balke Treadmill (Time) | Max $\dot{V}O_2$ (mL·kg⁻¹·min⁻¹) | 12-min Run (Miles) | 1.5-Mile Run (Time) |
| 99 | Superior | 25:00 | 51.1 | 10:09 | 1.73 | 21:30 | 46.0 | 1.59 | 11:22 |
| 95 | | 21:01 | 45.3 | 11:32 | 1.57 | 18:03 | 41.1 | 1.46 | 12:52 |
| 90 | Excellent | 20:00 | 43.9 | 11:58 | 1.53 | 17:00 | 39.5 | 1.46 | 13:24 |
| 85 | | 18:04 | 41.1 | 12:51 | 1.46 | 15:29 | 37.4 | 1.35 | 14:16 |
| 80 | | 17:05 | 39.7 | 13:22 | 1.42 | 15:00 | 36.7 | 1.33 | 14:34 |
| 75 | Good | 16:45 | 39.2 | 13:32 | 1.40 | 14:04 | 35.3 | 1.30 | 15:11 |
| 70 | | 16:00 | 38.1 | 13:58 | 1.37 | 13:30 | 34.5 | 1.27 | 15:35 |
| 65 | | 15:03 | 36.7 | 14:32 | 1.33 | 12:59 | 33.7 | 1.25 | 15:58 |
| 60 | | 14:45 | 36.3 | 14:44 | 1.32 | 12:30 | 33.0 | 1.23 | 16:21 |
| 55 | Fair | 14:01 | 35.2 | 15:13 | 1.29 | 12:00 | 32.3 | 1.21 | 16:46 |
| 50 | | 13:46 | 34.9 | 15:24 | 1.28 | 11:29 | 31.6 | 1.19 | 17:13 |
| 45 | | 13:01 | 33.8 | 15:57 | 1.25 | 11:01 | 30.9 | 1.17 | 17:38 |
| 40 | | 12:30 | 33.0 | 16:21 | 1.23 | 10:30 | 30.2 | 1.15 | 18:07 |
| 35 | Poor | 12:00 | 32.3 | 16:46 | 1.21 | 10:01 | 29.5 | 1.13 | 18:37 |
| 30 | | 11:18 | 31.3 | 17:22 | 1.18 | 9:40 | 29.0 | 1.12 | 18:59 |
| 25 | | 10:40 | 30.4 | 17:58 | 1.16 | 9:00 | 28.0 | 1.09 | 19:44 |
| 20 | | 10:00 | 29.4 | 18:38 | 1.13 | 8:20 | 27.0 | 1.07 | 20:32 |
| 15 | Very poor | 9:10 | 28.2 | 19:32 | 1.10 | 7:35 | 25.9 | 1.03 | 21:31 |
| 10 | | 8:08 | 26.7 | 20:47 | 1.06 | 6:46 | 24.8 | 1.00 | 22:43 |
| 5 | | 7:00 | 25.1 | 22:22 | 1.01 | 5:35 | 23.1 | 0.95 | 24:42 |
| 1 | | 5:00 | 22.2 | 25:49 | 0.93 | 3:43 | 20.4 | 0.88 | 28:39 |
| | | $n = 6{,}709$ | | | | $n = 4{,}539$ | | | |

**Total _n_** = 11,248

(continued)

### Table 15.3  Fitness Categories for Maximal Aerobic Power for Men and Women by Age (continued)

**WOMEN**

| % | | Age 60-69 | | | | Age 70-79 | | | |
|---|---|---|---|---|---|---|---|---|---|
| | | Balke Treadmill (Time) | Max V̇O₂ (mL · kg⁻¹ · min⁻¹) | 12-min Run (Miles) | 1.5-Mile Run (Time) | Balke Treadmill (Time) | Max V̇O₂ (mL · kg⁻¹ · min⁻¹) | 12-min Run (Miles) | 1.5-Mile Run (Time) |
| 99 | Superior | 20:00 | 43.9 | 1.53 | 11:58 | 20:00 | 43.9 | 1.53 | 11:58 |
| 95 | | 15:47 | 37.8 | 1.36 | 14:05 | 15:01 | 36.7 | 1.33 | 14:34 |
| 90 | Excellent | 14:30 | 35.9 | 1.31 | 14:53 | 12:30 | 33.0 | 1.23 | 16:21 |
| 85 | | 13:31 | 34.5 | 1.27 | 15:35 | 11:43 | 31.9 | 1.20 | 17:00 |
| 80 | | 12:30 | 33.0 | 1.23 | 16:21 | 11:00 | 30.9 | 1.17 | 17:38 |
| 75 | Good | 12:00 | 32.3 | 1.21 | 16:46 | 10:23 | 30.0 | 1.15 | 18:14 |
| 70 | | 11:19 | 31.3 | 1.18 | 17:21 | 10:01 | 29.5 | 1.13 | 18:37 |
| 65 | | 11:00 | 30.9 | 1.17 | 17:38 | 10:00 | 29.4 | 1.13 | 18:38 |
| 60 | | 10:25 | 30.0 | 1.15 | 18:12 | 9:05 | 28.1 | 1.10 | 19:38 |
| 55 | Fair | 10:00 | 29.4 | 1.13 | 18:38 | 8:59 | 28.0 | 1.09 | 19:44 |
| 50 | | 9:46 | 29.1 | 1.12 | 18:52 | 8:37 | 27.4 | 1.08 | 20:11 |
| 45 | | 9:16 | 28.4 | 1.10 | 19:25 | 8:01 | 26.6 | 1.05 | 20:56 |
| 40 | | 8:41 | 27.5 | 1.08 | 20:06 | 7:33 | 25.9 | 1.03 | 21:34 |
| 35 | Poor | 8:09 | 26.8 | 1.06 | 20:46 | 7:01 | 25.1 | 1.01 | 22:20 |
| 30 | | 7:43 | 26.1 | 1.04 | 21:20 | 6:49 | 24.8 | 1.00 | 22:38 |
| 25 | | 7:05 | 25.2 | 1.01 | 22:14 | 6:29 | 24.4 | 0.99 | 23:10 |
| 20 | | 6:45 | 24.7 | 1.00 | 22:44 | 6:07 | 23.8 | 0.98 | 23:46 |
| 15 | Very poor | 6:15 | 24.0 | 0.98 | 23:32 | 5:15 | 22.6 | 0.94 | 25:20 |
| 10 | | 5:33 | 23.0 | 0.95 | 24:46 | 4:30 | 21.5 | 0.91 | 26:51 |
| 5 | | 4:45 | 21.9 | 0.92 | 26:19 | 3:15 | 19.7 | 0.86 | 29:51 |
| 1 | | 3:07 | 19.5 | 0.86 | 30:13 | 1:17 | 16.8 | 0.78 | 36:12 |
| | | | | | | | | | |
| | | *n* = 1,313 | | | | *n* = 187 | | | |

**Total *n* = 1,500**

Adapted with permission from *Physical Fitness Assessments and Norms for Adults and Law Enforcement*. The Cooper Institute, Dallas, Texas, 2009. For more information: www.cooperinstitute.org

| Table 15.4 | Approximate Energy Requirements in METs for Horizontal and Grade Walking | | | | | |
|---|---|---|---|---|---|---|
| mph | 1.7 | 2.0 | 2.5 | 3.0 | 3.4 | 3.75 |
| % Grade $m \cdot min^{-1}$ | 45.6 | 53.6 | 67.0 | 80.4 | 91.2 | 100.5 |
| 0 | 2.3 | 2.5 | 2.9 | 3.3 | 3.6 | 3.9 |
| 2.5 | 2.9 | 3.2 | 3.8 | 4.3 | 4.8 | 5.2 |
| 5.0 | 3.5 | 3.9 | 4.6 | 5.4 | 5.9 | 6.5 |
| 7.5 | 4.1 | 4.6 | 5.5 | 6.4 | 7.1 | 7.8 |
| 10.0 | 4.6 | 5.3 | 6.3 | 7.4 | 8.3 | 9.1 |
| 12.5 | 5.2 | 6.0 | 7.2 | 8.5 | 9.5 | 10.4 |
| 15.0 | 5.8 | 6.6 | 8.1 | 9.5 | 10.6 | 11.7 |
| 17.5 | 6.4 | 7.3 | 8.9 | 10.5 | 11.8 | 12.9 |
| 20.0 | 7.0 | 8.0 | 9.8 | 11.6 | 13.0 | 14.2 |
| 22.5 | 7.6 | 8.7 | 10.6 | 12.6 | 14.2 | 15.5 |
| 25.0 | 8.2 | 9.4 | 11.5 | 13.6 | 15.3 | 16.8 |

From American College of Sports Medicine. *ACSM's Guidelines for Exercise Testing and Prescription.* 7th ed. Philadelphia (PA): Lippincott Williams & Wilkins; 2006. p. 292.

| Table 15.5 | Approximate Energy Requirements in METs for Horizontal and Grade Jogging/Running | | | | | | |
|---|---|---|---|---|---|---|---|
| mph | 5 | 6 | 7 | 7.5 | 8 | 9 | 10 |
| % Grade $m \cdot min^{-1}$ | 134 | 161 | 188 | 201 | 214 | 241 | 268 |
| 0 | 8.6 | 10.2 | 11.7 | 12.5 | 13.3 | 14.8 | 16.3 |
| 2.5 | 9.5 | 11.2 | 12.9 | 13.8 | 14.7 | 16.3 | 18.0 |
| 5.0 | 10.3 | 12.3 | 14.1 | 15.1 | 16.1 | 17.9 | 19.7 |
| 7.5 | 11.2 | 13.3 | 15.3 | 16.4 | 17.4 | 19.4 | |
| 10.0 | 12.0 | 14.3 | 16.5 | 17.7 | 18.8 | | |
| 12.5 | 12.9 | 15.4 | 17.7 | 19.0 | | | |
| 15.0 | 13.8 | 16.4 | 18.9 | | | | |

From American College of Sports Medicine. *ACSM's Guidelines for Exercise Testing and Prescription.* 7th ed. Philadelphia (PA): Lippincott Williams & Wilkins; 2006. p. 292.

| Table 15.6 | **Approximate Energy Requirements in METs during Leg Cycle Ergometry** | | | | | | |
|---|---|---|---|---|---|---|---|
| | | Power Output (kg · m · min⁻¹ and W) | | | | | |
| Body Weight | | 300 | 450 | 600 | 750 | 900 | 1,050 | 1,200 (kg · m · min⁻¹) |
| kg | lb | 50 | 75 | 100 | 125 | 150 | 175 | 200 (W) |
| 50 | 110 | 5.1 | 6.6 | 8.2 | 9.7 | 11.3 | 12.8 | 14.3 |
| 60 | 132 | 4.6 | 5.9 | 7.1 | 8.4 | 9.7 | 11.0 | 12.3 |
| 70 | 154 | 4.2 | 5.3 | 6.4 | 7.5 | 8.6 | 9.7 | 10.8 |
| 80 | 176 | 3.9 | 4.9 | 5.9 | 6.8 | 7.8 | 8.8 | 9.7 |
| 90 | 198 | 3.7 | 4.6 | 5.4 | 6.3 | 7.1 | 8.0 | 8.9 |
| 100 | 220 | 3.5 | 4.3 | 5.1 | 5.9 | 6.6 | 7.4 | 8.2 |

From American College of Sports Medicine. *ACSM's Guidelines for Exercise Testing and Prescription.* 7th ed. Philadelphia (PA): Lippincott Williams & Wilkins; 2006. p. 292.

The limitation of using these tables is that they restrict the workout options. For example, for the walking table, only certain grade and speed options are presented. Box 15.4 provides an example of how to use these tables to determine exercise workload ranges for a hypothetical client.

In summary, anytime a workload is determined using oxygen consumption, the Personal Trainer must consider the client's individual differences in skill and efficiency. The Personal Trainer should also always monitor the client's response to the exercise (including HR or rating of perceived exertion [RPE]) and make adjustments to workload based on the individual's response to the exercise load (7). If the Personal Trainer needs to determine workload for a more diverse range of activities (*e.g.,* cleaning the house, hunting, or specific sports activities), other tables (1,8) are available.

A Personal Trainer should monitor the client's response to the exercise (including HR, rating of perceived exertion, and any other signs or symptoms of overexertion).

| Table 15.7 | **Approximate Energy Requirements in METs during Arm Cycle Ergometry** | | | | | |
|---|---|---|---|---|---|---|
| | | Power Output (kg · m · min⁻¹ and W) | | | | |
| Body Weight | | 150 | 300 | 450 | 600 | 750 | 900 (kg · m · min⁻¹) |
| kg | lb | 25 | 50 | 75 | 100 | 125 | 150 (W) |
| 50 | 110 | 3.6 | 6.1 | 8.7 | 11.3 | 13.9 | 16.4 |
| 60 | 132 | 3.1 | 5.3 | 7.4 | 9.6 | 11.7 | 13.9 |
| 70 | 154 | 2.8 | 4.7 | 6.5 | 8.3 | 10.2 | 12.0 |
| 80 | 176 | 2.6 | 4.2 | 5.8 | 7.4 | 9.0 | 10.6 |
| 90 | 198 | 2.4 | 3.9 | 5.3 | 6.7 | 8.1 | 9.6 |
| 100 | 220 | 2.3 | 3.6 | 4.9 | 6.1 | 7.4 | 8.7 |

From American College of Sports Medicine. *ACSM's Guidelines for Exercise Testing and Prescription.* 7th ed. Philadelphia (PA): Lippincott Williams & Wilkins; 2006. p. 293.

| Table 15.8 | Approximate Energy Requirements in METs during Stair Stepping | | | | | |
|---|---|---|---|---|---|---|
| **Step Height** | | **Stepping Rate Per Minute** | | | | | |
| in | m | 20 | 22 | 24 | 26 | 28 | 30 |
| 4 | 0.102 | 3.5 | 3.8 | 4.0 | 4.3 | 4.5 | 4.8 |
| 6 | 0.152 | 4.2 | 4.6 | 4.9 | 5.2 | 5.5 | 5.8 |
| 8 | 0.203 | 4.9 | 5.3 | 5.7 | 6.1 | 6.5 | 6.9 |
| 10 | 0.254 | 5.6 | 6.1 | 6.5 | 7.0 | 7.5 | 7.9 |
| 12 | 0.305 | 6.3 | 6.8 | 7.4 | 7.9 | 8.4 | 9.0 |
| 14 | 0.356 | 7.0 | 7.6 | 8.2 | 8.8 | 9.4 | 10.0 |
| 16 | 0.406 | 7.7 | 8.4 | 9.0 | 9.7 | 10.4 | 11.1 |
| 18 | 0.457 | 8.4 | 9.1 | 9.9 | 10.6 | 11.4 | 12.1 |

From American College of Sports Medicine. *ACSM's Guidelines for Exercise Testing and Prescription.* 7th ed. Philadelphia (PA): Lippincott Williams & Wilkins; 2006. p. 293.

### Heart Rate and Heart Rate Reserve

Often, a Personal Trainer will not have access to information on oxygen consumption. Because HR and oxygen consumption have a linear relationship, in the absence of oxygen consumption information, HR can be used. When HR is used to determine intensity, ACSM recommends a range of between 64% and 76% up to 95% of $HR_{max}$ (7). The following calculation can be used to determine the exercise target HR based on a percentage of $HR_{max}$:

$$\text{Target HR (lower end of range)} = (\text{maximal HR}) \times 0.64$$

$$\text{Target HR (upper end of range)} = (\text{maximal HR}) \times 0.95$$

For example, for a 20-year-old with an estimated $HR_{max}$ of 200 (220 − 20 = 200 bpm), the range will be 128–190 bpm. However, the resulting target HR range may be so wide that it is not helpful to guide the client's exercise session. The Personal Trainer must therefore consider the client's health history and fitness goals to narrow the range. For apparently healthy individuals, the range is often narrowed to 70% to 85% of $HR_{max}$ (7). Therefore, for the 20-year-old, moderately active client, the target HR range will be 140–170 bpm. If a client is very deconditioned or unfit, then a lower percentage will be used (*e.g.*, 55%–70%).

Using HR in prescribing intensity can be helpful as it represents a client's physiological response, but it too has shortcomings. Accuracy can be compromised when estimations of $HR_{max}$ are used or when medications are taken, which may influence HR (*i.e.*, β-blockers, a drug that suppresses HR at rest and during exercise). Medication use can be identified within the initial health history and should be updated as needed when changes in medications occur. When an actual measured $HR_{max}$ taken during a graded exercise test is unavailable, the Personal Trainer commonly uses an age-predicted estimate (220 − Age). Be aware that there are some controversies over using this method to estimate $HR_{max}$. The concern with this method (7) is the wide range of HR variability for a given single age (1 *SD* equals ± 10–12 bpm). Thus, a 20-year-old may not have an $HR_{max}$ of 200 as predicted by this formula, but instead, his or her estimate could be as low as 188 or as high as 212. Some population-specific equations for estimating $HR_{max}$ are available (7). These may be superior to the "220 − Age" equation, at least in some individuals, although they are not recommended for

| **Box 15.4** | **Example for Use of MET Tables** |
|---|---|

Client: Joe
Characteristics:

Age = 40 yr                   Weight = 175 lb (80 kg)                   Height = 70 in (1.78 m)

$\dot{V}O_{2max}$ = 45 mL · kg$^{-1}$ · min$^{-1}$

To calculate $\dot{V}O_2R$, use the following formula:

$$\text{Target } \dot{V}O_2 = [(\text{percentage}) \times (\dot{V}O_{2max} - \dot{V}O_{2\,rest})] + \dot{V}O_{2\,rest}$$

Because Joe's $\dot{V}O_{2max}$ puts him at approximately the 75th percentile (Table 15.3), he is considered to be in the good category. As a result, his Personal Trainer decides to prescribe a range of 60%–75% $\dot{V}O_2R$. To determine the target $\dot{V}O_2$ range, the calculations for Joe are as follows:

$$\text{Target } \dot{V}O_2 \text{ (lower end)} = [(0.60) \times (45 - 3.5)] + 3.5 = 28.4 \text{ mL} \cdot kg^{-1} \cdot min^{-1}$$

$$\text{Target } \dot{V}O_2 \text{ (upper end)} = [(0.75) \times (45 - 3.5)] + 3.5 = 34.6 \text{ mL} \cdot kg^{-1} \cdot min^{-1}$$

Thus, the workouts will range between 28.4 and 34.6 mL · kg$^{-1}$ · min$^{-1}$.
Joe indicates that he wants to use the treadmill as well as a stationary bike.
Joe's Personal Trainer will convert the oxygen consumption from units of mL · kg$^{-1}$ · min$^{-1}$ to METs. This is accomplished by dividing the lower and upper ends of the target zone by 3.5 as shown below.

$$28.4 \text{ mL} \cdot kg^{-1} \cdot min^{-1} / 3.5 = 8.1 \text{ MET}$$

$$34.6 \text{ mL} \cdot kg^{-1} \cdot min^{-1} / 3.5 = 9.9 \text{ MET}$$

Using Table 15.4, the Personal Trainer can determine a walking intensity on the lower end of the range (~8.1 MET). Note that many options are available at the 8.1-MET target, including walking at 1.7 mph (2.7 km · h$^{-1}$) with 25% grade (8.2 MET level) or walking at 2.5 mph (4 km · h$^{-1}$) with a 15% grade (8.1 MET). However, these would be a rather awkward workload due to the very steep grade. Therefore, the Personal Trainer would discuss with Joe various options. Joe indicated that he likes walking on incline when exercising on the treadmill and thus the Personal Trainer suggests 3.4 mph with a 10% grade.

For the upper end of the workload range (9.9 MET), Joe indicated he would rather jog on a level treadmill. Using Table 15.5, the Personal Trainer sees that 6 mph (9.6 km · h$^{-1}$) with no grade will be approximately 10 MET (*i.e.*, 10.2 MET). Joe will be instructed to monitor his heart rate and RPE as well to make adjustments to these workloads as he becomes accustomed to the exercise.

Joe also requested guidance on determining appropriate settings on a stationary bike. To use Table 15.6 (leg cycle ergometry), the Personal Trainer must know Joe's body weight. Body weight is 175 lb (80 kg). Going across the row for 80 kg in Table 15.6, the workloads approximating 8.1 MET and 9.9 MET are slightly over 900 kp · m · min$^{-1}$ (150 W) and 1,200 kp · m · min$^{-1}$ (200 W). These settings will provide Joe with guidance on what workloads to begin his exercise.

universal application (7). Table 15.9 provides the commonly used equations for estimating HR$_{max}$ for various populations. Although directly measured HR$_{max}$ is preferred to estimated methods, when this is not feasible, an estimation using one of these methods is acceptable. When estimating HR$_{max}$, choose an equation that most represents the client population.

Heart rate reserve (HRR) is the difference between HR$_{max}$ and HR$_{rest}$. Exercise intensity can be determined from HRR in a similar manner as $\dot{V}O_2R$. This method is often referred to as the Karvonen method (7).

$$\text{Target HR (lower end of range)} = [(0.40) \times (HR_{max} - HR_{rest})] + HR_{rest}$$

$$\text{Target HR (upper end of range)} = [(0.85) \times (HR_{max} - HR_{rest})] + HR_{rest}$$

| Table 15.9 | Commonly Used Equations for Estimating Maximal Heart Rate | |
|---|---|---|
| **Study** | **Equation** | **Population** |
| Fox (1971) | $HR_{max} = 220 - Age$ | Small group of men and women |
| Astrand (1952) | $HR_{max} = 216.6 - (0.84 \times Age)$ | Men and women ages 4–34 yr |
| Tanaka (2001) | $HR_{max} = 208 - (0.7 \times Age)$ | Healthy men and women |
| Gellish (2007) | $HR_{max} = 207 - (0.7 \times Age)$ | Men and women participants in an adult fitness program with broad range of age and fitness levels |
| Gulati (2010) | $HR_{max} = 206 - (0.88 \times Age)$ | Asymptomatic middle-aged women referred for stress testing |

$HR_{max}$, maximal heart rate.
Adapted with permission from American College of Sports Medicine. *ACSM's Guidelines for Exercise Testing and Prescription.* 9th ed. Philadelphia (PA): Lippincott Williams & Wilkins; 2013.

Selection of the intensity range must be made with the client's fitness, health status, and fitness goals in mind.

For example, when using this method for a 20-year-old client who has an $HR_{rest}$ of 75, the range will be 125–181 bpm. This range is too wide to be a useful intensity for exercise prescription. Thus, changes must be made based on the client's fitness. If the client is moderately active, using a range of 60%–80% may be appropriate, whereas, if the client is deconditioned, a range of 40%–50% may be more appropriate.

### Rating of Perceived Exertion

RPE is used to subjectively rate overall feelings of exertion during exercise and so can be helpful in guiding exercise intensity (7,8). Commonly used is a 6- to 20-point scale (7). Table 15.10 lists the Borg RPE scale. The threshold level for cardiorespiratory benefits appears to be at an RPE between 12 and 16 (8). The verbal descriptors for this range include "somewhat hard" to "hard." When using RPE, the Personal Trainer should keep in mind the variability between individuals (*e.g.*, the RPE value will not necessarily correspond directly with a particular percentage of $HR_{max}$ or percentage of HRR) and then make adjustments as needed (7).

RPE is often recommended for determining exercise intensity in older adults and is helpful for individuals having difficulty assessing their HR or who are taking medications which influence HR. Although older adults are encouraged to attain similar amounts of physical activity related to days per week and time per session as younger people (11), given the wide range of fitness levels in older adults, using a perceived exertion scale (*i.e.*, a moderate or 5- to-6-level rating of exertion on a 10-point scale) to gauge intensity is often more preferable than standard activity descriptions. For example, for some older adults, moderate-intensity activity may be a slow walk, whereas for others, it may be a brisk walk or jog.

### Talk Test

A very simple way to consider intensity is the "talk test" (13). This simply means that as clients exercise, they should be able to speak (have a conversation) with someone. When comfortable speech is not possible (*e.g.*, gasping for breath after every word or two), it may indicate that the intensity is moving above the level typically prescribed. Thus, the goal is to exercise as close as possible to the point at which speech first becomes difficult.

| Table 15.10 | Category Scale for Rating of Perceived Exertion |
| --- | --- |
| | **Category Scale** |
| 6 | No exertion at all |
| 7 | Extremely light |
| 8 | |
| 9 | Very light |
| 10 | |
| 11 | Light |
| 12 | |
| 13 | Somewhat hard |
| 14 | |
| 15 | Hard (heavy) |
| 16 | |
| 17 | Very hard |
| 18 | |
| 19 | Extremely hard |
| 20 | Maximal exertion |

Copyright Gunnar Borg. Reproduced with permission. For correct use of the Borg scales, it is necessary to follow the administration and instructions given in Borg G. *Borg's Perceived Exertion and Pain Scales.* Champaign (IL): Human Kinetics; 1998.

## Exercise Type or Mode

The mode of exercise needs to be selected with consideration for the client's fitness, health, skill, and interests. During the consultation with a client, it is best to discuss what activities are most enjoyed as well as those that are accessible. Enjoyability and access may seem obvious but are important to consider when selecting an exercise mode for best possible adherence.

Typically, cardiorespiratory exercises are those that involve the use of large muscle groups in a repetitive, or rhythmic, fashion. Some activities are weight-dependent, meaning that body weight is moved during the exercise (*e.g.*, walking, running). In other activities, body weight is not a factor because the body is supported (*e.g.*, cycling, swimming). These activities are referred to as weight-bearing and nonweight-bearing exercises, respectively (8). Use of non–weight-bearing exercises may be useful in avoiding injuries of the lower limbs due to overuse (8). ACSM has classified a number of cardiorespiratory endurance activities into four groups (7) (Table 15.11). The groups do not necessarily represent the recommended or optimal progression of activity but rather present the Personal Trainer with a structure of the characteristics of different exercise modes that should be considered when selecting activities.

Group A includes endurance activities that require minimal skill or fitness to perform. Walking would be an example. Group A activities easily accommodate individual fitness levels and thus are recommended for all adults (7). Group B activities are those that require minimal skill but, in contrast to Group A activities, are typically performed at a more vigorous intensity. Jogging and

| Table 15.11 | Grouping of Cardiorespiratory Exercise and Activities | | |
| --- | --- | --- | --- |
| **Exercise Group** | **Exercise Description** | **Recommended for** | **Examples** |
| A | Endurance activities requiring minimal skill or physical fitness to perform | All adults | Walking, leisurely cycling, aqua-aerobics, slow dancing |
| B | Vigorous-intensity endurance activities requiring minimal skill | Adults (per the preparticipation screening guidelines Chapter 11) who are habitually physically active and/or at least average physical fitness | Jogging, running, rowing, aerobics, spinning, elliptical exercise, stepping exercise, fast dancing |
| C | Endurance activities requiring skill to perform | Adults with acquired skill and/or at least average physical fitness levels | Swimming, cross-country skiing, skating |
| D | Recreational sports | Adults with a regular exercise program and at least average physical fitness | Racquet sports, basketball, soccer, downhill skiing, hiking |

Adapted with permission from American College of Sports Medicine. *ACSM's Guidelines for Exercise Testing and Prescription.* 9th ed. Philadelphia (PA): Lippincott Williams & Wilkins; 2013.

running are examples. Group B activities are appropriate for those who exercise regularly and who have at least an average level of fitness. Examples of Group C exercises are swimming and cross-country skiing. This group reflects activities that have a high relationship between skill and energy expenditure (7). For example, an experienced swimmer may be able to easily swim at a constant intensity, whereas a person with poor swimming skill would be very inefficient and would struggle to swim at an appropriate and constant intensity to receive cardiorespiratory benefits.

Recreational sports like basketball, soccer, tennis, and other racquet sports are classified as Group D activities (7). These activities are typically vigorous and intermittent. The nature of these activities does not lend themselves to constant, controlled intensity levels. This is even more true when competition is involved. As a result, Group D activities should be used with caution for clients with low fitness or who are at high risk or symptomatic of disease unless modifications to rules are implemented (7). Group D activities are generally recommended as ancillary activities that are added to a regular fitness program (7).

The Personal Trainer should use these activity groupings to guide their selection of an appropriate exercise mode for their client. As noted previously, Group A activities are appropriate to use with any client, but especially for clients beginning an exercise program. Group B activities are recommended for most or all regular exercisers with at least an average fitness level. Group C activities may be included but will require discussion with the client regarding their skill levels for the activities in question. Group D activities may best be included as additional activity after a fairly good level of fitness is achieved. The Personal Trainer and the client must maintain open lines of communication regarding the selection of exercise modes. In some situations, individuals will be satisfied with continuing with various Group A activities. Other clients may have goals to move to Group B, have the skills or desire to learn new skills to include Group C activities, or enjoy the variety and challenge of Group D activities.

The Personal Trainer should also always instruct clients about proper posture and body alignment during cardiorespiratory training. Having a client perform these exercises in a proper biomechanical position is just as important with cardiorespiratory exercise as when clients are performing resistance

The Personal Trainer should also instruct clients about proper posture and body alignment while participating in cardiorespiratory training.

training exercises, as discussed in Chapter 14. Typical concerns with treadmill exercise include leaning forward, uneven or unnatural gait, and excessive gripping on the handrails. Proper upright posture, body alignment, and normal gait with the use of handrails only for balance should be encouraged. Similarly, with stair steppers or other cross-training machines, upright posture should be maintained rather than allowing forward head protrusion, rounded shoulders, or poor alignment. The biggest challenge with cycle ergometry is determination of appropriate seat height. Seat height should be adjusted to allow for 5°–10° of knee flexion at the bottom of the pedal stroke. Figures 15.1 through 15.4 show examples of proper exercise postures.

## Time or Exercise Session Duration

Exercise duration and intensity are typically inversely related. As one increases, the other decreases. Thus, intensity of the exercise must be considered when determining the duration. ACSM recommends 30–60 minutes per day (150 min $\cdot$ wk$^{-1}$) of moderate-intensity exercise, 20–60 minutes per day (75 min $\cdot$ wk$^{-1}$) of vigorous exercise, or a combination of both to improve cardiorespiratory fitness (7). This duration can be in one exercise session or could be accomplished intermittently. If the exercise is done intermittently, then the minimum time should be 10 minutes for each interval (3). Sedentary individuals should begin with very short bouts (*i.e.*, 5–10 min $\cdot$ d$^{-1}$) of low-intensity exercise. Time and intensity should then be gradually increased while always being mindful of the client's fatigue level. The rate of progression will vary depending on the health status and age of the individual. Longer durations of exercise ($\geq$60–90 min $\cdot$ d$^{-1}$) are recommended for weight control especially for those who are otherwise sedentary (4). This time frame does not include warm-up and cool-down, both of which should be completed in addition to the time spent at the target exercise program (6).

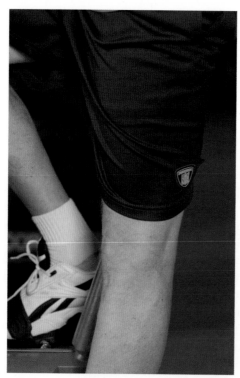
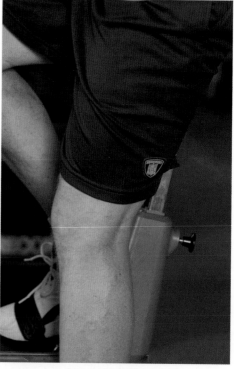

**A**   Full extension   **B**   5° to 10° bend

**FIGURE 15.1.** Personal Trainers should instruct clients to adjust seat heights to maintain a 5°–10° bend in the knee before reaching full extension to reduce compression on the joint structure. Full extension of knee while pedaling on the stationary bike is not recommended.

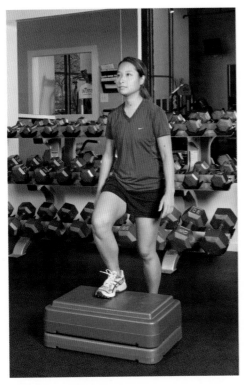

**FIGURE 15.2.** Stepping activity.

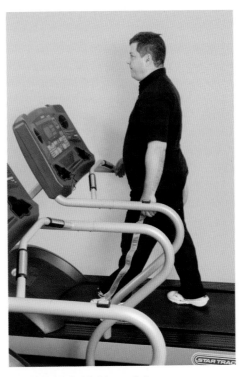

**FIGURE 15.3.** Walking activity.

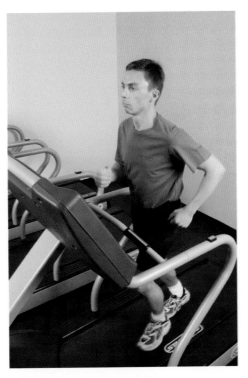

**FIGURE 15.4.** Jogging activity.

## Box 15.5 Calculation of MET, MET-min, and kcal · min$^{-1}$

A shortcoming of caloric expenditure estimates includes the influence of coordination and skill. An experienced swimmer, for example, will expend less energy to swim the same pace as someone with an inefficient stroke patterns. Even though they are at the same pace and theoretically doing a similar amount of work, the inexperienced swimmer will expend more calories than those expended by the experienced swimmer. Thus, the Personal Trainer needs to understand that interindividual differences limit the precision of this estimation.

ACSM recommends expending 150–400 kcal in physical activity each day (7). Sedentary individuals need to begin on the lower end of the range and progress upward. Expenditures of approximately 1,000 kcal · wk$^{-1}$ are associated with decreases in the risk of all-cause mortality (7) and values of $\geq$500–1,000 MET-min · wk$^{-1}$ are consistently associated with lower rates of cardiovascular disease and premature mortality (7) Therefore, a recommended exercise volume for decreasing risk of premature mortality is an exercise volume of $\geq$500–1,000 MET-min · wk$^{-1}$.

Selection of frequency, intensity, and duration determines the calories expended during the activity.

The following equation can be used to approximate the number of calories expended per minute of a given activity (7):

$$\text{Calories per min} = (\text{MET} \times 3.5 \times \text{body weight in kilograms}) / 200$$

The attraction of using this approach is it includes both time and intensity of the prescribed exercise mode. For example, if a client runs on the treadmill at 0% grade at 7 mph for 45 minutes, the Personal Trainer can "summarize" the caloric expenditure of the workout by using this formula and the MET level for 7 mph which is 11.7 MET. If the client weighs 150 lb (68.2 kg), then the number of calories expended for the total workout can be determined as follows:

$$(11.7 \times 3.5 \times 68.2) / 200 = 14 \text{ kcal} \cdot \text{min}^{-1}$$

$$14 \text{ kcal} \cdot \text{min}^{-1} \times 45 \text{ min} = 630 \text{ kcal for the workout}$$

ACSM recommends a minimum goal of $\geq$500–1000 MET-min · wk$^{-1}$ (7). To determine if a person who walks 3 mph (about 3.3 MET) for 30 minutes on 5 days of the week is getting a sufficient volume of exercise, use the following calculation:

$$30 \text{ min at this intensity} = 3.3 \text{ MET} \times 30 \text{ min} = 99 \text{ MET-min} \cdot \text{d}^{-1}$$

$$\text{Volume for 5 d of activity} = 99 \times 5 = 495 \text{ MET-min} \cdot \text{wk}^{-1}$$

Thus, this person is just under the recommended volume. The Personal Trainer should encourage that this person increase time, intensity, or frequency to meet the guidelines. Weekly volume for someone exercising at a higher intensity, for example, jogging 5 mph for 20 minutes 3 days per week would be

$$5 \text{ mph} = 8.6 \text{ MET}$$

$$20 \text{ min at this intensity} = 8.6 \times 20 = 172 \text{ MET-min} \cdot \text{d}^{-1}$$

$$\text{Volume for the 3 d of activity} = 172 \times 3 = 516 \text{ MET-min} \cdot \text{wk}^{-1}$$

Thus, this person is within the recommended weekly volume range. Calculating MET-min · wk$^{-1}$ is especially useful when individuals combine activities of different intensity levels (*e.g.*, walking and jogging in the same week). For example, the MET-min · wk$^{-1}$ for a person walking 2 days per week at 3 mph for 30 minutes and jogging at 5 mph for 2 days per week for 20 minutes would be determined as follows:

$$3 \text{ mph} = 3.3 \text{ MET and 5 mph} = 8.6 \text{ MET}$$

$$30 \text{ min at 3 mph} = 3.3 \text{ MET} \times 30 \text{ min} = 99 \text{ MET-min} \cdot \text{d}^{-1}$$

$$\text{Volume for 2 d of activity} = 99 \times 2 = 198 \text{ MET-min} \cdot \text{wk}^{-1}$$

*(continued)*

| Box 15.5 | Calculation of MET, MET-min, and kcal · min⁻¹ *(continued)* |
| --- | --- |

$$20 \text{ min at } 5 \text{ mph} = 8.6 \times 20 = 172 \text{ MET-min} \cdot d^{-1}$$

$$\text{Volume for 2 d of activity} = 172 \times 2 = 344 \text{ MET-min} \cdot wk^{-1}$$

$$\text{Total volume for 4 d} = 198 + 344 = 542 \text{ MET-min} \cdot wk^{-1}$$

MET values for select activities are shown in Tables 15.2 and 15.4–15.6 (these values are gross MET values which reflect exercise plus rest to determine net METs for the activity alone simply subtract 1 from the numbers in the table). For a more extensive list, please see the updated *Compendium of Physical Activities* (1) or http://sites.google.com/site/compendiumofphysicalactivities/home. Note that the MET values in various tables may differ slightly as these are approximations.

## Volume or Amount (Calories Expended)

Exercise volume is the product of frequency, intensity, time (duration), and type (FITT) of exercise. Exercise volume is used to estimate the gross energy expenditure of an individual's exercise program. Determining exercise volume is important in realizing health/fitness outcomes, particularly with respect to body composition and weight management. Exercise volume is typically expressed in $kcal \cdot day^{-1}$, $kcal \cdot wk^{-1}$, or $MET\text{-}min \cdot wk^{-1}$. Box 15.5 provides definitions and calculations for MET, MET-min, and $kcal \cdot min^{-1}$. These then can be used to calculate volume in $MET\text{-}min \cdot wk^{-1}$ and $kcal \cdot wk^{-1}$ to evaluate whether the exercise program is at the appropriate overload volume.

## Progression

Progression as a component of the exercise prescription ensures that the overload is not applied in a manner that exceeds the cardiorespiratory system's ability to adapt. Any or all of the FITT components need to be increased to continually overload and challenge the cardiorespiratory system. Similarly, all should be adjusted to attain the goals of the client. When and how much to increase each component will depend on the client's initial fitness level, his or her progress, health status, and goals. Intensity and duration of the exercise bout are usually increased first with duration increases ranging from 5 to 10 minutes for a couple of weeks before intensity is increased. Frequency may be increased from 3 days a week to 5 days a week depending on the exercise responses and goals of the client. Volume of exercise is therefore gradually progressed during the course of the exercise prescription until goals are reached. Intensity, duration, and frequency of the exercise endurance phase are gradually increased which results in a gradual progression of the volume of exercise performed. As noted previously, if there is a decrease in the overload such as an injury, travel, or unexpected work obligations, the system will de-adapt and fitness gains will be lost. Therefore, the Personal Trainer must work with the client to anticipate periods of decreased physical activity and plan for a safe "reentry" back into the exercise program. To avoid an overuse injury, clients should refrain from "jumping back" into the same level of activity after more than a few days off.

> Intensity, duration, and frequency of the exercise endurance phase are gradually increased which results in a gradual progression of the volume of exercise performed.

## Sample Cardiorespiratory Endurance Training Programs

Tables 15.12 and 15.13 include examples of cardiorespiratory endurance programs for various types of activities (*e.g.*, walking/jogging program and a typical mix of activities which may be available at a health club). For each, an overall scheme of a 6-month training progression is shown

| Table 15.12 | Sample Walking and Jogging Program | | | |
|---|---|---|---|---|
| **Status** | **Time Point** | **Warm-Up** | **Workout**[a] | **Cool-Down** |
| Beginner | First week | Slow, easy walking pace for a couple of minutes | Walk at a pace that gives a light level of exertion (level 3 or 4) for 10 min at least twice a day for a total of 20 min each day (3 d · wk$^{-1}$). Your weekly total should be 60 min. | Slow, easy walking pace for a couple of minutes |
| | Progression, part 1 | Slow, easy walking pace for 5 min | Each week add 15 min to your weekly total until you reach 120 min of activity (e.g., 30 min 4 d · wk$^{-1}$). Stay at this duration and increase your intensity over the next couple of weeks from light (level 3 or 4) to moderate (level 5 or 6). Once you are comfortable with this time and intensity for a couple of weeks, continue to add 10–15 min · wk$^{-1}$ until you reach 150 min. | Slow, easy walking pace for 5 min |
| | Progression, part 2 | Easy walking pace for 5–10 min | Walk at a pace that gives a moderate level of exertion (level 5 or 6); continue to add 10–15 min each week to progress from 150 min · wk$^{-1}$ to a total of 200 min. | Easy walking pace for 5–10 min |
| | Final week | Easy walking pace for 5–10 min | Walk at a pace that gives a moderate level of exertion (level 5 or 6) for 30–60 min (3–5 d · wk$^{-1}$). Your weekly total should be 200 min. | Easy walking pace for 5–10 min |
| Intermediate | Initial week | Easy walking pace for 5–10 min | Walk at a pace that feels moderate (level 5 or 6) for 30–60 min (3–5 d · wk$^{-1}$). Your weekly total should be 200 min. | Easy walking pace for 5–10 min |
| | Progression | Easy walking pace for 5–10 min | Continue to increase exercise duration by 10–15 min · wk$^{-1}$ to approach 300 min of moderate activity accumulated on a weekly basis. Another option is to introduce a more vigorous activity, such as jogging, realizing that the time needed will be less (typically 2 min of moderate activity equals 1 min of vigorous activity). | Easy walking pace for 5–10 min |
| | Final week | Easy walking pace for 5–10 min | Walk at a pace that feels moderate (level 5 or 6) for 45–90 min (3–5 d · wk$^{-1}$). Your weekly total should be 300 min (moderate intensity). OR Combine moderate and vigorous walking on alternate days. Your weekly total should be equivalent amounts of moderate and vigorous activity (e.g., 200 min of moderate plus 50 min of vigorous). | Easy walking pace for 5–10 min |

| Table 15.12 | | Sample Walking and Jogging Program *(continued)* | | |
|---|---|---|---|---|
| **Status** | **Time Point** | **Warm-Up** | **Workout**[a] | **Cool-Down** |
| Established | Continue/ maintain | Easy walking pace for 5–10 min | Walk at a pace that feels moderate (level 5 or 6). Your weekly total should be a minimum of 300 min (moderate intensity). OR Jog (at level 7 or 8). Your weekly total should be a minimum of 150 min (vigorous intensity). OR Combine moderate and vigorous walking on alternate days. Your weekly total should be equivalent amounts of moderate and vigorous activity (*e.g.,* 200 min of moderate plus 50 min of vigorous). | Easy walking pace for 5–10 min |

[a]Level of exertion is on a scale of 0–10 (sitting at rest is 0 and your highest effort level is 10).
Adapted with permission from American College of Sports Medicine. *ACSM's Complete Guide to Fitness and Health.* Champaign (IL): Human Kinetics; 2011. p. 396.

for an apparently healthy client. Use of the terms *beginner, intermediate,* and *established* to describe the fitness level of the client is somewhat subjective. For some individuals, even the beginner stage may present too much of a challenge. If so, starting out with only 5–10 minutes of exercise may be more appropriate. The progression should not be too aggressive. Do not focus on achieving target goals quickly but rather to gradually increase the overall workload to establish compliance and promote adherence. Progression should be individualized on the basis of the client's initial fitness level, health status, age, and individual goals.

For each stage, a range rather than a single number is included for frequency, intensity, and duration. The role of a Personal Trainer is to assist the client with the appropriate balance based on individual responses. Frequency of exercise progresses gradually over the 6-month period outlined from 3 days per week up to a target of 3–5 days per week. Intensity increases from relatively low to a target of 70%–85% HRR. By slowly increasing the intensity, the client is able to adapt to the higher levels of exercise without becoming discouraged or experiencing retrogression (*i.e.,* a reversal of gains due to excessive overload). The duration of the exercise session also increases in small steps to allow for appropriate adaptations. Finally, the Personal Trainer can consider changing the mode of exercise to provide more variety in the program.

Progression should be individualized on the basis of the client's initial fitness level, health status, age, and individual goals.

Recall that the activities are classified by group. Walking is a Group A activity and is appropriate for anyone. The progression found in Table 15.12 could also be used with swimming or other aquatic exercises, which are Group C activities and require skill to maintain an appropriate intensity for a sufficient period of time. For each activity, the sequence in time, intensity, and frequency as well as progression of the different types of activities should be noted. When designing a program, occasionally including new modes of exercise can provide much-appreciated variety but should be introduced gradually so that appropriate adjustments can be made (*i.e.,* appropriate overload). Most importantly, remember that the overall training program must match the goals of the client.

| Table 15.13 | Sample Cross-Training Program at a Health Club | | | | |
|---|---|---|---|---|---|
| **Status** | **Time Point** | **Warm-Up** | **Workout**[a] | | **Cool-Down** |
| Beginner | First week | Slow, easy walking pace for a couple of minutes | Pick one activity each day at a light level of exertion (level 3 or 4) for 10 min at least twice a day for a total of 20 min each day (3 d · wk$^{-1}$). Select from walking on the treadmill or stationary biking. Your weekly total should be 60 min. | | Slow, easy walking pace for a couple of minutes |
| | Progression, part 1 | Slow, easy walking pace for 5 min | Each week add 15 min to your weekly total until you reach 120 min of activity (*e.g.*, 30 min 4 d · wk$^{-1}$). Potential activities include treadmill walking, stationary biking, and using a stair climber. Stay at this duration and increase your intensity over the next couple of weeks from light (level 3 or 4) to moderate (level 5 or 6). Once you are comfortable with this time and intensity for a couple of weeks, continue to add 10–15 min · wk$^{-1}$ until you reach 150 min. | | Slow, easy walking pace for 5 min |
| | Progression, part 2 | Easy walking pace for 5–10 min | Exercise at an intensity that gives a moderate level of exertion (level 5 or 6); continue to add 10–15 min each week to progress from 150 min · wk$^{-1}$ to a total of 200 min. | | Easy walking pace for 5–10 min |
| | Final week | Easy walking pace for 5–10 min | Exercise at an intensity that gives a moderate level of exertion (level 5 or 6) for 30–60 min (3–5 d · wk$^{-1}$). Activities may include treadmill walking; stationary biking; or using a stair climber, elliptical trainer, rowing machine, or Nordic ski machine. Your weekly total should be 200 min. | | Easy walking pace for 5–10 min |
| Intermediate | Initial week | Easy walking pace for 5–10 min | Exercise at a level that feels moderate (level 5 or 6) for 30–60 min (3–5 d · wk$^{-1}$) using a treadmill, stationary bike, stair climber, elliptical trainer, or Nordic ski machine. Your weekly total should be 200 min. | | Easy walking pace for 5–10 min |
| | Progression | Easy walking pace for 5–10 min | Continue to increase exercise duration by 10–15 min · wk$^{-1}$ to approach 300 min of moderate activity accumulated on a weekly basis. Another option is to introduce more vigorous activity a couple of days per week, such as jogging on the treadmill, taking a spinning class, or taking a step aerobics class, realizing that the time needed will be less (typically, 2 min of moderate activity equals 1 min of vigorous activity). | | Easy walking pace for 5–10 min |

| Status | Time Point | Warm-Up | Workout[a] | Cool-Down |
|---|---|---|---|---|
| | Final week | Easy walking pace for 5–10 min | Exercise at a level that feels moderate (level 5 or 6) for 45–90 min (3–5 d · wk$^{-1}$). Your weekly total should be 300 min (moderate intensity). OR Combine moderate and vigorous walking on alternate days. Your weekly total should be equivalent amounts of moderate and vigorous activity (*e.g.*, 200 min of moderate plus 50 min of vigorous). | Easy walking pace for 5–10 min |
| Established | Continue/ maintain | Easy walking pace for 5–10 min | Exercise at an intensity that feels moderate (level 5 or 6). Your weekly total should be a minimum of 300 min (moderate intensity). OR Exercise at a higher intensity (level 7 or 8). Your weekly total should be a minimum of 150 min (vigorous intensity). Or Combine moderate and vigorous walking on alternate days. Your weekly total should be equivalent amounts of moderate and vigorous activity (*e.g.*, 200 min of moderate plus 50 min of vigorous). | Easy walking pace for 5–10 min |

Table 15.13 **Sample Cross-Training Program at a Health Club** (continued)

[a]Level of exertion is on a scale of 0–10 (sitting at rest is 0 and your highest effort level is 10).
Adapted with permission from American College of Sports Medicine. *ACSM's Complete Guide to Fitness and Health*. Champaign (IL): Human Kinetics; 2011. p. 396.

## Weight Loss

Many clients are interested in losing weight and often consult Personal Trainers. The ACSM Position Stand, "Appropriate Physical Activity Intervention Strategies for Weight Loss and Prevention of Weight Regain for Adults" (2) indicates that increasing activity levels above the baseline of 150 minutes per week of moderately intense exercise is important to assist with weight loss or to help maintain weight loss. In these situations, the recommended duration of exercise is 50–60 minutes per day (this can be divided into multiple shorter exercise sessions), or 250–300 minutes per week (8). More information about exercise and weight loss is provided in Chapter 20.

## Implementing Cardiorespiratory Endurance Training Programs

Implementation of effective cardiorespiratory endurance training programs requires the Personal Trainer to have knowledge of the current scientific basis of exercise. This chapter has reviewed the ACSM guidelines (3,7) regarding the FITT-VP components of exercise prescription (*i.e.*, frequency, intensity, time, type, volume, and progression). These guidelines provide

Implementation of effective cardiorespiratory endurance training programs requires the Personal Trainer to have knowledge of the current scientific basis of exercise.

a framework to structure the exercise program rather than a rigid checklist. The Personal Trainer must evaluate each client individually for health status and disease risks (see Chapter 11) and conduct individual fitness assessments (see Chapter 12), which are used to determine an appropriate initial level of exercise.

In some ways, the professional Personal Trainer creates an exercise prescription like a master chef designs a gourmet meal. Unlike a novice chef, who would be tied to a recipe, the master chef is able to take knowledge of various ingredients to create individualized, appealing dishes. In a similar manner, a qualified Personal Trainer does not try to fit all clients into a single set prescription (*i.e.,* recipe approach) but rather applies a solid understanding of all the ingredients (*i.e.,* frequency, intensity, mode, and duration) to customize a combination of components into a healthy "meal" for the client.

## SUMMARY

Cardiorespiratory endurance training is an essential part of a client's overall exercise program. Other important components include resistance and flexibility training, which are detailed in Chapters 14 and 16, respectively. Each cardiorespiratory endurance training session includes three basic parts: warm-up, endurance phase, and cool-down. A cardiorespiratory endurance program or prescription requires the FITT-VP components: frequency, intensity, duration, mode, volume, and progression. The Personal Trainer must balance the FITT-VP components with the client's characteristics (*e.g.*, health status, initial fitness), life situations (*e.g.*, work schedule, availability of exercise time), goals (*e.g.*, general fitness, weight loss, competition), and preferences.

## REFERENCES

1. Ainsworth BE, Haskell WL, Herrmann SD, et al. 2011 Compendium of Physical Activities: a second update of codes and MET values. *Med Sci Sports Exerc.* 2011;43(8): 1575–81.

2. American College of Sports Medicine. American College of Sports Medicine Position Stand. Appropriate physical activity intervention strategies for weight loss and prevention of weight regain for adults. *Med Sci Sports Exerc.* 2009;41:459–71.

3. American College of Sports Medicine. American College of Sports Medicine Position Stand. Quantity and quality of exercise for developing and maintaining cardiorespiratory, musculoskeletal, and neuromuscular fitness in apparently healthy adults: guidance for prescribing exercise. *Med Sci Sports Exerc.* 2011;43(7):1334–59.

4. American College of Sports Medicine. American College of Sports Medicine Position Stand. The recommended quantity and quality of exercise for developing and maintaining cardiorespiratory and muscular fitness, and flexibility in healthy adults. *Med Sci Sports Exerc.* 1998;30(6):975–91.

5. American College of Sports Medicine. American College of Sports Medicine Position Stand. The recommended quan-

tity and quality of exercise for developing and maintaining fitness in healthy adults. *Med Sci Sports.* 1978;10:vii–x.

6. American College of Sports Medicine. *ACSM's Complete Guide to Fitness and Health.* Champaign (IL): Human Kinetics; 2011. 408 p.

7. American College of Sports Medicine. *ACSM's Guidelines for Exercise Testing and Prescription.* 10th ed. Philadelphia (PA): Wolters Kluwer; 2018.

8. American College of Sports Medicine. *ACSM's Resource Manual for Guidelines for Exercise Testing and Prescription.* 6th ed. Philadelphia (PA): Lippincott Williams & Wilkins; 2010. 896 p.

9. Haskell WL, Lee IM, Pate RR, et al. Physical activity and public health: updated recommendations for adults from the American College of Sports Medicine and the American Heart Association. *Med Sci Sports Exerc.* 2007;39(8): 1423–34.

10. Kraus H, Hirschland RP. Muscular fitness and health. *JOHPER.* 1953;24:17–9.

11. Nelson ME, Rejeski WJ, Blair SN, et al. Physical activity and public health in older adults: recommendations from the American College of Sports Medicine and the American

Heart Association. *Med Sci Sports Exerc.* 2007;39(8): 1435–45.

12. Pate RR, Pratt M, Blair SN, et al. Physical activity and public health: a recommendation from the Centers for Disease Control and Prevention and the American College of Sports Medicine. *JAMA.* 1995;273(5):402–7.

13. Persinger R, Foster C, Gibson M, Fater DC, Pocari, JP. Consistency of the talk test for exercise prescription. *Med Sci Sports Exerc.* 2004;36:1632–6.

14. Pollock ML. The quantification of endurance training programs. *Exerc Sport Sci Rev.* 1973;1(1):155–88.

15. U.S. Department of Health and Human Services. *2008 Physical Activity Guidelines for Americans* (ODPHP Publication No. U0036) [Internet]. Washington (DC): U.S. Department of Health and Human Services; [cited 2017 Mar 2]. Available from: www.health.gov/paguidelines

16. U.S. Department of Health and Human Services. *Physical Activity and Health: A Report of the Surgeon General.* Atlanta (GA): U.S. Department of Health and Human Services, Public Health Service, Centers for Disease Control and Prevention, National Center for Chronic Disease Prevention and Health Promotion; 1996.

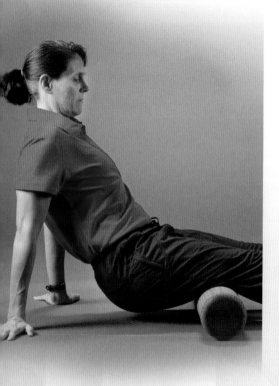

## OBJECTIVES

**Personal Trainers should be able to:**

- Describe the factors influencing flexibility.
- Understand the benefits and risks of flexibility training.
- Determine how to evaluate flexibility.
- Understand various methods of stretching.
- Be aware of precautions for individuals with health concerns.
- Develop a flexibility program based on the FITT-VP principles.

# INTRODUCTION

Flexibility refers to the degree to which a joint moves throughout a normal, pain-free range of motion (ROM). As most physical activities and sports consist of numerous multijoint movements, it is essential that musculoskeletal function not be compromised by inadequate flexibility. Stretching is the method used most commonly to increase joint ROM. American College of Sports Medicine (ACSM's) current position stand on exercises to develop and maintain fitness and flexibility in adults recommends the inclusion of general stretching exercises emphasizing the major skeletal muscle groups at least 2–3 days a week (4). Like body composition, cardiorespiratory fitness, or muscular strength, flexibility is classified as a health-related dimension of fitness (17). This means that flexibility contributes to an overall improved quality of life in athletes and the general public alike.

The purpose of this chapter is to present flexibility as an essential ingredient of health-related fitness and to provide Personal Trainers with a basic understanding of how to properly incorporate flexibility training into the exercise programs of healthy individuals.

## Determinants of Flexibility

Hamill, Knutzen, and Derrick (35) suggest that several factors determine flexibility. These factors include joint structure, health of soft tissue around the joint, length of antagonist muscles, and temperature of the tissues being stretched in addition to the viscoelastic ("rubber band-like") properties of the tissues surrounding the joint. Not surprisingly then, flexibility is largely determined by how well these factors facilitate movement.

Figure 16.1 depicts a typical human knee joint. To better understand the importance of the properties of the tissues surrounding the joint, study the anterior view (*panel A*) and the cross-sectional view (*panel C*) of Figure 16.1. Notice that the knee is padded with fat and is secured into place by ligaments. These tissues influence knee ROM both at the joint itself and elsewhere in the lower extremity. For example, tightness of the ligaments as illustrated in Figure 16.1 or excessive fat surrounding the thigh could inhibit knee ROM during flexion. In fact, one belief about bodybuilders is that they are "muscle bound" and possess a more limited joint ROM as a result of the additional bulk. This is true to a certain extent because thick skeletal muscles can certainly limit ROM. Thus, if the training demands of an athlete or the natural (healthy) body composition of a client predispose them toward greater muscle bulk rather than flexibility, there may be a trade-off such that a more limited joint ROM may be appropriate.

As can be seen from Figure 16.1, contraction of the quadriceps femoris muscles will produce leg extension if the knee is bent at the start of the movement. However, tight quadriceps femoris muscles (perhaps as a result of soreness or poor conditioning) can restrict full leg extension and limit joint flexibility. Notice too from Figure 16.1 that the joint is restricted by the very architecture of the bones themselves. Leg extension is limited by what are termed "bony blocks," which consist of the ends of the femur and tibia resisting hyperextension during full leg extension. It is also possible that injury, disease, and poor soft tissue integrity can contribute to hypermobility or excessive ROM in a joint. The possibility of hypermobility can also be imagined when studying Figure 16.1.

It is possible that injury, disease, and poor soft tissue integrity can contribute to hypermobility or excessive ROM in a joint.

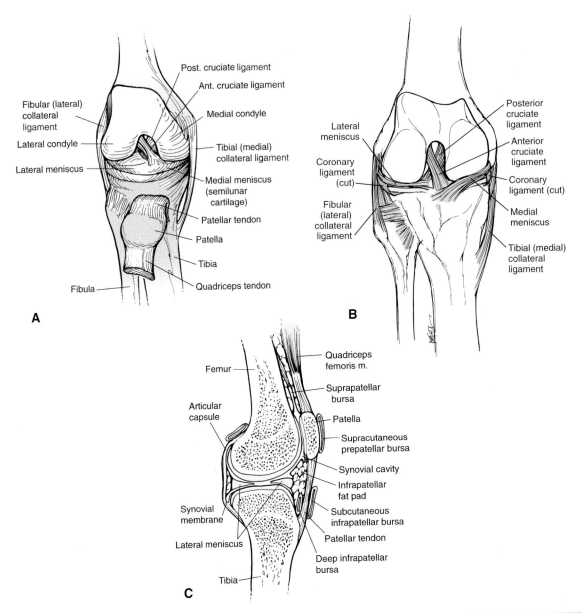

| Ligament | Insertion | Action |
|----------|-----------|--------|
| Anterior cruciate | Anterior intercondylar area of tibia to medial surface of lateral condyle | Prevents anterior tibial displacement; resists extension, internal rotation, flexion |
| Arcuate | Lateral condyle of femur to head of fibula | Reinforces back of capsule |
| Coronary | Meniscus to tibia | Holds menisci to tibia |
| Medial collateral | Medial epicondyle of femur to medial condyle of tibia and medial meniscus | Resists valgus forces; taut in extension; resists internal, external rotation |
| Lateral collateral | Lateral epicondyle of femur to head of fibula | Resists varus forces; taut in extension |
| Patellar | Inferior patela to tibial tuberosity | Transfers force from quariceps to tibia |
| Posterior cruciate | Posterior spine of tibia to inner condyle of femur | Resists posterior tibial movement; resists flexion and rotation |
| Posterior oblique | Expansion of semimembranosus muscle | Supports posterior, medial capsule |
| Transverse | Medial meniscus to lateral meniscus in front | Connects menisci to each other |

**FIGURE 16.1.** Typical joint anatomy: **(A)** anterior, **(B)** posterior, and **(C)** lateral. (Reprinted with permission from Hamill J, Knutzen KM. *Biomechanical Basis of Human Movement.* 3rd ed. Philadelphia [PA]: Lippincott Williams & Wilkins; 2009. p. 212.)

Clearly, joints have inherent structural properties that determine full ROM. Not surprisingly, these properties differ by joint and among individuals, which often explains the large variability in joint ROM values observed in instances such as testing and performance. Although the anatomical structure of the joint clearly influences ROM, there are other influences such as age, sex, and physical activity history that also play a role in determining ROM.

## Age

With increasing age, the ability to move through a full ROM becomes compromised with an overall loss of flexibility of approximately 25%–30% by age 70 years (9,21,30,34). The decreases in flexibility that one may experience will depend on the joint itself. Brown and Miller (13) determined a 30% loss in hamstring flexibility from the age of 20–29 years to 70+ years, whereas Germain and Blair (30) found a 15% loss in shoulder flexion from the age of 20–30 years to 70+ years.

Loss of ROM within a joint may have several causes. With age, changes occur in the framework of the connective tissue collagen fibers as demonstrated by increased rigidity of the tissue (5). This increased rigidity is attributed to tighter cross-linkage within and between collagen fibers, which makes the joint more resistant to bending (43,66). There is also a reduction of elastin as well as a deterioration of the cartilage, ligaments, tendons, synovial fluid, and muscles with age, which may decrease joint ROM (1,14,56). Physiological changes are not the only suspect in the age-related loss of flexibility. Decreased physical activity appears to accelerate the age-related loss of ROM (14,49).

## Sex

Numerous studies suggest that females are more flexible than males owing to a different pattern of skeletal architecture and connective-tissue morphology and certain hormonal differences (10,27,29,67). The differences in ROM between sexes may result from differences in joint and bone structures (2). For example, females typically have broader and shallower hips than males have, which creates the possibility of a greater ROM in the pelvic region (2). Gelabert (29) also suggested that females generally have a greater range of extension in the elbow because of a shorter upper curve of the olecranon process of the elbow than males. Females may also have greater potential for flexibility in trunk flexion after puberty because of a comparatively lower center of gravity and shorter leg length (16).

## Physical Activity History

An individual's history of physical activity has an impact on his or her joint ROM. Studies have shown that an individual who is physically active is also more likely to have a greater ROM than a sedentary individual (18,37,39). Cornu et al. (18) demonstrated that volleyball players exhibited greater flexibility in wrist extension than sedentary individuals. In another sport-related study, Jaeger et al. (37) found that elite field hockey players had significantly greater hip ROM than sedentary individuals. Studies have not been limited to sport activity, though. In a study by Voorrips et al. (63) that examined different habitual physical activity of older women, it was found that the more active older women had significantly greater flexibility in the hip and spine than moderately active and sedentary older women.

# Benefits and Risks of Flexibility Training

As with other forms of physical training, flexibility training has both benefits and risks. These benefits and risks are frequently described from the anecdotal and personal experiences of coaches, clinicians, and exercise leaders rather than from sound research or understanding of the science of human anatomy, physiology, and biomechanics. Unfortunately, the existing science of

The existing science of flexibility training often presents fitness professionals with more questions than answers regarding the benefits and risks of stretching.

flexibility training often presents fitness professionals with more questions than answers regarding the benefits and risks of stretching. The following two sections will provide the Personal Trainer with a short review of the scientific evidence supporting the benefits and risks associated with flexibility training.

## Benefits

### Improved Range of Motion in Selected Joints

Flexibility training has been shown to improve an individual's joint ROM (42,48,63). In a long-term study on the effects of flexibility exercise on shoulder and hip ROM by Misner et al. (48), it was found that the flexibility program used produced significant increases in shoulder extension (5.7%), shoulder transverse extension (10.4%), hip flexion (13.3%), and hip rotation (6.3%). A minor improvement (5.5%) was also observed in shoulder flexion. Improvements in flexibility could be seen in a relatively short time period. Kerrigan et al. (39) recorded improved ROM values in both static and dynamic hip extension when participants followed the program twice daily for 10 weeks. Kukkanen and Malkia (42) also found improvements in spinal ROM and greater hamstring flexibility after subjects followed a 3-month program.

### Improved Performance for Activities of Daily Living

The extent to which individuals can live independently in the community depends on their ability to perform basic daily tasks such as self-care and essential household chores. These tasks are formally termed "activities of daily living" (ADLs). Balancing ability and postural control are critical aspects of performing ADLs (62). In fact, the ability to perform ADLs has been highly correlated with joint mobility (60). In other words, ADLs are easier to perform when an individual possesses an acceptable ROM within the joint. In addition, flexibility exercises can significantly aid balance and postural stability, particularly when combined with resistance exercise (11,19). Thus, flexibility training can improve ADL functioning both directly through enhancing ROM and indirectly through its effect on postural control (31,33,40).

## Risks

### Joint Hypermobility

Although it is suggested that certain individuals or athletes (*e.g.*, gymnasts) may possess extraordinary joint ROM, there is insufficient scientific evidence to link hypermobility to flexibility training.

Hypermobility syndrome is known as "congenital laxity" of ligaments and joints. This condition is characterized by extreme ROM accompanied by mild- to moderate-intensity pain (25). Although it is suggested that certain individuals or athletes (*e.g.*, gymnasts) may possess extraordinary joint ROM, there is insufficient scientific evidence to link hypermobility to flexibility training.

### Decreased Strength

There is some evidence to suggest that static stretching may contribute to decreased muscular strength. In a recent study, Nelson et al. (51) found that muscle strength and endurance performance reduced after short-term static stretching in physical education college students. Fowles et al. (26) found similar results after prolonged stretching of the ankle plantar flexors. This voluntary strength deficit persisted for up to an hour after stretching. In addition, Kokkonen et al. (41) demonstrated that stretching prior to the execution of a one repetition maximum decreased the performance of the lift. A review by McHugh and Cosgrave (47) indicates that acute preparticipation stretching will decrease the ability to generate a maximal force, but if these stretches are part of other activities used in a warm-up, then performance is not seriously affected. In fact, in activities such as gymnastics that require large ROM movements, it is necessary to perform preparticipation activity to achieve the required ROM for the performance (47). Thus, although these studies suggest that maximal strength or performance may be compromised following an acute stretching bout, it is possible that if preperformance stretching is accompanied by other warm-up movements, performance is not negatively impacted. However, because flexibility exercises may acutely reduce power and strength, it is recommended that flexibility exercises be performed after exercise and sports where strength and power are important for performance.

> Because flexibility exercises may acutely reduce power and strength, it is recommended that flexibility exercises be performed after exercise and sports where strength and power are important for performance.

### Ineffective for Preventing Injury

Flexibility training is often promoted as a means of reducing injury risk. However, the research does not show a consistent link between performing regular flexibility training and a reduction in musculotendinous injuries (4,47,59,65). Reviews published regarding injury prevention and flexibility have generally been unable to conclude whether or not stretching before or after exercise contributed to injury prevention among competitive or recreational athletes (59). McHugh and Cosgrave (47) suggested that there is some evidence that preparticipation stretching may reduce the incidence of muscle strains, but that it does not prevent overuse injuries. Finally, Witvrouw et al. (65) concluded that the type of sport activity in which an individual participates is critical when determining the value of flexibility training to reduce injury. They found that the more explosive the skills involved in an activity, the more likely stretching may be needed to decrease injury.

> The more explosive the skills involved in an activity, the more likely stretching may be needed to decrease injury.

### Temporary Effects

Interestingly, the duration of time that increased flexibility lasts after stretching may not be as long as what Personal Trainers may think. Increased flexibility following acute stretching is extremely short-lived. DePino et al. (20) recruited 30 male subjects and found that the improvements in knee ROM following static stretching of the hamstrings lasted less than 3 minutes. These authors further suggest that athletes who statically stretch and then wait longer than 3 minutes before activity can expect to lose any ROM gained as a result of the preceding bout of stretching. Spernoga et al. (58) tested 30 male subjects using proprioceptive neuromuscular facilitation (PNF) on the hamstring muscles and found that ROM improvements lasted only 6 minutes after the stretching protocol ended. Although this does not seem like a significant improvement, it was also found that hip flexion passive range of motion (pROM) was significantly increased after 12 weeks of stretching (53). In fact, it was concluded that "ACSM flexibility training recommendations are effective for improving hip flexion ROM" (53, p. 389). Although it seems as though stretching has little acute impact, it may be that longer duration training is effective for increasing ROM.

## Evaluating Flexibility

Assessment of clients' ROM is an essential component of developing their exercise program.

Assessment of clients' ROM is an essential component of developing their exercise program. Goniometry assessment provides the fitness professional with several important pieces of information. These include the following:

- Initial ROM prior to the start of the exercise program
- Baseline measurements from which plans can be made for future exercise goals
- Immediate ROM feedback
- Identification of muscular imbalances

Chapter 12 provides a more comprehensive discussion on evaluating flexibility.

## Types of Stretching

Several methods exist to improve flexibility and increase joint ROM, and nearly all of them involve some form of stretching (examples of most of the types of stretching are presented in Figs. 16.2 through 16.40). Stretches can be performed by the clients (active stretching) themselves or with the help of the Personal Trainer (passive stretching). Although passive stretching can be very helpful for improving flexibility, it should only be performed by a Personal Trainer with adequate knowledge and experience to prevent injury to the client. There are generally three types of stretching that can be performed using active or passive techniques to improve flexibility: static, dynamic, and PNF. Table 16.1 provides an overview of various types of stretching and their appropriate use.

There are generally three types of stretching that can be performed using active or passive techniques to improve flexibility: static, dynamic, and proprioceptive neural facilitation or PNF.

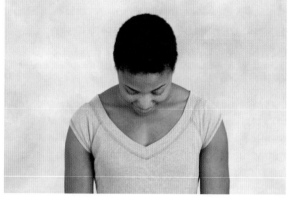
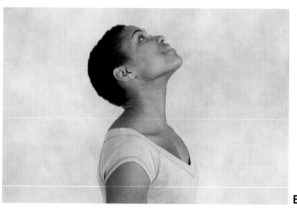

**FIGURE 16.2.** Forward flexion and extension. **A.** Facing forward, move head forward to tuck chin into chest, hold. Then move slowly from this flexion position to extension. **B.** Extension should involve looking up to ceiling until a 45° angle is reached and hold. Avoid dropping head back onto the upper back.

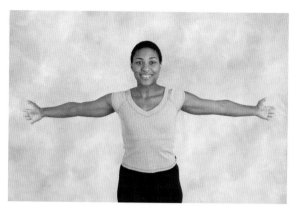

**FIGURE 16.3.** Chest stretch: Shoulders should be relaxed, not elevated. Move extended arms to the back and keep arms at or a little below shoulder height. A good cue for this stretch is "open arms wide."

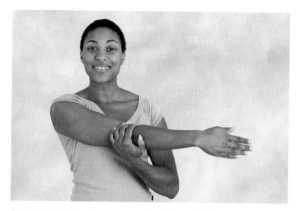

**FIGURE 16.4.** Arm across the chest: Facing forward, extend the right arm and draw across the chest. Arm should be as straight as possible, with gentle tension developed on the right shoulder. Grasp right elbow with the left hand. Apply gentle pressure with the left hand to increase tension on the right shoulder and repeat with the other arm/other side.

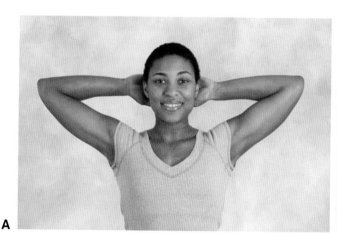

A

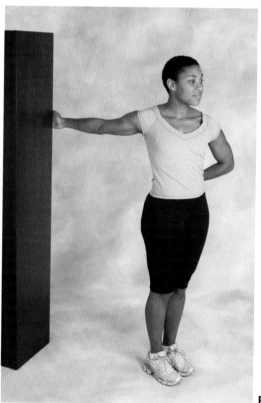

B

**FIGURE 16.5.** Chest stretch (progression). **A.** Place the palms of the hand on the back of the head and bring elbows back. **B.** Place extended arm against an open doorway and lean forward, feeling gentle tension develop across the chest.

**FIGURE 16.6.** Elbow behind the head: Facing forward, bring left arm up, bend from the elbow, and drop the hand behind the head. Try to reach right shoulder with left hand. Repeat with other arm/other side. Bring right hand to left shoulder and gently pull left elbow rightward to increase tension on left arm (triceps brachii).

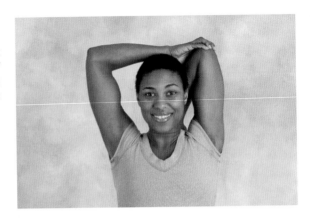

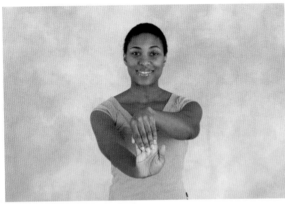

**A**

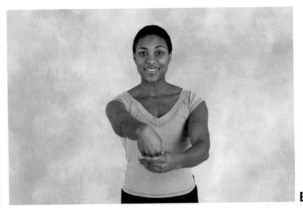

**B**

**FIGURE 16.7.** Palm up/palm down. **A.** This exercise can be performed while standing or seated. Extend right arm perpendicular to the body. Extend wrist so the palm faces away from the body. Gently pull right hand (fingertips) toward body until tension develops in the forearm flexors. Repeat with other arm/other side. **B.** This exercise can be performed while standing or seated. Extend right arm perpendicular to the body. Flex wrist so the palm faces the body. Gently pull right hand with left hand until tension develops in the forearm extension.

**FIGURE 16.8.** Arm hug: Cross the arms around the body, elbows pointing forward. Let the upper body round.

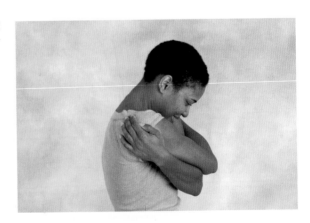

Visit thePoint to watch video 16.1, which demonstrates the kneeling cat.

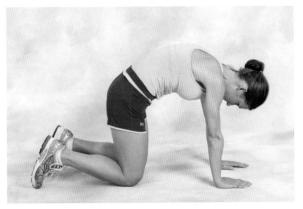

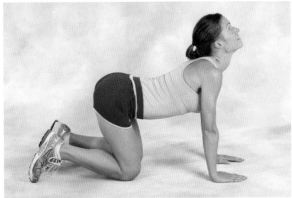

**FIGURE 16.9.** Kneeling cat: Kneel in quadruped position. Draw in abdominals and contract the gluteals, round throughout the entire spine.

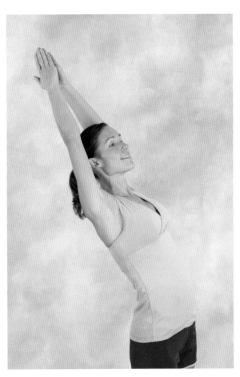

**FIGURE 16.10.** Pillar/overhead reach: Facing forward, stand erect and extend arms above head, keeping shoulders in neutral position. Place hands together and use the palms to press upward. Stretch can also involve the trunk muscles (torso) by moving in frontal plane to one side of the body and back. Hold when tension is developed in the torso on the side opposite reach.

Visit thePoint to watch video 16.2, which demonstrates the modified cobra.

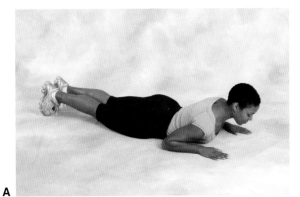

A

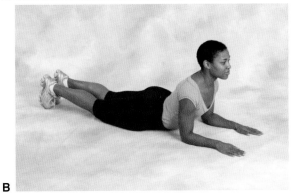

B

**FIGURE 16.11.** Modified cobra. **A.** Lie prone on the floor with the head resting on the forearms and the legs extended. Place the elbows directly under the shoulders with the hands facing forward. **B.** Press into the forearms and raise the upper body, keeping the hips on the floor.

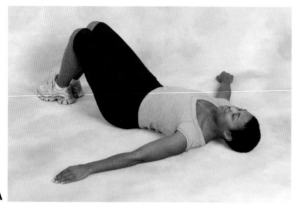

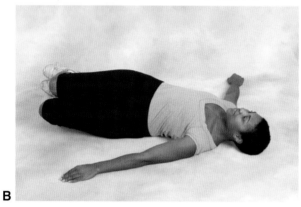

**FIGURE 16.12.** Supine rotational stretch. **A.** Lie face up on the floor. Bend knees so that the feet are flat on the floor. Then extend arms across the floor to stabilize upper body with movement. **B.** Slowly move both legs with the knees bent to the left side of the body. Maintain upper back against the floor and the abdomen oriented toward the ceiling. Repeat by moving the legs to the right side.

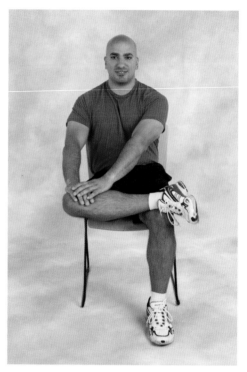

**FIGURE 16.13.** Seated hip rotator stretch level I: Sit upright on a sturdy, nonmovable chair. Cross right ankle onto bent left knee. Gently press down on right knee until tension develops in the outer portion of the right thigh. Repeat with the opposite side.

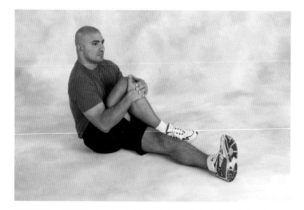

**FIGURE 16.14.** Seated hip rotator stretch level II: Sit upright on the floor, with left leg extended and right knee bent. Place the right foot over the left leg. Hug the knee toward the chest. Repeat on other side.

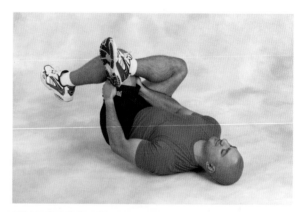

**FIGURE 16.15.** Supine hip rotator stretch (progression from seated): Lie face up on floor with knees bent so feet are flat on the floor. Cross right ankle onto bent left knee. Lift left foot off the floor. Wrap hands around the left leg and draw into the body. Focus on opening up the right knee until tension develops in the outer portion of the right thigh. Repeat on the opposite side.

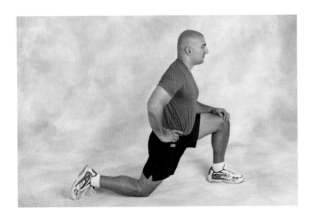

**FIGURE 16.16.** Kneeling hip flexors stretch: Kneel on knees with upper body lifted. Plant the left foot on the floor until a 90° angle is reached with both the front and back legs. Shift the weight forward while keeping the upper body lifted.

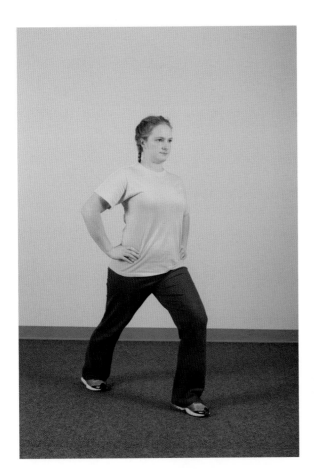

**FIGURE 16.17.** Standing hip flexor stretch: Stand erect and keep hands on the hips. Step forward with left foot into a lunge position; right heel may be elevated to facilitate this movement. Shift the hips forward. Maintain this position, feeling tension develop in hips, quadriceps, and buttocks. Repeat with the opposite side.

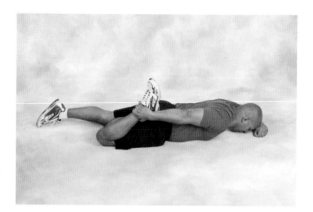

**FIGURE 16.18.** Prone quadriceps stretch: Lie prone on the floor with legs extended and draw right heel back toward the gluteals.

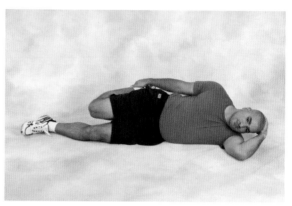

**FIGURE 16.19.** Side-lying quadriceps stretch (progression): Lie on floor with left side of the body; the trunk should be perpendicular to the floor. Bend right knee, keeping knees and hips stacked. Reach with the right hand across the front of the right foot. Gently pull thigh back slightly using the right arm. Allow the left arm to stabilize the torso. Repeat with the left thigh by positioning the body with the right side against the floor.

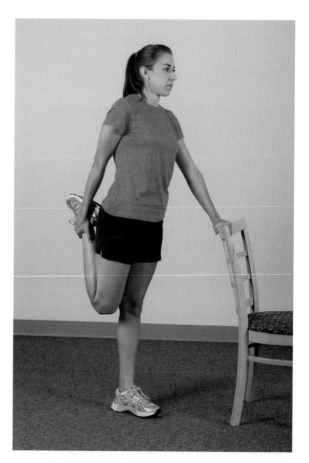

**FIGURE 16.20.** Standing quadriceps stretch (progression): While in a standing position (a chair may be used to hold onto for support), bend the right knee toward the gluteals. Grasp the right ankle with the right hand and gently pull thigh back slightly using the right arm.

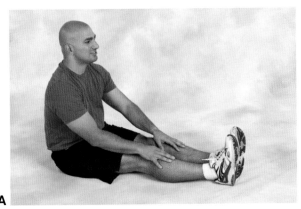

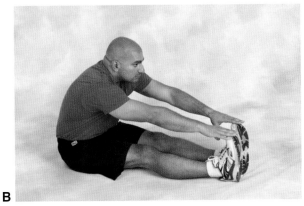

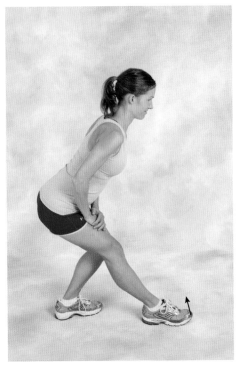

**FIGURE 16.21.** Seated hamstring stretch. **A.** Sit upright on the floor with both legs extended and hands resting on the quadriceps. **B.** Slowly walk the hands forward toward the feet, keeping the chest lifted.

**FIGURE 16.22.** Standing hamstring stretch (progression): Standing upright, bring the right foot slightly ahead of the left foot. Slowly draw the hips back while slightly bending the left knee and extending the right knee. Bring the toes of the right foot off the floor and toward the body, hold, and then return to the starting position. Repeat with the opposite leg.

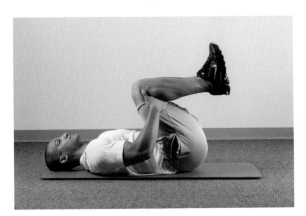

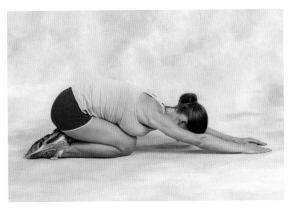

**FIGURE 16.23.** Supine knees to chest: Lie supine on the floor and hug the knees to the chest. This can be done with one leg or two legs.

**FIGURE 16.24.** Child's pose: Kneel in a quadruped position and sit back onto heels with arms extended.

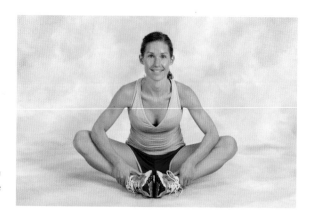

**FIGURE 16.25.** Butterfly stretch: Sit upright on the floor with the soles of the feet together. Draw the knees to the floor and lean forward from the hips.

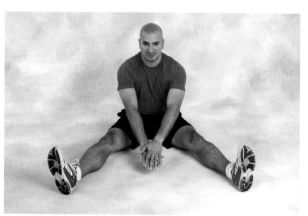

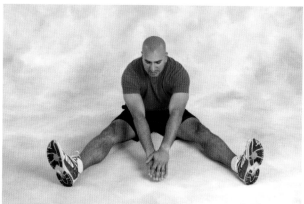

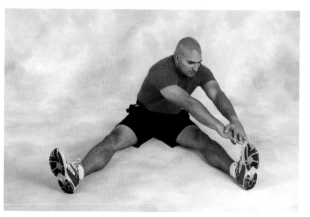

**FIGURE 16.26.** Straddle: Sit upright on floor with both legs extended. Slowly spread legs apart so that feet are as far from each other as possible and gently reach toward center or alternate reach from right to left.

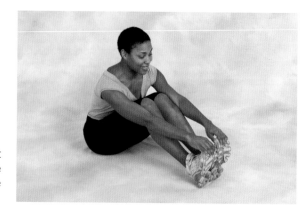

**FIGURE 16.27.** Seated calf stretch: Sit upright with both legs extended. Turn the toes toward the ceiling and draw the tops of the toes toward the upper body.

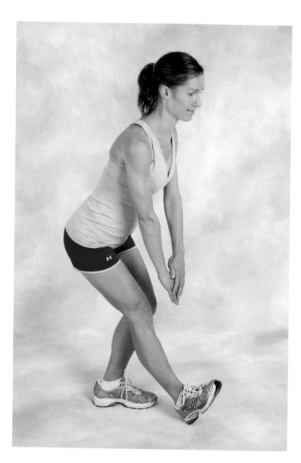

**FIGURE 16.28.** Standing calf stretch: Place body weight on the left leg, with the right leg forward and heel on the ground. Grasp banister or handrail for support if necessary. Bring the toes of the right foot toward the body and sit back slightly onto the left leg. Feel the stretch develop in the right calf and slowly return to the starting position and repeat with the opposite side.

**Visit thePoint to watch video 16.3, which demonstrates dynamic arm circles.**

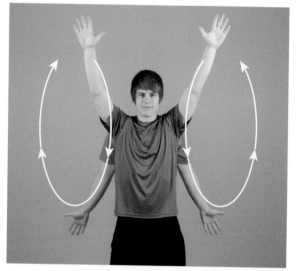

**FIGURE 16.29.** Dynamic arm circles: Stand with feet shoulder width apart and knees slightly bent. Raise both arms to the side at shoulder height, with palms facing down, and make small circles with the arms extended, gradually increasing the size of the circles.

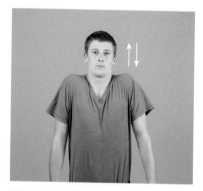

**FIGURE 16.30.** Shoulder shrugs: Lift both shoulders toward the ears and then lower away from the ears.

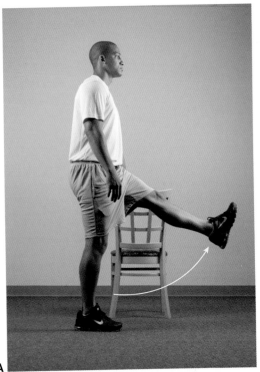
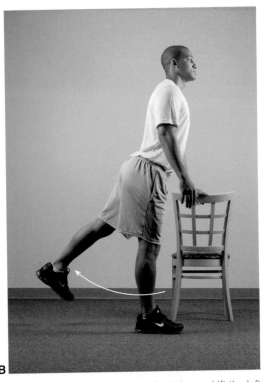

**FIGURE 16.31.** Pendulum leg swings (front to back): Place a hand on the back of a chair for balance. Lift the left leg and swing the leg forward (in front of the body) and backward (behind the body). Begin with small swings and progress to larger swings. Switch to the opposite leg.

**Visit thePoint to watch video 16.4, which demonstrates front to back and side to side leg swings.**

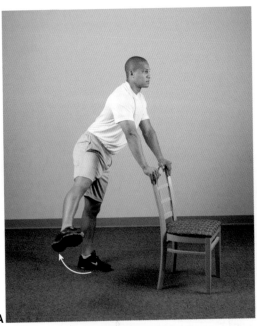
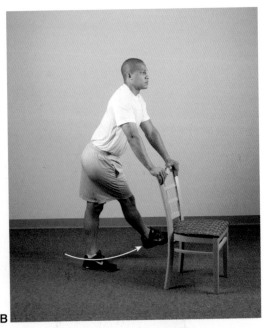

**FIGURE 16.32.** Pendulum leg swings (side to side): Place both hands on the back of a chair for balance. Swing the right leg out to the right and back across the body to the left. Begin with small swings and progress to larger swings. Switch to the opposite leg.

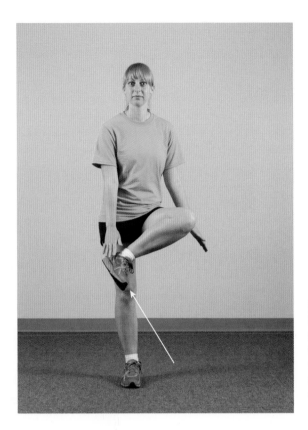

**FIGURE 16.33.** Dynamic external hip rotation: Stand upright with feet shoulder width apart. Raise the left foot in front of the body and allow the knee to rotate outward. Tap the inside of the left heel with the right hand. Switch and raise the right foot and rotate knee outward. Tap the inside of the right heel with the left hand. Alternate tapping each foot and progress to walking forward while alternating feet.

**Visit thePoint to watch video 16.5, which demonstrates dynamic internal and external hip rotation.**

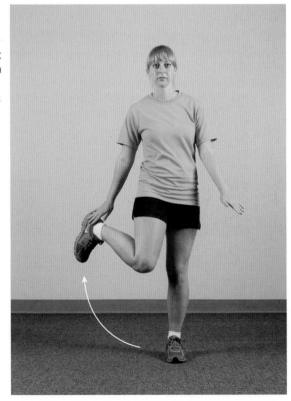

**FIGURE 16.34.** Dynamic internal hip rotation: Stand upright with feet shoulder width apart. Raise the right foot toward the side of the body and tap the outside of the right heel with the right hand, allowing the knee to rotate inward. Switch and tap the outside of the left heel with the left hand. Alternate tapping each foot and progress to walking forward while alternating feet tapping.

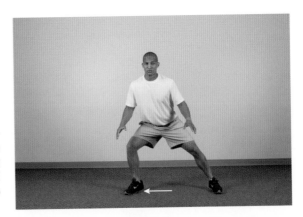

**FIGURE 16.35.** Side shuffle: Stand with feet shoulder width apart and knees slightly bent. Take one step to the right with the right foot and then bring the left foot in to meet the right foot. Begin with small steps, progress to larger steps, and then progress to a shuffle. Switch to the opposite direction.

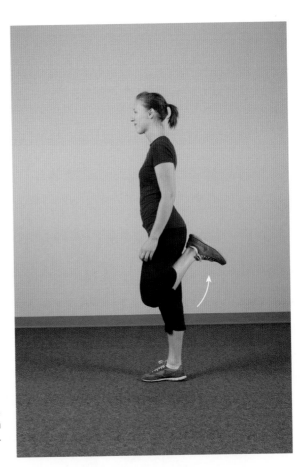

**FIGURE 16.36.** Butt kicks: Begin marching in place. Pull the heel in closer toward the buttocks with each step and progress to moving forward (walking or jogging) while kicking the buttocks.

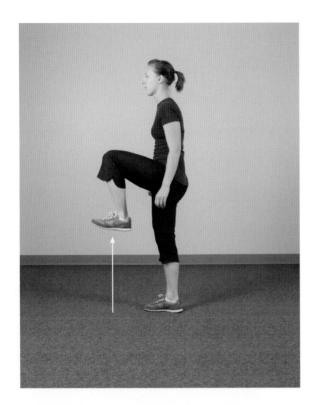

**FIGURE 16.37.** High knees: Begin marching in place. Raise the knees higher and higher with each step and progress to moving forward (walking or jogging) with high knees (keep posture upright).

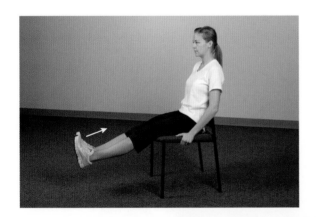

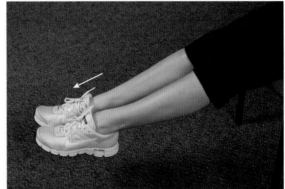

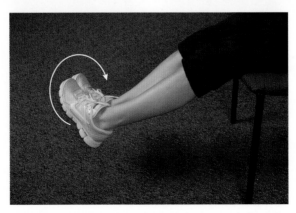

**FIGURE 16.38.** Dynamic foot ROM: Sit upright in a chair with both legs extended together. Pull toes toward the body and then point toes away from the body and pull toes toward the body. Rotate feet clockwise and counterclockwise. Can be done one foot at a time.

**Visit thePoint to watch video 16.6, which demonstrates the soldier walk.**

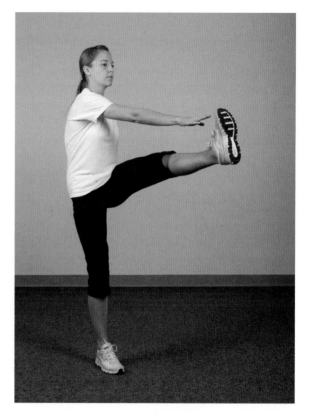

**FIGURE 16.39.** Soldier walk: Simultaneously rotate the right arm forward and raise the left leg (straight). Reach the right hand toward the left lower leg and toes and switch to the opposite side. Alternate to the opposite side. Progress to walking while alternating sides (keep posture upright).

**Visit thePoint to watch video 16.7, which demonstrates the wood chop.**

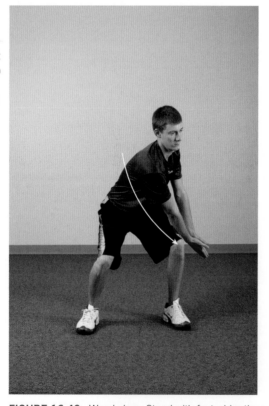

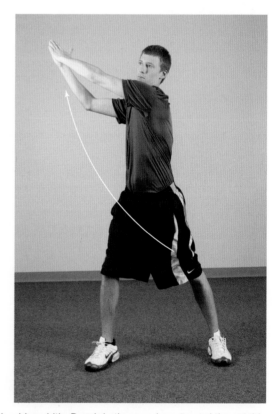

**FIGURE 16.40.** Wood chop: Stand with feet wider than shoulder width. Reach both arms down toward the outside of the left foot while bending the knees slightly. Move the arms diagonally across the body and end reaching above the right shoulder. Switch to the opposite side.

| Table 16.1 | Overview of Stretching Technique and Appropriate Use | | |
|---|---|---|---|
| **Technique** | **Definition** | **Exercise Design** | **Appropriate Use** |
| Static stretching | This is the most common method used to improve flexibility. Static stretching consists of slowly moving to minor discomfort and then holding that stretch. | All major muscle groups should be targeted at least 2–3 d · wk$^{-1}$. Hold each static stretches for 10–30 s, 30–60 s for older adults. ACSM recommends stretches be repeated 2–4 times to accumulate a total of 60 s for each flexibility exercise. | Appropriate for use following a thorough warm-up (a thorough warm-up consists of 5–10 min of light to moderate multijoint, large muscle group movements) or during the cool-down period |
| Dynamic stretching | Dynamic stretching involves moving parts of your body through a full ROM while gradually increasing the reach and/or speed of movement in a controlled manner. These exercises are very rhythmic in nature. Dynamic stretching is often incorporated in the "active" phase of the group exercise warm-up due to their similarity to the movements or patterns that will be used during the conditioning period. | Begin gradually with a small ROM progressing to larger ROM, repeating each activity 5–12 times. | Appropriate for use during the warm-up or as part of the cool-down |
| PNF | PNF stretching involves both the stretching and contraction of the targeted muscle group. Although there are several ways to employ PNF, the most common technique is termed *contract-relax*. Following the preliminary passive stretch, the muscle is isometrically contracted for 6 s, relaxed for 2–3 s, and then passively moved into the final stretch which is held for 10–30 s. This method is most effective with the use of a trainer to assist the client through the stretch. | All major muscle groups should be targeted at least 2–3 d · wk$^{-1}$. A 3- to 6-s muscle contraction at 20%–75% maximum intensity is followed by 10–30 s of assisted stretching. A total of 60 s of stretching time should be achieved per targeted muscle group. | Appropriate for use following a through warm-up or during the cool-down period. Appropriate for certified fitness professionals to use with clients if properly educated on the technique |
| Passive stretching | The client is not actively involved in this type of stretching. The client assumes a position and then either holds it with some other part of the body (*i.e.*, arm) or with the assistance of a partner or some other apparatus (*i.e.*, stretching strap). The goal is to slowly move the client into the stretch in order to prevent a forceful action and possible injury. | Exercise design would follow the static stretching protocol. | Appropriate for use following a thorough warm-up or during the cool-down period. Appropriate for certified fitness professionals to use with clients if properly educated on the technique |

*(continued)*

| Table 16.1 | Overview of Stretching Technique and Appropriate Use *(continued)* | | |
|---|---|---|---|
| **Technique** | **Definition** | **Exercise Design** | **Appropriate Use** |
| Ballistic stretching | This approach involves a bouncing or jerky type movement to reach the muscle's ROM limits. This bouncing motion may produce a powerful stretch reflex that counteracts the muscle lengthening and could possibly lead to tissue injury. Although ballistic stretch is not common practice for the general population, its use in training and rehabilitation of athletes where explosive movements are critical, it may have a justifiable role. | Exercise design would be determined by activity-specific needs on an individual basis. | Not appropriate for the general population; may be suitable for athletes involved in ballistic sport skills |

PNF, proprioceptive neuromuscular facilitation; ROM, range of motion.

## Static

Static stretching is undoubtedly the method used most commonly to improve flexibility. Static stretching can be performed actively and passively and consists of slow movements into position and holding the position for a few seconds at peak tension. For example, to actively stretch the sternocleidomastoid (neck) muscles, the client would perform a lateral flexion of the neck as depicted in Figure 16.41. This position would be held at peak tension for 10–30 seconds before returning the head upright. Static stretches can be modified too, as depicted in Figure 16.41, so that the

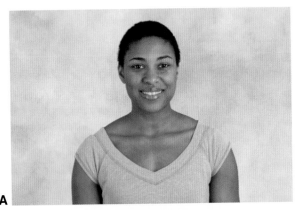

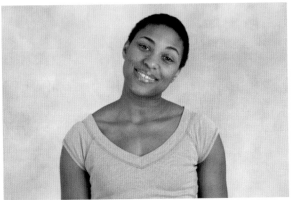

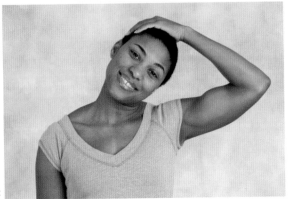

**FIGURE 16.41** Progression of a static stretch. **A.** Facing forward, tilt head to the left, moving only in the frontal plane. Hold and then return to the starting position. **B.** Repeat with the other side. A good cue for this exercise is "right ear to right shoulder." **C.** Reach with one arm in opposite direction from head tilt. With or without a partner, pull from top of head toward the direction of stretch, applying gentle pressure only.

client can better hold at peak tension or truly achieve peak tension via self-assistance and support. Furthermore, lateral flexion of the neck also serves as a good example of how static stretches can be passive stretches. Through careful movements, the Personal Trainer could also guide the client's head into position and hold at peak tension for a designated period.

Despite the popularity of static stretching, little agreement has been reached among experts with respect to how long the static stretch should be held at peak tension. The American College of Sports Medicine suggests a hold range of 10–30 seconds (3). Data from Nelson and Bandy (52) supports this recommendation when they concluded that static stretches of 30 seconds, 3 days a week, for 6 weeks, significantly improved hamstring flexibility in high school–aged males than in unstretched controls. Interestingly, Sainz de Baranda and Ayala (53) reported that no particular single duration (15, 30, or 45 s) of static stretching was better with regard to its effect on ROM. Thus, the Personal Trainer should advise his or her clients to hold static stretches for 10–30 seconds. ACSM recommends stretches be repeated two to four times to accumulate a total of 60 seconds for each flexibility exercise (*e.g.*, if each stretch is held for 15 s, each would be repeated four times) (3). Box 16.1 provides an example of static flexibility stretches and training.

## Dynamic

Dynamic stretching is a form of stretching that incorporates movement along with muscle tension development. Dynamic stretches should be performed only as active stretches. In the broadest sense, dynamic stretches are built into every mode of exercise and physical activity.

---

### Box 16.1    Sample Static Flexibility Training Program

**Client:** A 40-year-old woman who has been medically cleared to begin a consistent exercise program
  Height = 168 cm (5′ 6″)
  Weight = 68 kg (150 lb)
  No history of orthopedic problems; mild chronic back pain
**Objectives:** Improve flexibility as measured by goniometry
**Session:** 15-minute warm-up using a NordicTrack CX 1055 elliptical trainer (average heart rate: 108 bpm)

| Body Region | Exercise | Comments |
| --- | --- | --- |
| Neck | Lateral flexion | Begin as an active stretch; move head slowly to prevent dizziness. |
| Shoulders | Arms across chest | Avoid bending the elbow as the arm is brought across the chest. |
| Chest | Chest stretch | Maintain relaxed shoulders. |
| Arms | Elbow extension | |
| Back | Kneeling cat | Discontinue stretch if it produces immediate back pain. |
| Torso | Modified cobra | Discontinue stretch if it produces immediate back pain. |
| Hips | Seated hip rotator, level I | Progress to level II exercise when level I was performed for 30 s without pain. |
| Thigh (anterior) | Prone quadriceps | Maintain upright posture and natural spinal curves. |
| Thigh (posterior) | Seated hamstring | Maintain upright posture and natural spinal curves. |
| Calves | Standing calf stretch | Maintain upright posture and natural spinal curves. |

*Trainer's Notes*: Be sure to follow the FITT-VP guidelines for flexibility training suggested in this chapter, keeping in mind that they can be adapted to the individual needs of the client. If one or more of the recommended parameters do not seem to be effective, adapt as needed. This program can and should be progressed as the client achieves greater low-back ROM. Remeasure with the goniometer every 4–6 weeks. By following the stretches listed in this chapter, this client will be able to progress from these basic stretches to more complex ones. The order of exercises performed during a session is not important.

Dynamic stretching has been characterized as being very similar to a sport- or function-specific warm-up (38). The goal is to move the specific joint in a controlled manner within a normal ROM in order to minimize the risk of injury. It is important to progressively introduce dynamic stretches into the stretching program, particularly if the client is not accustomed to this type of stretching. Dynamic stretches should begin gradually with a small ROM progressing to larger ROM, repeating each activity 5–12 times (23,55). An example of this is arm circles; begin with small, slow circles and gradually progress into larger and faster circles until a full ROM is reached for the shoulder joint. It is difficult to depict examples of dynamic stretching on paper. Consider the movements of a boxer in the ring prior to a fight. Jabs he makes with the upper extremities and quick turns of the torso all serve as good examples of dynamic stretch. Tae Bo movements and stereotypical medicine ball exercises provide further examples of dynamic stretching. Ideally, dynamic stretches incorporate movements that are specific to sport movements of interest, but excellent dynamic stretches can also be developed on the basis of the flexibility needs of the medically cleared population at large. Box 16.2 provides an example of dynamic flexibility stretches and training.

Sometimes, dynamic stretching is confused with another form of movement termed "ballistic stretching." Ballistic stretching refers to the use of the momentum of the moving body segment to produce a bouncing or jerky movement that is done to obtain a peak muscle tension or stretch. For example, a client seated upright on the floor could extend his or her arms forward in an effort to

---

**Box 16.2 — Sample Dynamic Range of Motion Training Program**

**Client:** A 25-year-old male, medically cleared to begin consistent exercise program
Height = 191 cm (6′ 3″)
Weight = 95 kg (215 lb)
No history of injury or orthopedic problems
**Objectives:** Improve sports performance and prevent injury through increasing joint ROM and warming up prior to conditioning phase of activity
**Session:** 5-minute warm-up using a treadmill (average heart rate, 110 bpm)

| Body Region | Exercise | Comments |
| --- | --- | --- |
| Shoulders | Arm circles | Start with small circles and progress to a larger ROM. |
| | Shoulder shrugs | |
| Hips and buttocks | Pendulum leg swings (front/back, side/side) | Begin with small swings and progress to larger swings. |
| | Hip internal/external rotation | Progress to walking forward while alternating feet. |
| | Side shuffle | This exercise can start in a stationary position and then progress to a walk or light jog. |
| Quadriceps | Butt kicks | This exercise can start in a stationary position and then progress to a walk or light jog. |
| Hamstrings | High knees | Progress to walking while alternating sides. |
| Ankles | Dynamic foot ROM | |
| Full body | Soldier walk | |
| | Wood chop | |

*Trainer's Notes*: Full-body dynamic ROM exercises should be performed after the completion of exercises of individual muscle groups. Many dynamic ROM exercises can be progressed by adding forward or lateral movement in the phases of walking, jogging, and then running (*e.g.*, butt kicks and high knees). Progressions should be given to clients only when they have demonstrated control of movement in a stationary position.

## Box 16.3    Ballistic Stretching — Understanding the Controversy

Some flexibility experts fail to distinguish dynamic stretching from another form of movement termed *ballistic stretching*. Unfortunately, this misunderstanding has resulted in a great deal of confusion by fitness professionals, so much so Personal Trainers often discourage clients from performing dynamic stretches. Almost all physical movements impose some type of dynamic stretch on the soft tissues that bring about these movements. In contrast, ballistic stretching refers to the bouncing or jerky stretching action or movement that is done to obtain a peak muscle tension. For example, a client seated upright on the floor could extend his or her arms forward in an effort to reach the toes. By moving slowly into that position and holding for a few seconds at peak tension, the client would be performing an active static stretch. However, if in an attempt to touch the toes the client pushed forward repeatedly with short, successive, bouncing flexions at the hip, he or she would be performing a ballistic stretch.

The claim is often made that ballistic stretching is unsafe or at least ineffective for improving flexibility. It

is thought that each successive "bounce" movement in ballistic stretching may impose too rapid a stretch on muscles while they are in the process of contracting making them susceptible to muscle injury. In fact, Smith et al. (57) found that similar bouts of static and ballistic stretching induced increases in delayed-onset muscle soreness (DOMS) in 20 male subjects unaccustomed to such exercise. Importantly, though, these researchers concluded that the static stretching actually induced significantly more DOMS than did ballistic stretching. In terms of performance, Nelson and Kokkonen (50) concluded that acute ballistic muscle stretching inhibited maximal strength performance, but Unick et al. (61) found no statistically significant difference in vertical jump performance as a result of static or ballistic stretching among actively trained women.

No attempt is being made here to settle the controversy surrounding ballistic stretching. Personal Trainers should recognize that both dynamic and ballistic stretching movements are normal components of sport activity and may have legitimate roles in the training and rehabilitation of athletes (46).

reach the toes. By moving slowly into that position and holding for a few seconds at peak tension, the client would be performing an active static stretch. However, if in an attempt to touch the toes the client pushed forward repeatedly with short, successive, bouncing flexions at the hip, he or she would be performing a ballistic stretch. Ballistic stretching is controversial. It has often been considered a "contraindicated" movement, but in fact, when properly performed, ballistic stretching may be done safely in adults, particularly in individuals who perform ballistic movements such as those found in basketball. Ballistic stretching can be equally effective as static stretching in increasing joint ROM (4). Box 16.3 provides a discussion on the controversy regarding the use of ballistic stretching.

## Proprioceptive Neuromuscular Facilitation

Visit thePoint to watch video 16.8, which demonstrates PNF stretching.

Proprioceptive neuromuscular facilitation or PNF involves both active and passive techniques designed to improve joint ROM. Several muscle groups can be trained when PNF techniques are properly used. This form of stretching requires an experienced Personal Trainer and a cooperative client. PNF stretching should be performed only by competent and trained practitioners, as overstretching is possible if the technique is not fully understood. PNF techniques involve a dual process where an isometric contraction is followed by a static stretch in the same muscle/tendon group (*i.e.*, contract–relax). PNF stretching is commonly believed to elicit a relaxation response from the neuromuscular system. This response can occur in the prime mover (agonist), synergist, and antagonist muscles across a particular joint. With a stretch-induced reduction in muscle tone, joint ROM increases during subsequent stretches and eventually during physical activity. However, a review by Chalmers (15) refutes this rationale and points to studies that suggest that PNF improves ROM

PNF stretching should be performed only by competent and trained practitioners, as overstretching is possible if the technique is not fully understood.

mainly because of changes in the ability to tolerate stretching and/or changes in the viscoelastic properties of the stretched muscle. Although the mechanism for ROM change with PNF continues to be studied, it is clear that PNF techniques have long been shown to increase joint ROM.

## Rationale for Flexibility Training

Despite the importance of full, pain-free joint ROM for sport and physical activity, the justification for certain flexibility training techniques is controversial. Moreover, little scientific evidence exists to support either continuing or discontinuing even the most common stretching habits designed for injury prevention among competitive or recreational athletes (59). Not surprisingly, the Personal Trainer is bound to be confused with respect to the inclusion or omission of flexibility exercises in the overall conditioning of clients.

One approach to this problem involves conducting a thorough fitness assessment of the client to determine the extent to which inflexibility limits sport and/or general physical performance. Should ROM deficiencies be evident in the client, then the Personal Trainer is justified in prescribing the basic stretching techniques described in this chapter. These stretches (static, dynamic, and PNF) are most commonly known to improve flexibility. It is reasonable to employ these techniques and continue to monitor the flexibility needs of the client. Although at least one early study (44) found significant improvements in flexibility with all three methods, Personal Trainers are encouraged to select an approach that best suits the needs, limitations, and abilities of the client while continuing to monitor joint ROM and its ultimate impact on sport and physical activity performance.

## Designing a Flexibility Training Program

There are three preliminary training guidelines unique to the design of flexibility programs. These involve warm-up, breathing, and posture.

There are three preliminary training guidelines unique to the design of flexibility programs. These involve warm-up, breathing, and posture.

### Warm-Up

Although stretches can be performed at the start, in the middle, and/or at the finish of the workout, it is common to precede stretching with a brief, aerobic exercise warm-up. An active warm-up reduces the resistance to stretch (64). It has been established that increasing the temperature of a muscle increases the elastic properties or the ability to stretch (28,32,54,66). Warm muscle tissue responds less stiffly than cold muscle tissue. Little evidence suggests that the exercise warm-up should be altered to accommodate flexibility training exclusively. Typical warm-up exercises include stationary cycling, treadmill walking/running, or rowing. It is often recommended that stretching be done at the end of the workout after the muscles are warm.

### Breathing

Proper breathing techniques are often helpful in relaxing the client and allowing movement into position more comfortably. Flexibility training is no time to perform a Valsalva maneuver (air expiration against a closed glottis). Purposeful and controlled breathing that accompanies relaxing exercise may help reduce stress levels and decrease voluntary muscle tension. Remind exercisers to exhale slowly as they move toward the end point of a stretch and inhale as they return to the starting position.

## Posture

In the design of a flexibility training program, Personal Trainers should understand the proper positioning of the stretch to target the appropriate muscle group. Focus on maintaining proper body alignment during the execution of the exercises. For example, consider the stretch depicted in Figure 16.20. Posture can be greatly improved by using the "free hand" (the hand *not* grasping the ankle) to hold a railing or the back of a chair to maintain balance. The Personal Trainer should emphasize that one should avoid pressing the elevated foot to the gluteals (*i.e.*, hyperflexion at the knee) or leaning into the stretch for additional force development. Some reminders for correct postural alignment are listed in the following text:

- Maintain neutral position of the spine (characterized by having a slight inward curve at the cervical and lumbar spines and a slight outward curve of the thoracic spine).
- Shoulders should remain back and away from the ears.
- Hips should be in a neutral and level position (see Figs. 16.22 and 16.28 for examples of proper hip placement).

## Precautions for Individuals with Health Concerns

There is little reason to avoid flexibility training in the apparently healthy individual. However, there are several common health conditions that require special attention and may present challenges to the Personal Trainer in regard to flexibility training. Four of these conditions are arthritis, muscular imbalance, osteoporosis, and hip fracture/replacement. Although Chapter 20 provides specific guidelines about exercise programming for these special populations, this section will present information to consider when designing flexibility training programs for individuals who may have these conditions.

> There is little reason to avoid flexibility training in the apparently healthy individual.

### Arthritis

Over 50 million Americans suffer from arthritis or other joint pain and inflammation, with a higher prevalence found in women compared to men. Arthritis is believed to limit physical activity in both normal weight and obese adults (8). Arthritis is defined as an inflammation of a joint resulting in damage to the joint structure. There are more than 100 different types of arthritis, with the two most common types being osteoarthritis and rheumatoid arthritis (61). Osteoarthritis is a chronic degenerative condition that develops over time and is believed to result from either abnormal or excessive wear on "normal" cartilage or normal wear on "abnormal" cartilage. Rheumatoid arthritis is classified as an autoimmune disease in which the body attacks and destroys the joint surface. In either case, individuals with arthritis tend to limit movement because of pain and stiffness, which may result in an increased loss of flexibility and joint motion. Fortunately, flexibility and joint range can be improved in an individual with arthritis through training (45). In addition, training may assist in pain reduction, fatigue, and inflammation (3). Consider the following guidelines when flexibility training an individual with arthritis (3,61):

- Avoid strenuous exercises during acute flare ups and periods of inflammation. However, it is appropriate to gently move joints through their full ROM during these periods.
- Encourage individuals with arthritis to stretch during the time of day when pain is typically least severe and/or in conjunction with peak activity of pain medications.
- If the client experiences greater joint pain following a training session, the session may have been too intense and may need to be modified.
- Avoid overworking individuals who have taken anti-inflammatory medications (*e.g.*, aspirin, ibuprofen, and naproxen sodium); these drugs can temporarily lessen musculoskeletal pain and make it possible for a client to do too much.

- Discuss with clients the importance of wearing shoes that have good shock absorption and stability.
- Functional activities such as sit-to-stand, step-ups, and stair climbing are good exercises that assist in ADLs.

### Muscular Imbalance

Many people have muscular imbalances of the body, which may create postural alignment issues and injury. Repetitive movements, poor posture, and weak or tight muscles can cause these muscular imbalances. Consider a baseball or tennis player who consistently trains and plays with joint dominance. When the body experiences an imbalance in muscular forces on opposite sides of a joint, ROM of that joint may be affected (2). The obvious goal to correct the muscular imbalance would be to strengthen the weak muscles and stretch the shorter muscle if ROM is compromised.

### Osteoporosis

Osteoporosis is a disease in which bone mineral density (BMD) is reduced, bone microarchitecture deteriorates, and the bone becomes fragile and very susceptible to fracture. Osteoporosis afflicts more than 50% of the population aged 50 years and older (22). Both men and women lose bone steadily after about age 35 years; however, at menopause, women often have an accelerated loss of bone due to hormone changes. The most common sites for bone loss include spine, hips, and wrists. Flexibility exercises for those with osteopenia (low bone mass) or diagnosed osteoporosis should be designed to minimize the chance for fracture. When possible, it may be helpful to have the client use a chair or handrail for support when needed. Examples of exercises to avoid include those that involve twisting, bending, or compression of the spine or those that stress the wrists or hips. Specifically avoid the following:

- Bending forward (*e.g.*, forward fold pose)
- Supine spinal rotation or twists
- Plough pose
- Back extension (*e.g.*, cobra pose)

### Hip Fracture or Replacement

For individuals who have recently had a hip fracture or hip replacement, it is recommended to avoid flexibility exercises that involve excessive

- Internal rotation of the hip (turning the foot inward)
- Hip adduction (crossing the legs beyond the midline)
- Hip flexion (thigh more than parallel to floor)

##  Flexibility Program Development

The ACSM recognizes that joint ROM is important and can be improved by engaging in flexibility training (4). Flexibility programs should follow the same FITT-VP principles (*i.e.*, Frequency, Intensity, Type, Time, Volume, and Progression) of exercise prescription as resistance training (see Chapter 14) or cardiorespiratory endurance (see Chapter 15). In this section, the ACSM FITT-VP guidelines are outlined. Unless otherwise indicated, the guidelines apply to all three of the stretching examples presented in Figures 16.2 through 16.40. Also as noted previously, flexibility exercises are most effective when the muscles are warm; thus, low-to-moderate intensity warm-up activities should be done preceding all stretching.

## Frequency

It is currently recommended that stretches be performed at least 2–3 days a week, but stretching exercises are most effective when performed daily, including two to four stretch repetitions per muscle group. Bandy et al. (7) found no increase in hamstring flexibility in 93 female and male subjects when the frequency of stretching was increased from one to three times per day. Little research exists to refute the practice of stretching daily whether followed by other physical activity or not.

## Intensity

Moving into position of tightness or mild discomfort before holding a stretch is the current recommendation on static flexibility training intensity. This subjective feeling of discomfort will vary from client to client. Individual effort can be standardized in the laboratory using maximal voluntary isometric contractions. Feland and Marin (24) found that a submaximal form of PNF produced comparable gains in hamstring flexibility to those produced by maximal voluntary isometric contractions in 72 male subjects aged 18–27 years. These authors concluded that PNF stretching using submaximal contractions might reduce injury risk associated with PNF stretching. Because most Personal Trainers will not have access to isokinetic equipment, it is recommended that fitness professionals employ a Borg Rating of Perceived Exertion scale (12) and suggest that clients position themselves for (static) stretching at an intensity that corresponds to a 13–15 (*somewhat hard* to *hard*) range.

## Time

Current recommendations involve stretch hold times of 10–30 seconds for active static stretches. Times of 10–30 seconds are also recommended for PNF techniques when preceded by a 3- to 6-second active contraction. However, with older adults, an increase to 30–60 seconds for the stretch hold time is recommended. There seems to be little additional flexibility benefit to static stretch hold times that exceed 30 seconds in the younger adult (6).

## Type

It is recommended that a general stretching routine be used to best improve flexibility. This means that stretches should involve the major muscle and tendon groups of the body. Some of the more commonly performed static stretches and dynamic stretches are presented in this chapter. For an example of how these parameters can be incorporated into a flexibility training program, see Box 16.2. Because PNF techniques require advanced skill and experience, only Personal Trainers who have advanced training and practice should attempt employing these stretches. For more information about PNF techniques, readers are referred to Houglum (36).

## Volume

A total of 60 seconds of flexibility exercises per joint is recommended. This goal may be accomplished by repeating each exercise two to four times (*e.g.*, two 30-s stretches or three 20-s stretches or four 15-s stretches) of the same joint.

## Progression

Recommendations for optimal progression are unknown. It is recommended that low- to moderate-intensity aerobic activities be done as a warm-up or that moist heat packs or hot baths be used to passively warm the area prior to stretching. Flexibility exercises may acutely reduce power and strength, so it is recommended that flexibility exercises be performed after any exercise or sport where strength and power are important for performance.

## SUMMARY

The purpose of this chapter was to present flexibility as an essential ingredient of health-related fitness and to provide Personal Trainers with a basic understanding of how to properly incorporate flexibility training into the exercise programs of healthy individuals. Although the science of flexibility training may seem confusing and at times conflicting, Personal Trainers are urged to continue to keep pace with the changes in the scientific literature as it develops.

# REFERENCES

1. Adrian MJ. Flexibility in the aging adult. In: Smith EL, Serfass RC, editors. *Exercise and Aging: The Scientific Basis.* Hillside (NJ): Enslow Publishers; 1981. p. 45–57.

2. Alter MJ. *Science of Flexibility.* 3rd ed. Champaign (IL): Human Kinetics; 2004. 368 p.

3. American College of Sports Medicine. *ACSM's Guidelines for Exercise Testing and Prescription.* 10th ed. Philadelphia (PA): Wolters Kluwer; 2018.

4. American College of Sports Medicine. American College of Sports Medicine Position Stand. Quantity and quality of exercise for developing and maintaining cardiorespiratory, musculoskeletal, and neuromuscular fitness in apparently healthy adults: guidance for prescribing exercise. *Med Sci Sports Exerc.* 2011;43(7):1334–59.

5. Bailey AJ. Ageing of the collagen of the musculoskeletal system. *Int J Sports Med.* 1989;10:S86–90.

6. Bandy WD, Irion JM. The effect of time on static stretch on the flexibility of the hamstring muscles. *Phys Ther.* 1994;74(9):845–52.

7. Bandy WD, Irion JM, Briggler M. The effect of time and frequency of static stretching on flexibility of the hamstring muscles. *Phys Ther.* 1997;77(10):1090–6.

8. Barbour KE, Helmick CG, Theis KA, et al. Prevalence of doctor-diagnosed arthritis and arthritis-attributable activity limitation-United States, 2010-2012. *MMWR Morb Mortal Wkly Rep.* 2013;62(44):869–73.

9. Bassey EJ, Morgan K, Dallosso HM, Ebrahim SBJ. Flexibility of the shoulder joint measured as range of abduction in a large representative sample of men and women over 65 years of age. *Eur J Appl Physiol Occup Physiol.* 1989;58:353–60.

10. Bell R, Hoshizaki T. Relationships of age and sex with joint range of motion of seventeen joint actions in humans. *Can J Appl Sports Sci.* 1981;6:202–6.

11. Bird M, Hill KD, Ball M, Hetherington S, Williams AD. The long-term benefits of a multi-component exercise intervention to balance and mobility in healthy older adults. *Arch Gerontol Geriatr.* 2011;52:211–6.

12. Borg G. *Borg's Perceived Exertion and Pain Scales.* Champaign (IL): Human Kinetics; 1998. 104 p.

13. Brown DA, Miller WC. Normative data for strength and flexibility of women throughout their life. *Eur J Appl Physiol Occup Physiol.* 1998;78:77–82.

14. Buckwalter JA. Maintaining and restoring mobility in middle and old age: the importance of the soft tissues. *Instr Course Lect.* 1997;46:459–69.

15. Chalmers G. Re-examination of the possible role of Golgi tendon organ and muscle spindle reflexes in proprioceptive neuromuscular facilitation muscle stretching. *Sports Biomech.* 2004;3(1):159–83.

16. Corbin CB. *A Textbook of Motor Development.* 2nd ed. Dubuque (IA): Brown; 1980. 315 p.

17. Corbin CB, Welk GJ, Corbin WR, Welk KA. *Fundamental Concepts of Fitness and Wellness.* 2nd ed. Boston (MA): McGraw-Hill; 2006. 302 p.

18. Cornu C, Maisetti O, Ledoux I. Muscle elastic properties during wrist flexion and extension in healthy sedentary subjects and volley-ball players. *Int J Sports Med.* 2003;24(4):277–84.

19. Costa PB, Graves BS, Whitehurst M, Jacobs PL. The acute effects of different durations of static stretching on dynamic balance performance. *J Strength Cond Res.* 2009;23(1):141–7.

20. DePino GM, Webright WG, Arnold BL. Duration of maintained hamstring flexibility after cessation of an acute static stretching protocol. *J Athl Train.* 2000;35(1):56–9.

21. Einkauf DK, Gondes ML, Jensen MJ. Changes in spinal mobility with increasing age in women. *Phys Ther.* 1987;67:370–5.

22. Facts and Statistics [Internet]. Nyon (Switzerland): International Osteoporosis Foundation; [cited 2017 Feb 22]. Available from: https://www.iofbonehealth.org/facts-statistics#category-23

23. Faigenbaum AD, McFarland JE, Schwerdtman JA, Ratamess NA, Kang J, Hoffman JR. Dynamic warm up protocols, with and without a weighted vest, and fitness performance in high school female athletes. *J Athl Train.* 2006;41(4):357–63.

24. Feland JB, Marin HN. Effect of submaximal contraction intensity in contract-relax proprioceptive neuromuscular facilitation stretching. *Br J Sports Med.* 2004;38(4):E18.

25. Finsterbush A, Pogrund H. The hypermobility syndrome: musculoskeletal complaints in 100 consecutive cases of generalized joint hypermobility. *Clin Orthop.* 1982;168:124–7.

26. Fowles JR, Sale DG, MacDougall JD. Reduced strength after passive stretch of the human plantarflexors. *J Appl Physiol.* 2000;89(3):1179–88.

27. Gabbard C, Tandy R. Body composition and flexibility among prepubescent males and females. *J Hum Move Stud.* 1988;14(4):153–9.

28. Garrett WE, Best TM. Anatomy, physiology, and mechanics of skeletal muscle. In: Buckwalter JA, Einhorn TA, Simon SR, editors. *Orthopaedic Basic Science Biology and Biomechanics of the Musculoskeletal System.* 2nd ed. Rosemont (IL): American Academy of Orthopaedic Surgeons; 2000. p. 684–716.

29. Gelabert RR. *Gelabert's Anatomy for the Dancer.* New York (NY): Danad; 1966. 57 p.

30. Germain NW, Blair SN. Variability in shoulder flexion with age, activity and sex. *Am Correct Ther J.* 1983;37:156–60.

31. Gersten JW, Ager C, Anderson K, Cenkovich F. Relation of muscle strength and range of motion to activities of daily living. *Arch Phys Med Rehabil.* 1970;3:137–42.

32. Gillette T, Holland GJ. Relationship of body core temperature and warm-up to hamstring range of motion. *J Orthop Sports Phys Ther.* 1991;13(3):126–31.

33. Guralnik JM, Simonsick EM. Physical disability in older Americans. *J Gerontol.* 1993;48:3–10.

34. Hageman PA, Blanke DJ. Comparison of gait in young women and elderly women. *Phys Ther.* 1986;66:1382–7.

35. Hamill J, Knutzen KM, Derrick TR. Neurologic considerations for movement. In: Hamill J, Knutzen KM, Derrick TR, editors. *Biomechanical Basis of Human Movement.* 4th ed. Philadelphia (PA): Lippincott Williams & Wilkins; 2015. p. 99–128.

36. Houglum PA. *Therapeutic Exercise for Musculoskeletal Injuries.* 2nd ed. Champaign (IL): Human Kinetics; 2005. 1005 p.

37. Jaeger M, Freiwald J, Englehardt M, Lange-Berlin V. Differences in hamstring musclestretching of elite field hockey players and normal subjects. *Sportverletz Sportschaden.* 2003;17(2):65–70.

38. Jeffreys I. Warm-up and stretching. In: Baechle TR, Earle RW, editors. *Essentials of Strength Training and Conditioning.* 3rd ed. Champaign (IL): Human Kinetics; 2008. p. 296–324.

39. Kerrigan DC, Xenopoulos-Oddsson A, Sullivan MJ, Lelas JJ, Riley PO. Effect of hip flexor-stretching program on gait in the elderly. *Arch Phys Med Rehabil.* 2003;84(1):1–6.

40. Klein DA, Stone WJ, Phillips WT, et al. PNF training and physical function in assisted-living older adults. *J Aging Phys Act.* 2002;10:476–88.

41. Kokkonen J, Nelson AG, Cornwell A. Acute muscle stretching inhibits maximal strength performance. *Res Q Exerc Sport.* 1998;69(4):411–5.

42. Kukkanen T, Malkia E. Effects of a three-month therapeutic exercise programme on flexibility in subjects with low back pain. *Physiother Res Int.* 2000;5(1):46–61.

43. LaBella FS, Paul G. Structure of collagen from human tendon as influenced by age and sex. *J Gerontol.* 1965;20:54–9.

44. Lucas RC, Koslow R. Comparative study of static, dynamic, and proprioceptive neuromuscular facilitation stretching techniques on flexibility. *Percept Mot Skills.* 1984;58(2):615–8.

45. MacDonald CW, Whitman JM, Cleland JA, Smith M, Hoeksma HL. Clinical outcomes following manual physical therapy and exercise for hip osteoarthritis: a case series. *J Orthop Sports Phys Ther.* 2006;36(8):588–99.

46. Mahieu NN, McNair P, De Muynck M, et al. Effect of static and ballistic stretching on the muscle-tendon tissue properties. *Med Sci Sports Exerc.* 2007;39(3):494–501.

47. McHugh MP, Cosgrave CH. To stretch or not to stretch: the role of stretching in injury prevention and performance. *Scand J Med Sci Sports.* 2010;20:169–81.

48. Misner JE, Massey BH, Bemben M, Going S, Patrick J. Long-term effects of exercise on the range of motion of aging women. *J Orthop Sports Phys Ther.* 1992;16(1):37–42.

49. Munns K. Effects of exercise on the range of joint motion in elderly subjects. In: Smith EL, Serfass RC, editors. *Exercise and Aging: The Scientific Basis.* Hillside (NJ): Enslow Publishers; 1981. p. 167–78.

50. Nelson AG, Kokkonen J. Acute ballistic muscle stretching inhibits maximal strength performance. *Res Q Exerc Sport.* 2001;72(4):415–9.

51. Nelson AG, Kokkonen J, Arnall DA. Acute muscle stretching inhibits muscle strength endurance performance. *J Strength Cond Res.* 2005;19(2):338–43.

52. Nelson RT, Bandy WD. Eccentric training and static stretching improve hamstring flexibility of high school males. *J Athl Train.* 2004;39(3):254–8.

53. Sainz de Baranda P, Ayala F. Chronic flexibility improvement after 12 week of stretching program utilizing the ACSM recommendations: hamstring flexibility. *Int J Sports Med.* 2010;31(6):389–96.

54. Sapega AA, Quedenfeld TC, Moyer RA, Butler RA. Biophysical factors in range-of-motion exercise. *Phys Sports Med.* 1981;9(12):57–65.

55. Sekir U, Arabaci R, Akova B, Kadagan SM. Acute effects of static and dynamic stretching on leg flexor and extensor isokinetic strength in elite women athletes. *Scand J Med Sci Sports.* 2010;20:268–81.

56. Shepard RJ. *Physical Activity and Aging.* Chicago (IL): Yearbook Medical Publishers; 1978. p. 45–8.

57. Smith LL, Brunetz MH, Chenier TC, et al. The effects of static and ballistic stretching on delayed onset muscle soreness and creatine kinase. *Res Q Exerc Sport.* 1993;64(1):103–7.

58. Spernoga SG, Uhl TL, Arnold BL, Gansneder BM. Duration of maintained hamstring flexibility after a one-time, modified hold-relax stretching protocol. *J Athl Train.* 2001;36(1):44–8.

59. Thacker SB, Gilchrist J, Stroup DF, Kimsey CD Jr. The impact of stretching on sports injury risk: a systematic review of the literature. *Med Sci Sports Exerc.* 2004;36(3):371–8.

60. Thompson CJ, Osness WH. Effects of an 8-week multimodal exercise program on strength, flexibility, and golf performance in 55- to 79-year-old men. *J Aging Phys Act.* 2004;12(2):144–56.

61. Unick J, Kieffer HS, Cheesman W, Feeney A. The acute effects of static and ballistic stretching on vertical jump performance in trained women. *J Strength Cond Res.* 2005;19(1):206–12.

62. Vermeulen J, Neyens JCL, van Rossum E, Spreeuwenberg MD, de Witte LP. Predicting ADL disability in community-dwelling elderly people using physical frailty indicators: a systematic review. *BMC Geriatr.* 2011;11:33.

63. Voorrips LE, Lemmink KA, van Heuvelen MJ, Bult P, van Staveren WA. The physical condition of elderly women differing in habitual physical activity. *Med Sci Sports Exerc.* 1993;25(10):1152–7.

64. Wenos DL, Konin JG. Controlled warm-up intensity enhances hip range of motion. *J Strength Cond Res.* 2004;18(3): 529–33.

65. Witvrouw E, Mahieu N, Danneels L, McNair P. Stretching and injury prevention. *Sports Med.* 2004;34:443–9.

66. Wright V, Johns RJ. Observations on the measurement of joint stiffness. *Arch Rheum.* 1960;3:328–40.

67. Youdas JW, Krause DA, Hollman JH, Harmsen WS, Laskowski E. The influence of gender and age on hamstring muscle length in healthy adults. *J Orthop Sports Phys Ther.* 205;35(4):246–52.

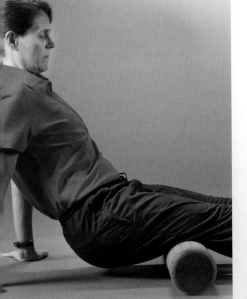

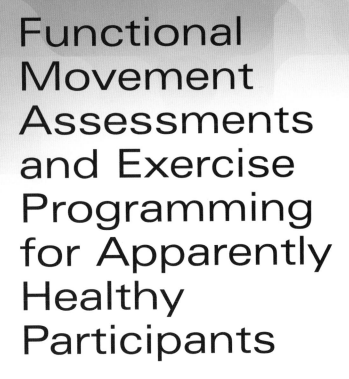
# Functional Movement Assessments and Exercise Programming for Apparently Healthy Participants

## OBJECTIVES

**Personal Trainers should be able to:**

- Understand the integration of the motor system and the sensory system in developing motor patterns.

- Examine the importance of stability, mobility, and proprioception within the context of progressive exercise programing.

- Understand the relevance of optimizing posture for improved neuromuscular function.

- Identify the muscles commonly affected by neuromuscular imbalances.

- Describe appropriate assessments and exercise prescription and self-myofascial release strategies to improve movement potential.

# INTRODUCTION

One of the most salient features of successful strength and conditioning programs is progressively overloading the body to the extent that adaptation occurs. This progression is optimized when three fundamental features are present: sensory acuity, optimal stabilization strategies, and mobility. There are, however, a number of pervasive issues, including obesity and overweight, sedentary lifestyles, poor posture, improper training and aging that are known to compromise these preconditions of progression. With knowledge of biomechanics, motor control, and optimal alignment, the Personal Trainer is in a position to make the necessary program adjustments and offer lifestyle recommendations to accommodate for these ever-present issues. Ultimately, these accommodations can lay the foundation for optimal gains in functional capacity, strength, and performance.

 **Sensorimotor Control**

## Motor Learning

During early phases of motor learning, performance is largely under conscious control, meaning a great deal of focus and concentration is needed in order to successfully perform the movement. Upon repeated practice, control of individual movements becomes integrated into motor patterns. These motor patterns are stored in the central nervous system (CNS), not unlike saving a document on a computer. Once motor patterns are integrated and stored, they become automatic and are fine-tuned by unconscious sensory feedback. The saving of motor patterns makes the neuromuscular system more efficient when the body is exposed to similar demands in the future. For this reason, after sufficient practice, we do not really have to think about riding a bike, hitting a golf ball, or performing a clean and jerk. The problem lies in the saving of faulty motor patterns, as once stored, motor patterns can be challenging to correct.

## Proprioception

The sensory system and the motor control system, collectively known as the sensorimotor system, work together to control movement, balance, posture, and joint stability (15,24,31). Essentially, in order for optimal movement to occur, the body requires the brain to process afferent sensory information from multiple sources. Dr. Charles Sherrington (53) was the first to characterize this input as proprioception. Currently, proprioception is understood to be the sense of knowing where one's body is in space and is composed of static (joint position sense) and dynamic (kinesthetic movement sense) (16). Proprioception enables us, with closed eyes, to estimate the size of our feet, describe the width of our pelvis, and scratch our noses. Table 17.1 describes common movements that are derived from proprioceptive acuity. This sensory input is gathered from specialized nerve endings, termed mechanoreceptors, that are located within the skin, muscles, fascia, and joints (49). Information collected from visual and vestibular centers further supports proprioception, and when taken together, the result is precise body awareness and well-adapted motor actions (Fig. 17.1).

Proprioception is an important mediator of joint stability and mobility and ultimately the calibration of movement (18). It follows that this sensory acuity is central to safely perform many of the resistance training exercises that are included in conventional exercise programs.

| Table 17.1 | Salient Features of Proprioceptive Acuity |
|---|---|
| **Characteristic** | **Example** |
| Postural control | Maintaining balance during perturbations (a force, such as a gentle tap or vibration, that is applied with the intention of altering balance) |
| Precise calibration of limb position in space | Threading a needle |
| Maintenance of steady muscle force production/movement amplitudes | Unbroken, smooth motion during the eccentric and concentric phases of a dumbbell chest press |
| Discrimination of object weight | Tailoring the effort required to lift a 5-lb weight and a 25-lb weight |
| Production of coordinated gait patterns | Biomechanically efficient walking; running |
| Controlling the timing of muscular contraction for dynamic stabilization and multisegmental movement | Executing a tennis serve or a clean and jerk |
| Feedback and feed-forward motor control | Reaction time and anticipatory responses in a soccer game |

If there are disturbances in proprioception, reactive (feedback) and preparatory/anticipatory (feed-forward) motor control and stability will be altered, increasing the risk of injury (48). It is also important to note that problems with stability and/or mobility issues will perpetuate proprioceptive deficits. Figure 17.2 describes the afferent and efferent pathways involved in the sensorimotor system.

## Key Point

Motor control is developed through enhancing proprioceptive acuity and grooving proper movement patterns through practice.

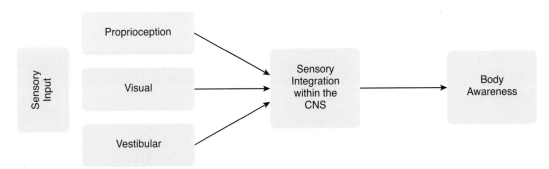

**FIGURE 17.1.** Sensory input from vestibular, visual, and proprioception are integrated within the central nervous system resulting in relatively keen body awareness.

**FIGURE 17.2.** The sensorimotor system integrates all sensory (afferent) and muscular (efferent) activity. Afferent activity is indicated by the dotted lines, whereas the solid lines indicate efferent activity. (Adapted from Riemann BL, Lephart SM. The sensorimotor system, part I: the physiologic basis of functional joint stability. *J Athl Train.* 2002; 37[1]:71–9.)

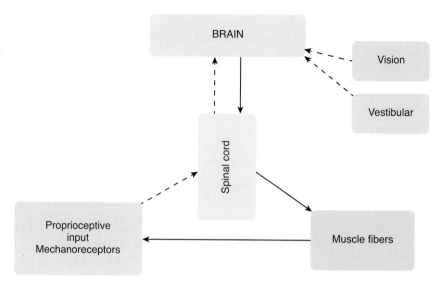

## Stability and Mobility

There is a good reason why we prefer driving a car with aligned tires, lug nuts tightened, and fan belts secured. For example, if the fan belt is secured (stability), it can move at a very high speed (mobility) for many miles without wear and tear. If these requisite features are not present, we can expect to shell out money for repairs far sooner than the manufacturer originally predicted. We might also expect far-reaching changes to the overall structure and function of the car. The factors that contribute to the mechanical efficiency and the long life of our cars are akin to the features needed for optimal function in the body, stability, and mobility.

Stability has been defined as the state of remaining unchanged, even in the presence of forces that would normally change the state or condition (26). Others have defined stability as the state of a joint remaining or promptly returning to proper alignment through an equalization of forces (47). Joint stabilization then occurs through coordinated muscle coactivation, creating a suitable amount of stiffness to maintain joint alignment (35).

Stabilization strategies are managed at the subcortical level, where the generation of stability is somewhat automatic and requires quality proprioceptive input. For example, a tennis player does not consciously consider the use of the rotator cuff muscles (glenohumeral stabilizers) while serving, rather the player is more focused on the voluntary actions of the ball toss and the service motion. Ideally, the muscles of the rotator cuff perform the job of joint centration (keeping the humeral head in an optimal position within the glenoid fossa) in an anticipatory manner, described as glenohumeral stabilization (37). To this end, the sensorimotor system is responsible for providing awareness,

## Key Point

Optimal stabilization strategies require

1. A stable base from which forces are transferred
2. Adequate muscular capacity (strength and endurance)
3. CNS motor programming (integration of sensory input) that produces synchronous activation of the muscles

| Table 17.2 | Muscle Classification | |
|---|---|---|
| **Mobilizers** | **Stabilizers** | |
| Upper trapezius | Deep cervical flexors | |
| Levator scapulae | Lower trapezius | |
| Pectoralis major and minor | Serratus anterior | |
| Deltoids | Rotator cuff (infraspinatus, supraspinatus, teres minor, subscapularis) | |
| Erector spinae | Middle and lower trapezius | |
| Iliopsoas | Transversus abdominis | |
| Quadriceps | Multifidus | |
| Rectus abdominis | Gluteus medius and maximus | |

coordination, and feedback to maintain optimal positioning of the shoulder joint, thereby enhancing the quality of movement and reducing the chance of injury (22,59). Conversely, if the stabilizing rotator cuff muscles are not recruited with proper timing and speed and proper muscle patterns, the humeral head is subject to the pulling forces of the deltoid muscles, which can cause the humeral head to shift upward within the socket. The upward translation is problematic in that several musculotendinous structures (*e.g.*, biceps tendon and rotator cuff tendons) that are located in this area can become impinged between the acromion process and the head of the humerus. Other illustrations of the automation of healthy stabilization strategies are the anticipatory bracing that occurs when a dog unexpectedly pulls on the leash, the bracing of the neck and trunk when cyclist rides over a pothole, or the postural adjustments that are made during abrupt change directions on the tennis court.

Some researchers have categorized muscles as two distinct, yet interdependent systems, stabilizers or mobilizers (6,46). Categorization is largely based on their relative contributions to movement and maintaining posture, and position in the body (Table 17.2).

Classifying muscles in this way is beneficial for the Personal Trainer, as stabilizing muscles have unique characteristics (Table 17.3) that require specialized training approaches, which will

| Table 17.3 | Mobilizer and Stabilizer Characteristics | |
|---|---|---|
| **Mobilizers** | **Stabilizers** | |
| Fast twitch | Slow twitch | |
| Fatigues easily | Resistant to fatigue | |
| Superficial | Deep | |
| Relatively small proprioceptive role | Major contributor to proprioception | |
| High force production | Low force production | |
| Prone to hold excess tension/shorten | Prone to inhibition/weakness | |
| Concentric | Isometric/eccentric | |
| Gross movement | Joint stabilization | |

## What Is the Core?

Perhaps the most common discussion of stabilization relates to core function. This is because the hips and the trunk serve as our center of mass and attempts to centralize the strength and coordination of the core are believed to yield optimal force production through the limbs. The principle of core stability can be illustrated in a simple comparison, shooting a canon off of a canoe versus a stable surface. To date, there is no universally accepted definition of the core, where some researchers describe the core as a muscular cylinder with the abdominals comprising the front, the multifidus and gluteals the back, the diaphragm as the roof, and the pelvic floor as the base of the cylinder (6–8,35). Tse et al. (60) defined the core as all muscles of the trunk and pelvis that contribute to maintaining a stable spine. Other researchers suggest that the core is an integrated system composed of passive structures (*e.g.*, ligaments and bone), the active spinal muscles and thoracolumbar fascia, and the neural control unit (40,41). Precise definition notwithstanding, there is universal agreement that the core is central to all kinetic chains, and that upper and lower extremity movement is optimized in conditions where there is sufficient endurance and neuromuscular control of the core (6–8). Moreover, proper core function improves the spine's ability to withstand the various loads and directional forces that it encounters during daily activities, sport and exercise.

be described later in this chapter. Generally speaking, mobilizing muscles are superficially located and responsible for controlling locomotion, alignment, and balancing forces imposed on the spine. Stabilizing muscles are more centrally located and largely function to create stiffness across joints. These muscles are shorter in length and respond to changes in posture and extrinsic loads. Conversely, mobilizers, or global muscles, comprise long lever arms, allowing greater force production, torque and gross multiplanar movements.

 ## Mediators of the Proprioception, Mobility, and Stability

### Overweight and Obesity and Physical Inactivity

Overweight and obesity is a worldwide epidemic and is associated with elevated risk for a number of chronic diseases such as diabetes, hypertension, and the metabolic syndrome. Among adult men and women, obesity and overweight has been shown to be associated with alterations in motor function and postural control, possibly due to reductions in muscular strength and endurance, postural distortion, discomfort with movement, and the perception of stiffness (29,54). Unfortunately, associations of poor motor control and elevated BMI have also been reported in children and adolescents (11,13,14). Moreover, obesity and overweight in growth and developmental stages is believed to contribute to aberrant motor patterning, which extends to adulthood (54).

### Propensity for Inhibition of Stabilizing Muscles

Dr. Vladimir Janda, a key figure in 20th century rehabilitation and one of the first to characterize the sensorimotor system, suggested that certain muscles had an inherent propensity for weakening or inhibition, while other muscles were prone to hypertonicity (24). Ultimately, the tendencies of certain muscles to weaken or tighten may lead to postural distortion and alterations in motor control (24). This altered regulation of the sensorimotor system may occur due to participation in sports involving repetitive actions, overtraining, poor ergonomics, sedentary lifestyle, trauma, or disease.

## Previous Injury and Pain

Disturbances in the motor control system often follow injury and leave residual effects (45,56). In other words, although the client is pain-free, mobility and stability problems and sensory deficits remain. This sets the stage for a perpetuating cycle of motor control impairment and mobility and stability limitations. Specifically, these alterations lead to inappropriate magnitudes of muscle forces and stiffness across joints, allowing for a joint to buckle or undergo shear translation (as described in the rotator cuff example earlier) (35). The loss of stability may be due to damage incurred to the passive structures of the joint (*e.g.*, tendons, ligaments) where they can no longer support joint integrity. Additionally, sensory receptors within the joints may be compromised, which will result in the delayed action of stabilizing muscles (56). The delay in action changes the order of muscle activation that is necessary for joint centration (20,46).

## Everyday Posture and Limited Variety of Movement

Sahrmann (33) proposes that movement impairment stems from a biomechanical cause. In which case, repeated movements in one direction or sustained postures result in the remodeling of sarcomeres, whereby muscle lengths adaptively shorten or lengthen. The adaptive shortening represents a loss of sarcomeres, whereas muscle lengthening represents the addition of sarcomeres in series, taken together results in overall muscle imbalance (33). In effect, we stray from a neutral position and begin to adopt the posture that we are in most of the time (51). The muscle length adaptations then influence length tension and force-coupling relationships, motor control, and ultimately how we are able, or in many cases unable, to move (51). This set of circumstances is often seen in individuals that are sedentary, where the muscles of the anterior torso, and internal rotators of the shoulder tend to shorten. Athletes are also susceptible to development of faulty stabilization strategies and mobility, particularly those who perform repeated unvaried or unidirectional movement patterns (*e.g.*, cyclists, runners, golfers, overhead athletes).

From a performance standpoint, a tight and shortened agonist (prime mover) has a lowered activation threshold and is described as hypertonic. This simply means that it will not take much stimulus to activate the muscle. In which case, hypertonic muscles suppress (decrease neural activity via reciprocal inhibition) the activity of lengthened antagonists and cause further weakening of that muscle (61). For example, hypertonic iliopsoas muscles often result from repeated hip flexion as seen in long distance cycling or running, or from prolonged seated postures. The hypertonicity of the hip flexors then contributes to the progressive weakening of the gluteus maximus via reciprocal inhibition. The gluteus maximus is an important hip extensor; thus, when forceful hip extension is necessary, the hamstrings (a synergist of the gluteus maximus) will compensate for the weakened gluteus maximus. This compensatory pattern is problematic for two main reasons. First, the pattern overworks the synergists (in the example, the hamstrings), which increases the risk for injury. Second, this compensatory pattern becomes etched within the sensorimotor system and will alter quality proprioception, mobility and stability. These alterations then tend to perpetuate further postural distortion. For example, when the hamstrings become hypertonic (also due to sedentary posture), they exert a downward force upon the proximal attachment site at the ischial tuberosity of the pelvis. This force rotates the pelvis posteriorly, which reduces the neutral curvature of the lumbar spine (flattens the low back) (51).

## Joint Structure

Mobility and stability are partly derived from the articular geometry, or the shape and depth of joints. It is important to realize that some clients will present with structural anomalies that will prohibit full range of motion (ROM) on certain exercises. For example, an individual's hip joint may have a capsular structure that prevents performing a deep squat with the feet pointed in a neutral alignment. In such cases, the Personal Trainer should encourage movement that is most comfortable for the client and not attempt to stretch through this nonmodifiable limitation.

## Age

The adverse effects of aging on proprioception, stability and mobility are well established (18,62). This is particularly relevant for the Personal Trainer, as the percentage of individuals over the age of 60 years continues to increase and the risk of falls, due to diminished kinesthesia and postural control, increases with age. These factors highlight the functional significance of balance and stability training in older populations. The reasons behind proprioceptive decline in the elderly include a reduction in the number of joint mechanoreceptors, changes to the structure and sensitivity of mechanoreceptors, inadequate processing of proprioceptive input within the CNS (1,2,17,23).

---

### Key Point

Alterations in movement quality can stem from multiple factors including obesity and overweight, sedentary behavior, poor postures, unvaried movement, joint structure, propensity for certain muscles to become inhibited, and age. It follows that fitness practitioners must consider each of these omnipresent factors when designing exercise programs.

---

 ## What Is Neutral Position and Why Is It so Important?

Panjabi (41) describes neutral position as "the posture of the spine in which the overall internal stresses in the spinal column and muscular effort to hold the posture are minimal." A nice illustration of mechanical importance of neutral can be seen in a tent that has supporting wires equally tight around the structure. Conversely, if one set of support wires is tighter in comparison to the

---

### Implications for Personal Trainer

**Context for the Principles of Overload, Specificity, and Other Training Variables**

The principle of overload is a fundamental construct of resistance training design (30). The overload principle suggests that in order to enhance muscular fitness, the body must exercise at an intensity that exceeds what it is normally accustomed to. It is important to recognize that overload represents a specific threshold that must be met in order for adaptation to occur. The way in which we introduce overload, however, must consider a superseding principle, which is quality movement should not be compromised, as flawed motor patterns can be easily ingrained and are difficult to correct once they take hold. To put it another way, overload should not outpace the client's sensory awareness, capacity to stabilize, and ability to move through a full ROM without compensation.

The principle of specificity suggests that specific adaptations occur upon application of specific demands. Accordingly, to improve proprioceptive acuity, sensory-specific training is necessary. More to the point, strength training is not the most effective way to improve sensory deficits.

In summary, fundamental principles of exercise prescription must be taken within context of quality movement. This means the adjustment of resistance training variables, including exercise selection, velocity of movement, and the number of repetitions and sets, should all be based on the client's sensorimotor capacity.

other side, the tent will likely collapse. In humans, maintaining neutral is important because it organizes the body into its most biomechanically efficient posture (40,41). More specifically, neutral position (a) optimizes ideal muscle length-tension and force-coupling relationships, (b) minimizes compressive and shear forces imposed on the joint, and (c) optimizes the timing and speed of contraction of stabilizing muscles.

 # Assessment and Prescription

## Establishing a Movement Baseline

A widely held belief is that simple bodyweight movement is an appropriate place to begin a strength and conditioning program. This logic is based on the assumption that the client already has sufficient proprioceptive acuity, mobility, and appropriate command of the stabilizing muscles to maintain optimal alignment. Given the pervasive contributors of muscle imbalance described earlier, this assumption is a chancy supposition, whereby further exploration into the client's true movement baseline is likely needed (51).

Considering the majority of fitness assessments will take place in fitness centers, gyms, and studios, without the use of sophisticated laboratory equipment, the most pragmatic strategies for the Personal Trainer are left to observation of static and dynamic postures and symmetry of movement. It is important to note that if pain is present during any of the following assessments or exercises, the Personal Trainer should recommend a medical exam by a qualified medical professional.

### Assessment of Static Neutral Posture

Although static posture does not necessarily capture how an individual moves, it does provide the Personal Trainer some insight regarding specific muscle imbalances. This information can then be used in the selection of stabilization exercises and stretching and self-myofascial release (SMR) strategies. Static postural assessments also help clients develop an awareness of neutral posture, which holds great relevance when clients are performing dynamic movements that require maintenance of neutral while under load (*e.g.*, squat, lunge, deadlift, farmer's carries).

#### PLUMB LINE ASSESSMENT

Use of a plumb line or a static posture app is useful in identifying deviations from a neutral position. Clients should be barefoot, wear form-fitting clothing that enables the assessor to identify bony landmarks, and be encouraged to assume their everyday, relaxed posture during the assessment. Table 17.4 describes a basic plumb line postural assessment.

#### WALL TEST

In addition to the plumb line assessment, a wall assessment of normal lumbar curvature and forward head posture is helpful. Instruct the client to stand with his or her back against a wall and feet approximately 6 in from the wall. Ideally, the back of the head should be positioned against the wall and the assessors hand should be able to fit snuggly in between the wall of the client's lumbar spine and the wall. Taken together, these static postural assessments expose areas of tightness and/or weakness. There are occasions where simply drawing the client's attention to the postural distortion and offering verbal cues will prove helpful (Table 17.5). Additionally, Table 17.5 offers specific stretching targets that correspond to the listed postural deviations.

#### PROGRESSIVE APPROACH TO DEVELOPING POSTURAL AWARENESS

Unfortunately, due to various sensory, mobility, and stability limitations, the ability to distinguish neutral spine may be challenged. To begin, the Personal Trainer should cue the client,

| Table 17.4 | Basic Plumb Line Static Postural Assessment | |
|---|---|---|
| View | Setup for Assessment | Alignment Checkpoints (the plumb line should pass through these anatomical landmarks) |
| Sagittal | Client should stand sideways to the plumb line, with the line positioned slightly anterior to the client's ankle (lateral malleolus) | External auditory meatus (ear canal)<br>Acromioclavicular joint<br>Greater trochanter of the femur<br>Tibial tuberosity |
| Anterior | Client should stand facing the plumb line, with feet equidistant from the line. Align the plumb line with the pubis. | Navel<br>Sternum<br>Chin<br>Nose<br>Eyes are equidistant from the line.<br>Additionally, the shoulder girdle should be level. |

Adapted from Kendall FP. *Muscles: Testing and Function with Posture and Pain.* 5th ed. Baltimore (MD): Lippincott Williams & Wilkins; 2005. 560 p.

both manually and verbally, to arch the low back and then flatten the low back (see Table 17.6 for progressive postural staging of this process). This should be repeated several times, upon which the client should be asked to find the middle of the two extremes. Once neutral alignment is found, the client should be instructed to hold this posture for several seconds and then lose neutral by arching or flattening the low back, only to regain neutral position again. The client should begin performing each stage with eyes open and then eyes closed. When more dynamic movements, such as hip hinging and squatting, are introduced a dowel placed along the spine provides valuable tactile feedback for the client. The client should be encouraged to maintain three points of contact with the dowel: the back of the head, the upper thoracic spine, and the pelvis.

| Table 17.5 | Postural Corrective Suggestions | |
|---|---|---|
| Postural Deviation | Suggestive Verbal Cues | Stretching Target |
| Forward head posture | "Tuck the chin." | Pectoralis major and minor; latissimus dorsi; abdominals |
| Increased thoracic curvature | "While tucking your chin, stand or sit as tall as possible." | Pectoralis major and minor; latissimus dorsi; abdominals |
| Internal rotation of the shoulders | "Create as much width between your shoulders." | Pectoralis major and minor; latissimus dorsi |
| Posterior pelvic tilt | "Align your rib cage over your pelvis." | Hamstrings; abdominals |
| Hyperextension of lumbar spine | "Gently contract your glute muscles."<br>"Lock your ribcage on top of your pelvis." | Erector spinae; quadratus lumborum; quadriceps; iliopsoas |

| Table 17.6 | Progressive Stages for Neutral Posture |
|---|---|
| Stage 1 Lying on the ground | |
| Stage 2 Seated | |
| Stage 3 Standing | |
| Stage 4 Standing and adding in hip hinging | |
| Stage 5 Farmer carries with bilateral loading | |
| Stage 6 Farmer carries with unilateral loading | |

## Integrative Assessments and Corrections

As muscles rarely work in isolation, assessments that consider the body as an integrated system, involving various segments of the body responding to movements in a synchronous coordinated fashion, are quite valuable (60). Although the following patterns may seem rudimentary, keep in mind that poor posture, fatigue, repeated asymmetrical movements, stress, and poor exercise practices have the potential to corrupt even the most primal motor patterns (24,28,32,35,51). Reclaiming these basic patterns then feeds the reflexive and intentional stabilization strategies needed for more functional movements such as the deadlift, squat, lunges etc. (9,38).

### WALL PLANK-AND-ROLL

The wall plank-and-roll (WPR) is not only an assessment of lumbar stability but can also serve as an exercise to enhance lumbar torsional (anti-rotational) control (63). The client should be instructed to face a wall, with feet positioned approximately 2 ft from the wall. The client's elbows should be positioned on the wall, with forearms lying one on top of the other. The client should then be instructed to "brace" or stiffen the trunk (35), and pivot on the balls of their feet while pulling one elbow off the wall ending in a side plank position. The client should be encouraged to rotate the entire body as a single unit. No lumbar or pelvic motion should be observed while pivoting from side to side. Once the client demonstrates sufficient stability for the wall roll, progressions include side planks on the floor, initially performed on the knees and ultimately performed in a full body side plank position. Of practical relevance, in order to optimize the effectiveness of isometric endurance exercises such as the side plank (also called the side bridge), Dr. Stuart McGill recommends performing repeated sets of short-duration holds (8–10 s) rather than having the client perform one set of a prolonged (>30 s) (35).

### TEACHING HOW TO BRACE

With respect to teaching clients how to brace, a few concepts are important to emphasize. First, the client should be instructed to precontract, or brace, the abdominal wall prior to performing isometric exercises such as a plank or isotonic movements such as squatting movements. Stuart McGill (35) suggests the use of the simple cue of "pretend you are about to be hit in the stomach." It is worth mentioning that the "hit" is not necessarily a full force strike to the stomach, rather only intended to create the image of creating sufficient stability to maintain neutral alignment but not too much stiffness where motion is prevented (35). In other words, *the intensity of the brace should be tailored to the **relative intensity** of the exercise*, where the resultant coactivation of the trunk muscles is ample to protect the spine during lifting tasks but does not encumber proper mobility. For example, a client performing a bodyweight squat may require a low level of bracing intensity; however, when performing a one repetition maximum (1-RM) squat, the client should be encouraged to brace with closer to a maximal effort to maintain spinal integrity.

### Diaphragmatic Breathing Assessment and Corrective Methods

Evaluation of diaphragmatic control is important for several reasons. First, the diaphragm muscles are not only the prime muscles of respiration but they are also a vital muscle of core stabilization. To this end, if proper diaphragmatic control is not present, the generation of intra-abdominal pressure required to stabilize the spine during lifting tasks can be compromised (27,38). Second, breathing pattern problems have been shown to result in muscular imbalance, motor control alterations, and chronic low back pain (12,35,38). Third, as with proper conditioning of any muscle in the body, improving the endurance of the respiratory muscles enables these muscles to perform at higher capacities, ultimately leading to improved work capacity and prolonged time to fatigue (34). Fourth, those who tend to breathe at quicker rates, described as hyperventilation, exceed the gas exchange needs of metabolism. To this end, over-breathing has the potential to drastically lower carbon dioxide ($CO_2$) levels, which can raise pH levels (34). Not only is this a performance limiting issue, if hyperventilation is severe enough, light-headedness and possibly unconsciousness can result. Finally, alterations in breathing mechanics have been correlated with low scores on the Functional Movement Screen (9), an evaluation of movement quality that explores seven different movement patterns.

Healthy breathing patterns, or diaphragmatic breathing, involve the expansion of the rib cage and abdomen and involves proper recruitment and endurance of the diaphragm muscles (43). Conversely, altered breathing involves breathing from the upper chest, as shown by rib cage elevation, and often involves shallow and quick breathing rates (12). The Hi-Lo Assessment is a simple assessment of proper diaphragmatic control during breathing and is detailed in Table 17.7.

Ideally, the hand on the upper abdomen should rise before the hand on the chest. Additionally, the hand on the chest should move slightly forward and not upward toward the chin (12). Conveniently, this simple assessment also serves as a means to correct the breathing pattern problem. The basic approach, detailed in Table 17.8, involves the client practicing a diaphragmatic breathing pattern while progressing through more challenging postures and movements. Clients demonstrating improper breathing habits should be encouraged to regularly practice breathing (using the same hand positions) that is focused on expansion of the rib cage and upper abdomen prior to any chest movement and to increase the length of each breath, in particular the client should be encouraged to fully exhale. Routine follow-up breathing pattern assessment should be performed to monitor for changes and to emphasize the relevance of diaphragmatic breathing patterns in optimizing core stability and overall health.

| Table 17.7 | Hi-Lo Assessment |
|---|---|
| Client places one hand on his or her sternum and one hand on his or her upper abdomen. | |
| The client is then instructed to perform 10 breathing cycles. | |
| The client reports which hand moved first at the beginning of the inhalation phase during the majority of the assessment. In addition, the practitioner should observe the hand movements of the client. | |

Adapted from Chaitow L. Breathing pattern disorders, motor control, and low back pain. *J Osteopath Med.* 2004;7(1):33–40.

| Table 17.8 | Diaphragmatic Breathing Pattern Progression | |
|------------|---------------------------------------------|--|
| **Stage** | **Description** | **Postural Progression** |
| Static | Maintenance of postural stability while breathing diaphragmatically | Supine on stable surface<br>Seated<br>Standing |
| Dynamic | Simultaneous limb movement while maintaining postural stability and diaphragmatic breathing patterns | Supine on floor with arm or leg movement<br>Supine on foam roller with arm or leg movement<br>Seated with arm or leg movement<br>Standing with arm or leg movement |
| Advanced | Increase ventilation by performing any type of aerobic exercise | Immediately stop the aerobic exercise and perform an isometric exercise (*e.g.*, side-plank, bird dog, curl-up). This will assist in improve the coordination of the diaphragm during tasks of core stabilization. Note: For these low loading challenges, abdominal bracing should occur in concert with diaphragmatic breathing. |

Adapted from Nelson N. Diaphragmatic breathing: the foundation of core stability. *Strength Cond J*. 2012;34(5):34–40; McGill SM. *Low Back Disorders: Evidence-Based Prevention and Rehabilitation*. 2nd ed. Champaign (IL): Human Kinetics; 2007. 328 p.

## ROLLING PATTERNS: ASSESSMENT AND CORRECTION

Although infants can roll with relative efficiency by 6–8 months of age, the pattern may become altered later in life due to mobility deficits or insufficient core stabilization patterning (21). More specifically, demonstration of efficient rolling patterns reveals proper recruitment sequencing of the core stabilizing muscles (*i.e.*, initiated with the deeper trunk stabilizers, including the transversus abdominis, multifidus, diaphragm and pelvic floor, and followed by recruitment of the more superficial or global muscles including the internal and external obliques, rectus abdominis, quadratus lumborum, erector spinae). However, given the lack of variety of daily movement among many individuals (including athletes performing motions in one direction), symmetrical rotational efficiency may be altered. The objective of the assessment is to observe the rolling strategy of the client in eight different patterns, leading from all four quadrants of the body. Ideally, the client should be able to roll with equal ease in all directions. When first performing the rolling assessments, use limited cues (Table 17.9), as the goal is to observe their movement plan and "cheating" methods.

There are times where clients will have difficulty completing rolling patterns. In which case, Table 17.10 and Figures 17.3–17.8 provide some of the common associated mobility and stability limitations and corresponding corrections. The rolling pattern itself can also be modified by placing a foam roller under one side of the trunk (just lateral to the spine); this will assist the client in rolling away from the bolstered side.

The client should be encouraged to practice each of the patterns (particularly the patterns where coordination and symmetry of movement was poor) while keeping the cues offered in Table 17.11 in mind.

## Addressing Alignment Issues

It is essential for the Personal Trainer to be able to critically appraise the quality of movement during an exercise session. In the fitness center setting, this evaluation will often rely on observing

| Table 17.9 | Assessment of Rolling Patterns | |
|---|---|---|
| **Rolling Direction**[a] | **Beginning Position** | **Cues** |
| Supine to prone leading with the right or left arm | Supine, legs straight, and slightly abducted; arms overhead and slightly abducted; when looking down at the client, they should resemble an "X." | "With no help from the legs, roll onto your belly." |
| Supine to prone leading with the right or left leg | Supine, legs straight, and slightly abducted; arms overhead and slightly abducted | "With no help from your arms, roll onto your belly." |
| Prone to supine leading with the right or left arm | Prone, legs straight, and slightly abducted; arms overhead and slightly abducted | "With no help from your legs, roll onto your back." |
| Supine to prone leading with the right or left leg | Prone, legs straight, and slightly abducted; arms overhead and slightly abducted | "With no help from your arms, roll onto your back." |

[a]Each pattern should be performed right to left and left to right, totaling eight patterns.

| Table 17.10 | Correctives for Those Who are Initially Unable to Perform Rolling Patterns |
|---|---|
| **Exercise Progression for Rolling Patterns** | |
| **Strength or mobility limitation** | **Corrective stretch or exercise** |
| Thoracic spine mobility | Modified cobra stretch (Fig. 17.3); doorway pectoralis major stretch |
| Gluteus maximus weakness | Bird dog (Fig. 17.4) or quadruped exercises; glute bridges (Fig. 17.5) |
| Gluteus medius weakness | Lateral band walks (Fig. 17.6); clam shell exercises (Fig. 17.7) |
| Core endurance | Wall plank-and-roll; side plank performed on knees (Fig. 17.8) |

| Table 17.11 | Verbal Cues for Rolling Patterns |
|---|---|
| **Rolling Direction**[a] | **Verbal Cues** |
| Supine to prone leading with the right arm | "Begin by looking to the left, lead with the eyes and head; lift the right arm; look into the left shoulder and roll over like a rag doll." |
| Supine to prone leading with the right leg | "Flex the hip and then cross the right leg over the left and roll." |
| Prone to supine leading with the right arm | "Lift the right arm, look up and over the opposite shoulder and roll." |
| Prone to supine leading with the right leg | "Bend the right knee, lift the foot toward the ceiling, cross the right leg over the left and roll." |

[a]These sample cues are for rolling from right to left. Simply reverse the cuing when rolling from left to right.
Adapted from Hoogenboom BJ, Voight ML, Cook G, Gill L. Using rolling to develop neuromuscular control and coordination of the core and extremities of athletes. *N Am J Sports Phys Ther.* 2009;4(2):70–82.

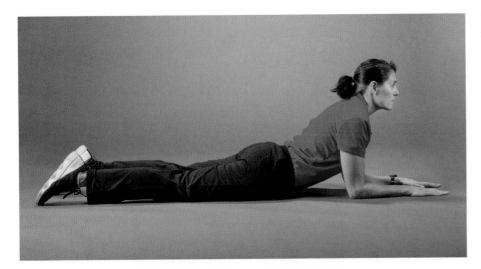

**FIGURE 17.3.** Modified cobra stretch.

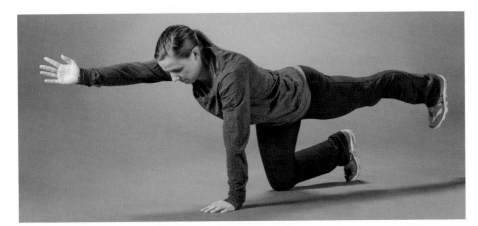

**FIGURE 17.4.** Bird dog.

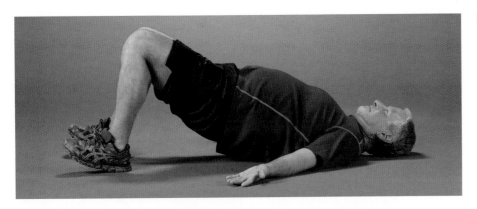

**FIGURE 17.5.** Glute bridge.

**FIGURE 17.6.** Lateral band walks.

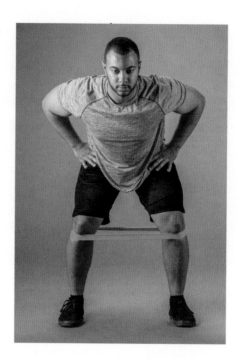

**FIGURE 17.7.** Clam shell.

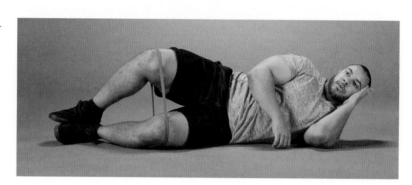

**FIGURE 17.8.** Side plank performed on the knees.

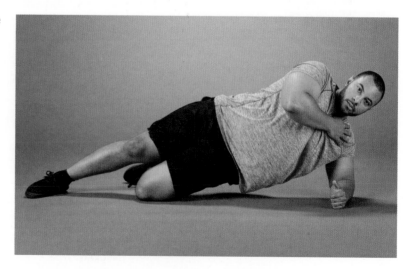

| Table 17.12 | **Alignment Fault Checklist** |
|---|---|

Loss of cervical neutral — head positioned in front of the body or tilting up or down

Loss of thoracic extension — rounding of the thoracic spine

Internal rotation of the shoulders

Posterior pelvic tilt — loss of neutral lordosis in the lumbar spine or flattening of lumbar spine

Anterior pelvic tilt — excessive arching of low back

Knee valgus — knees collapsing inward

any alignment faults that may present during the performance of an exercise (Table 17.12). Many times, verbal and manual cuing can correct the problem; however, there are occasions where alignment faults are the result of low endurance, timing issues of the stabilizing muscles, and/or tightness in the mobilizing muscles that were outlined earlier in this chapter (Table 17.13).

The training goal is to improve the endurance and functional stabilization capacity of these muscles. In which case, a good place to start is incorporating isometric exercises applied at various joint specific angles for the weakened or inhibited muscles (3), with short duration hold and relax cycles (5–8 s). For example, if weakness is noted in the rhomboid muscles (demonstrated by excessive thoracic kyphosis), an effective approach might involve the following:

- Instruct the client to maintain a tall neutral posture while retracting and depressing the scapula, holding this position for 5–8 seconds and then relaxing.
- Progression 1: Have the client perform multiple sets of this exercise, still using 5- to 8-second holds.
- Progression 2: Have the client perform the same isometric hold against light resistance tubing.

| Table 17.13 | **Common Alignment Faults Along with Corresponding Inhibited or Weak Stabilizing Muscles** | |
|---|---|---|
| **Alignment Fault** | **Associated Weak or Inhibited Muscles** | **Suggested Corrective Exercises** |
| Loss of cervical neutral | Deep cervical flexors (longus colli, capitis) | Chin tucks (Fig. 17.9); isometric cervical exercise (*e.g.*, using hands on forehead resisting neck flexion effort) |
| Loss of thoracic extension | Middle and lower trapezius | Scapular retraction with no weight (Fig. 17.10); progressing to seated rows |
| Internal rotation of the shoulders | External rotators of the shoulder (infraspinatus) | Band or dumbbell shoulder external rotation (Fig. 17.11) |
| Posterior pelvic tilt | Gluteus medius and maximus; multifidus | Glute bridges; quadruped or bird dog |
| Anterior pelvic tilt | Gluteus medius and maximus; transversus abdominis | Curl-up; side plank/bridge |
| Knee valgus | Gluteus medius and maximus | Lateral band walks; clam shells; glute bridges; bird dog |

**FIGURE 17.9.** Chin tucks.

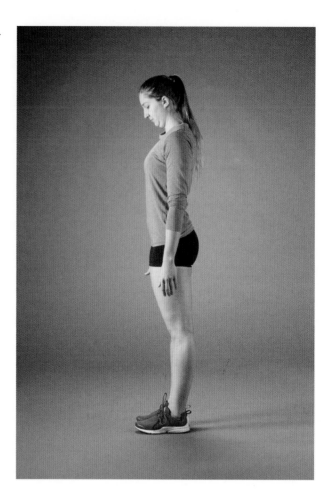

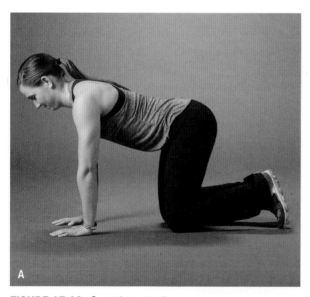

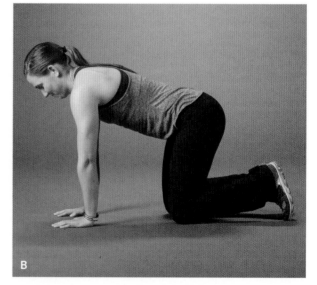

**FIGURE 17.10.** Scapular retraction.

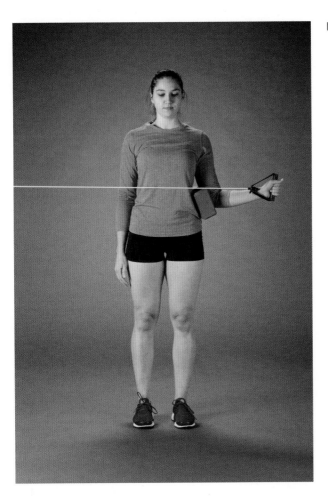

**FIGURE 17.11.** Band external rotation.

- Progression 3: As the client develops endurance and greater recruitment efficiency of the rhomboids, introduce more dynamic movements, such as a seated row or single arm dumbbell row. In this case, repetitions schemes should be focused on enhancing muscular endurance (12–15 repetitions).

### INSTABILITY TRAINING

Instability training is a method of training that challenges a client's ability to maintain balance while challenging the client's center of gravity. This is often accomplished by narrowing the client's base of support (*e.g.*, by moving the legs closer together, maintaining single leg postures, or performing exercises on unstable surfaces). By challenging posture in this way, instability training is thought to improve feed-forward and feedback mechanisms, ultimately improving stability and proprioception. It is worth noting that the goal of instability training is to improve stability and sensory acuity, not necessarily to improve strength in the extremities, thus should involve low load tasks. When planning instability training, it is essential to tailor the difficulty of the exercise to the client's relative functional capacity. In effect, the client should be able to demonstrate some level of postural control, but at the same time, the exercise should require a great deal of concentration. Once the client has mastered one level, the client should progress to the next level of difficulty. Table 17.14 illustrates a systematic approach to instability training. Once the client can adequately perform the exercise on the floor, the next stage would involve having the client perform the same sequence of exercises, only on an unstable surface, such as a cushioned surface or an Airex pad.

| Table 17.14 | Instability Training Progression Example | |
|---|---|---|
| **Exercise** | **Position** | **Demonstration of Mastery** |
| A1. Wide staggered stance on the floor Eyes open (Fig. 17.12) | Client stands on the floor with one foot in front of the other, wide stance to increase the base of support. | Maintains optimal alignment without significant swaying for 30 s |
| A2. Wide staggered stance on the floor Eyes closed | Client stands on the floor with one foot in front of the other, wide stance to increase the base of support. | Maintains optimal alignment without significant swaying for 30 s |
| A3. Wide staggered stance on the floor with weight shift Eyes closed | Client stands on the floor with one foot in front of the other, wide stance to increase the base of support. Instruct client to shift majority of weight onto front foot then to back foot. | Maintains optimal alignment without significant swaying for 30 s |
| B1. Narrow staggered stance Eyes open | Client stands on the floor with one foot directly in front of the other as if standing on a balance beam. | Maintains optimal alignment without significant swaying for 30 s |
| B2. Narrow staggered stance Eyes closed | Client stands on the floor with one foot directly in front of the other as if standing on a balance beam. | Maintains optimal alignment without significant swaying for 30 s |
| B3. Narrow staggered stance Eyes closed with weight shift | Client stands on the floor with one foot directly in front of the other as if standing on a balance beam. Instruct client to shift majority of weight onto front foot then to back foot. | Maintains optimal alignment without significant swaying for 30 s |
| C1. Single-leg stance Eyes open | Client stands on one foot on the floor. | Maintains optimal alignment without significant swaying for 30 s |
| C2. Single-leg stance Eyes closed (Fig. 17.13) | Client stands on one foot on the floor. | Maintains optimal alignment without significant swaying for 30 s |
| C3. Single-leg stance with reach | Client stands on one foot on floor and reaches with opposite hand to a specific target. | Able to perform several reaches without losing balance |

The next stage might incorporate the use of a wobble board or Bosu trainer, as the client performs functional challenges such as medicine ball tosses or sport specific tasks (Figs. 17.14 and 17.15).

## Self-Myofascial Release and Stretching

Another important component of a well-rounded exercise prescription is managing hypertonic muscles and soft tissue restriction that compromise mobility. Although stretching approaches such as proprioceptive neuromuscular facilitation (PNF), and static stretching are known to improve ROM, several reviews have reported significant deleterious effects on neuromuscular performance when done prior to activity (5,25). Conversely, several recent investigations have shown that SMR elicits improvements in ROM without concomitant performance decrements when done prior to activity (19,42,55).

SMR is based on a form of manual therapy believed to alleviate the discomfort associated

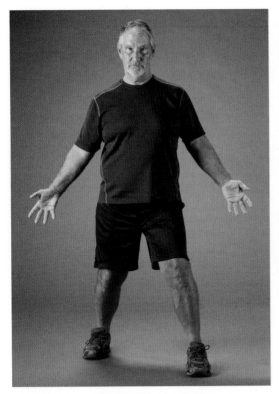

**FIGURE 17.12.** Wide staggered stance, eyes open.

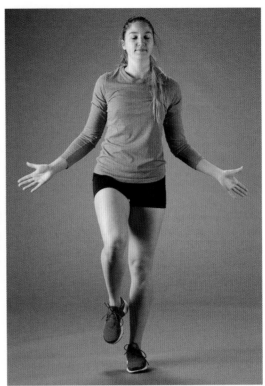

**FIGURE 17.13.** Single-leg stance, eyes closed.

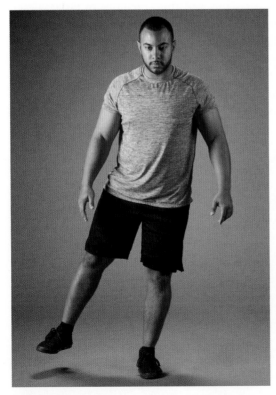

**FIGURE 17.14.** Progression option: one leg on floor.

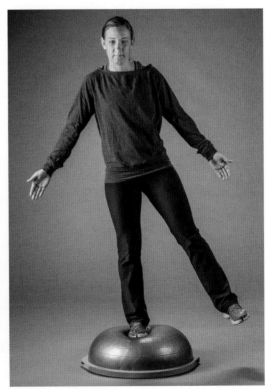

**FIGURE 17.15.** Progression option: one leg on Bosu.

**FIGURE 17.16.** Lacrosse ball on upper back.

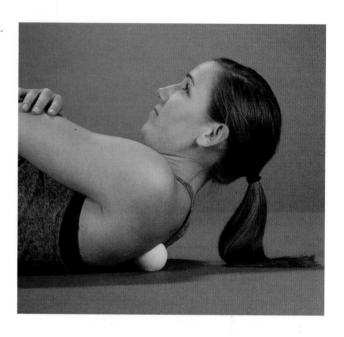

with tender spots within the myofascia, known as trigger points (10,58), and relax hypertonic areas within soft tissue (36). SMR involves the compression of soft tissue using tools such as foam rollers, roller massagers, or tennis balls and is performed by the individual rather than by a therapist (Figs. 17.16 and 17.17). Currently, the mechanisms behind SMR are unclear, although prevailing theories suggest that the compressive forces imposed on the myofascia stimulate various mechanoreceptors that reduce muscle-firing rates (50,52,57). Additionally, mechanical pressure induced by SMR may improve the viscous and fluid qualities of fascia, described as thixotropism (52). Other theories have proposed that the myofascia becomes restricted due to local inflammation (4). Although it is unclear how SMR might reduce inflammation, there is evidence indicating that SMR transiently increases local blood flow (39,44). To this end, the increased blood flow may aid in the reduction of inflammation. Table 17.15 includes a few suggested SMR and stretching targets for common alignment issues.

**FIGURE 17.17.** Foam rolling hamstrings.

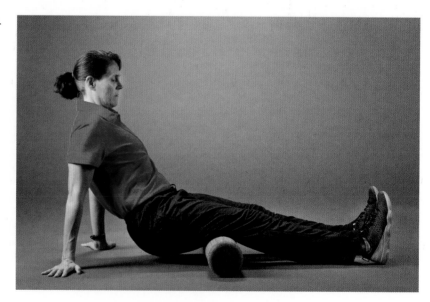

| Table 17.15 | Alignment Issues and Soft Tissue Targets |
| --- | --- |
| **Alignment Fault** | **Self-Myofascial Release and Stretching Targets** |
| Excessive kyphosis of the thoracic spine | Pectoralis major and minor; latissimus dorsi; abdominals |
| Internal rotation of the shoulders | Pectoralis major and minor; latissimus dorsi |
| Posterior pelvic tilt | Hamstrings (see Fig. 17.17); abdominals |
| Hyperextension of the lumbar spine | Quadratus lumborum; quadriceps; iliopsoas |

## Lifestyle Recommendations

Stability, mobility, and sensory issues develop over long periods of time and are often mediated by lifestyle habits. Although exercise sessions are a critical piece of the repatterning process, the Personal Trainer should also offer recommendations that address lifestyle issues known to perpetuate muscle imbalance. Suggestions might include improving the ergonomics of the work environment, setting a recurring alarm to serve as a reminder to stand and walk around the office, practice of diaphragmatic breathing, and foam rolling while watching television.

## SUMMARY

Although progressive overload is essential for improvements in strength and endurance outcomes, it should not come at the expense of proper movement patterning. To this end, it is critical for the Personal Trainer to recognize that stability, mobility, and proprioception are requisite features of motor patterning and collectively serve as the foundation for strength and functional development. Unfortunately, pervasive issues such as sedentary behavior, obesity and overweight, and limited variety in movement impair these foundational components of fitness. If insufficient stabilizing strategies, lack of mobility, and low proprioceptive acuity are observed, Personal Trainer must incorporate a systematic, progressive approach to improve baseline function prior to advancing the client into more conventional exercise prescription.

## REFERENCES

1. Adamo D, Martin B, Brown S. Age-related differences in upper limb proprioceptive acuity. *Percept Mot Skills.* 2007;104(3 Pt 2):1297–309.
2. Aydog S, Korkusuz P, Doral M, Tetick O, Demirel H. Decrease in the numbers of mechanoreceptors in rabbit ACL: the effects of aging. *Knee Surg.* 2006;14(4):325–9.
3. Baechle TR, Earle RW. *Essentials of Strength Training and Conditioning.* 2nd ed. Champaign (IL): Human Kinetics; 2000. 672 p.
4. Bednar DA, Orr FW, Simon GT. Observations on the pathomorphology of the thoracolumbar fascia in chronic mechanical back pain: a microscopic study. *Spine.* 1995;20(10):1161–4.
5. Behm DG, Chaouachi A. A review of the acute effects of static and dynamic stretching on performance. *Eur J Appl Physiol.* 2011;111(11):2633–51.
6. Bergmark A. Stability of the lumbar spine: a study in mechanical engineering. *Acta Orthop Scand.* 1989;230(Suppl):20–4.
7. Bliss L, Teeple P. Core stability: the centerpiece of any training program. *Cur Sports Med Rep.* 2005;4(3):179–83.
8. Borghuis J, Hof A, Lemmink K. The importance of sensory-motor control in providing core stability. *Sports Med.* 2008; 38(11):893–916.
9. Bradley H, Esformes J. Breathing pattern disorders and functional movement. *Int J Sports Phys Ther.* 2014;9(1): 28–39.

10. Bron C, Dommerholt JD. Etiology of myofascial trigger points. *Curr Pain Headache Rep*. 2012;16(5):439–44.

11. Cattuzzo MT, dos Santos H, Ré A, et al. Motor competence and health related physical fitness in youth: a systematic review. *J Sci Med Sport*. 2016;19(2):123–9.

12. Chaitow L. Breathing pattern disorders, motor control, and low back pain. *J Osteopath Med*. 2004;7(1):33–40.

13. Đokic Z. Relationship between overweight, obesity and the motor abilities of 9-12 year old school children. *Phys Cult*. 2013;67(2):91–102.

14. Duncan MJ, Stanley M, Wright SL. The association between functional movement and overweight and obesity in British primary school children. *BMC Sports Sci Med Rehabil*. 2013;5(1):1–8.

15. Franklin DW, Wolpert DM. Computational mechanisms of sensorimotor control. *Neuron*. 2011;72(3):425–42.

16. Gandevia SC, Refshauge KM, Collins DF. Proprioception: peripheral inputs and perceptual interactions. *Adv Exp Med Biol*. 2002;508:61–8.

17. Goble DJ, Brown SH. Task-dependent asymmetries in the utilization of proprioceptive feedback for goal-directed movement. *Exp Brain Res*. 2007;180(4):693–704.

18. Goble DJ, Coxon JP, Wenderoth N, Van Impe A, Swinnen SP. Proprioceptive sensibility in the elderly: degeneration, functional consequences and plastic-adaptive processes. *Neurosci Biobehav Rev*. 2009;33(3):271–8.

19. Healey KC, Hatfield DL, Blanpied P, Dofrman LR, Riebe D. The effects of myofascial release with foam rolling on performance. *J Strength Cond Res*. 2014;28(1):61–8.

20. Hodges PW, Richardson CA. Altered trunk muscle recruitment in people with low back pain with upper limb movement at different speeds. *Arch Phys Med Rehabil*. 1999;80(9):1005–12.

21. Hoogenboom BJ, Voight ML, Cook G, Gill L. Using rolling to develop neuromuscular control and coordination of the core and extremities of athletes. *N Am J Sports Phys Ther*. 2009;4(2):70–82.

22. Ionta S, Heydrich L, Lenggenhager B, et al. Multi-sensory mechanisms in temporo-parietal cortex support self-location and first-person perspective. *Neuron*. 2011;70(2):363–74.

23. Iwasaki T, Goto N, Goto J, Ezure H, Moriyama H. The aging of human Meissner's corpuscles as evidenced by parallel sectioning. *Okajimas Folia Anat*. 2003;79(6):185–9.

24. Jull GA, Janda V. Muscles and motor control in low back pain: assessment and management. In: Twomey LT, Taylor JR, editors. *Physical Therapy of the Low Back*. New York (NY): Churchill Livingstone; 1987. p. 253–78.

25. Kay AD, Blazevich AJ. Effect of acute static stretch on maximal muscle performance: a systematic review. *Med Sci Sports Exerc*. 2012;44(1):154–64.

26. Kersey R. Taber's Cyclopedic Medical Dictionary, 20th ed. *Athl Ther Today*. 2006;11(3):47.

27. Key J. 'The core': understanding it, and retraining its dysfunction. *J Bodywork Movement Ther*. 2013;17(4):541–59.

28. Kibler WB, Press J, Sciascia A. The role of core stability in athletic function. *Sports Med*. 2006;36(3):189–98.

29. Ková čiková Z, Svoboda Z, Neumannová K, Bizovská L, Cuberek R, Janura M. Assessment of postural stability in overweight and obese middle-aged women. *Acta Gymnica*. 2014;44(3):149–53.

30. Kraemer WJ, Ratamess NA. Fundamentals of resistance training: progression and exercise prescription. *Med Sci Sports Exerc*. 2004;36(4):674–88.

31. Lephart S, Riemann F, Fu F. *Proprioception and Neuromuscular Control in Joint Stability*. Champaign (IL): Human Kinetics; 2000. 439 p.

32. Lin YH, Li CW, Tsai LY, Liing R. The effects of muscle fatigue and proprioceptive deficits on the passive joint senses of ankle inversion and eversion. *Isokinet Exerc Sci*. 2008;16(2):101–5.

33. MacIntosh BR, Gardiner P, McComal AJ. *Skeletal Muscle: Form and Function*. 2nd ed. Champaign (IL): Human Kinetics; 2006. 432 p.

34. McArdle WD, Katch FI, Katch VL. *Exercise Physiology: Nutrition, Energy, and Human Performance*. 8th ed. Baltimore, MD: Wolters Kluwer; 2015. 1088 p.

35. McGill SM. *Low Back Disorders: Evidence-Based Prevention and Rehabilitation*. 2nd ed. Champaign (IL): Human Kinetics; 2007. 328 p.

36. McKenney K, Elder AS, Elder C, Hutchins A. Myofascial release as a treatment for orthopaedic conditions: a systematic review. *J Athl Train*. 2013;48(4):522–7.

37. Myers J, Wassinger C, Lephart S. Sensorimotor contribution to shoulder stability: effect of injury and rehabilitation. *Man Ther*. 2006;11(3):197–201.

38. Nelson N. Diaphragmatic breathing: the foundation of core stability. *Strength Condition J*. 2012;34(5):34–40.

39. Okamoto T, Masuhara M, Ikuta K. Acute effects of self-myofascial release using a foam roller on arterial function. *J Strength Cond Res*. 2014;28(1):69–73.

40. Panjabi MM. The stabilizing system of the spine. Part I. Function, dysfunction, adaptation, and enhancement. *J Spinal Disord*. 1992;5(4):383–9.

41. Panjabi MM. The stabilizing system of the spine. Part II. Neutral zone and instability hypothesis. *J Spinal Disord*. 1992;5(4):390–7.

42. Peacock CA, Krein DD, Silver TA, Sanders GJ, Carlowitz KA. An acute bout of self-myofascial release in the form of foam rolling improves performance testing. *Int J Exerc Sci*. 2014;7(3):202–11.

43. Pryor JA, Prasad SA. *Physiotherapy for Respiratory and Cardiac Problems*. Edinburgh (United Kingdom): Churchill Livingstone; 2002. 618 p.

44. Quere N, Noel E, Lieutaud A, d'Alessio P. Fasciatherapy combined with pulsology touch induces changes in blood turbulence potentially beneficial for vascular endothelium. *J Bodywork Movement Ther*. 2009;13(13):239–45.

45. Richardson C, Jull G, Hodges P, Hides J. *Therapeutic Exercise for Spinal Segmental Stabilisation in Low Back Pain*. Edinburgh (United Kingdom): Churchill Livingstone; 1999. 192 p.

46. Richardson C, Hodges PW, Hides J. *Therapeutic Exercise for Lumbopelvic Stabilization : A Motor Control Approach for the Treatment and Prevention of Low Back Pain*. 2nd ed. Edinburgh (United Kingdom): Churchill Livingstone; 2004. 271 p.

47. Riemann BL, Lephart SM. The sensorimotor system, part I: the physiologic basis of functional joint stability. *J Athl Train*. 2002;37(1):71–9.

48. Röijezon U, Clark NC, Treleaven J. Proprioception in musculoskeletal rehabilitation. Part 1: basic science and principles of

assessment and clinical interventions. *Man Ther.* 2015;20(3): 368–77.

49. Rothwell J. *Control of Human Voluntary Movement.* London (United Kingdom): Chapman and Hall; 1994. 325 p.

50. Roylance DS, George JD, Hammer AM, et al. Evaluating acute changes in joint range-of-motion using self-myofascial release, postural alignment exercises, and static stretches. *Int J Exerc Sci.* 2013;6(4):310–319.

51. Sahrmann S. *Diagnosis and Treatment of Movement Impairment Syndromes.* St. Louis (MO): Mosby; 2002. 384 p.

52. Schleip R. Fascial plasticity — a new neurobiological explanation: part 1. *J Bodywork Movement Ther.* 2003;7(1):11–9.

53. Sherrington C. *The Integrative Action of the Nervous System.* New Haven (CT): Yale University Press; 1906. 128 p.

54. Shultz S, Byrne N, Hills A. Musculoskeletal function and obesity: implications for physical activity. *Curr Obes Rep.* 2014;3(3):355.

55. Sullivan KM, Silvey D, Button DC, Behm DG. Roller-massager application to the hamstrings increases sit-and-reach range of motion within five to ten seconds without performance impairments. *Int J Sports Phys Ther.* 2013;8(3):228–36.

56. Switlick T, Kernozek TW, Meardon S. Differences in joint-position sense and vibratory threshold in runners with and without a history of overuse injury. *J Sport Rehab.* 2015;24(1):6–12.

57. Tozzi P. Selected fascial aspects of osteopathic practice. *J Bodyw Mov Ther.* 2012;16(4):503–19.

58. Travell JG, Simons DG, Simons DG. *Myofascial Pain and Dysfunction: The Trigger Point Manual.* Baltimore (MD): Williams & Wilkins; 1983. 628 p.

59. Tripp B, Yochem E, Uhl T. Functional fatigue and upper extremity sensorimotor system acuity in baseball athletes. *J Athl Train.* 2007;42(1):90–8.

60. Tse MA, McManus AM, Masters RSW. Development and validation of a core endurance intervention program: implications for performance in college-age rowers. *J Strength Cond Res.* 2005;19(3):547–55.

61. Whittle MW. *Gait Analysis: An Introduction.* 4th ed. Edinburgh (Scotland): Butterworth Heineman Elsevier; 2007. 255 p.

62. Wingert JR, Welder C, Foo P. Age-related hip proprioception declines: effects on postural sway and dynamic balance. *Arch Phys Med Rehabil.* 2014;95(2):253–61.

63. Yoon C, Lee J, Kim K, Chan Kim H, Chung SG. Original research: quantification of lumbar stability during wall plank-and-roll activity. *PM R.* 2015;7(8):803–13.

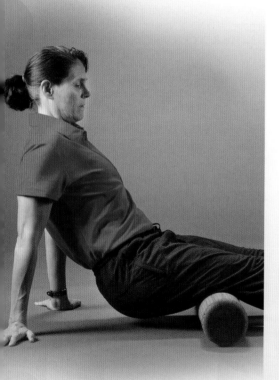

# 18 Personal Training Session Components

## OBJECTIVES

**Personal Trainer should be able to:**

▪ Understand how to organize training sessions.

▪ Apply basic customer service skills as they are applied in a fitness facility and during a personal training session.

▪ Understand communication skills necessary to promote client adherence and motivation.

▪ Use goal-setting techniques and client accountability to promote adherence.

▪ Understand criteria for an optimal personal training session.

▪ Develop a checklist for professional behavior.

## INTRODUCTION

What actually takes place in a typical personal training session? How does a Personal Trainer decide what will happen within a particular client's scheduled workout time? How is the session organized? What would an optimal session look like? How would the ideal Personal Trainer behave in order to have the greatest impact on a client's well-being and fitness? These questions, and more, will be addressed in this chapter, which will specifically address the needs and typical activities of Personal Trainers.

In most facilities, Personal Trainers will encounter a diverse clientele, including older adults, middle-aged professionals, young athletes, fit or unfit, those with injuries and disabilities and those without, clients who are extremely motivated, and clients who do not want to work hard. A skilled Personal Trainer is able to communicate effectively with all types of people, provide motivation, and move clients toward their goals through implementation of individualized exercise programs.

 ## Optimal Client Care and Customer Service

Before sequencing and motivational information is presented, a discussion of optimal customer service is in order. This is because effective customer service is the primary responsibility of every Personal Trainer.

Personal Trainers should keep in mind that every person they come in contact with throughout their work day, who is not on staff, is considered a "customer."

Personal Trainers should keep in mind that every person they come in contact with throughout their work day, who is not on staff, is considered a "customer." This includes all training clients, facility members, and guests (prospective clients). This section presents basic customer service skills that every Personal Trainer should strive to perfect.

### Client Safety

Personal Trainers are responsible for client safety. For example, all Personal Trainers should understand mechanisms of injury for the major joints of the body. Knees, shoulders, and spines are more likely to get hurt in certain positions and during certain moves, so a competent Personal Trainer will avoid these positions and moves whenever possible (for additional information, see Chapters 3 and 4 as well as the activity-specific Chapters 15–17). In addition, it is extremely important that Personal Trainers provide exercises and programs that are appropriate for each individual client. A hallmark of a skilled Personal Trainer is the ability to provide personalized, individualized programs; in other words, no one client's program should look the same as any other client's program. Knowledgeable Personal Trainers need to know hundreds, if not thousands, of exercises, variations, and modifications. In this way, the Personal Trainer is always able to provide the right exercise at the right time for the right client. For example, not every client can, or should, do a traditional overhead (military) press. If a client complains of shoulder pain while performing this exercise, what should the Personal Trainer do? Consider ways to modify the overhead press, and if the client still reports pain, the Personal Trainer should select an easier, safer exercise for the deltoids (such as a front raise or isometric shoulder abduction or shoulder flexion against a wall). Of course, if the client still reports pain, deltoid exercises should be discontinued and the client should be asked to consult his or her physician. A primary duty of a Personal Trainer is to listen to and observe the client in order to find the safest, most effective exercise or variation at that point in time.

It is imperative that the Personal Trainer know the client's physical limitations as ascertained from the health history and fitness evaluation prior to designing a program. However, the reality is that a client's needs can change from day to day, making it critical to modify and adjust the program or a specific exercise on the spot.

## Plan Each Workout

Prior to each session, the Personal Trainer should review the client's short- and long-term goals, any health issues or injuries, and the details of the last few sessions. In this way, the Personal Trainer can plan the most appropriate workout for each client, always keeping in mind the recommendations specified by current American College of Sports Medicine (ACSM) guidelines (2). How will overload be created? Changing the frequency, intensity, duration, or type of exercise are all proven strategies. Rest time, speed of movement, balance, core challenge, coordination, agility, and more can all be manipulated by changing the specific exercise, the equipment utilized, the sequencing of exercises, and the way the program is put together. However, the Personal Trainer should always be ready to alter and adapt the plan, depending on the client's needs and current status. Checking with a client regarding their physical and mental readiness to begin the exercise session is crucial.

## Utilize Proper Charting

Proper charting is a "must-have" — not only from a customer service perspective but also from an ethical and liability standpoint. Documenting all activities and events will help the Personal Trainer provide optimal service while limiting liability risk. All workout specifics should be recorded, such as weight/reps/sets used, training heart rate (HR) and/or rating of perceived exertion (RPE), blood pressure (BP) responses or changes (if BP cuff is available), and signs and/or symptoms that may have occurred during a session, including any pain that occurred with exercise and what action was taken accordingly. Relevant subjective comments made by the client should also be noted. The Personal Trainer should chart ideas and goals for the next workout. If another staff member will be training that client next, any special exercise or program should be carefully detailed in order to prevent confusion. The purpose of keeping good notes is to

- Keep track of exercise programs, so that their effectiveness can be evaluated at the time of the next fitness assessment
- Share program information if more than one Personal Trainer will be working with a client
- Reinforce long-term and short-term objectives
- Keep track of the client's workout over time so that progression can be appropriately applied
- Provide evidence of professionalism in the event of a lawsuit

A Personal Trainer should be sure to update the fitness program chart as soon as any change in medical or structural condition (*e.g.*, musculoskeletal injury) presents itself. In addition, the Personal Trainer should take the appropriate steps, speak to the client regarding those conditions that affect the program, and ask the client's permission to contact his or her physician if warranted.

## Be Attentive

Attentiveness begins the moment the client walks onto the exercise floor and finishes with the Personal Trainer saying goodbye to the client. Attention to every detail within the workout is important. Pertinent details include the following:

- Monitor all signs and symptoms of cardiovascular disease.
- Provide water and a towel, if appropriate.
- Modify or progress exercises based on the client's ability.

Attention to every detail within the workout is important.

- Make certain the client trains within the desired target training zone.
- Ensure proper breathing, alignment, and technique during all exercises.
- Adhere to fitness program–specific recommendations.
- Listen to the client and ask for feedback.

## Maintain Professional Conduct in the Training Facility

A Personal Trainer who is training a client must focus on that client alone (Fig. 18.1). Watching TV monitors, chatting with staff or other members, looking at oneself in the mirror, and talking or texting on a cell phone all show disrespect for the client. Aside from the safety factor, if a client perceives that his or her Personal Trainer is disinterested and uncaring, the quality of the workout will be compromised. Body language is important; a Personal Trainer should always face the client and, whenever possible, physically be on the same level. For example, if the client is lying supine on the floor performing abdominal crunches, the Personal Trainer should also be nearby on the floor, either in a sitting or in a kneeling position. Standing above a supine client and talking down to him or her may be intimidating and is impersonal. Finally, Personal Trainers should maintain professionalism even during potentially challenging work environments (*e.g.*, competition for clients among other Personal Trainers).

## Maintain a Professional Appearance

The Personal Trainer's appearance must be neat and professional. Personal Trainers who are not required to wear a uniform might consider developing their own to create a consistently professional image. Like effective branding does for any product on the shelf, a consistently professional appearance will speak volumes about a Personal Trainer. First impressions are important, and it is up to the Personal Trainer to portray a professional appearance that will produce the desired impression for every client and prospective client.

First impressions are important, and it is up to the Personal Trainer to portray a professional appearance that will produce the desired impression for every client and prospective client.

## Work on Self-Improvement

Personal Trainers should set short- and long-term career goals for themselves and make a concerted effort to reach those goals. Reading related literature; attending clinics, workshops, and conferences; and sharing information with other Personal Trainers will enhance knowledge, skills, and abilities. Networking with other trainers and allied exercise and health care professionals, such as dietitians,

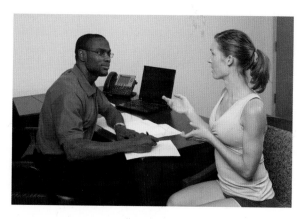

**FIGURE 18.1.** Proper body language is critical to success in the Personal Trainer. (From Ratamess N. *ACSM's Foundations of Strength Training and Conditioning.* Philadelphia [PA]: Lippincott Williams and Wilkins; 2012.)

physical therapists, and exercise physiologists, allows Personal Trainers to refer when necessary and helps promote the profession from within. It is highly recommended that Personal Trainers work to attain a college degree in a fitness or health-related field; this may be critical if and when state licensure is mandated, although the potential degree requirements are not known. Additionally, acquiring certifications in specialty areas, such as martial arts, yoga, Pilates, older adults, pregnancy, and diabetes, will increase a Personal Trainer's knowledge and enhance his or her ability to attract a wide variety of clients (for more information on ACSM speciality certifications, see Chapter 1).

## Help Keep the Facility Clean

During nontraining time, check the facility to make sure that all is in order, the weights are put back, and the facility looks presentable. Personal Trainers should make periodic checks of the changing rooms and locker room facilities, going out of their way to make sure the areas are inviting and comfortable to clients.

 # Personal Training Session Criteria for Appropriate Sequencing

## Session Components

A Personal Trainer must include appropriate workout components in the personal training session (Table 18.1). A typical hour spent with a client should include some or all of the following components:

- Greeting
- Appropriate warm-up
- Cardiorespiratory aerobic or anaerobic interval work
- Cool-down phase
- Muscular strength/endurance component: traditional exercises and functional exercises
- Core work for stability
- Condition-specific exercises (*e.g.*, orthopedic protocols, pregnancy protocol)
- Neuromotor training (promotion of balance, agility, and coordination)
- Flexibility component
- Goal setting and farewell
- Charting

## Continuity and Planning

The "flow" of the personal training session should proceed in a continuous, uninterrupted manner. Making efficient use of floor space and choice of exercise modality when the training floor is crowded is also important. It is up to the Personal Trainer to be creative and make alternative choices of exercises when necessary, particularly if the preferred equipment is already in use by other members of the facility. Additionally, prior to the session, the Personal Trainer should prepare the client's program for the day, set up equipment if possible, review the client's short- and long-term goals, any health issues or injuries, and the details of the last few sessions.

## Greeting and Punctuality

The Personal Trainer should greet the client in an appropriate manner. A friendly, professional greeting with a handshake and a smile goes a long way to setting the tone and building rapport with the client. Rapport is developed over time through empathetic listening, being trustworthy, and establishing repeated positive interactions with a client (for more information on listening

| Table 18.1 | Personal Training Session Evaluation Criteria/Checklist |
|---|---|
| Greeting | ▪ Personal Trainer's appearance is neat and professional.<br>▪ Provide appropriate greeting and reception.<br>▪ Pick up client on time.<br>▪ Display good client rapport.<br>▪ Ask how the client feels and on what he or she would like to focus. |
| Warm-up phase | ▪ Utilize appropriate cardiorespiratory equipment.<br>▪ Consider any musculoskeletal or metabolic limitations.<br>*Relevant to goals and/or structure of workout*<br>▪ A minimum of 5 min in length.<br>▪ Appropriate intensity (*i.e.*, at low end of training zone). |
| Cardiorespiratory phase | Monitor and document intensity responses (HR, RPE).<br>Follow ACSM guidelines.<br>▪ Monitor HR, RPE, talk test, and/or breathlessness at the various stages of the workout.<br>▪ Use RPE for any *hypertensive clients* on medication that affects HR. RPE is to be monitored throughout workout with *pregnant clients*. Perceptual signs/signals (such as ataxia [unsteadiness of gait] or other physical signs of fatigue) should be monitored in conjunction with HR, BP, and RPE, and exercise is modified accordingly. This is especially important in clients who have a tendency to work hard and underestimate their RPE. |
| Cool-down phase | ▪ A slow decrease in exercise intensity occurs at the end of the CV bout, any hard bout of exercise, or at any point within the workout, prior to final flexibility and abdominal work.<br>▪ The postexercise cool-down activity should be 5–10 min in length; it is dependent upon the exercise intensity, exercising time, and client-specific conditions (*e.g.*, provide hypertensive client and less fit clients a longer cool-down period to allow for HR and BP to return toward preexercise levels without blood pooling or orthostatic hypotensive responses). |
| Muscular strength and endurance component | Follow ACSM guidelines.<br>*Exercise selection takes the following into account:*<br>▪ Client's goals (long term and short term)<br>▪ Overall training program and program components<br>▪ Client's skill and fitness levels<br>▪ Any musculoskeletal or metabolic conditions and subsequent health care provider recommendations<br>▪ Any day-to-day considerations (*i.e.*, client is tired, sore, had recent illness, inconsistent attendance, hasn't trained in over 1 mo)<br>▪ Availability of equipment and other activities occurring within fitness center.<br>▪ The client's need for foundational training, traditional resistance exercise, and/or functional training<br>▪ Previous exercise sessions<br>*Spotting and cueing:*<br>▪ Always ask permission before hands-on spotting.<br>▪ The hands-on interaction is based upon the client, the exercises utilized, the appropriate feedback needed, and their overall program.<br>▪ Properly monitor the range of motion on resistance training exercises; give feedback on speed of movement; ensure client safety. |

*(continued)*

| Table 18.1 | Personal Training Session Evaluation Criteria/Checklist (continued) |
|---|---|
| Muscular strength and endurance component (continued) | ■ Free weights: Appropriate spotting occurs *at all times* with all clients. Personal Trainer is in a position to assist the clients with the weights if they are not able to maintain good form or are unable to complete the activity. Personal Trainer positions his or her body in such a way that the client is comfortable, safe, and experiences an improved workout.<br>■ Teaching cues are safe, accurate, and appropriate for the client. Provide a variety of cues: alignment, safety, educational, and motivational. Use a positive style of cueing.<br>■ Incorporate a "setup" phase, when needed, to help the client achieve proper alignment and technique.<br>*Equipment use:*<br>■ Use a variety of equipment during the workout.<br>■ Return all equipment and maintain them in a neat, orderly condition. |
| Core work for stability | ■ Focus on appropriate core stability exercises for the neck, scapulae, spine, and pelvis. |
| Condition-specific protocols | ■ Do not exceed scope of practice and follow the licensed health care provider's recommendations.<br>■ Know what *not* to do as well as what to do.<br>■ Seek medical clearance for all pregnant women. |
| Neuromotor training | ■ Include exercises for balance, agility, and enhanced proprioception. |
| Flexibility component | ■ Occurs after client is thoroughly warmed up<br>■ Static stretches are held for 30–60 s, proprioceptive neuromuscular facilitation stretches can be held for 6–7 s.<br>■ Include stretches for the major muscle groups, any specific areas highlighted within the fitness assessment, or muscle groups emphasized during the workout.<br>■ Incorporate relaxation and/or stress-management techniques, if appropriate. |
| Goal setting and farewell | ■ Help client set a short-term goal and/or give "homework" at end of session, if appropriate.<br>■ Thank client for a good workout.<br>■ Farewell should be friendly, positive, and affirmative. |
| Charting | *The client's session should include specific information regarding*<br>■ New exercises/machines utilized, how the client felt and performed the exercises<br>■ Client's subjective comments<br>■ Any particular changes in the client's fitness level as noted on a specific machine (*e.g.,* "ran 0.3 m farther than usual today;" "wasn't able to complete usual distance due to hard workout")<br>■ Relevant observations made by Personal Trainer<br>■ Any pain or discomfort that occurred during the session<br>■ Any notes for the next workout |
| Innovation and problem-solving skills | *Ability to improvise and modify any aspect of client's workout based on*<br>■ Other activities occurring within the fitness center<br>■ Specific injuries, limitations, or complaints of pain/discomfort<br>■ Equipment availability |

Adapted from American College of Sports Medicine. American College of Sports Medicine position stand. Progression models in resistance training for healthy adults. *Med Sci Sports Exerc.* 2009;41(3):687–708.

and communication, see Chapter 9). Personal Trainers should make every effort to improve communication skills; ability to listen and communicate well is essential for the development of client rapport and motivation. Inappropriate language (*i.e.,* demeaning comments; racial, ethnic, or sexist epithets; or "locker-room talk") has no place in a Personal Training session and can damage rapport. The relationship between a Personal Trainer and a client is a professional one and thus personal conversation should generally be kept to a minimum. A Personal Trainer should focus completely on the client's needs from the moment of greeting the client to the farewell at the end of the session. At the beginning of the session, an inquiry should be made about the client's status and include any of the following: how he or she feels, any aches or pains, how the client felt after the last session, and what the client would like to work on that day.

In addition, the Personal Trainer should always start the session on time. Starting a session late is unprofessional and indicates to the client that the Personal Trainer does not value the client's time.

## Warm-Up Phase

The Personal Trainer must help the client select an appropriate warm-up modality that

- Considers any musculoskeletal or metabolic limitations
- Is relevant to the goals and/or structure of the workout
- Is a minimum of 5 minutes in length
- Is an appropriate intensity (*i.e.,* low intensity, increasing toward the low end of training zone)
- Includes monitoring of RPE and/or HR

In many cases, when a client is experienced and has worked with the Personal Trainer for an extended period of time, the client arrives early and completes the warm-up prior to the actual training session.

## Cardiorespiratory Phase

The Personal Trainer is responsible for helping design an appropriate cardiorespiratory and/or anaerobic interval program for each client; ACSM guidelines for the development of cardiorespiratory fitness should be followed (2). The Personal Trainer should also monitor HR or RPE throughout the various stages of the entire workout.

The client's HR may be monitored by palpating the pulse, either at the radial or carotid arteries, or by using an HR monitor (for information on measuring HR, see Chapter 12). If using the HR method, the Personal Trainer should be aware of disadvantages associated with this method, including its potential inaccuracy due to the assumption that any one maximal HR formula fits all. Also, several extraneous factors, such as heat, humidity, illness, cigarette smoking, and stress, may affect HR. Clients should also be monitored for ataxia (unsteadiness of gait) or other physical signs of fatigue or stress (2).

RPE is frequently recommended as another way to assess exercise intensity (2). The Borg 6–20 RPE scale (see Table 15.10) or a simple 0–10 scale may be used (see Chapter 15). With new clients, it is helpful to have an actual RPE chart visible while explaining proper intensity, but eventually, most clients can understand and apply the RPE scale effectively without a visible chart. For more information on monitoring exercise intensity, see Chapter 15.

In practice, many Personal Trainers design cardiorespiratory programs for their clients but eventually encourage clients to perform this part of the workout on their own. In this way, for many clients, the actual session is reserved for the more various and complicated muscle conditioning exercises. If the Personal Trainer is not actually supervising the cardiorespiratory workout, the Personal Trainer should nevertheless always ask the client about his or her adherence to the workout and about program variables such as duration, frequency, intensity, and mode.

## Cool-Down Phase after Cardiorespiratory Exercise

The cool-down portion of the workout should be 5–10 minutes in length, depending on the intensity and duration of the workout and client-specific conditions (*i.e.*, less-fit clients should be allowed a longer cool-down period to allow HR and BP to decrease). Ideally, HR and/or RPE should be monitored during the cool-down.

## Muscular Strength/Endurance Component

Many clients seek a Personal Trainer's advice because they are unsure of what exercises to do in the weight room; they want a program that gets results. Additionally, they often want a Personal Trainer to help make certain they are exercising correctly with safe and effective form and technique. Therefore, in addition to following ACSM guidelines for resistance training, Personal Trainers should be familiar with a large number of exercises and know how to properly teach, spot, and cue each exercise in such a way that clients understand and follow through with correct performance.

### Exercise Selection and Programming

The Personal Trainer must take several factors into account when deciding which exercises to give a client. These factors include the following:

- Client's goals and attitude
- Client's fitness and skill level
- Any musculoskeletal issues or injuries
- Any recommendations from the client's health care providers
- Considerations on the particular training day (*e.g.*, client is tired, sore, has been ill, has not trained regularly, has not trained in over a month)
- Availability of equipment and other activities occurring within the fitness center

A skilled Personal Trainer should know a large number of traditional exercises for each muscle group, including single-joint and multijoint exercises utilizing machines as well as free weights and other equipment. It may be useful to organize the vast number of possible exercises along a continuum from easiest to hardest (see Fig. 18.2); such a continuum provides a practical way to think about exercise selection (6).

To be even more specific, the left, easy, or foundational side can provide a starting point for new clients. At the beginning of a program, it is wise to select basic exercises that promote core stability and mobility, thus helping to create a strong and safe foundation for harder and more complex exercises. Examples might include supine abdominal hollowing, supine heel slides, quadrupeds (bird dogs), hip hinging, and scapular depression and retraction exercises. These foundational exercises help prepare the client for more challenging work and can be used to educate him or her about

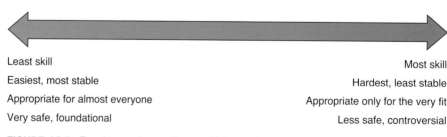

| Least skill | Most skill |
| --- | --- |
| Easiest, most stable | Hardest, least stable |
| Appropriate for almost everyone | Appropriate only for the very fit |
| Very safe, foundational | Less safe, controversial |

**FIGURE 18.2.** Exercise session continuum. (Adapted from Ratamess N. *ACSM's Foundations of Strength Training and Conditioning*. Philadelphia [PA]: Lippincott Williams and Wilkins; 2012. p. 319.)

safety, proper alignment, and injury prevention. As a client progresses, exercises may be selected from the traditional weight room repertoire and include the use of variable resistance machines, cable column setups, and free weights. Progression often moves from single-joint exercises to multijoint exercises and from open kinetic chain to closed kinetic chain movements.

Eventually, many clients may progress to less traditional exercises — now often labeled under the heading of functional training — such as woodchoppers, reverse woodchoppers, lunges with a pickup, and other moves that incorporate balance, core, and coordination challenges (see Chapter 17). Compared with traditional weight training, these moves often utilize a lighter weight held farther from the trunk and help to improve biomechanical efficiency and neuromuscular control (5). On the far right side of the exercise continuum are sport-specific moves that prepare an athlete for performance (see Chapter 19 for more specifics on advanced program options). Because functional exercises and, especially, sport-specific moves require a high degree of fitness, skill, balance, coordination, and core stability, Personal Trainers should not select these exercises until the client is able to perform them safely and correctly. In fact, many clients have no desire to progress all the way to the sport-specific/performance end of the continuum. It's important to realize that many people want to exercise for health, fitness, and wellness benefits and that this does not necessarily include sports performance or aggressive, very difficult moves or routines. The Personal Trainer should emphasize the muscle groups and movements that are specific to the client's individual goals and objectives. Finally, the Personal Trainer should attempt to select exercises according to the initial or follow-up fitness evaluations and interviews.

## Spotting: Hands-On Interaction

The Personal Trainer should provide appropriate spotting during all aspects of the exercise session. Legally, it is a Personal Trainer's job to ensure client safety. The Personal Trainer should monitor ranges of motion and prevent the client from moving into extreme and unsafe positions, such as extreme shoulder horizontal abduction in a supine dumbbell fly. As a general rule, when a client lifts a heavy weight, the Personal Trainer needs to spot the weight for safety (keeping hands on or near the weight). If the client is a novice, or is performing an exercise for the first time, or is lifting a light weight, the Personal Trainer may need to spot specific joints or actions, instead of the weight. For example, if a client is performing a squat for the first time (in which case the weight would be either light or nonexistent), the Personal Trainer may need to kneel and spot the client's knees, helping the client to find and feel the correct knee position while moving. During core, balance, and agility work, the Personal Trainer should assist the client and help ensure proper alignment and technique. Personal Trainers should properly position themselves to prevent the client from falling and should provide adequate support for the client during balance-training drills. During stretching, the Personal Trainer may spot the client as needed to help ensure proper form and alignment.

The hands-on interaction that occurs during the workout should be based on the client, the exercises used, the appropriate feedback needed, and the overall program. Always consider the client's safety, alignment, and comfort level with touch. Because not all clients are comfortable with hands-on techniques, the Personal Trainer must always ask permission before touching.

> The Personal Trainer must always ask permission before touching the client.

Do not touch a client if he or she says no, or seems uncomfortable in any way, and stay away from gender-specific areas of the body. Additionally, the Personal Trainers should be aware of their body position. It is usually best to be on the same level as the client. For example, if the client is on the floor performing supine abdominal work, the Personal Trainer should not be standing over them shouting down commands. Instead, kneel or sit near the client in order to facilitate hands-on spotting if necessary, increase client comfort, and maintain an appropriate speech volume.

A good technique for teaching clients proper form is to have a "setup" phase prior to the performance of each exercise. During the setup, the Personal Trainer carefully ensures that the client is focused and properly aligned and the core is stabilized. Only then does the client actually begin to move and perform the exercise.

### Cueing

Proper cueing during a client's session is critical. It is the Personal Trainer's job to help the client perform each segment of the workout, and each exercise, correctly. This can be accomplished with skillful spotting and cueing. There are many different types of cues, including educational, safety, alignment, and motivational cues. In addition, cues may be delivered visually, orally, and through touch (tactile cues). Because a majority of individuals are primarily visual learners, the Personal Trainer needs to be adept at exercise demonstration as well as visual cueing. Another useful cueing technique is the right/wrong method. This method can be very effective for clients who are having difficulty with proper positioning. For example, if a client is having trouble maintaining a neutral pelvis, the Personal Trainer may demonstrate a misaligned pelvis versus a neutral pelvis. In other words, show the client the incorrect position and then the correct position. Many clients find this type of teaching technique very helpful. Remember to phrase all cues positively, as in "Make sure to always keep a slight bend in your knees" instead of "Don't lock your knees." Constant use of the word "don't" sounds negative and pejorative. In general, it's best to avoid monotonous counting; clients already know how to count! Instead, the Personal Trainer should make certain he or she is providing detailed information and cues that will ensure the safety and efficacy of each exercise.

### Equipment Use

The Personal Trainer should use a variety of equipment during the workout. Any equipment used during the workout must be returned to a neat, orderly condition during the course of the workout to maintain safety and not interfere with any other workouts that are occurring within the same time frame. Personal Trainers have many equipment and exercise options, and as a client progresses and becomes more skilled, variety may become more and more important. Machines, free weights, cable columns, stability balls, BOSU balance trainers, TRX suspension devices, kettlebells, medicine balls, foam rollers, and elastic tubing and bands are all common in many facilities. Personal Trainers should first be familiar with a wide variety of exercises on all types of equipment and then select the most appropriate exercise for each client depending on the client's level of fitness, skill, goals, musculoskeletal and/or metabolic issues, exercises performed in the previous session, and equipment availability.

The Personal Trainer should use a variety of equipment during the workout.

## Core Work for Stability

All clients, both novice and experienced, need to be able to maintain neck, scapular, spinal, and pelvic stability in order to perform exercises with good alignment and to minimize the risk of injury. The Personal Trainer should therefore make time in the session to focus on core exercises such as abdominal hollowing, pelvic tilts, and scapular depression and retraction; these may be performed supine or standing against a wall. Scapular awareness can also be promoted in the prone "prop" position (up on the elbows) because gravity pulls the torso downward and the scapulae tend to elevate. Many clients find it challenging to maintain the prone prop position for even 30–60 seconds while keeping the scapulae depressed. The quadruped/all fours/bird-dog position is another excellent way to teach core stability of the neck, scapulae, spine, and pelvis; many movement variations exist, such as holding the opposite arm and leg parallel to the floor, or slowly lifting arm and leg up and down without moving the core. The plank, and all its variations, is yet another way to challenge core stability and, depending on the variation (*e.g.*, a side plank), can be quite advanced.

## Condition-Specific Protocols

Most Personal Trainers will occasionally work with clients with special conditions; these conditions can include pregnancy as well as a large number of musculoskeletal issues such as low back pain, tennis elbow, rotator cuff tendonitis, hip bursitis, lateral knee pain, and more. Although a Personal Trainer must never exceed his or her scope of practice and should always refer a client with active musculoskeletal pain to a medical practitioner, the reality is that many clients want to stay active and will continue working with their trainer, even with an injury. If the Personal Trainer agrees to continue training a client with a history of musculoskeletal pain, it is incumbent upon the Personal Trainer to adhere to the recommendations of the client's licensed health care provider. In other words, the Personal Trainer must know what NOT to do as well as what to do. For example, a client who has finished a regimen of physical therapy sessions for tennis elbow may have a specific exercise protocol that he or she need to continue postrehab (provided by the physical therapist), which may then be incorporated into the personal training session. Likewise, when training pregnant women, it is recommended that a woman past her first trimester of pregnancy avoid exercising in the supine position, particularly if she is symptomatic. The Personal Trainer should make certain to include alternate abdominal exercises that are not in the supine position and should also seek a medical clearance for all pregnant women (1,2). Such condition-specific protocols will need to be sequenced into the personal training session.

> The Personal Trainer must follow the recommendations of the client's licensed health care provider.

## Neuromotor Training

Neuromotor training includes training for balance, coordination, gait, agility, and enhanced proprioception. Neuromotor training is recommended as part of a comprehensive exercise program, particularly for older adults who are at an increased risk of falling (2,3). Younger and middle-aged adults involved in physical activities that involve agility, balance, and other motor skills may also benefit, although research in this area is still limited (2). Balance exercises may be either static (such as standing on one leg while incorporating upper body movements) or dynamic. A dynamic balance exercise involves transferring body weight from one foot to the other; for example, pretending to walk along a "tightrope," or a line on the floor, with one foot directly in front of the other can be challenging for some clients. Personal Trainers should make an effort to include both types of balance exercises in the exercise session whenever possible.

## Flexibility Component

A flexibility component can be included anytime the muscles have been warmed up. Flexibility exercises can be included at the end of the personal training session. The Personal Trainer should teach his or her client a basic stretching routine that addresses all active muscles and all joints with a decreased range of motion. Muscles that have been vigorously challenged or repetitively utilized during the workout should be stretched. This final segment can also be a good time to incorporate relaxation techniques such as deep breathing, progressive muscle relaxation, and positive imagery. Many clients are unfamiliar with stress management "quick fixes" and will be grateful for any tips and strategies from the Personal Trainer. Details on stretching and developing flexibility are found in Chapter 16.

**FIGURE 18.3.** Personal Trainer reviewing goal setting with a client. (Adapted from Ratamess N. *ACSM's Foundations of Strength Training and Conditioning.* Philadelphia [PA]: Lippincott Williams and Wilkins; 2012. p. 319.)

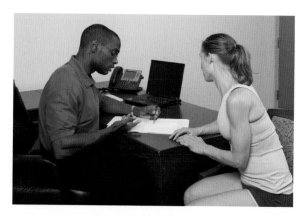

## Goal Setting and Farewell

Goal setting is critical for success (Fig. 18.3). The Personal Trainer can ask his or her client to set a short-term goal at the end of each session. The goal should ideally be relatively easy to attain, positive, and doable for the client. Some sample short-term goals include the following: "Take a 10-minute walk after lunch every day for the next 3 days," "Go for a 1-hour walk in the park on Saturday with the kids," and "Stand up and pace during every phone call on Friday." Another suggestion is for the Personal Trainer to assign "homework" for the client. Examples of homework include the following: "Every night at dinner, sit on the edge of the chair and maintain a perfectly neutral spine for 60 seconds," "Twice a day, stand against a wall and make certain the spine and neck are in neutral," "While making coffee every morning, stand on one foot and balance for 20 seconds," and so on. Goals should always be set by the client, whereas "homework" may be assigned by the Personal Trainer. In either case, let clients know that they will be asked about the goal or the homework at the next session. Small steps help promote long-term behavior change. Upon completion of the session, thank the client for a good workout. Always end the session with a positive and affirmative farewell, with plans for the next meeting.

## Charting

Proper charting was discussed earlier in the chapter. The Personal Trainer needs to allow enough time after the session to record all workout details, client goals, and ideas for the next session.

# Education and Motivation

## Client Education

Most clients have a specific area of concern. In order to make the session more meaningful, Personal Trainers can gear the workout to address these concerns. Some clients, for example, want to "tone up" their hips and thighs. The Personal Trainer can take this opportunity to educate the client about the meaning of "toning up" and include information about muscle-specific exercises such as hip extensions and hip abduction and adduction movements. The effectiveness of multimuscle exercises such as squats and lunges should be discussed. Additionally, the Personal Trainer might educate the client about the importance of increasing lean body mass while also promoting cardiorespiratory exercise as a way to burn large numbers of calories and reduce excessive body fat.

The Personal Trainer should talk to each client about how the routine he or she has designed relates to the client's goals and training objectives. When prudent, appropriate postrehab protocols

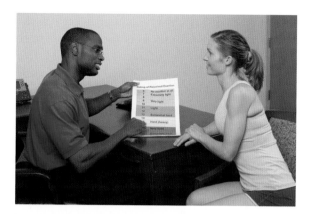

**FIGURE 18.4.** Personal Trainer explaining the use of the RPE chart to a client.

should be implemented and explained as to how they will be integrated into the client's program to improve or prevent further injury.

Another important area for client education is proper breathing technique. The client should never hold his or her breath during any contraction. This increases intrathoracic pressure and as a result increases BP, which may or may not be dangerous for a specific client but is certainly unnecessary. As a general rule, the client should inhale before starting the lift, exhale when performing the concentric contraction, and inhale during the eccentric phase.

Many clients hire trainers primarily for guidance in the weight room. However, the Personal Trainer should educate the client about all the components of fitness and should also provide a suitable program for cardiorespiratory conditioning. Typically, many clients will perform their cardiorespiratory workout before or after the actual supervised session. This will depend on the client's overall physical condition, daily schedule, and specific training goals and objectives. The Personal Trainer should make sure that clients understand how to operate their preferred aerobic equipment and that they can either take their own HR or gauge RPE effectively, before they exercise without supervision. It is important to ask clients what additional activities they are performing outside of the facility. This will assist the Personal Trainer in designing training sessions and can provide additional opportunities for education. The Personal Trainer should teach each client the physiological basis of the RPE scale and explain how this will assist in monitoring exercise intensity and how it will make the sessions more efficient (Fig. 18.4).

In light of the current obesity epidemic, Personal Trainers need to provide most clients with strategies for increasing their physical activity throughout the day, and the risks of constant sitting should be discussed. Help clients with tips for incorporating more nonexercise movement into their day. Encourage them to stand more and sit less, to take movement breaks during TV commercials, and to be "inefficient" when doing household chores — making more trips than necessary, in order to burn more calories and keep the body active.

Another important area for client education involves low back care and the maintenance of proper posture throughout the day. Personal Trainers can help reduce the incidence of back pain by teaching clients how to adjust their chairs and sit correctly, how to bend and lift, and how to find ideal spinal alignment in activities of daily living.

## Client Motivation

The ideal Personal Trainer is also a great motivator. What does this mean? A great motivator makes each workout as interesting and as varied as possible. Most clients are motivated by a trainer who is also a good role model, someone who practices what he or she preaches. Personal Trainers who are enthusiastic and passionate about fitness and wellness can be inspiring. Good motivators are genuine, empathetic, and caring and let clients know that they believe in the clients' ability to succeed at their goals. Many novice exercisers hire a Personal Trainer because they need extrinsic motivation. Extrinsic motivation is the type of motivation that comes from the outside; for example, a client who adheres to a program because he or she wants to win a reward, such as a free 6-month club membership, is extrinsically motivated. A client may be motivated to keep exercising because of positive feedback from the Personal Trainer — another example of extrinsic motivation, where the concern may be more about the outcome instead of the process.

However, people are more likely to adopt healthy lifestyles and fitness regimens for the long run if they are intrinsically motivated. Intrinsic motivation comes from within. Clients with intrinsic motivation continue to exercise simply because they enjoy it and they feel better when they do; exercise becomes its own reward. Personal Trainers can help clients become more intrinsically motivated by bringing attention to feelings of well-being after an exercise session and by helping clients discover the benefits of exercise for themselves. Exercise sessions should be productive yet fun and enjoyable.

A motivating Personal Trainer also helps clients achieve feelings of self-efficacy. Self-efficacy has been defined as the confidence a person has that they can perform a given task well (4). In the fitness setting, this means that a client eventually knows what to do and is comfortable doing it. A client with self-efficacy, for example, is able to walk into the cardiorespiratory training room and/or the weight room and feel a sense of mastery in terms of some or all of the equipment. Such a client knows how to adjust the machines for his or her own use and understands how to perform the chosen exercises properly. An important task of the Personal Trainer is to enable clients to have this type of mastery and competence in the exercise environment. Most clients find that having a sense of self-efficacy with regard to fitness and wellness is very motivating and helps ensure long-lasting adherence. Chapters 7, 8, and 9 can assist you in developing your client's self-efficacy regarding exercise.

> The Personal Trainer should help promote the client's self-efficacy, or sense of mastery and competence, in the exercise environment.

## SUMMARY

The Personal Trainer must strive to deliver the highest level of client care and customer service. This includes focusing on safety, appropriate planning and charting the client's program and progress, being attentive to the client, and always behaving professionally. All components of a training session should be administered sequentially and closely observed, from warm-up through to the cool-down, and standard exercise guidelines should be followed. Personal Trainers should acknowledge that they are role models, educators, and motivators of clients and therefore continue to challenge themselves in these areas.

## REFERENCES

1. American College of Obstetricians and Gynecologists. Exercise during pregnancy and the postpartum period. ACOG Committee Opinion No. 267. *Obstet Gynecol.* 2002; 99:171–3.

2. American College of Sports Medicine. *Guidelines for Exercise Testing and Prescription.* 10th ed. Philadelphia (PA): Wolters Kluwer; 2018.

3. American College of Sports Medicine, American Heart Association. Joint position stand. Exercise and physical activity for older adults. *Med Sci Sports Exerc.* 2009;41(7): 1510–30.

4. Bandura A. *Social Foundations of Thought and Action: A Social Cognitive Theory.* Englewood Cliffs (NJ): Prentice-Hall; 1986. 544 p.

5. Beckham SE, Harper M. Functional training: fad or here to stay? *ACSM's Health Fitness J.* 2010;14(6):24–30.

6. Yoke M, Kennedy C. *Functional Exercise Progressions.* Monterey (CA): Healthy Learning; 2003. 126 p.

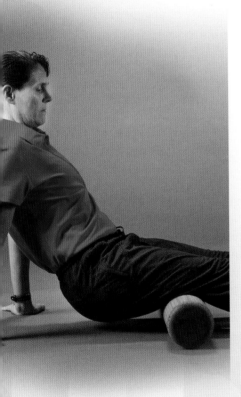

# 19 Advanced Program Options

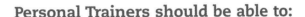

## OBJECTIVES

**Personal Trainers should be able to:**

- Identify the roles and proficiencies of Personal Trainers whose clients consist mostly of competitive athletes and/or those with advanced training goals.

- Discuss how to maximize performance by improving one or more health- and skill-related fitness components.

- Identify ACSM recommendations for advanced resistance training.

- Identify various advanced resistance training techniques (including the use of strength implements and ballistic resistance training) used to maximize muscle strength, hypertrophy, power, and endurance and how they may be used in a training program.

- Understand recommendations for plyometric, sprint, agility, and anaerobic conditioning program design.

# INTRODUCTION

The Personal Training profession has evolved rapidly and accommodated numerous segments of the population. Not only have Personal Trainers rendered services to previously sedentary as well as novice and moderately trained individuals, but a growing number of athletes and highly fit individuals have hired Personal Trainers in the quest to maximize performance. Although several sports teams may have a full-time strength and conditioning coach on staff, some athletes at the elite and professional levels prefer to hire a Personal Trainer for individualized training. Athletes may work with their strength coaches during in-season and preseason training and may hire a Personal Trainer for off-season training. The Personal Trainer may serve as part of a team of specialists that includes sport coaches, strength and conditioning coaches, nutritionists, physicians, athletic trainers, physical therapists, massage therapists, and chiropractors and may provide training camps for athletes. For example, several athletes attend off-season speed-and-agility training camps and many college football players attend strength and conditioning camps prior to combine testing in preparation for the National Football League (NFL) draft. As the Personal Training profession includes clientele with advanced fitness levels, the roles and proficiencies of the Personal Trainer will expand. Box 19.1 presents examples of educational foundations and proficiencies important to a Personal Trainer. The scope of this chapter is to provide Personal Trainers with advanced anaerobic training recommendations.

> Not only have Personal Trainers rendered services to previously sedentary as well as novice and moderately trained individuals, but a growing number of athletes and highly fit individuals have hired Personal Trainers in the quest to maximize performance.

The motivation, coaching, instruction, and direct supervision provided by the Personal Trainer are instrumental for athletes and highly fit individuals. Not only does supervised training result in less injuries and better technique, but abilities may be enhanced. Personal Training poses several advantages to the athlete/client targeting progression. Research has shown supervision results in greater strength gains (27,33) and the

| Box 19.1 | Professional Educational Foundations and Proficiencies of a Personal Trainer |
|---|---|
| Anatomy, physiology, and kinesiology | Weight and implement training |
| Bioenergetics | Aerobic endurance training |
| Exercise/sports biomechanics | Plyometric, speed, and agility training |
| Sports nutrition | Balance and functional training |
| Supplements and ergogenic aids | Strength, power, and ballistic training |
| Overtraining and detraining | Flexibility training |
| Periodization and recovery | Muscle endurance and hypertrophy training |
| Weight loss/body fat reduction | Sport-specific demands and conditioning |
| CPR administration and first aid | Advanced program design |
| Injury prevention | Skills assessment |

self-selection of greater training loads (33). Although athletes are supervised to a large extent by the coaching staff, often, a few coaches must monitor several athletes simultaneously. Personal Trainers offer the advantage of one-on-one instruction for an entire workout.

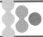

## Advanced Training Status

Advanced training necessitates the client's desire to maximize specific components of fitness, whereas Personal Trainers who work in the general health and fitness domain train clients primarily to improve health and get in better shape; advanced clients train rigorously with the aim of improving (or maximizing) one or more fitness components. The *needs analysis* for advanced clientele reveals training needs to be focused on maximizing performance as well as on injury prevention (12,17,23,32). A breakdown of the metabolic and biomechanical aspects of the sport guides the Personal Trainer to designing an appropriate program. Exercises are selected and the short-term program variables are manipulated in a way to achieve training goals. Greater specificity is needed for goal attainment, and the training program is periodized (*e.g.*, broken down into training phases) to reflect priorities given to multiple fitness components. Fitness components may be categorized as health related or skill related. Health-related components of fitness include muscle strength and endurance, aerobic endurance, flexibility, and body composition. Skill-related components of fitness include power, speed, agility, balance, reaction time, and coordination. Both of these components are critical to improving performance. Although athletic success is related to skill level, conditioning traits can differentiate athletes of different caliber (15,16). Elite athletes possess greater strength, power, speed, and jumping ability compared with athletes of lesser rank (15). For example, Division I football players have greater maximal strength, vertical jump height, fat-free mass, lower percent body fat, and faster 40-yd dash times than Division II players have (13). Thus, health- and skill-related components of fitness appear to contribute to athletic success and are of value to anyone with advanced training goals.

Advanced training is a culmination of the individual's goals and training status. Maximizing fitness is a goal commonly shared by athletes and individuals who strive for fitness improvements in a noncompetitive manner. Training status encompasses a continuum of factors such that fitness level, training experience, and genetic endowment each make a contribution. One may designate an advanced client as one who has at least 1 year of consistent progressive training and has experienced a substantial level of adaptation. Those who truly excel may attain elite status in which they rank highly in one or more components of fitness. Skill level increases as one progresses to advanced training status. Training advanced to elite clients can pose a challenge to Personal Trainers. Some of the largest rates of fitness improvements take place in untrained individuals where the window of adaptation is high while trained individuals may show a slower rate of progression (1). Therefore, the Personal Trainer must be creative and must design advanced training programs based on the scientific principles of progressive overload, variation, and specificity (discussed in Chapters 13 and 14). This chapter provides an introduction to a number of advanced training options; additional instruction and experience in implementing the various techniques should be gained prior to personal training any clients.

### Competitive Training Goals

Advanced clients train for competition or the satisfaction of improving fitness and performance. Personal Trainers can provide an advantage to all athletes whether they compete in aerobic or anaerobic sports, or in "hybrid" sports, which include both aerobic and anaerobic aspects. Athletes may seek the services of Personal Trainers for strength training or assistance in their sport-specific training or off-season conditioning. This may entail the integration of weight training with speed, agility, flexibility, and/or plyometric training. The Personal Trainer may work in tandem with the athlete's coaching staff or may play a pivotal role in one-on-one training of athletes in lifting sports. The major competitive lifting sports include *weightlifting, powerlifting, bodybuilding,* and *strength competitions* each with numerous local, state, national, and international competitions, as well as federations, for an athlete to participate. Personal Trainers with the appropriate background may assist bodybuilders with weight training and cardiovascular training in preparation for the athlete's on-stage competition; assist power lifters with weight training programs targeting maximal performance of the squat, deadlift, and bench press exercises; and assist strength athletes with sport-specific strength training targeting events commonly contested in "strongman" or "strongwoman" competitions. Other athletes who require a mixture of anaerobic strength, power, and endurance as well as sufficient cardiovascular endurance may call on Personal Trainers to play a role in off-season weight, speed, agility, flexibility, and plyometric training and/or possibly with some pre- or in-season conditioning (depending on the sport and coaching staff).

# Advanced Program Design

Advanced training programs consist of systematic manipulation of the acute program variables. The manipulation of these variables becomes more critical because of the smaller window of adaptation shown in advanced or elite athletes. The level of variation is greater than that seen in beginning and intermediate programs. A basic program may improve several components of fitness simultaneously in an untrained or moderately trained individual. However, this same program may only improve one or two fitness components in a trained individual. Advanced training is characterized by greater specificity and requires periodization in the program (12,16,17,21,32,38) (see Chapter 14). Training cycles are common, and each cycle may target a few components of fitness. Exercise selection increases are based on training and program goals along with enhanced motor coordination. An analogy can be drawn to martial arts. In martial arts, individuals begin learning basic movements, master these movements, and progress to more challenging movements and complex series of movements toward progression to a black belt. Training is similar in that it is important to keep the program simple at first but increase complexity with progression. Advanced training requires the optimal integration of training modalities. A strength/power athlete may simultaneously perform resistance, sprint, agility, and plyometric training in a preseason training phase, and an endurance athlete may simultaneously perform aerobic endurance, interval, and some resistance training (RT). Although training basics have been discussed in previous chapters, this chapter focuses on the applied concepts of advanced program design of resistance, plyometric, sprint, and agility training.

## Resistance Training

American College of Sports Medicine (ACSM) has been instrumental in providing Personal Trainers with guidelines and recommendations for RT. Early position stands focused mostly on untrained populations. However, in 2002, ACSM first published RT guidelines targeting progression from novice to advanced training status for those individuals striving to increase muscle strength, power, endurance, and hypertrophy (1). In 2009, ACSM extended these guidelines by publishing an evidenced-based position stand (2). The basic elements of ACSM RT guidelines were discussed in Chapter 14. ACSM recommendations for advanced RT are presented in Table 19.1. The Personal Trainer can use these recommendations when prescribing the client exercise selection, sequence, intensity, volume, muscle actions, rest intervals, frequency, and lifting velocity. The Personal Trainer needs to prescribe an

> The Personal Trainer can use ACSM recommendations for resistance training when prescribing the client exercise selection, sequence, intensity, volume, muscle actions, rest intervals, frequency, and lifting velocity.

| Table 19.1 | American College of Sports Medicine Recommendations for Advanced Resistance Training (1,2) | | | |
|---|---|---|---|---|
| | **Muscle Strength** | **Hypertrophy** | **Muscle Endurance** | **Power** |
| Muscle action | CON, ECC, and ISOM | CON, ECC, and ISOM | CON, ECC, and ISOM | CON, ECC, and ISOM |
| Intensity and repetitions | Cycling loads of 80%–100% of 1-RM. | A loading range of 70%–100% of 1-RM be used for 1–12 repetitions per set in periodized manner such that the majority of training is devoted to 6–12 RM and less training devoted to 1–6 RM loading. | Various loading strategies (10–25 repetitions or more) in periodized manner | Heavy loading (85%–100% of 1-RM) for ↑ force, light-to-moderate loading (30%–60% of 1-RM for upper body exercises, 0%–60% of 1-RM for lower body exercises) performed at an explosive velocity for ↑ RFD, 1–6 repetitions in periodized manner |
| No. sets per exercise | Multiple sets (3–6) | Multiple sets (3–6) | Multiple sets (3–6) | Multiple sets (3–6) |
| Exercises | Unilateral and bilateral single- and multiple-joint exercises should be included with emphasis on multiple-joint exercises. Emphasis be placed on free-weight exercises with machine exercises used to compliment program needs. | Unilateral and bilateral single- and multiple-joint free weight and machine exercises | Unilateral and bilateral multiple- and single-joint free weights and machine exercises | Unilateral and bilateral multiple-joint free weight exercises |
| Exercise order | Large muscle group exercises before small muscle group exercises, multiple-joint exercises before single-joint exercises, higher intensity exercises before lower intensity exercises, or rotation of upper and lower body or opposing exercises | Large muscle group exercises before small muscle group exercises, multiple-joint exercises before single-joint exercises, higher intensity exercises before lower intensity exercises, or rotation of upper and lower body or opposing exercises | Various sequencing combinations | Similar to strength training |

*(continued)*

| Table 19.1 | American College of Sports Medicine Recommendations for Advanced Resistance Training (1,2) (continued) | | | |
|---|---|---|---|---|
| | **Muscle Strength** | **Hypertrophy** | **Muscle Endurance** | **Power** |
| Rest intervals | At least 2–3 min for structural exercises using heavier loads. For assistance exercises, a shorter rest period length of 1–2 min may suffice. | Correspond to goals of each exercise: 2–3 min may be used with heavy loading for structural exercises, and 1–2 min may be used for other exercises of moderate-to-moderately high intensity. | Short rest periods, for example, 1–2 min for high-repetition sets (15–20 repetitions or more), <1 min for moderate (10–15 repetitions) sets. For circuit training, rest periods should correspond to time needed to get from one exercise to another. | At least 2–3 min for structural exercises when intensity is high; shorter rest interval (1–2 min) for assistance exercises |
| Repetition velocity | A continuum of velocities from unintentionally slow to fast CON velocities and should correspond to the intensity. | Slow, moderate, and fast repetition velocities depending on the load, repetition number, and goals of the exercise | Intentionally slow with moderate repetition number (10–15); moderate to faster with large number of repetitions (15–25 or more) | Fast |
| Frequency | 4–6 d · wk⁻¹ | 4–6 d · wk⁻¹ | 4–6 d · wk⁻¹ | 4–5 d · wk⁻¹ |

ECC, eccentric; CON, concentric; ISOM, isometric; RFD, rate of force development.
Adapted with permission from American College of Sports Medicine. *ACSM's Guidelines for Exercise Testing and Prescription.* 9th ed. Philadelphia (PA): Lippincott Williams & Wilkins; 2013.

appropriate set structure when multiple-set programs are used. For example, constant load/repetition (keeping load and repetition number the same for each set), heavy-to-light (decreasing weight each set while maintaining or increasing repetition number), light-to-heavy (increasing weight each set while maintaining or decreasing repetition number), and undulating (integrated) systems are all effective for progression (17,28,32). Thus, it is up to the personal preference of the Personal Trainer and client as to which one or combination of systems will be used.

Key elements of advanced RT involve the planning of training and potential use of advanced techniques. Advanced RT involves periodization of the acute program variables, primarily the volume, intensity, and exercise selection. Training phases target different fitness components and the volume and intensity, especially for the critical structural exercises, will be prescribed accordingly. The Personal Trainer may assess the client's RT progress periodically via one repetition maximum (1-RM) testing (see Chapter 12) or multiple repetition maximum (RM) testing. Multiple RM testing involves lifting a weight multiple times and then doing some mathematical calculations to estimate 1-RM (see reference [32] for a list of commonly used equations). Common exercises assessed include the bench press, squat, deadlift, and power clean, although any exercise can be assessed depending on program priorities. Multiple RMs can be assessed and used for testing high-intensity muscle endurance or can be used to predict 1-RM strength (22,32).

Periodic strength testing (~3 mo or more) not only can be used to measure progress but also is instrumental for determining training loads for some structural exercises that are prescribed based on a percentage of 1-RM. In addition, advanced RT techniques provide additional overload and can assist advanced clients in overcoming training plateaus (32). Although intermediate clients can benefit from their use, they are best reserved for advanced trainees.

Examples of advanced RT techniques include heavy and forced negatives, functional isometrics, partial repetitions, variable resistance, forced repetitions, breakdown sets, combining exercises, discontinuous sets, quality training, and spectrum repetition/contrast loading combinations.

## Advanced Resistance Training Techniques

Advanced RT techniques are based on program variables and exercise range of motion (ROM). Techniques discussed in this chapter include heavy and forced negatives, functional isometrics, partial repetitions, variable resistance, forced repetitions, breakdown sets, combining exercises, discontinuous sets, quality training, and spectrum repetition/contrast loading combinations.

### HEAVY AND FORCED NEGATIVES

Heavy negatives target the eccentric (ECC) phase with a slow cadence (>3–4 s) using heavy to supramaximal loading in the presence of capable spotters or a power rack with the pins set at appropriate height. Concentric (CON) phases are performed with assistance from a spotter or the Personal Trainer. Variations include performing a bilateral exercise with a moderate weight and then lowering/returning the weight with only one limb and/or using a machine with multiple loading capacities that enable greater ECC loading. Repetitions during traditional sets can be enhanced with force applied to ECC phase via the Personal Trainer (*forced negatives*). Heavy ECC training should be used with caution (4- to 6-wk training cycles, one or two times per year) to reduce muscle damage and the risk of overtraining and/or injury. For example, the client may perform three or four sets of the bench press and then perform one or two additional sets of heavy negatives for two or three repetitions (32). This is a technique seen in advanced strength and hypertrophy training (12).

### FUNCTIONAL ISOMETRICS

Functional isometrics (ISOM) involve lifting a barbell in a power rack a few inches until it is pressed or pulled against the rack's pins. The client continues to push/pull maximally for ~2–6 seconds with a high rate of force development. The rack's pins are set in two places (when not beginning from the floor): at the starting position and at the targeted area of the ROM. Because skeletal muscles produce more force during ISOM actions, the rationale is to target specific areas of the ROM to increase dynamic strength to a greater extent. Functional ISOM can be performed in multiple areas of the ROM but are effective when performed near the sticking region (or weak point) of the exercise (28,32). For example, the client may set the pins slightly above the parallel position for the barbell squat and perform three to five sets of three to five repetitions with a moderate load. This is an effective strength and power training technique. Some commonly targeted exercises are the bench press, deadlift, squat, and clean pull and can be easily integrated into an RT program.

### PARTIAL REPETITIONS

Partial repetitions are performed in a limited ROM with the intent to enhance ROM-specific strength and potentially full exercise ROM strength. Most often, the repetitions are performed in either the area of maximal strength or near the sticking point. Partial repetitions can be used in different ways. Some clients may use them for hypertrophy and muscle endurance enhancement by extending sets beyond exhaustion when a full ROM repetition can no longer be performed unassisted. Some athletes (mostly bodybuilders) have integrated partial repetitions into dynamic sets with full ROM repetitions. Often, partial repetitions are performed in the area of maximal strength with heavy to supramaximal loading. Strength expression varies throughout the ROM yielding a parabolic curve for single-joint exercises and a linear curve for multiple-joint exercises. Ascending strength curves (where force increases as exercise ROM progresses) are expressed for "pushing" exercises, whereas descending curves (where force decreases as exercise ROM progresses) are expressed for "pulling" exercises (see Fig. 14.3). For a pushing exercise like the bench press, maximal force is produced near the lockout phase. Supramaximal loads may be lifted in this ROM (29). Strength athletes such as power lifters may benefit from including partial ROM lifts into strength peaking mesocycles. Often, one to three sets of partial repetitions are performed following completion of the full ROM exercise, for example, the client may perform four sets of traditional squats followed by one to three sets of partial squats. A power rack is recommended as the pins prevent bar movement below the inferior segment of the lift.

### Variable Resistance Training

Variable resistance training (VRT) is performed by altering the loading throughout the ROM. Common ways for clients to perform VRT is through specific machines, elastic bands, or by altering free weight exercises via bands and/or chains. The latter is more commonly seen in advanced RT of strength and power athletes. Variable resistance machines modify loading via cams that vary in length and change the mechanics based on ascending/descending strength curves for single-joint exercises. Many athletes have used bands and chains for multiple-joint VRT individually and have added them to barbells to create free weight VRT (32,36). Bands and chains come in different sizes and provide a variety of resistance levels. The bench press is also commonly used. Chains are applied to both ends of the bar while it is in the racked position with much of the chain links suspended in the air. Upon liftoff, the client supports the majority of chain weight. As the bar descends, more chain links are supported by the floor, thereby reducing the load. Upon ascent of the bar, progressively more loading is encountered as the chain links are lifted from the floor. Loading depends on the weight and size (5–7 ft) of the chain, and the distance of the bar from the floor. Chains oscillate which increases the stabilization requirement. A similar effect is gained through elastic bands attached to the floor (or rack) and bar (with less oscillation). The farther the band is stretched, the more resistance applied to the bar.

### Forced Repetitions

Forced repetitions are those completed with assistance of a spotter or via self-spotting (for exercises like the leg press or unilateral arm exercises) beyond one's normal capacity. The rationale is to extend a set beyond failure with hopes of providing greater increases in muscle strength, endurance, and hypertrophy (12,32). The Personal Trainer should apply minimal assistance allowing up to approximately one to four repetitions. Forced repetitions can be used exclusively as a set with heavy to supramaximal loading or can be used to extend a set when failure has occurred. As a result, forced repetitions elicit higher levels of fatigue than traditional repetitions. Although forced repetitions are used in novice and intermediate RT, they are best utilized for advanced training as they provide a potent neuromuscular stimulus and need to be used with caution.

### Contrast Loading

Contrast loading involves inclusion of low, moderate, and high repetitions (with concomitant changes in loading) within a session. Heavy weights are usually lifted first followed by light/moderate weights, or are alternated. For example, a client may perform six sets of an exercise. The first two sets may be performed with heavy weights for five repetitions; the next two sets may be performed with moderate weights for 10 repetitions; and the last two sets may be performed with light weights for 20 repetitions. Multiple fitness components are stressed. The goal is to recruit as many muscle fibers as possible with heavy weights then stimulate circulatory/metabolic growth factors with low-to-moderate weight and high repetitions (32). This technique is used mostly by bodybuilders to increase muscle hypertrophy.

## BREAKDOWN SETS

Breakdown (or descending) sets involve a rapid reduction in weight with minimal rest thereby allowing the client to extend a set by performing additional repetitions. The rationale is when failure occurs, there is still potential to perform more repetitions beyond fatigue with less weight. Single or multiple breakdowns may be used and are most effective when a spotter or the Personal Trainer is present to remove weights or change pins on machine weight stacks quickly (28). Breakdown sets are traditionally used to enhance muscle hypertrophy and endurance. However, breakdown sets can be used to target muscle strength if a heavy weight is lifted for a few repetitions, 5%–10% of the load is reduced allowing one to two additional repetitions are performed, etc., until the targeted number of repetitions are completed.

## COMBINING EXERCISES

Combining exercises involves performing two or more exercises consecutively or simultaneously with minimal rest and are primarily used for increasing muscular endurance and hypertrophy, especially if the client is attempting to minimize workout duration. Muscle strength can increase, but it is a secondary goal as the weight lifted for each exercise is less than what would typically be used if the exercise was performed alone (and dependent on the weakest of the exercises). The metabolic demands of a workout can be greater when combination exercises are used due to the longer duration of each set and potential for greater workout continuity (32). For example, multiple exercises can be combined to form a single exercise (combination lifts). This is common when using Olympic lifts, for example, a clean from the floor, a front squat, and a push press to finish for a series of repetitions, and traditional exercises. Combination exercises such as the lunge with rotation, dumbbell squat with shoulder press, and the burpee with push-up (to name a few) have become popular in recent years especially when included in metabolic circuit programs that have increased in popularity. It is important for the Personal Trainer to select a weight that can be tolerated for the weakest of the exercises in sequence when nonbody weight exercises are performed.

Another strategy is to perform all repetitions for one exercise followed by consecutive performance of one or more exercises with minimal rest in between exercises. Because the client is performing exercises in succession, weights can be selected that match each exercise. These include (a) supersets (consecutive performance of two exercises either for the same or different muscle groups), (b) tri-sets (consecutive performance of three exercises), and giant sets (consecutive performance of four or more exercises separate from circuit training). Often bodybuilders use supersets, tri-sets, and giant sets of exercises that stress similar muscle groups. Some strength athletes use supersets to increase muscle strength, but do so using exercises that stress opposing or unrelated muscle groups (to allow adequate recovery with use of heavier weights).

## QUALITY TRAINING

Quality training involves reducing rest interval lengths within specific loading/volume parameters as training progresses. Although mostly used to increase muscle endurance and hypertrophy, recent evidence shows it can be used for strength increases (37). For example, a client currently training the squat for four sets of 10 repetitions with 275 lb using 2.5 minutes in between sets may gradually reduce rest intervals by 10–20 seconds on a weekly or biweekly basis until a targeted value (*e.g.*, 1.5 min) is reached and performance is maintained. Subsequently, the client may add weight, increase rest interval length, and begin the process once again.

## DISCONTINUOUS SETS

Sets that include rest intervals in between repetitions are discontinuous sets. The goal is to increase the quality of effort for each repetition by maximizing acute force and power output. Peak force and velocity decrease as a continuous set is prolonged. Including an intra-set rest interval may limit fatigue and increase repetition quality. Inserting a rest interval in between repetitions results in more repetitions performed and higher force/power output (6). One variation, *rest-pause training*, allows more repetitions to be performed with maximal or near-maximal weights. For example, a client may target five repetitions with a 3-RM load. The client performs three repetitions without assistance, racks the weight, and rests for 10–15 seconds. The client then proceeds to perform one additional repetition with the same load, rests for 10–20 seconds, and performs one additional repetition totaling five altogether. The length of the rest interval, volume, and resistance can be altered depending on the goals of the set. A variation used by some elite power lifters is the *dynamic method* (36). The way this method has been commonly used is by having the individual perform 8–10 sets of a structural exercise for two or three explosive repetitions with moderate loading (~60% of 1-RM) with 45 seconds to 1 minute rest in between sets. Although the repetitions are performed consecutively, the large set number coupled with substantial rest illustrates a variation of rest-pause training. The use of multiple repetitions is advantageous for those lifters who attain peak force or power on the second or third repetition rather than the first. A variation used successfully by Olympic weightlifters is *cluster training*. Typically, 10–45 seconds rest intervals are used in between repetitions of the Olympic lifts and variations to maximize bar velocity and power. Cluster sets can be structured in different ways. The load can be kept constant for all repetitions, or can be increased, decreased, or undulated.

## Motion-Specific Training

Motion-specific training, also known as functional training, involves the use of exercises that train specific movements. Motion-specific training involves adding resistance to movements, many of which stress the entire body or core musculature to a large extent. The intent is to improve athletic performance, balance, and coordination and to provide a link between strength gained through traditional RT and motion-specific strength. Exercises consist of multiplanar movements sometimes performed in unstable environments with various pieces of equipment such as bands, medicine balls, dumbbells, stability balls, kettle bells, ropes, TRX (for suspension training), and other devices. Exercises performed in unstable environments often require the client use less loading. The goal is to increase primarily core (stabilizer) muscle strength and not the prime movers per se (although there could be a secondary strength-building effect). For example, a client will be able to use heavier dumbbells when performing the bench press on a flat bench (*e.g.*, stable environment) versus a stability ball (*e.g.*, unstable environment). The flat bench press will have a better strength-building effect for upper body musculature, whereas the stability ball bench press will have a stronger core component. Thus, unstable motion-specific training is best utilized when integrated into traditional RT programs. The combination can be used to optimize performance.

A staple of motion-specific training is the use of body weight exercises. Exercises such as body weight squats, lunges, push-ups, pull-ups, dips, reverse dips, sit-ups, crunches, leg raises, burpees, and hyperextensions all require the client to overcome one's body weight. In the absence of adding external weight, body weight exercises can be made more difficult by changing grip/stance width, leverage (moment arm of resistance), cadence, or by using unilateral versus bilateral contractions (one rather than two arms or legs). Basic knowledge of biomechanics is critical for the Personal Trainer to make exercises easier or more difficult in the absence of adding external resistance (32). Increasing the moment arm of resistance, size of the base support, amount of weight supported by musculature, and the center of gravity (COG) can change exercise difficulty dramatically (see Chapter 4 for more information on biomechanics). The push-up is a good example. It can be made easier by performing it on the knees (*modified push-up*) or more difficult by staggering hand spacing or by performing it with one leg in motion while suspended in the air (a *Spiderman push-up*). Performing a back extension or sit-up is more difficult with the hands overhead than crossed at chest level. Difficulty is increased by adding a rotation or unilateral (vs. central) loading. Some body weight exercises are extremely difficult and performed mostly by advanced clients.

Basic knowledge of biomechanics is critical for the Personal Trainer to make exercises easier or more difficult in the absence of adding external resistance.

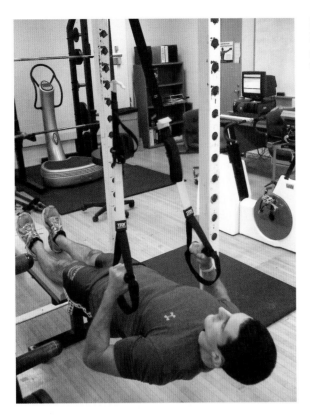

**FIGURE 19.1.** TRX inverted row. (From Ratamess N. *ACSM's Foundation of Strength Training and Conditioning.* Philadelphia [PA]: Wolters Kluwer/Lippincott Williams & Wilkins; 2012.)

Exercises such as one-arm push-ups, single-leg squats, and single-arm pull-ups are difficult for many. An exercise such as the pull-up press requires a great deal of strength. The client presses the body outward from the top pull-up position (with a wide pronated grip). Athletes such as gymnasts who train against body weight possess high levels of muscle strength and power.

Body weight training is aided by devices which allow body weight to be manipulated. For example, the TRX Suspension Trainer consists of two straps with adjustable handles and foot attachments that can be suspended or anchored from the ceiling, a door, beams, or a power rack (Fig. 19.1). It is based on a pendulum system where manipulation of the client's body position (distance from anchor, body angle relative to floor, height of the starting position and COG, and size of base support) dictates the percentage of body weight that needs to be overcome. For example, the more upright the body (feet back) the easier the exercise is (less weight to support) for some upper body exercises. The closer to the ground (feet closer to anchor) the more difficult the exercise is as a larger percentage of body weight must be overcome. Advanced clients benefit greatly from body weight training as does a beginner.

## Strength Implements

By definition, RT entails any method or form of exercise requiring the client to exert a force against a resistance. The source of the resistance may vary greatly. Although most advanced RT programs target free weights and machines, the use of other sources of resistance including body weight, medicine balls, movement-specific devices, bands/cables, and strength implements has increased in popularity among advanced trainees. Implements provide a different stress to the client than free weights as many implements provide unbalanced resistance and the gripping may be more difficult. Some exercises with implements cannot be replicated similarly with free weights. Table 19.2 presents some popular implements used in advanced strength and conditioning programs (see Ratamess [32] for additional information).

| Table 19.2 | Examples of Strength Implements Used in Resistance Training |
| --- | --- |
| **Implement** | **Characteristics** |
| KB | Weights with superior handle location; enhance grip strength due to thicker handles and leverage changes as KB moves; handle allows KB to swing freely; grasped off of COG due to position of handle |
| Sleds | Resist linear movements; provide strong stimulus to all major muscle groups, ↑ metabolic challenge; can be loaded with weights for pushing or pulling (with a harness); some sleds have multiple handles which allow pushing from low and high body positions; automobiles and trucks have been used in a similar manner |
| Kegs | Fluid (or sand)-filled drums; great balance requirement as fluid moves when kegs are lifted; require strong grip to hold in stable positions during lifting |
| Log bars | Have a mid-range grip support for lifting with a semi-pronated forearm position; some are filled with water to add resistance and balance requirements; vary in length based on strength level |
| Farmer's walk bars | Allows the athlete to grasp heavy weights and walk/run for a specified distance; great for grip strength/endurance training and total-body strength and conditioning |
| Thick bars | Bars with large diameters (2, 2¾, 3 in); used for grip strength training (34) |
| Super yoke | Device ~6 ft in length with a bar that is placed on rear shoulders supported by two beams that is loaded with weights; athlete must control yoke from swaying ↑ balance requirement. |
| Sledge hammers | Used for striking drills on tires; can be made more difficult by grasping the hammer closer to end of handle or more explosive by grasping the hammer closer to the head for speed and power |
| Tires | From trucks and heavy equipment for flipping; involves triple extension of hips, knees, and ankles for total-body strength, power, and conditioning |
| Stones | Lifted from the ground to various heights for total-body strength, power, and endurance; adjustable stands may be used for loading stones. |
| Sandbags | Bags of sand for lifting; some have handles making it easier to grasp and expands exercise selection; provides unbalanced resistance |
| Heavy bags | Punching bags used for exercises in addition to striking; can be thrown or lifted in multiple directions |
| Battling ropes | Ropes of various length and width used for various exercises during metabolic training |
| Chains | Added to BBs to provide variable resistance for multijoint exercises with ascending strength curves; oscillate during motion which increases stability requirement; can be used solely as a source of resistance |

KB, kettle bell; BB, barbell; COG, center of gravity.
Adapted with permission from U.S. Department of Health and Human Services. *Physical Activity Guidelines Advisory Committee Report, 2008.* Washington (DC): U.S. Department of Health and Human Services. American College of Sports Medicine. *ACSM's Guidelines for Exercise Testing and Prescription.* 9th ed. Philadelphia (PA): Lippincott Williams & Wilkins; 2013.

## Olympic Lifts

The Olympic lifts (snatch, clean, and jerk) and several variations are total-body resistance exercises that recruit most major muscle groups. They are the most complex resistance exercises to perform and are considered the most effective exercises for increasing total-body power (12). Because of the complexity of these lifts, Personal Trainers should have advanced training and instruction before using with clients. Repetitions are performed with fast movements of the lower body and trunk (as the arms serve as guides and assist the client in preparation for catching the bar) and the kinetics closely resemble jumping and several motor skills comprising many anaerobic sports. The *clean and jerk* is a two-staged exercise where the athlete lifts the bar from the floor to shoulder level and then to an overhead position. The power clean is used to assess maximal strength and power (Fig. 19.2). It results in larger amounts of weight lifted compared with the *snatch* which involves lifting the weight directly from the floor to an overhead position (Fig. 19.3). The snatch is considered more complex because the bar must be lifted a greater distance directly from the floor requiring greater bar velocity. Variations (*e.g.*, over-head squat, hang clean/snatch, Romanian deadlift, high pull) are related exercises that enhance specific performance aspects of the complete lift and are used for strength and power enhancement as several require fast force production and teach proper kinesthetic awareness needed to apply maximal force to the ground. Often, these exercises are taught in progressions starting with the clean and later the snatch as they are similar in movement during some phases. Olympic lifts should be performed on a wooden platform with bumper plates. However, some facilities may not have platforms so modifications can be made to create adequate space and the use of a matted surface may suffice. It is important to teach the

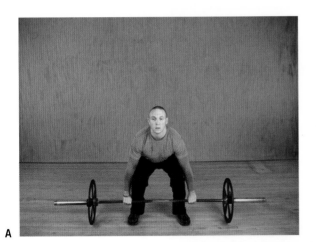
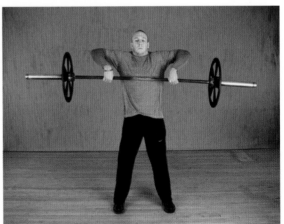
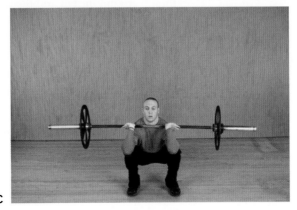

**FIGURE 19.2.** The power clean. **A.** The starting position. **B.** The second pull phase. **C.** The final position after catch when the client descends with the bar into the full front squat position. (Adapted from Ratamess N. *ACSM's Foundation of Strength Training and Conditioning.* Philadelphia [PA]: Wolters Kluwer/Lippincott Williams & Wilkins; 2012. p. 319.)

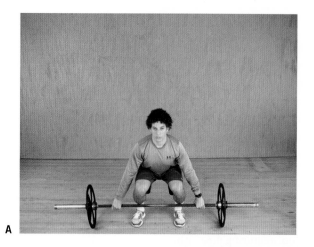
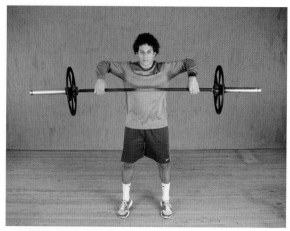

A

B

C

**FIGURE 19.3.** The snatch. **A.** The starting position. **B.** The second pull phase. **C.** The catch position where the client descends into the full overhead squat position. (Adapted from Ratamess N. *ACSM's Foundation of Strength Training and Conditioning.* Philadelphia [PA]: Wolters Kluwer/Lippincott Williams & Wilkins; 2012. p. 319.)

client how to properly drop the weights when learning the Olympic lifts. A missed lift could do more harm to the client if it is continued erroneously. Rather, it is safer to drop the bar in a controlled manner. Lastly, the Olympic lifts are ideally performed using a *hook grip*. The hook grip involves wrapping the thumb around the bar and then wrapping the first three fingers around the thumb and bar for added support. A strong grip is necessary, and this configuration allows for greater support during fast pulling movements. Although effective for grip support, the hook grip is uncomfortable and may take some time for the client to adjust to the technique.

> Because of the complexity of Olympic lifts, Personal Trainers should have advanced training and instruction *before* using with clients.

### Technical Aspects of Performing the Olympic Lifts

The Olympic lifts are technically challenging resistance exercises. Discussion of proper technique is best summarized by dissecting the lifts into phases. Because the clean and snatch have some similarities, they will be discussed together and their differences will be highlighted. The phases include the starting position, the first pull (barbell is pulled from the floor), a transition phase prior to the second pull, the second pull, the catch, and the finish. Boxes 19.2 and 19.3 discuss technical aspects of each of the phases of the clean and jerk and snatch exercises.

| Box 19.2 | Technical Aspects of Performing the Clean and Snatch |
|---|---|

**Phase** | **Correct Performance**

**Starting position**
- Feet are placed at hip width, toes pointed slightly outward, and bar is located on the floor near the shins.
- Hips and trunk are flexed to an angle of 25°–50° with the ground, with the hips positioned close to or slightly above the knees.
- Trunk is more upright and hips are higher during the clean because of the narrower grip width compared with the snatch.
- Shoulders are positioned directly over or slightly in front of bar with the COG over the middle of the foot.
- Low back is kept flat by hyperextending the lumbar spine and retracting the shoulder girdle.
- Head is straight or slightly upward and arms grasp bar with elbows extended out and wrists flexed.
- Wide grip width is used for snatch and shoulder width grip is used for clean.
- Snatch grip width may be determined by having the individual stand and abduct one arm laterally (to where it is parallel to the ground) while making a fist and measuring the length of the opposite shoulder to the fist (the length represents the snatch width) — the bar should be ~4–6 in above the head during the overhead squat.

**First pull**
- Bar is pulled toward the body (4–12 cm for the snatch; 3–10 cm for the clean) and is lifted off of ground to ~31% of height for the clean and ~35% for the snatch.
- Mostly knee extension and plantarflexion with little change in trunk angle and COG shifts toward heels (knee angle slightly greater for snatch than clean).
- Elbows remain extended, shoulders move in front of bar, and trunk angle may slightly increase by end of phase.
- Phase lasts ~0.50 s — bar is lifted ~1.5 m · s$^{-1}$ for snatch and ~1.2 m · s$^{-1}$ for clean.

**Transition**
- Adjustment phase characterized by unweighting
- Knee flexion (double knee bend) with an increase in trunk extension
- Bar reaches lower third of thigh for clean and middle of thigh for snatch.
- Postural realignment (vertical torso) occurs allowing a second pull to maximize force and power.

**Second pull**
- Bar is pulled upward and slightly away from body by extension of hips, knees, and ankles.
- Elbows remain extended throughout.
- Force applied to bar decreases at top as athlete prepares to pull him or her under the bar for the catch.
- Most explosive phase takes ~0.1–0.25 s with snatch requiring more time than clean.
- Bar velocities for snatch are ~10%–20% higher than the clean.
- Optimal bar trajectory (S-shaped pattern): (a) bar is pulled toward body during first pull, (b) bar is pulled slightly away from body during second pull, and (c) bar moves closer to body in preparation for catch.

**Catch**
- Involves optimal positioning to catch the bar after second pull while bar is rising
- Athlete pulls bar to max height (68%–78% of height for snatch, 55%–65% of height for clean) and descends underneath simultaneously.
- Arms pull body down under bar.
- For the snatch: Feet move out into a squatting position (wider than hip width).
- Arms pull body under bar while feet are moving.
- Elbows are wide, trunk is upright, wrists turnover, and bar rotates.
- Throughout descent athlete applies force to bar to support weight in full squat position.

*(continued)*

| Box 19.2 | Technical Aspects of Performing the Clean and Snatch *(continued)* |
|---|---|

| Catch *(continued)* | ■ Athlete flexes shoulders, pushes head forward, and extends hips into an overhead squat finish.<br>■ For the clean, feet move out into squat position.<br>■ Athlete pulls himself down forcefully and receives bar at shoulder position.<br>■ During foot landing, wrists rotate around bar, elbows push forward and upward creating a shelf to catch weight.<br>■ Bar is caught on shoulders and chest — loading forces athlete down into a deeper front squat position.<br>■ Upper arms are parallel to ground, knees are over feet, and athlete completes lift with a front squat. |
|---|---|

Performance of the Olympic lifts can be augmented by inclusion of several skill transfer exercises and variations. Some multiple-joint basic strength exercises enhance one or more phases of the Olympic lifts. For example, the deadlift, back squat, behind-the-neck press, and good morning are exercises that strengthen large muscles (*e.g.*, ankle, knee, and hip extensors, shoulder and elbow extensors) involved in the Olympic lifts, emphasize proper body position, and improve kinetics in a manner that may transfer to Olympic lift performance.

| Box 19.3 | Technical Aspects of Performing the Jerk |
|---|---|

| Phase | Correct Performance |
|---|---|
| Starting position | ■ Athlete begins in the front squat position.<br>■ Hips and shoulders are aligned over rear segment of the middle of the foot.<br>■ Feet are hip width with toes slightly pointed outward, head slightly back, and arms are relaxed (near parallel to floor) with elbows in front of bar (tensing the arms could result in bar moving forward instead of vertical). |
| Descent | ■ A countermovement before the upward explosive thrust<br>■ Knees flex and ankles dorsiflex in a vertical manner with COG shifting slightly forward<br>■ Duration is ~0.20–0.25 s |
| Braking | ■ Transition between end of final third countermovement and beginning of thrust and takes ~0.12 s<br>■ With descent, horizontal bar displacement should be minimal (<2–4 cm). |
| Thrust | ■ Explosive extension of hips, knees, and ankles driving the bar vertically upward with bar velocities of 1.2–1.8 m $\cdot$ s$^{-1}$<br>■ Final segment is brought about by forceful pushing of bar by arms to help with diving under the bar |
| Split | ■ Most common position, although some prefer the squat when diving under bar<br>■ One hip flexes (front) and other extends (back) to form a stable base, the back leg lands before the front leg as feet leave the ground (taking ~0.20–0.28 s).<br>■ Back leg is nearly straight (~2-ft length from hip) and front knee flexes to >90° with shin perpendicular to floor (1-ft length in front of hip).<br>■ Bar is positioned slightly behind athlete's head in line with shoulders and hips, head is forward, and back is hyperextended. |
| Finish | ■ Weight is transferred to rear foot as front leg pushes backward. |

Exercises such as the front squat, overhead squat, and Romanian deadlift offer similar benefits and teach the client proper kinesthetic awareness and balance. Teaching the second pull during the clean and snatch may involve performing the high pull exercise (wide grip for snatch, shoulder-width grip for clean) from above the knee, below the knee, and from the floor. This allows the client to perform the pull rapidly from various levels without having to adjust body position for the catch. Some coaches and Personal Trainers begin these variations from the hang position. Many Olympic weightlifters perform variations known as the stop clean or stop snatch where the bar is lowered to the proper depth from the standing position and then subsequently lifted with high power output. Progression may continue to the catch and finish phases. Exercises such as the pressing snatch balance and heaving snatch balance teach descent under the bar for the snatch. The top position can be taught by progressing from the behind-the-neck press (snatch grip) to the overhead squat to the snatch balance. The first exercise teaches proper overhead proprioception. The second teaches the athlete to descend/ascend (squat) with the bar overhead. The third requires the athlete to descend into the overhead squat position rather than begin with it.

The primary goal of performing the Olympic lifts is to increase muscle power, speed, and strength. The Olympic lifts are performed at maximal velocity for usually one to six repetitions at the beginning of a training session. Intensity varies depending on the training phase. Heavy weights may be used during strength and power peaking phases and moderate to moderately heavy loads for other training phases. Peak power is produced at ~80% of 1-RM (19) so loading should encompass this intensity, in part, for advanced power training. Because of the need for high rate of force development and the exercise complexity, Olympic lifts should be performed early in a workout when fatigue is minimal. When multiple Olympic lifts and/or variations are performed, sequencing is based on complexity where the snatch takes precedence over the clean, both take precedence over the jerk, and variations are sequenced based on bar movement (*i.e.*, greater bar displacement means greater complexity and need for high velocity). For example, a hang clean would be performed before a high pull and a snatch below the knee would be performed before a snatch above the knee. Variations (skill transfer exercises) are performed after the full Olympic lifts in sequence. The frequency of Olympic lift inclusion in advanced training varies between 1 and 5 days per week. Among Olympic weightlifters frequencies as high as 18 workouts per week have been reported (43) with multiple short sessions per day. Box 19.4 depicts a sample program integrating multiple Olympic lifts focusing on the barbell snatch.

This type of program may be performed by an Olympic weightlifter or strength/power athlete as it emphasizes total-body power and snatch kinetics and technique. This program consists of five exercises sequenced from most complex to least complex for the Olympic lifts followed by three skill transfer exercises (variations). Each repetition is performed at high velocity for the Olympic lifts. Rest intervals are 3 minutes to allow adequate recovery in between sets.

| Box 19.4 | Sample Workout Emphasizing the Olympic Lifts | | |
|---|---|---|---|
| **Move** | **Repetitions** | **% of 1-RM** | **Rest Interval (min)** |
| Full snatch | 5 × 1–3 | 75–80 | 3 |
| Snatch pull | 5 × 3 | 85 | 3 |
| Overhead squat | 4 × 5 | 70 | 3 |
| Good morning | 3 × 5 | 85 | 3 |
| Romanian deadlift (snatch grip) | 3 × 5 | 75–80 | 3 |

# Plyometric Training

Plyometric training is a form of explosive exercise that targets power development. Historically, plyometric training was known as *shock training* and consisted mostly of depth jumps and variations where the intensity was ultra-high (39), but current plyometric training includes lower intensity exercises as well. Plyometric actions encompass the stretch-shortening cycle (SSC) where the lengthening or prestretching of skeletal muscles under loading enables a more forceful CON muscle action. The ECC phase plus the length of the brief ISOM phase between ECC and CON actions (coupling time) is the *amortization phase*. Minimizing the length of the amortization phase maximizes the use of elastic energy making for a more powerful effort. Although plyometric exercises are classified based on intensity (impact loading and complexity), they are still performed with maximal effort.

Plyometric training increases athletic performance (*e.g.*, jump height and power, sprinting ability, agility, and muscle strength) (7,18,24,26,31). Vertical jump performance may increase an average of 5%–9% (26). Plyometric training is most effective when combined with RT for increasing performance (9,35). For example, plyometric training 2 days per week can easily be integrated with RT. Plyometric training can be performed on separate days from weight training or on the same day. If performed on the same day, plyometric training may be given priority and performed first. If only the upper body is resistance trained that day, then lower body plyometrics can be performed uninhibited and the sequence can vary. It is not recommended that high-intensity lower body RT and lower body plyometric training be performed on the same day as the modality trained second would do so in a semifatigued state. Plyometric drills can be incorporated into a weight training workout (*e.g.*, complex training).

Plyometric exercises such as the vertical jump, standing broad jump, and ball chest pass (put) can be used for maximal power assessment. The maximal vertical jump (performed near a wall or using a VerTec) is one of the most common power assessments used for athletes. The higher the jump, the greater the power the client possesses. The standing broad jump is another example of power assessment, testing power during horizontal locomotion. For upper body power, often the medicine ball chest pass (or put) is used. The client is seated (or standing) with his or her back against a support (or wall) and chest passes the ball as far as possible. The farther the ball travels, the greater the power output. The Personal Trainer can easily incorporate these exercises into an assessment battery. Minimal equipment is needed. If the Personal Trainer does not have a VerTec, a tape measure can be used for both vertical and standing broad jump drills. Chalk can be used on the finger tips to mark superior position during the highest segment of the vertical jump. A medicine ball, tape measure, chalk, and a bench with back support (for the seated chest pass) are needed for the chest pass. Chalk is placed on the ball and the location is marked (in the center) when the ball lands on the ground. The distance is measured. Standards are available for the Personal Trainer (15,32) or the individual can develop their own data for comparison.

> The maximal vertical jump (performed near a wall or using a VerTec) is one of the most common power assessments used for athletes.

## Safety Considerations

Plyometric training is safe for clients of all ages provided it is properly supervised (11). The most common causes of injuries are violation of training guidelines, inadequate warm-up, progressing too fast in volume and intensity, poor technique, poor surface selection, and undisclosed predisposition. Progressing too quickly in volume and intensity could result in overreaching and subsequent of overtraining. Overtrained clients are more susceptible to injury. Inadequate warm-ups fail to prepare the client for intense exercise. Poor technique may limit exercise selection as sufficient coordination, balance, and strength are needed for moderate- to high-intensity plyometric exercises. Improper landing can place the client at greater risk of injury. Caution must be used with large clients. A prior injury or predisposition to injury can place the athlete at greater risk. Careful monitoring of clients is necessary. An injury may necessitate altering or temporarily discontinuing plyometrics until medical clearance has been obtained.

### Plyometric Program Design

Plyometric training variables include exercise selection, order, intensity, volume, frequency, and rest intervals. Designing a plyometric training program is multifactorial and should include planned progressive overload, specificity, and variation. Many factors need to be considered for plyometric training including the age/training status of the client, equipment availability, training surface, recovery in between workouts, nutrition, and the integration of plyometrics with other training modalities. Some critical factors include the following:

- Quality of training: Each repetition should be performed with maximal effort, minimal amortization, and maximal velocity.
- Exercise selection: The selection should be as specific to the demands of the sport/activity as possible comprising unilateral and bilateral drills.
- Plyometric training should take place in an area with sufficient space; for example, horizontal length of at least 30–40 yards and ceiling height (indoors) should be higher than maximal reach.
- Proper technique should always be instructed.
- Sufficient rest should be given when peak power is the goal.
- Gradual progression entails increases in intensity via the addition of complex exercises and some external loading. Low-intensity and moderate-intensity drills should be mastered before progressing to high-intensity drills.
- Volume can be increased with number of contacts and should be progressed gradually.
- High-intensity workouts require longer recovery period in between workouts.

Plyometric exercises consist of jumps-in-place, standing jumps, multiple hops/jumps, bounding, box drills, depth jumps, and throws preferably on a grass or matted surface (3). The surface should be yielding to reduce joint stress, but not too yielding to limit SSC activity. Jumps involve maximizing vertical or horizontal motion. Hops involve maximizing the repeated motion for a specific distance or pattern. Bounds are exaggerated horizontal drills with excessive stride length. Box drills involve jumping on or off boxes of different sizes. Depth jumps involve accentuating the ECC component by stepping off of a box prior to performing an explosive jump while spending minimal time on the ground. Intensity increases as drop height increases. Most often, drop heights of 20–115 cm are used (20–40 cm to begin with gradual progression) as the optimal depth jump height is debatable and individualized (32). Tosses and passes involve the upper torso and arms releasing the ball/object below or in front of the head. Throws involve the upper torso and arms releasing the ball or object above, over, or across the head. Some drills can be combined to form a more complex drill, that is, adding a sprint or multidirectional hop/jump to a depth jump.

To a certain extent, selection of plyometric exercises depends on equipment availability. Although plyometrics can be performed without equipment, some pieces of equipment are needed for some exercises. Common pieces of equipment include cones, boxes, jump ropes, mini-hurdles, bands, bags, weighted vests, medicine balls, slam balls, and core balls. Cones, bags, and hurdles are used as barriers for various hops and jumps. Boxes are used for box jumps, depth jumps, and variations. Jump ropes come in various forms and sizes with some designed for speed and some provide resistance. Bands provide resistance to jumping. Weighted vests can be used for additional resistance during plyometric drills. Medicine, core, and slam balls come in various sizes and are used for upper and lower body plyometrics.

Exercises are selected based on the client's training status and intensity. Plyometric programs begin with low- and moderate-intensity exercises for novice clients and progresses to high-intensity exercises over time. The intensity of plyometric exercises depends on several factors including complexity, loading (*e.g.*, body mass, external loading via vests, weights), velocity of impact, speed, and height and length of boxes or barriers used. Jumps-in-place are lowest in intensity, followed by standing jumps, multiple hops and jumps, bounding, box drills, and depth jumps (see reference Chu [3] for exercise explanations). Single-leg jumps are more intense than comparable double-leg jumps. Intensity is increased by using larger barriers or boxes or by setting cones/barriers farther apart (requiring the client to jump higher or farther). Exercises can be sequenced in numerous ways provided adequate recovery is given in between sets. Some strategies include the following:

- Low-intensity drills can be performed anywhere in sequence (at the beginning following a warm-up or later in the workout after pertinent moderate- and high-intensity drills).
- Moderate- and high-intensity drills are performed near the beginning (following appropriate warm-up and low-intensity drills) while fatigue is minimal.
- When upper body plyometric drills are included, the client may choose to alternate between lower and upper body drills to maximize workout efficiency.

The volume (number of sets and repetitions) of plyometric training varies and depends on intensity and frequency as well as the impact of other modalities, for example, RT and sprint/agility training. Plyometric volume and intensity are inversely related. Chu (3) has recommended volume guidelines for plyometric training (refer to the reference for specifics). Plyometric training typically takes place 1–4 days per week. High-intensity drills may necessitate a lower frequency when depth jumps are performed, and frequency may be lower when other modalities are included. Because of the intense nature of plyometric training, ~48–72 hours of recovery in between training sessions is recommended (3). Trained clients have greater tolerance and can perform high-intensity drills and a higher volume of exercise. Depth jump training requires fewer sets (two to four) of up to five to eight repetitions with long (2–10 min) rest intervals for 1–3 days per week (39). Lower plyometric volume and frequency is needed when training in-season athletes. Sports consist of plyometric actions so practice and competition are training stimuli.

Adequate rest intervals are needed during plyometric training. Rest interval lengths are exercise-specific and intensity-dependent. More rest is needed in between sets of high-intensity exercises (*e.g.*, box jumps, depth jumps) than low- or moderate-intensity exercises (*e.g.*, ankle hops). Work-to-rest ratios of 1:5 (for low- and moderate-intensity exercises) to 1:10 (for high-intensity exercises) are recommended (3). Intra-set rest intervals are used for noncontinuous jumps (*e.g.*, depth jump) or throws. Shorter rest intervals minimize recovery and target power endurance. Box 19.5 depicts a sample plyometric program. This workout trains the entire body and alternates between upper and lower body drills to increase efficiency.

| Box 19.5 | Sample Plyometric Training Program |
| --- | --- |
| General warm-up | 3- to 5-min jog |
| Dynamic ROM drills | 1 × 5 drills |
| Linear sprints | 3 × 20 yd (half speed) |
| Tuck jumps | 3 × 10 |
| Medicine ball side throw | 3 × 8 (each side) |
| Barrier jumps | 5 × 5 |
| Medicine ball back throw | 3 × 5 |
| Single-leg push-off | 3 × 6 (each leg) |
| Plyo push-up | 3 × 10 |
| Box jumps | 3 × 8 |
| Cool-down | Stretching |

## Ballistic Resistance Training

Ballistic RT is a plyometric modality aimed at increasing muscle power and strength. Traditional resistance exercises are performed in a full ROM where noticeable deceleration of the load occurs prior to completion of the CON phase. Deceleration is inevitable because the lifting action must then be reversed (*e.g.*, lowering the weight prior to lifting the weight for the next repetition). The length of the deceleration phase depends on the weight and velocity but may comprise more than 50% of the CON phase when lifting weights lower than 81% of 1-RM (10). However, this deceleration phase limits power development throughout the full ROM. Ballistic RT is designed to minimize deceleration by having the client maximally accelerate the bar throughout the full ROM. Maximal acceleration results in releasing the load (throwing the object) or having the client leave the ground (jump) during a squat-type exercise. Some common ballistic exercises include jump squats, bench press throws, and shoulder press throws. If a linear position transducer is available and attached to the barbell, these exercises may be used to assess peak power in clients (32). Caution must be used because the external load and participant's body weight must be absorbed prior to the next repetition. In lieu of these safety concerns, equipment has been designed using various braking systems to catch or decelerate the weight upon descent. Peak power is produced at loads corresponding to 15%–60% of 1-RM for the jump squat and bench press throw (20), although body weight alone may maximize power output during jump squats (5). Personal Trainers may incorporate ballistic training in various ways. It may be integrated into RT and/or plyometric training workouts. Because of the power component, ballistic exercises are prescribed in a similar manner to Olympic lifts in that they receive priority in sequencing. Loading may vary but tends to be moderate to enable fast lifting velocities. Another programming alternative is to use potentiation to enhance ballistic exercise performance. For example, a Personal Trainer may have the client perform three heavy sets of squats followed by three sets of jump squats. The heavy squats can facilitate recruitment of fast-twitch motor units so that in the absence of fatigue, the jump squats could be performed with greater power output. In addition to power development, ballistic RT can increase maximal strength (14,41) and augment maximal strength development for some exercises (25).

Ballistic resistance training is a plyometric modality aimed at increasing muscle power and strength.

## Speed and Agility Training

Speed and agility are essential athletic components. Speed is the change in distance over time. Maximal speed attainment takes ~20–40 m, so acceleration ability (ability to increase velocity) is a critical training component especially following a change of direction, deceleration, or from a static position. Sprints of at least 60–80 m involve acceleration, maximum speed maintenance, and speed endurance (deceleration). Acceleration is related to the ability to react to a stimulus with a quick first response. Obtaining and maintaining maximal speed are functions of conditioning. Agility comprises the ability to move rapidly while changing direction in response to a stimulus. Agility is complex and requires the optimal integration of several physiologic systems and fitness components. The client must coordinate several movements including the ability to react and start quickly, accelerate, decelerate, move in the proper direction, and maintain the ability to change direction as rapidly as possible while maintaining balance and postural control. The rapid change of direction occurs in a variety of stable or unstable positions (*e.g.*, standing [unilateral or bilateral], lying [prone or supine], seated, and/or kneeling positions).

Speed and agility are essential athletic components.

Sprint speed is the product of stride length and frequency (rate). Stride length is determined by leg length, leg strength and power, and sprinting mechanics. Stride frequency refers to the number of foot contacts per period of time. Maximal sprint speed occurs only at the optimal combination of stride length and frequency. Sprint, plyometric, strength, and ballistic training are the most effective ways to increase stride rate and frequency. An integrated approach is most effective where a combination of plyometric, sprint, flexibility, and RT is used. Sprint training increases acceleration and sprint speed and the combination of sprint and RT enhances maximal speed, speed endurance, power, and strength of the lower body.

Agility requires mobility, coordination, balance, power, SSC efficiency, stabilization, proper technique, strength, flexibility, body control, footwork, a rapid ability to accelerate and decelerate, anticipation, and scanning ability (40,42). Agility training includes multiple modalities including strength and power, sprint, specific agility, balance and coordination, and flexibility training. Exceptional balance is needed to control the COG. Stability is greatest when the COG is low, the base support is large, and the line of gravity is centered within the base support. Force production is greatest in stable body positions. Performing an exercise unilaterally instead of bilaterally, narrowing the base support, and performing an exercise on a stability ball, BOSU ball, balance disc, beam, and wobble board may improve balance. Performing an exercise with one's eyes closed, a combination exercise, or an exercise from an unstable position (*e.g.*, performing a shoulder press from a lunge position), in addition to sprint, plyometric, and agility drills are all ways to improve balance. Proper posture, foot contact with the ground, and arm action are needed during agility movements. Agility drills involve multiple movements including linear sprints, backpedalling, side shuffling, drop stepping, cariocas, cutting, pivoting, jumps, and cross-overs.

Sprint speed can be assessed using the 40-yd dash. Although other tests may be used, the 40-yd dash is common and standards are well-known. Multiple tests can be used to assess agility. Two of the more common assessments are the T-test and the pro-agility test (20-yd shuttle). For the T-test, four cones are needed. Three cones are aligned in a straight line 5 yd apart and a fourth cone is aligned with the second cone 10 yd apart, forming a "T." The client sprints forward 10 yd, shuffles left 5 yd to cone, shuffles right 10 yd to cone, shuffles left to middle cone, and backpedals to starting cone. For the pro-agility test, a football field may be used with parallel lines 5 yd apart. The client begins straddling the center line in a 3-point stance. Upon the start signal, the client sprints 5 yd to the line on the left, sprints right for 10 yd to furthest line, and sprints left for 5 yd to the center line. Both agility tests are timed with a stop watch and the client seeks completing each test in the fastest time as possible.

### Sprint and Agility Training Program Design

Sprint and agility training consists of drills aimed at targeting linear speed and multicapacity movement development (8). Personal Trainers should constantly monitor correct sprinting technique and be instructional to clients during agility drills. Clients should touch or run around cones in control, stay close to cones, have correct foot placement, lower the COG, decelerate and accelerate maximally, and have correct posture and approach angles. Cone lengths (and the number of cones) modulate the level of changing direction and pattern of acceleration/deceleration. Close distances force the client to change direction rapidly without large windows of acceleration, whereas large distances enable the client to accelerate over greater lengths which also creates an opportunity for deceleration management upon changing direction. Drills may be integrated to increase complexity. Agility training can be performed with zero (a lined field) or minimal equipment. The Personal Trainer can expand the client's exercise repertoire by having cones of various sizes, agility ladders, rings and agility dots, reaction balls, bags, tires, mini-hurdles, reaction belts, ropes, and/or agility poles. Speed and agility drills include the following:

- **Form drills:** drills used to improve technique and serve as general warm-up/dynamic ROM exercises such as arm swings, "butt kickers," high knees, ankling, marching, and pawing. Drills are usually performed for one to three sets for 20–30 yd.
- **Linear sprints:** sprints of various length. Short sprints (10–20 yd) are used for improving acceleration, moderate sprints (40–60 yd) are used for improving acceleration and maximal speed, and longer sprints (>60 yd) are used for improving all facets of sprinting especially speed endurance.

These sprints are performed with maximal effort. Other variations may be used. For example, a drill called *gears* can be used. The client may sprint for 100 yd. Cones could be set every 25 yd. The client runs ~50% intensity the first 25 yd, accelerates and runs faster upon reaching the second and third 25-yd markers, and will sprint maximally the last 25 yd. This helps improve acceleration ability from a running start and maximal speed. The drill falling starts can be used to improve acceleration from an unstable position. The client leans and falls forward (or can be pushed by a partner), braces, and subsequently sprints forward for the desired distance. Linear sprint drills are the most specific way to increase sprint speed.

■ **Overspeed training:** allows the client to attain supramaximal speed (by increasing stride length and frequency), or an assisted speed that is greater than maximal effort. Supramaximal speed can be achieved with a tail wind, downhill running (~1°–7° for ~50 m), towing, and high-speed treadmill running. The supramaximal velocity attained should not exceed a value >10% greater than the client's own ability or technical breakdowns could occur. Overspeed training is most effective when performed early in the workout where the client's energy levels are high and fatigue is minimal. For towing, elastic tubing (Bungee cord, latex tubing) can be used and attached around the client's waist. The opposite end can be attached to another athlete or a stationary object. The force of the tubing (from stretching) propels the client forward thereby allowing the client to increase stride length and frequency. If a stationary object is used, the client can attach the tubing in front, back up several yards, and begin running while being towed by the elastic tubing. The farther the distance, the greater the stretching of the tubing as more force will be applied to the client. The client may connect the other end of the tubing to another client or the Personal Trainer. The client can attach the tubing in front while the other client doing the towing can attach the other end of the tubing to their rear. The lead client begins sprinting and tows the rear client. Towing can be used for other drills such as backpedalling and side-to-side movements as well.

■ **Resisted sprint training:** The client sprints maximally against a resistance. Resistance may come in the form of wind (headwind), sleds, speed chutes, sand, weighted vests, harnesses, partner, stairs, and hills. Sleds are made of steel, have a handle and/or harness attachment, and have posts for plate loading. Loads of up to ~10% of body mass (for sprints of 10–50 yd) are typically used for speed training. A speed chute opens thereby increasing resistance as the client accelerates. Chutes come in different sizes and provide various levels of resistance especially at higher speeds of motion. Weighted vests are light, durable, and have the capacity for external loading (perhaps 10–20 lb or more). They are multipurpose and can be used for plyometric, agility, calisthenics, body weight, and sport-specific exercises. A harness can be used between two clients where the trailing client can provide resistance to the lead client. Enough resistance should be applied to allow the lead client to sprint to ~85%–90% of max speed. Some harnesses have a quick release mechanism which allows the cord to disengage enabling the lead client to continue sprinting without resistance. These can be used for other modalities besides linear sprinting, for example, backpedalling, lateral movements.

■ **Programmed agility drills:** those that are preplanned where the client is aware of the movements prior to beginning the drill. Some examples include the T-drill, square drill, 20-yd shuttle, figure-8 drill, and right triangle drill. There are numerous programmed drills that can be prescribed to a client. Drills should encompass the basic movements of linear sprints, accelerations/ decelerations, backpedalling, side and diagonal shuffling, cariocas, cutting, and pivoting.

■ **Reactive agility drills:** drills continued based on information from a Personal Trainer or object such as a ball. The client must react to a stimulus. Some examples include box jump with multidirection sprint, partner shadow or mirror drills, slap or tag drills, and drills that involve ball tosses and catching (*e.g.*, the blind partner toss).

■ **Quickness agility drills:** drills designed to produce fast movements and quick feet. Some examples include agility ladder drills, pop-up drills (from the ground), down-and-up drills (sprawl in wrestling, burpee), and the resisted let-go. Numerous ladder drills can be prescribed to the client. Some common ladder drills include ins and outs, hopscotch, two-in lateral shuffle, and the side rocker.

| Box 19.6 | Sample Combined Sprint and Agility Workout |
|---|---|
| General warm-up | 3- to 5-min jog |
| Dynamic ROM drills | 1 × 5 drills (callisthenic-type exercises to warm-up client in lieu of excessive static stretching) |
| High knees | 2 × 20 yd |
| Butt kickers | 2 × 20 yd |
| Backpedals | 2 × 20 yd |
| Side shuffles | 2 × 20 yd |
| Cariocas | 2 × 20 yd |
| Ladder ins and outs | 3 repetitions |
| 20-yd shuttle | 3 repetitions |
| Sprints | 6 × 40 yd |
| Flying sprints | 3 × 40 yd |
| Cool-down | Stretching |

Novice sprint and agility programs should focus on proper technique and footwork using basic drills. Basic drills have low levels of footwork complexity and change of directions. Complexity increases intensity. High-intensity agility drills include those with complex movement patterns, multiple directions, involve high rates of acceleration/deceleration, are reactive, and may incorporate some moderate-to-high plyometric drills in addition to basic agility movements. Similar to other modalities of training, variation of volume and intensity of sprint and agility is more conducive to progression rather than just increasing each over time. Box 19.6 depicts a sample combined sprint and agility workout that is an integrated approach, where both components are trained in a single workout. It is important to note that the Personal Trainer can prescribe and supervise independent sprint and agility workouts. In this case, the format may be similar except each workout comprises all speed or agility drills only.

## Anaerobic Conditioning

*Anaerobic conditioning* is a term that refers to high-intensity muscle endurance capacity (32). It comprises the ability to perform near-maximal to maximal exercise for an extended period of time. Anaerobic conditioning consists of exercises targeting speed, power, and strength endurance. Speed and agility endurance enhancement enables the client to maintain maximal speed and agility performance over time. Speed endurance training is characterized by longer sprints (30->300 yd for running and swimming, but possibly longer distances for cycling) and reduced rest intervals in between sets and repetitions of exercise ranging between 75%–100% of maximal speed (4). Drills consist of repeated sprints, interval sprints, and relays. Interval training allows the client to train at higher intensities while improving anaerobic and aerobic capacities. Low-intensity bouts of exercise interspersed in between high-intensity bouts allow the client to achieve higher net workout intensity. Intervals using a 1:1 ratio target aerobic capacity, whereas greater work-to-relief ratios (*e.g.*, 1:5 or 1:10) target anaerobic conditioning (ATP-PC and glycolysis energy systems; for more information on energy systems, see Chapter 5). Agility and plyometric drills can be used in standard set format (high repetitions, moderate set duration with rest intervals) or in circuit training format. For speed endurance training involving low- to moderate-intensity drills for moderate distances, 8–20 repetitions have been recommended for advanced clients and 5–12 for novice clients (30). For speed endurance training involving high-intensity drills for short to moderate distances, 4–12 repetitions have been recommended for advanced clients and 4–8 for novice clients (30).

Anaerobic conditioning can also be improved by inclusion of weight training, body weight, or implement training. Circuits allow the client to perform several exercises in a short period of time yielding substantial metabolic and cardiovascular responses that could improve aerobic capacity as well. Circuit progression entails increasing the load, repetitions, duration or length of drill, and reducing the total time needed to complete the entire circuit (*e.g., timed circuits*). Timed circuits are beneficial because they can enhance the power component. Fatigue results in slower repetitions and performance. Thus, a reduced time to complete a circuit indicates improved endurance as the client can maintain a better pace and movement velocity. Metabolic circuits have become popular among athletes and fitness enthusiasts to improve muscle endurance, aerobic capacity, and reduce percent body fat.

Anaerobic capacity can be assessed in many ways. Two common assessments include the 300-yd shuttle and the line drill. The 300-yd shuttle requires two parallel lines 25 yd apart. The client sprints as fast as possible from one line to other line and immediately sprints back to the starting line for six continuous round trips. For the line drill, a basketball court is typically used. The client begins at the baseline, sprints to the foul line and back, sprints from the baseline to the half-court line and back, sprints from the baseline to the far foul line and back, and sprints from the baseline to the far baseline and back continuously. Multiple trials can be given for each test and the best time or average of each test can be recorded. These are fatiguing tests, so plenty of rest (at least 3–4 min) should be given in between trials.

> Circuits allow the client to perform several exercises in a short period of time yielding substantial metabolic and cardiovascular responses that could improve aerobic capacity as well.

## SUMMARY

The Personal Training profession has evolved to accommodated athletes and those clients with advanced training status/goals. Personal Trainers have a unique niche in providing one-on-one individualized training services for advanced clients. Thus, Personal Trainers must have knowledge and proficiencies of advanced training concepts before implementing these techniques to maximize safety within client training programs Advanced training encompasses the potential prescription and supervision of periodized resistance, plyometric, sprint, agility, and anaerobic conditioning training programs to clients seeking to maximize several health- and skill-related components of fitness.

> For more details on training and testing of athletes, consult *ACSM's Foundations of Strength Training and Conditioning* (32).

## REFERENCES

1. American College of Sports Medicine. American College of Sports Medicine position stand. Progression models in resistance training for healthy adults. *Med Sci Sports Exerc.* 2002;34:364–80.

2. American College of Sports Medicine. American College of Sports Medicine position stand. Progression models in resistance training for healthy adults. *Med Sci Sports Exerc.* 2009;41:687–708.

3. Chu DA. *Jumping into Plyometrics*. 2nd ed. Champaign (IL): Human Kinetics: 1998. 177 p.

4. Cissik JM, Barnes M. *Sport Speed and Agility*. Monterey (CA): Coaches Choice; 2004. 256 p.

5. Cormie P, McCaulley GO, McBride JM. Power versus strength-power jump squat training: influence on the load-power relationship. *Med Sci Sports Exerc.* 2007;39:996–1003.

6. Denton J, Cronin JB. Kinematic, kinetic, and blood lactate profiles of continuous and intraset rest loading schemes. *J Strength Cond Res.* 2006;20:528–34.

7. de Villarreal ES, González-Badillo JJ, Izquierdo M. Low and moderate plyometric training frequency produces greater jumping and sprinting gains compared with high frequency. *J Strength Cond Res.* 2008;22:715–25.

8. Dintiman G, Ward B, Tellez T. *Sports Speed*: #1 Program for Athletes. 2nd ed. Champaign (IL): Human Kinetics; 1998. 224 p.

9. Dodd DJ, Alvar BA. Analysis of acute explosive training modalities to improve lower-body power in baseball players. *J Strength Cond Res.* 2007;21:1177–82.

10. Elliott BC, Wilson GJ, Kerr GK. A biomechanical analysis of the sticking region in the bench press. *Med Sci Sports Exerc.* 1989;21:450–62.

11. Faigenbaum AD, Kraemer WJ, Blimkie CJR, et al. Youth resistance training: updated position statement paper from the National Strength and Conditioning Association. *J Strength Cond Res.* 2009;23:S60–79.

12. Fleck SJ, Kraemer WJ. *Designing Resistance Training Programs.* 3rd ed. Champaign (IL): Human Kinetics; 2004. 377 p.

13. Garstecki MA, Latin RW, Cuppett MM. Comparison of selected physical fitness and performance variables between NCAA Division I and II football players. *J Strength Cond Res.* 2004;18:292–7.

14. Harris NK, Cronin JB, Hopkins WG, Hansen KT. Squat jump training at maximal power loads vs. heavy loads: effect on sprint ability. *J Strength Cond Res.* 2008;22:1742–9.

15. Hoffman J. *Norms for Fitness, Performance, and Health.* Champaign (IL): Human Kinetics; 2006. 232 p.

16. Hoffman J. Endurance training. In: *Physiological Aspects of Sport Training and Performance.* Champaign (IL): Human Kinetics; 2002. p. 109–19.

17. Hoffman JR, Ratamess NA. *A Practical Guide to Developing Resistance Training Programs.* 2nd ed. Monterey (CA): Coaches Choice Books; 2008. 200 p.

18. Holcomb WR, Lander JE, Rutland RM, Wilson GD. The effectiveness of a modified plyometric program on power and the vertical jump. *J Strength Cond Res.* 1996;10:89–92.

19. Kawamori N, Crum AJ, Blumert PA, et al. Influence of different relative intensities on power output during the hang power clean: identification of the optimal load. *J Strength Cond Res.* 2005;19:698–708.

20. Kawamori N, Haff GG. The optimal training load for the development of muscular power. *J Strength Cond Res.* 2004; 18:675–84.

21. Kraemer WJ. A series of studies-the physiological basis for strength training in American football: fact over philosophy. *J Strength Cond Res.* 1997;11:131–42.

22. Kraemer WJ, Fry AC, Ratamess NA, French DN. Strength testing: Development and evaluation of methodology. In: Maud PJ, Foster C, editors. *Physiological Assessments of Human Performance.* 2nd ed. Champaign (IL): Human Kinetics; 2006. p. 119–50.

23. Kraemer WJ, Ratamess NA. Fundamentals of resistance training: progression and exercise prescription. *Med Sci Sport Exerc.* 2004;36:674–88.

24. Lephart SM, Abt JP, Ferris CM, et al. Neuromuscular and biomechanical characteristic changes in high school athletes: a plyometric versus basic resistance program. *Br J Sports Med.* 2005;39:932–8.

25. Mangine GT, Ratamess NA, Hoffman JR, Faigenbaum AD, Kang J, Chilakos A. The effects of combined ballistic and heavy resistance training on maximal lower- and upper-body strength in recreationally-trained men. *J Strength Cond Res.* 2008;22:132–9.

26. Marcovic G. Does plyometric training improve vertical jump height? A meta-analytical review. *Br J Sports Med.* 2007;41:349–55.

27. Mazzetti SA, Kraemer WJ, Volek JS, et al. The influence of direct supervision of resistance training on strength performance. *Med Sci Sports Exerc.* 2000;32:1175–84.

28. McGuigan M, Ratamess NA. Strength. In: Ackland TR, Elliott BC, Bloomfield J, editors. *Applied Anatomy and Biomechanics in Sport.* 2nd ed. Champaign (IL): Human Kinetics; 2009. p. 119–54.

29. Mookerjee S, Ratamess NA. Comparison of strength differences and joint action durations between full and partial range-of-motion bench press exercise. *J Strength Cond Res.* 1999;13:76–81.

30. Plisk SS. Speed, agility, and speed-endurance development. In: Baechle TR, Earle RW, editors. *Essentials of Strength Training and Conditioning.* 3rd ed. Champaign (IL): Human Kinetics; 2008. p. 455–85.

31. Potteiger JA, Lockwood RH, Haub MD, et al. Muscle power and fiber characteristics following 8 weeks of plyometric training. *J Strength Cond Res.* 1999;13:275–9.

32. Ratamess N. *ACSM's Foundation of Strength Training and Conditioning.* Philadelphia (PA): Wolters Kluwer/ Lippincott Williams & Wilkins; 2012. 500 p.

33. Ratamess NA, Faigenbaum AD, Hoffman JR, Kang J. Self-selected resistance training intensity in healthy women: the influence of a personal trainer. *J Strength Cond Res.* 2008; 22:103–11.

34. Ratamess NA, Faigenbaum AD, Mangine GT, Hoffman JR, Kang J. Acute muscular strength assessment using free weight bars of different thickness. *J Strength Cond Res.* 2007; 21:240–4.

35. Ratamess NA, Kraemer WJ, Volek JS, et al. The effects of ten weeks of resistance and combined plyometric/sprint training with the Meridian Elyte athletic shoe on muscular performance in women. *J Strength Cond Res.* 2007;21:882–7.

36. Simmons L. What if? *MILO.* 1996;4:25–9.

37. Souza-Junior TP, Willardson JM, Bloomer R, et al. Strength and hypertrophy responses to constant and decreasing rest intervals in trained men using creatine supplementation. *J Int Soc Sports Nutr.* 2011;8:1–11.

38. Stone MH, Stone M, Sands WA. *Principles and Practice of Resistance Training.* Champaign (IL): Human Kinetics; 2007. 384 p.

39. Verkhoshansky Y, Siff M. *Supertraining.* 6th ed. Denver (CO): Supertraining International; 2009. 578 p.

40. Verstegen M, Marcello B. Agility and coordination. In: Foran B, editor. *High-Performance Sports Conditioning.* Champaign (IL): Human Kinetics; 2001. p. 139–65.

41. Vissing K, Brink M, Lønbro S, et al. Muscle adaptations to plyometric vs. resistance training in untrained young men. *J Strength Cond Res.* 2008;22:1799–810.

42. Young WB, Farrow D. A review of agility: practical applications for strength and conditioning. *Strength Cond J.* 2006;28:24–9.

43. Zatsiorsky V, Kraemer WJ. *Science and Practice of Strength Training.* 2nd ed. Champaign (IL): Human Kinetics; 2006. 264 p.

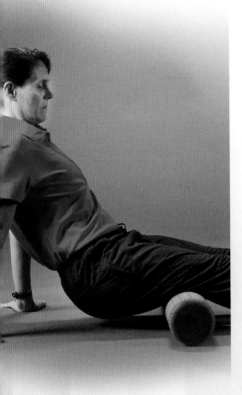

# Special Populations

## OBJECTIVES

**Personal Trainers should be able to:**

- Understand the value of physical activity for children and create age-appropriate exercise programs.

- Understand physiological changes with aging and create age-appropriate exercise programs for older adults.

- Describe exercise programming for clients with cardiovascular disease, diabetes, and hypertension.

- Describe exercise programming during pregnancy and postpartum.

- Describe exercise programming for obese clients.

- Understand how to create exercise programs for individuals with comorbidities.

## INTRODUCTION

According to the Centers for Disease Control and Prevention, less than one-third (30%) of U.S. adults report no leisure-time physical activity and almost 50% do not meet the 2008 Physical Activity Guidelines for adults (14). Physical inactivity is associated with numerous unhealthy conditions, including obesity, hypertension, gestational and Type 2 diabetes, and atherosclerotic cardiovascular disease (CVD) and contributes annually to 250,000 premature deaths (20,96). Overall, children are more active than their adult counterparts are; however, only the youngest children actually fulfill current physical activity guidelines. Older Americans are clearly the least physically active, with almost 40% reporting no leisure-time activity (14). Currently and over the next couple of decades, millions of baby boomers will continue to turn 65 years of age (91). In addition, current trends also show that although Americans are living longer, the number of individuals with chronic diseases continues to increase. Collectively, these factors make it increasingly likely that the Personal Trainer will be interacting with clientele who are other than apparently healthy adults. This chapter discusses the special considerations and scope of practice of exercise program design for the following subpopulations: children, older adults, cardiac disease, pregnancy, diabetes mellitus, obesity, hypertension, and individuals with comorbidities.

##  Programming for Children

*Physical Activity Guidelines* published in 2008 advocate for children to participate in at least 60 minutes per day of moderate- to vigorous-intensity physical activity and to include resistance exercise and bone-loading activity on at least 3 days per week (121).

Children and adolescents include individuals 6–17 years of age. *Physical Activity Guidelines* published in 2008 advocate for children to participate in at least 60 minutes per day of moderate- to vigorous-intensity physical activity and to include resistance exercise and bone-loading activity on at least 3 days per week (121). Unfortunately, after about age 10 years, most young people do not meet the physical activity guidelines.

Most young people are healthy, and thus, it is safe for them to initiate moderate-intensity activities without medical screening (5). Medical exams and exercise testing prior to participation generally are unnecessary in this population unless clinically indicated. The physiological responses to acute exercise in children are comparable to their adult counterparts with expected quantitative differences attributable to lean body mass and height disparities between the two populations (5). Table 20.1 indicates some of the key comparisons between adults and children. Children have lower anaerobic capacities compared with adults, which limits their potential for higher intensity exercise performance. When designing an exercise program for children and adolescents, the American College of Sports Medicine (ACSM) recommends three target areas: aerobic endurance, muscular strengthening, and bone strengthening activities (5). Regular endurance, resistance, and bone-loading exercise will confer favorable training adaptations in children, resulting in benefits to cardiovascular, metabolic, and skeletal health.

Regular endurance, resistance, and bone-loading exercise will confer favorable training adaptations in children, resulting in benefits to cardiovascular, metabolic, and skeletal health.

| Table 20.1 | Physiological Responses to Acute Exercise in Children Compared to Adults |
|---|---|
| **Variable** | **Difference** |
| Absolute oxygen uptake ($\dot{V}O_2$ in L · min$^{-1}$) | ↓ |
| Relative oxygen uptake ($\dot{V}O_2$ in mL · kg · min$^{-1}$) | ↑ |
| Cardiac output | ↓ |
| Heart rate | ↑ |
| Stroke volume | ↓ |
| Respiratory rate | ↑ |
| Minute ventilation (VE) | ↓ |
| Respiratory exchange ratio | ↓ |
| Systolic blood pressure | ↓ |
| Diastolic blood pressure | ↓ |

Adapted with permission from American College of Sports Medicine. *ACSM's Guidelines for Exercise Testing and Prescription.* 10th ed. Philadelphia (PA): Wolters Kluwer; 2018.

## Physical Activity for Children

As previously stated, many children do not meet current physical activity guidelines. Thus, a role of the Personal Trainer is to help identify a variety of age-appropriate activities for children that will safely and effectively develop aerobic, muscular, and bone strength. In addition, the Personal Trainer should work with parents/guardians to help develop and implement plans for their children to lessen the amount of time spent in sedentary activities (*e.g.*, watching television or movies, time on computer, or playing video games) while simultaneously increasing activities that encourages physical activity. Children who have been previously sedentary may be unable to initially achieve 60 minutes per day of physical activity. In these instances, it is prudent for the Personal Trainer to gradually progress the volume of physical activity upward over several months to ultimately achieve the 60-minute-per-day goal.

A role of the Personal Trainer is to help identify a variety of age-appropriate activities for children that will safely and effectively develop aerobic, muscular, and bone strength.

In general, the exercise prescription for children should follow the frequency, intensity, time, type, volume, and progression (FITT-VP) framework. Table 20.2 summarizes the youth physical activity guidelines (121). Personal Trainers should design physical activity programs for children with two primary goals in mind (4):

1. The program should fulfill the minimal amount of physical activity needed to achieve the health benefits associated with regular physical activity.
2. Children should be encouraged to participate in a variety of physical activities that are enjoyable and age-appropriate. Keeping activity fun and safe is important when working with children.

## Other Considerations for Children

Traditional resistance-training activities for children are generally safe and appropriate for children provided they receive proper instruction and supervision (5). By age 7 or 8 years, children should be physically and mentally mature enough to initiate a resistance-training program (49). The general

| Table 20.2 | Summary of Aerobic, Resistance, and Bone-Loading Activity Guidelines for Children | | |
|---|---|---|---|
| Parameter | Aerobic Activity | Resistance Activity | Bone-Loading Activity |
| Mode | Activities include running, hopping, swimming, dancing, and bicycling. | Can be unstructured (*e.g.*, playing on playground equipment, climbing trees, tug of war) or structured (*e.g.*, lifting weights, use of resistance bands) | Activities include running, jumping rope, basketball, tennis, and hopscotch. |
| Intensity | Moderate-intensity activity most days; corresponds to noticeable ↑ heart rate and breathing. Vigorous-intensity activity minimum of 3 d · wk$^{-1}$; corresponds to substantial ↑ heart rate and quick breathing | Use body weight as resistance or 8–15 submaximal repetitions to moderate fatigue all performed with good technique. | No specific recommendation; however, avoid extreme intensity. |
| Duration | ≥60 min · d$^{-1}$ | Included with the ≥60 min · d$^{-1}$ | Included with the ≥60 min · d$^{-1}$ |
| Frequency | Daily | ≥3 d · wk$^{-1}$ | ≥3 d · wk$^{-1}$ |

Adapted with permission from U.S. Department of Health and Human Services. *2008 Physical Activity Guidelines for Americans* [Internet]. Washington (DC): U.S. Department of Health and Human Services; [cited 2011 Mar 7]. Available from: http://www.health.gov/PAGuidelines /guidelines/default.aspx; American College of Sports Medicine. *ACSM's Guidelines for Exercise Testing and Prescription*. 10th ed. Philadelphia (PA): Wolters Kluwer; 2018.

resistance-training principles detailed earlier for adults (Chapter 14) can also be applied to children. However, it is critical that the Personal Trainer provide sufficient instruction on proper lifting technique and safety measures and closely supervise all training sessions. Modalities could include resistance machines, free weights (preferably dumbbells with younger ages), resistance bands, medicine balls, smaller kettle bells, cable machines, and body weight activities. If resistance machines are to be used, they should be designed to specifically fit children's body size to enhance the training response and decrease risk of injury. Therefore, employing adult-size machines in a child's resistance exercise program should be avoided. For younger children, unstructured muscle strengthening activities (*e.g.*, playing on playground equipment) can also be included within the 60 minutes per day of physical activity (5).

Children have underdeveloped thermoregulatory systems and subsequently are more prone to heat injuries than their adult counterparts (5). Personal Trainers should ensure that children remain properly hydrated and when possible encourage activity in thermoneutral environments.

Lastly, although most children are healthy, Personal Trainers may encounter children with health issues or disabilities such as asthma, Type 1 diabetes, or cerebral palsy. In this situation, Personal Trainers should consult with the child's medical team and familiarize themselves with the specific exercise recommendations for the disease or disability present in that child. Then, the Personal Trainer should adapt the physical activity program for these individuals according to their condition, symptoms, and functional capacity (4,90).

## Programming for Older Adults

Aging is a universal experience. Life expectancy in the United States has risen nearly 30 years since 1900 (37) and is 81.2 years for women and 76.4 years for men (11). Older adults are defined as men and women 65 years and older and/or adults age 50–64 years with clinically significant chronic conditions and/or functional limitations that impact movement ability, fitness, or physical activity (91). Each system in the body responds to aging differently. Thus, one's chronological age cannot be assumed equivalent to one's physiological or functional age. Individuals of similar ages can differ remarkably in functional capacity, which in turn will affect how they respond to exercise.

Although it is inevitable that physiological function declines with age, the rate and magnitude of change are dependent on a complex mixture of genetics, individual health, presence of disease/injury,

> Individuals of similar ages can differ remarkably in functional capacity, which in turn will affect how they respond to exercise.

and exercise history. Safe and effective exercise programming for older adults requires that Personal Trainers have knowledge of these age-related changes on physiological function at rest and throughout the exercise-intensity spectrum. A list of key physiological aspects of aging is presented in Table 20.3.

## Physiological Changes with Aging

Even though resting heart rate remains relatively unchanged (50), maximum heart rate declines steadily with increasing age (58). Maximum stroke volume (amount of blood pumped per heart beat) and maximum cardiac output (blood flow out of the heart per minute) likewise decline with age. Maximum stroke volume declines by 10% and maximum cardiac output declines by 20% in the three decades between age 30 and 60 years (114). These changes lead to reduced exercise capacity with declines in maximal volume of oxygen consumed per unit time ($\dot{V}O_{2max}$) of about 9% per decade in healthy sedentary adults, and this rate of decline progressively increases in old age

| Table 20.3 | Physiological Aspects of Aging | |
|---|---|---|
| **System** | **Parameter** | **Change** |
| Cardiovascular | Maximal heart rate and stroke volume | ↓ |
| | Maximal cardiac output | ↓ |
| | Resting and exercise blood pressure | ↑ |
| | Maximal oxygen consumption | ↓ |
| Environmental | Cold tolerance (heat production/blood redistribution) | ↓ |
| | Heat tolerance (sweat capacity/blood redistribution) | ↓ |
| Musculoskeletal | Lean body mass | ↓ |
| | Fat mass | ↑ |
| | Muscle strength | ↓ |
| | Bone mineral density | ↓ |
| | Flexibility | ↓ |
| Metabolic | Glucose tolerance | ↓ |
| | Insulin sensitivity | ↓ |
| Other | Balance | ↓ |
| | Reaction time | ↑[a] |

[a]Reaction time increases with age (*i.e.*, it will take longer to accomplish a task).
Adapted from American College of Sports Medicine. *ACSM's Guidelines for Exercise Testing and Prescription.* 10th ed. Philadelphia (PA): Wolters Kluwer; 2018.

(32,37,128). As a result, the functional capacity of the average sedentary person declines by 30% between the ages of 30 and 70 years (114).

Anaerobic capacity also declines with increasing age leading to a reduced ability to perform high-intensity exercise. Maximum blood lactate production, tolerance, and clearance rate after exercise decline (32,39). Blood vessels stiffen and become less able to expand when pulses of blood surge through leading to increased resting and exercise systolic blood pressure (37), making the heart work harder and increasing risk of CVD. The prevalence of hypertension greatly increases with age. For example, those with "normal" blood pressure at age 55 years have a 90% risk of developing hypertension over the remainder of their life (31,123). Blood vessels become longer and more convoluted, and their walls thicken, leading to a greater likelihood of impairment in the delivery of oxygen to tissues (64). Total body water declines with increasing age contributing to decreased blood volume and impaired thirst sensation. In males, total body water decreases about 0.3 kg per year after age 30 years, and in females, by 0.7 kg per year after age 70 years (37). These changes predispose the older person to reduced exercise capacity, dehydration, and impaired exercise tolerance in hot and humid weather (32).

Between age 45 and 85 years, there is a progressive decline in brain blood flow and a 20% decrease in brain weight, largely due to loss of fluid and nerve conduction velocity slows by 10%–15% causing slower reaction times and slower voluntary movements (114). These decrements in nerve conduction velocity are thought to contribute to some of the losses in muscular strength that occur with advancing age (88,110). However, the main culprit in decreased muscular strength with increasing age is a 30%–50% decrease in muscle mass between age 30 and 80 years due to decrease in the number of muscle fibers and greater atrophy of type II (fast-twitch) muscle fibers compared with type I fibers (10,37,77). As power is a function of both strength and speed of movement, these muscle fiber changes mean that power output declines at a faster rate than strength alone. Lower body strength declines more rapidly than upper body strength (32,64). Muscular endurance also declines with age, although it does not decrease as quickly as power (32). It isn't just the muscles that become weaker with advancing age. The connective tissue, ligaments, cartilage, tendons, and bones also weaken and become less flexible in old age (32,37). The weakening of bones (osteoporosis) occurs in both males and females; however, the problem is more prevalent in females, particularly after menopause. Females lose about 1% of bone density per year after 35 years of age, accelerating to 2%–3% per year for several years after menopause (32,37). Degeneration of the elastic components of connective tissue leads to a loss of mobility and stability in the joints. Even though muscles and bones become weaker through atrophy, body weight actually increases in the 30s, 40s, and 50s through a progressive accumulation of body fat, particularly in the abdominal region. After age 70 years, body weight starts to decline (32).

## Exercise Training Can Make a Difference

One might ask the question whether all these decrements are inevitably caused by biological aging or if exercise can counteract some of them. The answer is that only about 50% of the decrements noted earlier are due to actual aging, whereas the other 50% are due to sedentary living and can be altered with exercise (32,37,64,70). Thus, older adults should be counseled to avoid physical *inactivity* (79). Being regularly active throughout life not only significantly minimizes the normal age-related changes but also restores functional capacity in previously sedentary adults. Anaerobic, aerobic, and resistance-training exercise programs can increase aerobic capacity and muscular strength by 20%–30% or more, respectively, in older adults (32,65). These improvements are quite similar to those seen in young adults when compared based on relative change (relative to maximal capacity) and can occur at least into the 70s. Aerobic training may actually improve exercise efficiency to a greater extent in the elderly as compared with the young (130).

Older adults should be counseled to avoid physical inactivity (79).

## Successful Aging

Exercise not only improves quality of life but also increases the length of life. A meta-analysis of 38 studies found that regular physical activity at a mild to moderate intensity was strongly associated with a reduction in all-cause mortality in active compared with sedentary individuals (84). In everyday life, functional tasks like getting up out of a chair, climbing stairs, bringing in the groceries, and keeping the house clean require at least minimal levels of cardiovascular endurance, muscular strength, endurance and power, flexibility, and balance. Approaching or falling below these threshold levels has the effect of limiting participation in life and reducing independence. Regular involvement in aerobic, anaerobic, resistance, flexibility, and functional training is a key element of successful aging (32,36).

> Regular involvement in aerobic, anaerobic, resistance, flexibility, and functional training is a key element of successful aging (32).

## Exercise Testing in Older Adults

The likelihood is high that older adults will have clinically significant or underlying chronic disease. Thus, it is imperative that Personal Trainers complete a thorough preparticipation health screening and assessment (as detailed in Chapters 11 and 12) before beginning an exercise program with this population. A sedentary, asymptomatic older person can initiate low- to moderate-intensity exercise without medical evaluation (5). However, for sedentary older adults with known cardiovascular, metabolic, or renal disease and/or signs or symptoms suggestive of these diseases (see Chapter 11), a medical clearance is recommended before starting an exercise program (5). Exercise testing can determine functional capacity, help establish a safe exercise prescription and can enable monitoring of progress in an exercise program. ACSM (5) describes contraindications to exercise testing and participation in older individuals and provides detail on exercise testing. The main objective for working with older clients is to enhance and support "successful aging." Personal Trainers should design programs for older adults with three primary goals in mind:

1. Prevent or delay the progression of chronic diseases (and/or possibly "reverse" symptoms as in normalizing blood glucose).
2. Maintain or enhance cardiorespiratory fitness levels (*i.e.*, functional capacity).
3. Prevent functional limitations and disabilities.

## Design Considerations for Developing Cardiorespiratory Fitness in Older Adults

Cardiorespiratory fitness is arguably the most important goal of an exercise program for older adults. Low cardiorespiratory fitness contributes to premature mortality in middle-aged and older adults (51,128), and for every 10% improvement in cardiorespiratory fitness, one may expect a 15% reduction in overall mortality (16,43,92). Moreover, decreased cardiorespiratory fitness contributes to a reduction in physiological functional capacity and eventually can result in loss of independence (38,60). Sometimes because of the natural decline in function associated with aging, the Personal Trainer may need to interpret "no change" or "maintenance of function" as a successful outcome when working with older adults. For example, a Personal Trainer who works with an older client for 2–3 years and observes "no change" in the client's cardiorespiratory fitness level over that time can conclude that the program was effective. Why? The inevitable decline in physiological function, in this case cardiorespiratory fitness, has been delayed. In summary, normal age-related changes are minimized by being regularly active throughout life; additionally, a restorative function may be seen in cases where a sedentary lifestyle has been replaced by regular physical activity.

> Being regularly active throughout life not only significantly minimizes the normal age-related changes but also restores functional capacity in previously sedentary adults.

An exercise program should be based on exercise testing results, consider the person's preferences and capabilities, be individualized, and provide regular and meaningful feedback as support for long-term adherence. When working with an older client, plan warm-up (minimum of 5–10 min) with gentle dynamic stretching to gradually ease the person from rest to the chosen exercise intensity. A deliberate cool-down (minimum of 5–10 min) should gradually bring the person back to resting levels after exercise. In general, physical activity programs for older adults should be designed to meet the current recommendations of 30 minutes per day of moderate-intensity cardiorespiratory exercise on 5 days each week (or 150 min $\cdot$ wk$^{-1}$) or vigorous-intensity aerobic activity for a minimum of 20 minutes on 3 days each week (or 75 min $\cdot$ wk$^{-1}$) or an equivalent combination of both (5). When not feasible for older adults to fulfill these guidelines due to debilitating chronic conditions, Personal Trainers should encourage these individuals to be as physically active as their condition permits (5).

Exercise intensity for older adults is defined relative to individual fitness using a perceived physical exertion scale of 0–10 for which 0 is equivalent to sitting and 10 is maximal effort. Moderate-intensity activity is considered as a 5 or 6 and vigorous-intensity activity as a 7 or 8 (5). If moderate-intensity activities are included, then a target of 30 minutes per day (with even greater benefits for up to 60 min $\cdot$ d$^{-1}$) is recommended on at least 5 days per week. The exercise does not need to be continuous but can be accumulated in 10-minute bouts. Overall, on a weekly basis, 150–300 minutes per week of moderate-intensity physical activity is recommended (5). For those able and interested in engaging in vigorous-intensity activity, target at least 20–30 minutes per day on 3 or more days per week (total of 75–100 min $\cdot$ wk$^{-1}$) (5). An equivalent combination of moderate and vigorous activity can also be prescribed. Walking is the most common activity for older adults, although any activity that does not present excessive orthopedic stress can be included (5). In summary, the cardiorespiratory training principles detailed in Chapter 15 apply to older adults, although depending on the disease and functional status of the individual, the Personal Trainer must also consider medications, risk factor profile, and behavioral issues and modify the program accordingly. Table 20.4 outlines some of the program modifications that could be considered when working with older adults with functional impairments.

## Design Considerations for Developing Muscular Strength in Older Adults

Aging is associated with a reduction in muscle mass, which in turn contributes to decreased muscle strength and a decline in functional capacity. Undeterred, the process can ultimately result in reduced balance ability, mobility problems, and lack of independence for the older adult (99). Furthermore, decreased muscle mass plays a role in the development of glucose intolerance and Type 2 diabetes.

The Personal Trainer should recognize the importance of implementing a resistance-training program for older adult clients to attenuate the loss of muscle mass and protein (77,109). Muscle fiber size and performance, particularly the rate of force development, are consistently higher in older adults who are chronically exposed to strength training (1). Furthermore, some studies have suggested that resistance training can improve cognition, mood, self-confidence, and self-esteem (42,64,73,102).

When designing a resistance-training program for older individuals, the general resistance-training principles detailed earlier (Chapter 14) can be applied. In fact, in certain elderly clients, even explosive-type heavy resistance exercise has been shown to be safe and effective (26). However, it is critical that the Personal Trainer provide sufficient instruction on proper lifting technique and good posture. Initially, beginners may benefit from using weight training or resistance machines. Weight training machines leave less room for error in body position, and they safely enable larger absolute loads to be lifted. If weight-training machines are used with

| Table 20.4 | Aerobic Exercise Program Modifications for Older Adults |
|---|---|
| **Program Component** | **Program Modification** |
| Exercise mode | ■ Walking is an excellent mode of exercise for many older adults.<br>■ Modality should not impose excessive orthopedic stress.<br>■ Aquatic, stationary cycle, and recumbent stepper exercise may be preferable for clients with a diminished ability to tolerate weight-bearing exercise.<br>■ Modality should be accessible, convenient, and enjoyable to promote adherence.<br>■ A group setting may provide social reinforcement to adherence. |
| Exercise intensity | ■ To minimize complications and promote long-term compliance, intensity for inactive older adults should start low and progress according to client preference and tolerance. Initiating a program at <40% HRR or $\dot{V}O_2R$ is not unusual.<br>■ Many adults have clinically diagnosed conditions or likely have underlying chronic diseases; thus, a conservative approach to increasing intensity may be required.<br>■ Exercise need not be vigorous and continuous to be beneficial.<br>■ Measured peak heart rate is preferable to age-predicted peak heart rate because of the variability in peak heart rate in clients >65 yr and their greater risk for underlying CAD.<br>■ Activities performed at a given MET level represent greater relative intensities in older adults than in younger clients because of the decrease in peak METs with age (see Table 20.3).<br>■ Older adults are likely to be taking medications that can influence heart rate.<br>■ Intensity on a level of physical exertion should be 5–6 for moderate intensity and 7–8 for vigorous, on a scale from 0 to 10. |
| Exercise session duration | ■ To prevent injury, ensure safety, and promote adherence, older adults should increase exercise duration prior to intensity.<br>■ Duration need not be continuous to produce benefits. Clients who have difficulty sustaining exercise for 30 min or who prefer shorter bouts of exercise can be advised to exercise for 10-min bouts throughout the day.<br>■ A daily accumulation of 30 min moderate-intensity physical activity can provide health benefits.<br>■ Even greater benefits are possible with up to 60 min $\cdot$ d$^{-1}$ of moderate-intensity physical activity. |
| Exercise frequency | ■ Moderate-intensity exercise should be performed on 5 or more days per week, vigorous-intensity activity on 3 or more days per week, or a combination of moderate and vigorous on 3–5 d $\cdot$ wk$^{-1}$. |

HRR, heart rate reserve; CAD, coronary artery disease; MET, metabolic equivalent; $\dot{V}O_2R$, oxygen uptake reserve.
From American College of Sports Medicine. *ACSM's Guidelines for Exercise Testing and Prescription.* 10th ed. Philadelphia (PA): Wolters Kluwer; 2018.

small-framed or frail clients, care must be taken that they fit the individual properly. Other modalities such as free weights (*e.g.*, dumbbells), elastic bands, and body weight activities can offer different benefits for those older participants who are experienced in their use. A major advantage for these types of exercise modalities is that they are inexpensive, can be done at home, and take up minimal space. Another plus is they can promote kinesthetic awareness and help improve balance (102). Older participants should move through the full range of motion

(ROM) using proper form and avoid breath holding during the lifts. Intensity can be prescribed between moderate (5–6 on the 10-point exertion scale described previously) and vigorous (5). If the client's one repetition maximum (1-RM) is known, the target is 60%–70% 1-RM, although lower intensities (*e.g.*, 40%–50% 1-RM) are appropriate for beginners. Generally, one set of 10–15 repetitions is recommended when working with older adults (5). Eight to 10 exercises including the major muscle groups should be part of the resistance-training program (5). As with any resistance-training prescription, load should be increased when the number of repetitions that can be completed with proper form exceeds the initially prescribed number (*e.g.*, original prescription is 10 repetitions of 30 lb, and now the client can lift 12 repetitions with proper form and with a rating of perceived exertion (RPE) of 7 on a 10-point scale — then, it is appropriate to increase the load and decrease the number of repetitions back to 10).

In summary, although the resistance-training exercise prescription principles detailed in Chapter 14 are appropriate for many older individuals, they may need to be modified when working with those with functional limitations. Table 20.5 outlines modifications for resistance-training programs that could be considered when working with older adults.

## Design Considerations for Developing Flexibility in Older Adults

Flexibility is an essential component of fitness and decreases with age and physical inactivity. As was discussed in Chapter 16 with increasing age, the ability to move through a full ROM becomes compromised. Aging causes connective tissue to become stiffer, which makes the joint more resistant to bending (81,131). Additionally, the joint cartilage, ligaments, tendons, synovial

| Table 20.5 | Resistance-Training Guidelines for Older Adults |
|---|---|
| **Program Component** | **Program Modification** |
| Exercise mode | ■ Perform 8–10 exercises using the major muscle groups. <br> ■ Dynamic muscle strengthening activities include machine and free weights, weight-bearing calisthenics, resistance bands, and similar resistance exercises that use major muscle groups. |
| Exercise intensity | ■ Perform each lift or movement with a resistance that allows for 10–15 repetitions per exercise. <br> ■ Level of effort for muscle-strengthening activities should be light for beginners progressing to moderate to vigorous. On a 10-point scale, where no movement = 0, maximal effort = 10, moderate-intensity effort = 5 or 6, and high-intensity effort = 7 or 8. |
| Exercise session duration | ■ Complete at least one set of each exercise. <br> ■ Allow adequate rest between exercises to prevent carry-over fatigue. |
| Exercise frequency | ■ Resistance training should be performed on two or more nonconsecutive days per week. |

Adapted with permission from American College of Sports Medicine. *ACSM's Guidelines for Exercise Testing and Prescription.* 10th ed. Philadelphia (PA): Wolters Kluwer; 2018; Nelson ME, Rejeski WJ, Blair SN, et al. Physical activity and public health in older adults: recommendation for adults from the American College of Sports Medicine and the American Heart Association. *Med Sci Sports Exerc.* 2007;39:1435–45.

fluid, and muscles begin to deteriorate, which may decrease joint ROM (2,103). The loss of joint flexibility with aging has been reported to range from negligible to 57% with the majority of this loss occurring by age 65 years (37). Poor flexibility, coupled with decreased musculoskeletal strength, has been associated with a diminished ability to perform activities of daily living (ADLs) (32). Consequently, the beneficial effect of stretching on the achievement and maintenance of flexibility should not be overlooked.

Poor flexibility, coupled with decreased musculoskeletal strength, has been associated with a diminished ability to perform activities of daily living (32).

Over the last decade, much scientific inquiry has considered the topic of stretching. Collectively, the findings indicate that static stretching should only be done when muscles and joints are warm. In other words, static stretching itself should not be considered the "warm-up" prior to cardiorespiratory or resistance exercise. Static stretching done immediately prior to exercise could have potentially detrimental effects in some instances (*i.e.*, decreased muscle strength and endurance, impaired balance, and diminished reaction time) (104). The Personal Trainer should be mindful of this evidence when designing programs for older adult clients and consider sequencing the workout so that stretching follows the cardiorespiratory and/or resistance-training components. The exercise prescription principles for flexibility detailed in Chapter 16 are appropriate for older adults. To improve flexibility, older adults should gently increase the length of muscle beyond that used in everyday activities at least 2 days per week. This can be done dynamically, statically, or both. Static, held positions to stretch the muscles are to be held for 10–30 seconds and stretching should be employed for all the major muscle groups in the body. As noted in Chapter 16, guidelines for flexibility may need to be modified when working with those with functional limitations such as arthritis or osteoporosis.

## Design Considerations for Developing Balance in Older Adults

Fall incidence rates currently pose a serious health problem for older adults. In persons 65 years and older, it has been estimated that 35%–45% of otherwise healthy, community-dwelling adults fall at least once a year (59). Decreased balance with aging can be attributable to a series of declines in multiple physiological systems. These include decreases in joint and muscle flexibility (ROM), muscular strength, reduced central processing of sensory information, and slowed motor responses (59). With aging, myelin sheaths sometimes exhibit degenerative change and there is a loss of nerve fibers from the white matter in the brain (98). These changes contribute to a decline in sensory capability and cognitive function. Sensory capability is also affected by increasing age. Sight, hearing, taste, balance, vestibular function, and proprioception decline in old age leading to a greater risk of falling (37). Balance ability and postural control are critical factors for performing ADLs and participating in leisure-time activities (99). Balance and postural stability can be enhanced by combining flexibility with resistance exercise (13,35). Personal Trainers should therefore include balance exercises in older adults' exercise programs. Both static and dynamic balance activities should be employed at least twice a week. Progression should occur in a safe environment where a fall would not injure the participant (having spotters, having nearby secure objects to hang on to, and using mats). Progression can take place by steadily reducing the dynamic or static base of support (64). Although research has yet to identify the optimal frequency, duration, and type of balance exercises, balance training may be performed 3 days per week for 10–15 minutes each session (91). Balance training can be integrated into various phases of the exercise session, including warm-up, main component, or cool-down. Sample balance exercises and training progression (from simple to complex) are presented in Table 20.6 and are shown in Figures 20.1–20.3.

It is critical that Personal Trainers include balance exercises in older adults' exercise programs.

| Table 20.6 | Balance Exercises and Training Progression for Older Adults |
|---|---|
| **Position** | **Balance Exercise** |
| Sitting | ▪ Sit upright and complete progressions listed below. <br> ▪ Perform leg activities (heel, toe, or single-leg raises, marching). |
| Standing | ▪ "Clock" — balance on one leg (other leg at 45° or 90° angle), Personal Trainer calls out time, client moves nonsupport leg to the time called out (*i.e.*, 5 o'clock, 9 o'clock), alternate legs. <br> ▪ Perform leg activities (heel, toe, or single-leg raises — 45° or 90° angle, marching). <br> ▪ "Spelling" — balance on one leg, Personal Trainer asks the client to spell word working with nonsupport leg (*i.e.*, client's name, day of week, favorite food), alternate legs. |
| In motion | ▪ Heel-to-toe walking along 15-ft line on floor (first with and then without partner) <br> ▪ "Excursion" — alternating legs, lunge over a space separated by two lines of tape. Progress to hopping or jumping (using single-leg or double-leg) back and forth across the space. <br> ▪ Dribble basketball around cones that require the client to change direction multiple times. |
| Training progression | ▪ Arm progressions: use surface for support, hands on thigh, hands folded across chest <br> ▪ Surface progressions: chair, balance discs, foam pad, physioball <br> ▪ Visual progressions: open eyes, sunglasses or dim room lighting, closed eyes <br> ▪ Tasking progressions: single tasking, multitasking (*i.e.*, balance exercise + pass/ catch ball) |

Number of repetitions per exercise and rest intervals will be dependent on client conditioning and functional status.

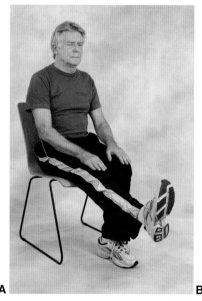
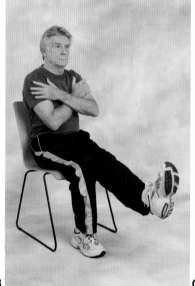
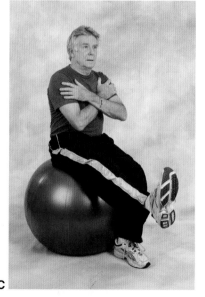

**FIGURE 20.1.** Sample progression of sitting balance exercises: **(A)** closed eyes, **(B)** arms crossed, and **(C)** physioball.

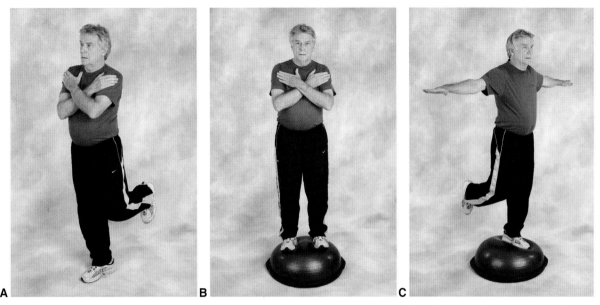

**FIGURE 20.2.** Sample progression of standing balance exercise, with arms crossed on floor **(A)**, and with arms crossed **(B)** and open **(C)** on balance training equipment.

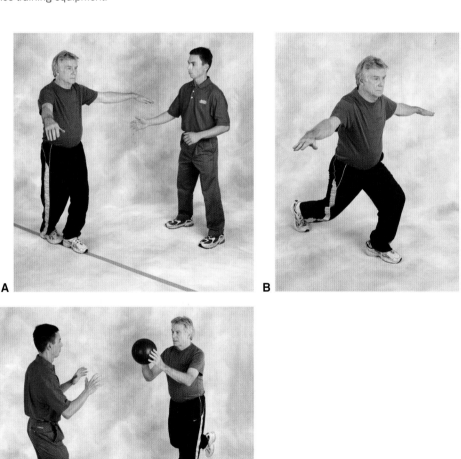

**FIGURE 20.3.** Sample progression of in-motion balance exercises: **(A)** heel-to-toe, **(B)** excursion, and **(C)** multitasking.

**Programming for Clients with CVD**

According to the American Heart Association, 82.6 million American adults (more than 1 in 3) have one or more types of CVD (89). Although the prevalence of CVD-related deaths has declined since the 1980s, it remains the leading cause of death in the United States (89). In fact, the most recent statistics from the American Heart Association indicated approximately 2,200 Americans die of CVD each day (89). Patterns of nutrient intake and physical inactivity underlie the global epidemic of chronic diseases, including obesity, hypertension, dyslipidemia, and Type 2 diabetes, which all serve as risk factors that contribute to the process of coronary artery disease (CAD). Clearly, a main goal of the Personal Trainer is to help clients with the primary prevention of atherosclerotic risk factors. Personal Trainers should know that individuals who are able to reach the age of 50 years with no CVD risk factors have markedly higher survival rates than those with any combination of risk factors (83). However, even those individuals who have only one risk factor at middle age are at a much higher risk for CVD and CAD than middle-aged people with no risk factors (83). Fortunately, exercise programs that can effectively stabilize and even reverse the process of atherosclerosis can be designed even for individuals with known CAD.

> Individuals who are able to reach the age of 50 years with no CVD risk factors have markedly higher survival rates than those with any combination of risk factors (83).

## Programming Goals for CVD

Positive risk factor modification is the primary goal of an aerobic exercise program for clients with heart disease. Scientific research has demonstrated that there is a dose-response relationship between exercise and multiple health outcomes, including risk of CAD and all-cause mortality, obesity, dyslipidemia, Type 2 diabetes, and perhaps most importantly, cardiorespiratory fitness (112,124). Cardiorespiratory fitness is an important marker for health outcomes and risk stratification (18). Studies have consistently demonstrated an inverse relationship between $\dot{V}O_{2max}$ values and CVD and total mortality in men and women across the lifespan (16–18,112). Moreover, it has been shown that risk for CVD is highest for individuals with low levels of cardiorespiratory fitness even when compared with those with traditional risk factors such as hypertension, dyslipidemia, or obesity (15). Each one metabolic equivalent (MET) increase (3.5 mL $\cdot$ kg$^{-1}$ $\cdot$ min$^{-1}$) in cardiorespiratory fitness can reduce the risk of CVD and all-cause mortality by 8%–17% (15,82). Based on the dose-response relationship between exercise and health outcomes, both the ACSM and U.S. Surgeon General have noted that the health benefits of a program are closely associated with total weekly energy expenditure (5,119). Recent studies have shown that exercise programs with energy expenditure of 14–23 kcal $\cdot$ kg$^{-1}$ $\cdot$ wk$^{-1}$ lead to significant improvements in cardiorespiratory fitness and other important risk factors for CAD, including dyslipidemia, body composition, and insulin sensitivity (45,66,78,107,112). In some patients with CVD, high-intensity aerobic interval training (AIT) may have potential for improving $\dot{V}O_2$ peak as compared with standard continuous moderate-intensity exercises (5,34). However, ACSM does not universally recommend using AIT with this population until further data regarding its safety and efficacy are available (5). Thus, when working with those with heart disease, the Personal Trainer should design an individualized aerobic exercise prescription conforming to the FITT-VP principles and parameters (frequency, intensity, time, type, volume, and progression) to fulfill total weekly energy expenditure levels that have been shown to elicit positive adaptations to CAD risk factors. Achievement of this objective will positively modify the process of atherosclerosis and subsequently reduce the likelihood of future cardiac events (117).

## Design Considerations for Cardiorespiratory Training for Clients with CVD

Exercise training is relatively safe for the majority of clients with CVD provided that appropriate assessment and screening is performed before beginning the program. The likelihood of an adverse event, although not entirely preventable, can be markedly reduced with baseline assessments, preparticipation screening, patient education, and client adherence to established exercise recommendations (5,53). All clients with CVD should have their cardiovascular risk assessed by their physician and gain physician clearance prior to participating in any exercise program. Individuals with cardiac disease may have previously participated in an outpatient cardiac rehabilitation exercise program. Personal Trainers should gain as much information as possible regarding client's participation in previous programs. Once it has been established that it is reasonably safe for the client with CVD to begin, the specific details of an exercise program can be formulated. Most of the cardiorespiratory assessments described in Chapter 12 can be provided to clients with CVD after proper screening and clinical evaluations including a recent clinical exercise test. Determining appropriate exercise intensity is dependent on the baseline cardiorespiratory fitness level. The Personal Trainer must recognize the critical importance of exercise intensity to the exercise prescription model, particularly for this population. Failure to meet minimal threshold values may result in lack of a training effect, whereas exceeding appropriate intensities can lead to overtraining at best and cardiac incident or death at worst. Also, working the client too hard can negatively impact their adherence to an exercise program (55), thereby undermining any positive changes previously made. For most previously sedentary clients with CVD, the threshold intensity for improving cardiorespiratory fitness approximates to 40%–80% of $\dot{V}O_2R$ or heart rate reserve (HRR) (113). Other exercise intensity considerations for those with CVD are presented in Table 20.7.

> For most previously sedentary clients with CVD, the threshold intensity for improving cardiorespiratory fitness approximates to 40%–80% of $\dot{V}O_2R$ or HRR (113).

An initial exercise program is to be designed to fulfill the threshold exercise intensity and total energy expenditure requirements (1,000 kcal $\cdot$ wk$^{-1}$ or 14 kcal $\cdot$ kg$^{-1}$ $\cdot$ wk$^{-1}$) necessary to modify the risk factors that mediate the process of atherosclerosis. Generally, this can be accomplished by prescribing moderate exercise intensity on 5–7 days per week for 20–60 minutes per session (5,85).

| **Table 20.7** | **Exercise Intensity Considerations for Clients with Cardiac Disease** |
|---|---|
| **Program Modification** | |
| Deconditioned and low–functional capacity clients may need to start at low intensities (20%–30% HRR or $\dot{V}O_2R$). | |
| Target exercise intensity should fall 10–15 bpm below a heart rate that has previously elicited abnormal clinical symptoms (*i.e.*, chest pain or other angina symptoms). | |
| β-Blockers and other heart rate–lowering medications will decrease the accuracy of exercise intensity prescription methods based on an age-predicted maximal heart rate. | |
| RPE levels of 11 (fairly light) to 13 (somewhat hard) typically correspond to the target heart rate for clients with CVD first initiating an exercise program. RPE can be progressed (14–16) after several months of training when conditioning has improved and no complications are present. | |

HRR, heart rate reserve; RPE, rating of perceived exertion.
Adapted with permission from American College of Sports Medicine. *ACSM's Guidelines for Exercise Testing and Prescription.* 10th ed. Philadelphia (PA): Wolters Kluwer; 2018.

The overarching goal of the aerobic exercise program is to have a steady progression of total weekly energy expenditure toward the upper end of the recommended range (*i.e.*, 3,000 kcal · wk$^{-1}$ or 23 kcal · kg$^{-1}$ · wk$^{-1}$).

## Designing Resistance-Training Programs for Clients with CVD

Resistance training in patients with CVD improves muscular strength and endurance, decreases cardiovascular demands of a given task, helps prevent/treat other chronic diseases (*e.g.*, osteoporosis, Type 2 diabetes), increases ability to perform daily activities, and improves self-confidence, among other benefits (5). Two primary goals of resistance training for those with CVD are as follows (99):

1. To maintain and improve muscular fitness levels for performing ADLs
2. To reduce the cardiovascular demands (*e.g.*, lower heart rate and blood pressure) associated with performing these tasks

The Personal Trainer should request that clients obtain physician approval before integrating resistance training into the exercise routine. Importantly, clients should inquire with the medical team about limitations the Personal Trainer should be aware of when designing the resistance-training program (*e.g.*, resistance training sooner than 3 mos post–bypass surgery is contraindicated). Clients with heart disease require careful monitoring for proper technique and breathing patterns. Straining, tight gripping of weight handles/bars, and the Valsalva maneuver should all be avoided. Progression of resistance training should be gradual, but often, the Personal Trainer may need to accept maintenance of strength as a more realistic objective. Exercise should be terminated if signs or symptoms such as dizziness, arrhythmias, unusual shortness of breath, or chest discomfort occur (5,127). General resistance-training guidelines for clients with CVDs are presented in Table 20.8.

| Table 20.8 | Resistance-Training Guidelines for Clients with Cardiac Disease |
|---|---|
| **Program Component** | **Program Modification** |
| Exercise mode | ▪ Perform 8–10 exercises using the major muscle groups. <br> ▪ Dynamic muscle strengthening exercises include machine and free weights, weight-bearing calisthenics, resistance bands, and similar resistance exercises that use major muscle groups. <br> ▪ Isometric exercise is not recommended for clients with CVD. |
| Exercise intensity | ▪ Begin program with a low weight for each exercise. <br> ▪ 10–15 repetitions per exercise to "moderate" fatigue, which approximately corresponds to an RPE range of 11–13 (light to somewhat hard) on the Borg 6–20 scale <br> ▪ The rate–pressure product (heart rate × systolic blood pressure) should not be greater than that prescribed during aerobic exercise. |
| Exercise session duration | ▪ Complete one set of each exercise initially; multiple sets can be introduced later as tolerated. <br> ▪ Allow adequate rest between exercises to prevent carry-over fatigue. |
| Exercise frequency | ▪ Resistance training should be performed on 2–3 nonconsecutive days per week. |
| Progression | ▪ Increase slowly as patient adapts (~2–5 lb · wk$^{-1}$ [1–2.3 kg] for upper body and 5–10 lb · wk$^{-1}$ [2.3–4.5 kg] for lower body). |

CVD, cardiovascular disease; RPE, rating of perceived exertion.
Adapted with permission from American College of Sports Medicine. *ACSM's Guidelines for Exercise Testing and Prescription*. 10th ed. Philadelphia (PA): Wolters Kluwer; 2018.

# Programming during Pregnancy and Postpartum

Pregnancy is associated with multiple anatomical and physiological changes. Originally, prevailing opinion was that physical activity should be discouraged during pregnancy because of the supposed increased maternal and fetal risk of untoward events (3). However, current research suggests that unless a specific obstetric or medical condition is present, the likelihood of adverse events or complications following acute exercise or chronic training in the mother and fetus is minimal (12). The Personal Trainer should recognize that similar to other populations, physical activities in people who are pregnant and those in postpartum period confer numerous benefits and should be encouraged. Collectively, the Personal Trainer, client, and obstetric health care provider can establish the following exercise program goals: Avoid excessive weight gain, reduce the risk of gestational diabetes, lower the incidence of low back pain, and prevent excessive decreases in cardiorespiratory and muscular fitness (12).

> Similar to other populations, physical activities in people who are pregnant and those in postpartum period confer numerous benefits and should be encouraged.

## Preparticipation Screening Exercise during Pregnancy and Postpartum

Prior to participation in an exercise program, pregnant women, regardless of physical activity history or lifestyle, should be evaluated by their obstetric provider to determine whether exercise is contraindicated. Having pregnant clients review the Physical Activity Readiness Medical Examination for Pregnancy (PARmed-X for Pregnancy) questionnaire (available at http://www.csep.ca) with their health care provider is recommended to help determine the appropriateness of participation in a fitness routine. This form can be signed by the obstetric provider to verify the safety of exercise and provide recommendations for cardiorespiratory and resistance-training activities. Personal Trainers who work with pregnant clients must be knowledgeable of, and able to educate clients on, the potential signs that would warrant the termination of exercise listed in Table 20.9.

## General Exercise Considerations during Pregnancy and Postpartum

Fatigue, nausea, and vomiting may limit exercise, especially during the first trimester. Importantly, the Personal Trainer should recognize the increased nutritional requirements of pregnant clients. Personal Trainers are encouraged to utilize the metabolic calculations presented in Chapter 15 to estimate the total energy expenditure of the client's exercise program. Pregnancy requires approximately an additional intake of 300 kcal per day to fulfill the increased metabolic demands of pregnancy (5).

| **Table 20.9** | **Warning Signs to Terminate Exercise during Pregnancy** |
|---|---|
| Vaginal bleeding | Muscle weakness affecting balance |
| Regular painful | Calf pain or swelling |
| Amniotic fluid leakage | Headache |
| Dyspnea prior to exertion | Chest pain |
| Dizziness | |

Pregnant women have diminished thermoregulatory control throughout pregnancy. Consequently, they need to be counseled to maintain adequate hydration, wear appropriate clothing that will facilitate heat dissipation, and avoid exercise in hot, humid conditions (3). Women should be encouraged to choose environmentally controlled indoor settings in these situations. Lastly, the Personal Trainer should remind clients that pregnancy is not a time to expect large improvements in fitness, and ultimately, throughout the gestational period, it is normal for numerous fitness parameters to decline (12).

The physiological changes associated with pregnancy persist for 4–6 weeks postpartum; however, women typically can gradually return to exercise provided the delivery was uncomplicated. Women who are nursing may elect to feed their babies prior to exercise to alleviate the discomfort of engorged breasts and to reduce the likelihood of feeding problems postexercise due to acidity in the breast milk (3).

## Aerobic Exercise Prescription during Pregnancy

The general cardiorespiratory training principles of exercise prescription detailed in Chapter 15 apply to pregnant and postpartum women, although the profound anatomical and physiological changes will require the Personal Trainer to make a number of special adaptations to the training program. Table 20.10 lists some of these exercise modifications for pregnancy. The consensus statement for regular physical activity from the U.S. Surgeon General (30 min of moderate-intensity

| Table 20.10 | Aerobic Exercise Program Modifications for Pregnant Women |
|---|---|
| **Program Component** | **Program Modification** |
| Exercise mode | ■ Walking and cycling may be easier to monitor for exercise intensity. <br> ■ Activities that increase the risk of falls (*e.g.*, skiing and skating), abdominal trauma (*e.g.*, basketball and softball), and rapid changes in movement that impact balance (*e.g.*, tennis) should be avoided and generally are not recommended. <br> ■ Activities at elevations >6,000 ft and scuba diving are contraindicated. |
| Exercise intensity | ■ Target heart rate (*e.g.*, %$HR_{max}$ or %HRR) should not be employed as a method to monitor exercise intensity due to the variability in maternal resting and maximal heart rate throughout pregnancy. Likewise, target $\dot{V}O_2$ (*e.g.*, %$\dot{V}O_2R$) is not a valid tool to monitor intensity due to the progressive decrease in cardiorespiratory fitness over the course of the pregnancy. <br> ■ RPE values of 12–13 (light to somewhat hard) on the 6–20 scale can be used to accurately and safely monitor exercise intensity. <br> ■ The talk test may also be used to monitor appropriate exercise intensity. Pregnant women should exercise at an intensity that permits conversation. Intensity should be decreased when conversation is not possible. |
| Exercise session duration | ■ Accumulating 30 min of exercise in 20–30 min intermittent bouts and adjusted as needed to a total of 150 min · $wk^{-1}$ of vigorous aerobic exercise. |
| Exercise frequency | ■ Moderate-intensity exercise should be regular rather than sporadic in nature. Exercise should be performed 3–5 d · $wk^{-1}$. |

$HR_{max}$, maximal heart rate; $\dot{V}O_2R$, oxygen uptake reserve; HRR, heart rate reserve; RPE, rating of perceived exertion.
Adapted with permission from American College of Obstetricians and Gynecologists. ACOG Committee Opinion No. 650. Physical activity and exercise during pregnancy and the postpartum period. *Obstet Gynecol*. 2015;126:e135–42; Artal R, O'Toole M. Guidelines of the American College of Obstetricians and Gynecologists for exercise during pregnancy and the postpartum period. *Br J Sports Med*. 2003;37:6–12; and American College of Sports Medicine. *ACSM's Guidelines for Exercise Testing and Prescription*. 10th ed. Philadelphia (PA): Wolters Kluwer; 2018.

physical activity on most, preferably all, days of the week) is an appropriate target aerobic exercise program for most women during uncomplicated pregnancies (96). Recreational and competitive athletes may train safely at higher intensities and volumes throughout pregnancy with the understanding that they are undergoing close obstetric supervision (12).

## Resistance Training and Flexibility Prescription during Pregnancy

The general resistance and flexibility training principles of exercise prescription detailed in Chapters 14 and 16, with several adjustments that account for morphological and physiological changes, apply to pregnant and postpartum women. After the first trimester, resistance and flexibility training exercises in the supine position should be avoided because of the potential obstruction of venous return and subsequent risk of orthostatic hypotension (3). Isometric or heavy resistance training may elicit a pressor response (sudden increase in heart rate and blood pressure) and is not recommended (12). Joint ROM will be enhanced during pregnancy because of increased circulating levels of relaxin, and therefore, the potential exists for ligament and joint capsule damage with an overly aggressive flexibility program (12). Consequently, Personal Trainers are encouraged to focus on maintaining normal joint ROM with slow, static stretching throughout pregnancy.

## Programming for Clients with Diabetes

Diabetes mellitus is a metabolic disorder stemming from abnormal pancreatic insulin production and/or diminished peripheral action of insulin. Diabetes is positively associated with the development of multiple diseases and disorders of the heart, vascular system (*e.g.*, stroke and hypertension), kidneys, eyes, and nervous system. Diabetes seriously compromises the heart and vascular system such that it is listed as the seventh leading cause of death in the United States (29). CVD mortality rates are up to 4 times higher in those individuals with diabetes mellitus compared with those without the disease (62). Looking at current data, it is clear that diabetes continues to be a significant problem in the United States. To date, 29.1 million American adults (9% of the U.S. adult population) have diabetes mellitus. Of that total, 21.1 million are diagnosed cases with 8.1 million undiagnosed cases for people 20 years and older reported in 2014 (29).

Two categories are used to classify individuals with diabetes: Type 1 and Type 2. Type 1 diabetes typically results from an autoimmune response whereby the body's own immune system mistakenly destroys the insulin-producing cells in the pancreas. Type 1 diabetes comprises approximately 5%–10% of all diagnosed cases of diabetes. This leaves 90%–95% of all diagnosed adults in the category of Type 2 diabetes. In general, the critical risk factors for Type 2 diabetes are associated with a sedentary lifestyle. Primary risk factors for Type 2 diabetes are age, family history, ethnicity, obesity, high alcohol intake, high fat diet, high blood triglycerides, high blood pressure and gestational diabetes or giving birth to a baby weight more than 9 lb (9). The most recent statistics indicate that 25.8% of individuals 65 years and older have diabetes with rate of new cases reported increasing across the lifespan (29,46). Moreover, it is estimated that approximately 81.5 million adult Americans have prediabetes (36.8% of the U.S. adult population), a condition in which blood glucose values are elevated beyond normal levels (*e.g.*, fasting blood glucose of 100–126 mg $\cdot$ dL$^{-1}$); these individuals have a markedly increased risk of developing Type 2 diabetes in their lifetime (8,62). Although Type 2 diabetes is more commonly associated with adults, it is now on the rise in children, fueled largely by inactivity and poor diets that lead to obesity. Therefore, Personal Trainers should recognize that diabetes prevention is appropriate for all populations, not only for the obese but also for the older adults and at-risk children.

Diabetes prevention is appropriate for all populations, not only for the obese but also for the older adults and at-risk children.

Because the growth of diabetes in the U.S. population is not slowing, the demand for competent Personal Trainers to provide appropriate exercise guidance and supervision to individuals with diabetes will continue to increase. Personal Trainers need to prepare to meet this challenge by continuing to enhance their ability to implement diabetes management and prevention programs.

## Pathophysiology of Diabetes

Normally, insulin is released in the pancreas in response to a rise in blood glucose following the intake and digestion of food. In Type 1 diabetes, pancreatic β-cells that produce insulin are destroyed by an autoimmune disorder, creating an absolute insulin deficiency (no insulin production) in the body. In Type 2 diabetes, insulin is produced but is ineffective at controlling blood glucose because of insulin resistance in body tissues. The pancreas increases insulin production to overcome this resistance, causing an excess of blood insulin in these individuals. Hyperinsulinemia (elevated blood insulin concentration) over time can contribute to a host of problems such as hypertension, hypercholesterolemia, excessive blood clotting, atherosclerosis, and kidney stones to name a few (29,33).

The main goal in the management of diabetes is adequately controlling blood glucose levels (5,8). Normal resting blood glucose level is less than $100 \text{ mg} \cdot \text{dL}^{-1}$. Diabetes is typically diagnosed when fasting blood glucose is $126 \text{ mg} \cdot \text{dL}^{-1}$ or greater on two or more occasions (4). Another important measurement of glucose control is the glycolated hemoglobin or hemoglobin A1c (HbA1C) measurement. Although blood glucose numbers describe the blood sugar at a single point in time, the HbA1C provides a better measure of glucose control over the last 2–3 months. In people without diabetes, a normal HbA1C value is somewhere between 3.5% and 5.5%. People with diabetes have higher HbA1C values because their bodies have consistently higher levels of blood glucose. A goal level for HbA1C for most people with diabetes is under 7% (4). Exercise, among other treatment strategies, can be used effectively to achieve this goal (8).

## Programming Goals for Those with Diabetes

Exercise training affects many subclinical health factors associated with diabetes and is critical for diabetes management. The main exercise programming goals for individuals with diabetes are to (4,8,21,22,69,105,108,122)

1. Improve insulin sensitivity and blood glucose control and decrease insulin requirements
2. Improve cardiorespiratory fitness
3. Improve blood lipid profiles
4. Reduce blood pressure
5. Improve muscular strength and endurance through enhancing skeletal muscle mass
6. Improve flexibility and joint ROM
7. Reduce body weight (particularly reduce intra-abdominal fat)
8. Assist with decreasing the risk of diabetic complications

Consistency in a daily routine is the major pillar in diabetes care. This regularity refers to when meals are eaten; the amount and type of food; when medications are taken; and frequency, intensity, and time (duration and time of day) of physical activity. Personal Trainers, when working with clients with diabetes, should maintain regular contact with the client's physician or other health care provider when designing or making changes to the exercise program. This will enable a more consistent and appropriate treatment plan for the client.

Consistency in a daily routine is the major pillar in diabetes care.

# Aerobic Training for Clients with Diabetes

The majority of research regarding exercise training and diabetes has been done in the area of aerobic exercise. A hallmark training adaptation to be expected from increased levels of aerobic activity is improved cardiorespiratory fitness; this positive outcome in particular carries tremendous benefit for clients with prediabetes or diabetes. Individuals with higher levels of cardiorespiratory fitness are at decreased risk of mortality from CVD compared with their counterparts with lower cardiorespiratory fitness levels regardless of body mass index (BMI) status (normal, overweight, or obese) (33,85). The positive effects of aerobic exercise on glucose metabolism and insulin sensitivity in clients with diabetes are known to be "subacute" changes, meaning that they are lost within a few days following the cessation of training (8). For Personal Trainers, this provides support for a consistent, almost daily training regimen for clients with diabetes. If these clients are to achieve the full benefits of aerobic exercise, the program must involve frequent exercise activities with adherence on a daily basis (118). Regular exercise in clients with diabetes assists in controlling blood glucose, enhancing insulin sensitivity, decreasing and managing body weight and blood pressure, improving lipid profiles, increasing cardiorespiratory fitness and exercise capacity, and managing some related conditions such as coronary heart disease or peripheral vascular disease (5,8,21,22,25,46,62,68,97).

## Frequency

ACSM recommends 3–7 days per week (5) with no more than 2 consecutive days between sessions of aerobic activity because of the relatively brief exercise-induced improvements in insulin action (57). Greater frequencies of physical activity have been shown to be more effective in improving glucose tolerance and insulin sensitivity with minimal exercise-induced complications (40). Personal Trainers should consider progressing clients to 5 days per week, or perhaps daily, with an appropriate mix of intensity and duration. Clients who are obese or are taking insulin may benefit most by a daily schedule as it allows for greater consistency and an opportunity for increasing caloric expenditure for purposes of weight management (8).

## Intensity

ACSM recommends a range of 40%–59% of $\dot{V}O_2R$ or HRR for clients with diabetes (5). Individual health status is an important consideration when selecting initial exercise intensity. In individuals who are regular exercisers, better blood glucose control may be achieved at higher exercise intensities ($\geq$60% $\dot{V}O_2R$) (5). The Personal Trainer may consider including high-intensity exercise within the exercise program for those individuals.

For clients who are overweight, sedentary, and/or more deconditioned, an appropriate starting point is 40% of $\dot{V}O_2R$ or HRR or slightly lower depending on the initial fitness level and tolerance to exercise. The decision to progress the client through the intensity range is to be made after taking into consideration the client's age, their ability to tolerate exercise, and their individual goals. In general, frequency and duration goals should be realized before implementing a significant progression in intensity (5).

Because some clients with a long history of diabetes may incur a condition that can affect the heart rate (and blood pressure) response to exercise (5), Personal Trainers are encouraged to use the RPE scale as an adjunct method for determining intensity, an RPE range of 11–13 (on the 6–20 scale) falls in line with the prescribed $\dot{V}O_2R$ and HRR values with adjustments made on the basis of the percentage values.

## Time

ACSM recommends a range of 20–60 minutes for clients with diabetes, continuous or accumulated in bouts of at least 10 minutes to total of 150 minutes per week (5). Once again, the Personal Trainer is given a great amount of room to adjust and progress within this large range. Recent research suggests a worthy minimal goal of 150 minutes per week to elicit positive changes in glucose tolerance and insulin sensitivity and potential changes in body weight (21,22,40). Greater benefits may be realized by increasing to 300 minute per week or more (5). This amount may seem high for the client who is overweight, deconditioned, or older. However, exercise may not need to be continuous to provide these benefits; therefore, using multiple bouts of exercise throughout the day (>10 min per bout) to achieve the overall exercise time goal is the recommended progression for these individuals (5,63). Progressing up to 30–40 minutes of continuous activity will help the client achieve his or her caloric expenditure goals. Because intensity may be relatively low in this population, frequency and duration are critical factors in determining caloric expenditure. If weight loss is a goal, and for many clients it will be, ACSM recommends 2,000 kcal per week or more and daily exercise (5).

### Type

Guidelines for choosing a mode of exercise are similar to those for an apparently healthy adult. In general, program adherence is improved if the client chooses an exercise modality that he or she enjoys. Walking is the most common form of exercise for clients with diabetes (8). However, there are some considerations to be made for clients with diabetes. For those clients who are obese or experience diabetic complications (peripheral neuropathy is one), Personal Trainers should minimize high-impact, weight-bearing activities or those that require greater balance and coordination (5). Therefore, alternating weight-bearing activities with non–weight-bearing activities, such as cycling, upper body ergometry, and swimming, may enhance the safety and appropriateness of the exercise program.

### Progression

Maximizing caloric expenditure is the highest priority in clients with Type 2 diabetes (5). Thus, the Personal Trainer should progressively increase exercise duration (either continuous or accumulated) and develop a program that promotes beneficial adaptations while combating boredom.

## Resistance Training for Clients with Diabetes

The ACSM resistance-training recommendations for healthy individuals (Chapter 14) are applicable for people with either prediabetes or Type 1 or Type 2 diabetes, with the understanding that unique contraindications to resistance exercise exist in this population — including retinopathy, neuropathy — and following recent treatments using laser surgery (5). A resistance-training program is essential for clients with diabetes to assist in managing their disease and associated complications as well as maintaining their physiological function through improving strength and endurance. Some believe that the increased risk of diabetes with increasing age is partly due to loss of muscle mass. This age-related muscle atrophy negatively impacts the ability to remain recreationally active, perform ADLs, and maintain independence (46). Significant research has demonstrated the effectiveness of circuit weight training for managing and preventing diabetes (46,47,86). Clients would be well advised to perform circuit weight training regularly to regulate blood glucose and prevent age-related muscle atrophy. In fact, for individuals with diabetic complications such as retinopathy, circuit training with fairly light workloads is recommended as blood pressure will not increase or spike as much as it does with higher loads. In summary, using resistance training to maintain skeletal muscle mass is known to be critical for managing and improving glycemic control and insulin sensitivity, decreasing HbA1C levels, reducing intra-abdominal fat, and improving the overall metabolic profile and quality of life in those with diabetes (8,21,23,27,44,47,69,97,115,118).

## Other Considerations for Clients with Diabetes

When creating individualized training programs for persons with diabetes, there are other health concerns that often accompany diabetes that need to be considered. Clients with diabetes should check their blood glucose before exercise. Ideally, blood sugar levels need to be between 100 and 250 mg $\cdot$ dL$^{-1}$. If they are lower than this, the client should eat a carbohydrate-rich snack. Clients with glucose levels above 250–300 mg $\cdot$ dL$^{-1}$ will need to check urine for ketones, and, if present, exercise should be delayed; if no ketones are present, exercise is okay but use caution.

Exercise has an insulin-like effect on circulating blood glucose, even in the absence of blood insulin. Thus, hypoglycemia (low blood glucose levels) is one of the most common but potentially serious complications that can occur during or after exercise in individuals with diabetes (5). The following strategies (5) may be helpful for minimizing a client's risk of developing hypoglycemia.

1. Know the warning signs of hypoglycemia and hyperglycemia (Table 20.11).
2. Avoid exercise during the time when hypoglycemic medication is working at its peak.
3. Client should eat 1–2 hours before exercise (perhaps, eat a snack during exercise if duration is prolonged).
4. Check blood glucose before exercise and if blood glucose is less than 100 mg $\cdot$ dL$^{-1}$ and then the client should eat a snack.
5. Client should exercise with a partner for safety reasons.
6. Have fruit juice or candy available if blood glucose gets too low.

Clients with diabetes are to work with their physician and/or registered dietitian for nutritional recommendations related to controlling blood glucose with exercise. Clients need to be cautioned against late night exercise as this could cause low blood glucose during sleep (nocturnal hypoglycemia) and inadvertently cause a potentially life-threatening situation. Thus, if late night exercise cannot be avoided, the clients should eat following exercise according to their physicians' or registered dietitians' guidelines. Personal Trainers who work with clients with diabetes should be knowledgeable of, and able to educate clients about, the warning signs of hypoglycemia. Table 20.11 includes a list of selected signs and symptoms of hyper- and hypoglycemia.

| Table 20.11 Selected Signs and Symptoms of Hyperglycemia and Hypoglycemia | |
|---|---|
| **Hyperglycemia (>300 mg $\cdot$ dL$^{-1}$)** | **Hypoglycemia (<70 mg $\cdot$ dL$^{-1}$ or rapid drop in glucose)** |
| Dry skin | Dizziness and headache |
| Hunger | Weakness and fatigue |
| Nausea/vomiting | Shaking |
| Blurred vision | Tachycardia (fast heart rate) |
| Frequent urination | Irritable |
| Extreme thirst | Confusion |
| Drowsiness | Sweating |
| Acetone breath ("fruity breath") | Slurred speech |
| | Anxious |
| | Hunger |

Adapted with permission from American College of Sports Medicine. *ACSM's Guidelines for Exercise Testing and Prescription.* 10th ed. Philadelphia (PA): Wolters Kluwer; 2018.

Clients need to be taught the exercise guidelines that are specific for proper management of diabetes. For example, warm-up and cool-down (5–10 min each) are particularly important in this population to avoid exercise-induced cardiovascular complications. Proper footwear is also critical for clients with diabetes, especially for those with or at risk for peripheral neuropathy and peripheral vascular disease. Clients need to be advised to maintain adequate hydration and avoid exercise in hot/humid environments, which will allow them to tolerate exercise better and will assist in proper blood pressure and body temperature regulation. Also, remember to recommend lighter resistance-training workloads to avoid high blood pressure spikes (especially in those with retinopathy).

In summary, the main programmatic considerations for Personal Trainers who work with clients with diabetes involve minimizing the risks involved with exercising while maximizing benefits. In cases where the individual has complications of diabetes such as diabetic retinopathy, peripheral neuropathy, or nephropathy, consult the client's physician before beginning the exercise program. These clients may need referral to a medically supervised environment if the condition limits overall exercise tolerance or if they have signs and/or symptoms of CVD.

 ## Programming for Obese Clients

Obesity is currently defined as having a BMI greater than $30 \text{ kg} \cdot \text{m}^{-2}$ (28). Looking back over the previous 20 years, there has been a substantial rise in the number of people who are obese. According to the National Health and Nutrition Examination Survey, more than one-third of U.S. adults and 17% of youth in 2011–2014 were considered obese. Compared to males, females had the highest prevalence and among ethnic groups, non-Hispanic black females were higher compared to Hispanic females (52,93). The most recent data indicate that the increases are not continuing at the same rate, but the overall prevalence of obesity remains high (52).

Reasons for the rising obesity levels are very complex and result from a number of factors including increased caloric consumption (overconsumption), decreased levels of physical activity, genetic predisposition, disease, and cultural/environmental (home, school, work, and community) influences (120). The close association of obesity with physical inactivity as well as to numerous chronic health issues such as Type 2 diabetes mellitus, CVD, hypertension, and certain types of cancers tend to obscure understanding its cause and may complicate treatment. Although obesity is linked to an increased risk of disability and all-cause mortality (28,72,94,126), it is not clear if this is a causal association or a result of inactivity (56). Personal Trainers who work with obese clientele should be prepared to interact and consult with a variety of professionals to design appropriate and effective exercise programming strategies.

 ## Programming Goals

Personal Trainers can make their greatest impact with obese clients by providing sound exercise programs that focus on promoting adherence to an active lifestyle that matches closely with appropriate dietary strategies. This is a challenge because it is common for overweight or obese individuals to have many deeply rooted negative attitudes and barriers to physical activity behavior that must be addressed before they can truly adhere to a program. The common exercise program goals for obese individuals are to (5,6,19,24,95,100,106,126)

1. Maximize caloric expenditure
2. Maintain or increase lean body mass to maintain resting metabolic rate
3. Improve metabolic profile
4. Lower the risk of comorbidities (*e.g.*, hypertension, diabetes, orthopedic problems)
5. Lower mortality risk
6. Promote appetite control
7. Improve mood state

## Aerobic Training for Obese Clients

The most recent ACSM Position Stand (6) recommends a minimum of 150 minutes per week of moderate-intensity physical activity for overweight and obese adults to improve health and to prevent significant weight gain. However, greater weight loss and enhanced prevention of weight regained will likely need much greater doses (approximately 250–300 min $\cdot$ wk$^{-1}$ or approximately 2,000 kcal $\cdot$ wk$^{-1}$) of moderate-intensity physical activity (6). Importantly, most evidence indicates that exercise alone (without dietary restriction) is fairly ineffective for weight loss (6), with an average of less than a 3% decrease.

> Most evidence indicates that exercise alone (without dietary restriction) is fairly ineffective for weight loss.

Extreme exercise or physical activity that results in a large negative energy balance will clearly result in weight loss. For example, it is well known that the intense energy demands of military training or mountain climbing will result in substantial weight loss, without restricting caloric intake. However, it is difficult for most individuals to achieve and sustain these high levels of physical activity. Therefore, most individuals who require substantial weight loss may need additional interventions (*i.e.*, energy restriction) to meet their weight loss goals. In terms of successful weight loss, diet with caloric restriction is the most important predictor. However, regular aerobic exercise should be used in concert with a low-calorie, low-fat, and high-fiber diet plan, thereby helping provide a negative caloric balance to achieve weight loss through maximizing energy expenditure (5). As long as the dietary restriction is not severe (*i.e.*, >500–700 kcal), adding physical activity to the diet has been shown to result in greater weight loss compared with diet alone (6). Most importantly, once weight loss has occurred, regular physical activity in the form of exercise is the most significant predictor of long-term weight management (5).

### Frequency

ACSM recommends a training frequency of 5 or more days per week to maximize energy expenditure in obese clients (5). Several studies have shown the effectiveness of a high-frequency exercise program on fat loss provided that the intensity is set appropriately (24,95,106).

### Intensity

Moderate- to vigorous-intensity aerobic activity is encouraged (5). Initial intensities should be determined based on current fitness level (*e.g.*, 40%–59% $\dot{V}O_2R$ or HRR). Later progression into more vigorous intensities (>60% $\dot{V}O_2R$ or HRR) may be appropriate for some obese clients but should be individualized on the basis of the client's goals and history. Past research supports moderate-intensity exercise as an effective method for supporting weight loss and successful weight management (6,100,106).

### Time

ACSM recommends a minimum of 30 minutes per day exercise duration progressing gradually to 60 minutes per day (5,6). This amount of exercise is consistent with past research and previous guidelines for weight loss and weight management strategies (6,24,41,101,106). However, some clients may be too severely deconditioned or have conditions that limit their ability to exercise for this long. In these cases, prescribing multiple bouts of exercise (10 min per session or more) may be best to begin with and gradually shift to more continuous exercise later in the program (5,6,63). Although this is more than the recommended level of exercise needed to support general health and prevent chronic disease, successful weight control may be more likely when obese clients are exercising 45–60 minutes per session (200–300 min $\cdot$ wk$^{-1}$), expending at least 300 kcal per session, and a total of 2,000 kcal or more per week (5,6).

### Type

Regular exercise is important for general health and not only for weight loss. Thus, any type of physical activity that the client will do regularly is recommended. However, the primary mode of exercise for large clients should involve large muscle groups and be aerobic in nature to provide the greatest caloric expenditure during exercise (5). Often, resistance exercise training is an appropriate adjunct mode of exercise for obese clients as it can be done without having to support the added weight of the body. This exercise should be in addition to an overall increase in leisure-time physical activity and decreased sitting time.

## Resistance Training for Obese Clients

Resistance-training programs are commonly treated as an adjunct to a regular, aerobic exercise program and generally should not be used in lieu of an aerobic program. However, resistance training is a critical component of the total exercise program for obese clients and should be incorporated into the program. The benefits of resistance training for clients who are obese are similar to the apparently healthy adult; thus, following the resistance-training guidelines highlighted in Chapter 14 is appropriate for obese and overweight clients.

Although there is little evidence that resistance training will reduce body weight without any modification of diet, resistance training has been associated with improvements in many chronic disease risk factors in the absence of significant weight loss (6,24). Resistance training has been shown to improve blood cholesterol, improve insulin sensitivity, reduce glucose-stimulated plasma insulin concentrations, and improve systolic and diastolic blood pressure (6). In addition, resistance training may also improve the maintenance of lean body mass in clients following a calorically restricted diet (24).

> Resistance training may also improve the maintenance of lean body mass in clients following a calorically restricted diet (24).

## Weight Loss Expectations

One major barrier to increasing exercise behavior in obese clients is an unrealistic weight loss expectation. Most people do not understand that exercise alone is not very effective for reducing weight. The Personal Trainer should explain that exercise is beneficial even if weight loss goals are not met. The ACSM recommends that overweight and obese individuals try to reduce their body weight by a minimum of 5%–10%, a value that is associated with initial improvements in risk factors. However, 150 minutes per week may only elicit up to 3% weight loss (6). Thus, much higher doses of physical activity combined with diet restriction are typically necessary to elicit significant weight change. For example, those in the National Weight Control Registry, who have lost and maintained a substantial amount of weight, report expending the energy equivalent to walking 25–30 miles per week (or more than 400 min $\cdot$ wk$^{-1}$) regularly (76).

Unfortunately, sometimes, the unrealistic expectations of clients are fostered by Personal Trainers themselves. In a survey of 500 health and fitness professionals (61), 87% responded that they felt "very competent" to prescribe exercise programs for weight loss. In other words, Personal Trainers believe that they can prescribe the amount of energy expenditure necessary for one to lose weight. However, other research indicates that Personal Trainers cannot deliver on their weight-loss promises and that obese clients are extremely dissatisfied with their performance (54,67,71). Dissatisfaction with treatment results runs deep among persons seeking help for obesity (54). For example, obese clients who were asked about potential weight loss results indicated that a minimum of 25% weight loss was acceptable but not ideal. In addition, they noted that 17% weight loss "could not be viewed as successful in any way" (54, p. 2133). Clearly, there is no exercise prescription that the Personal Trainer can suggest that will elicit a 20% or greater weight loss. This amount of weight loss requires careful caloric restriction that should be done under the supervision of a registered dietitian. Thus, Personal Trainers need to be mindful of the inconsistency between reality and expectation when working with obese clients. Thus, whereas obese clients need to understand that exercise is not a quick fix, Personal Trainers also need to understand that obesity is not caused by a simple imbalance in energy expenditure. Obesity is a heterogeneous condition, which requires a multifocal treatment plan, and there is wide variability in weight loss outcomes in obese people, regardless of program design. There is no singularly appropriate weight-loss treatment plan for all obese people.

Personal Trainers are obligated to educate obese clients that inactivity may be the problem not body weight per se. Trainers should instruct their clients that exercise and increasing physical activity will improve health but may not cure obesity. The exercise threshold required to improve one's health may be far below the exercise threshold required for weight loss (56,71). In other words, exercise is good for them regardless of whether or not they lose much weight. Lastly, Personal Trainers need to make sure that obese clients also understand the potential risks of sudden, extreme, or cyclical weight loss (56).

Personal Trainers are advised to not generalize that obese individuals lack self-control (116) or rationalize that weight-loss failure is solely a consequence of poor client compliance. As stated previously, obesity is a complex issue and successful long-term behavior change takes a multidimensional approach. Personal Trainers are encouraged to obtain further experience in motivational counseling, goal-setting strategies, and determining readiness for change before planning to work with obese clients (67).

## Other Considerations for Working with Obese Clients

First, obese clients do not regulate their body temperature as effectively as leaner clients (5). Therefore, Personal Trainers should educate their clients on proper exercise clothing, hydration, environmental issues (hot/humid environments), and signs of heat exhaustion/stroke. Second, obese clients are at greater risk of experiencing orthopedic injuries because of greater stress on joints due to their overall weight (5). Personal Trainers should keep this in mind during program design, in particular with the intensity portion. Considerations should also be made to include non–weight-bearing modalities when appropriate to minimize orthopedic stress. Also, Personal Trainers should be prepared to modify the exercise program on the basis of the presence of other conditions (diabetes, CAD, hypertension, etc.) that may require an adjustment from the prescription given earlier. Lastly, because of size limitations, some exercise machines may not be able to accommodate an obese client. Personal Trainers may need to be creative in their exercise planning and utilize equipment that can accommodate their particular clients (5). Table 20.12 includes some additional recommendations to follow for weight loss programs.

> Personal Trainers should be prepared to modify the exercise program on the basis of the presence of other conditions (*e.g.*, diabetes, CAD, hypertension).

| Table 20.12 | Additional Recommendations for Weight-Loss Programs |
| --- | --- |
| Gradual weight loss of 1 kg · wk$^{-1}$ or less | |
| Daily, negative caloric balance should not exceed 500–1,000 kcal. | |
| Goal for long-term weight loss of at least 5%–10% of total weight | |
| Employ behavioral modification strategies to enhance adherence | |
| Dietary intake should not be <1,200 kcal · d$^{-1}$. | |
| Balanced diet with fat intake <30% of total calories consumed | |

Adapted with permission from American College of Sports Medicine. *ACSM's Guidelines for Exercise Testing and Prescription.* 10th ed. Philadelphia (PA): Wolters Kluwer; 2018.

# Programming for Clients with Hypertension

With more than 76.4 million adults (1 in 3) with hypertension, it remains the most prevalent risk factor for CVD in the United States (89). Hypertension is the major contributor to the risk of stroke and is also related to the development of CAD (leading to myocardial infarction), heart failure, kidney disease, peripheral vascular disease, and blindness (5). Hypertension is often called the "silent killer" because of the lack of noticeable signs or symptoms of the disease until the development of serious problems. The current definition of hypertension is an elevated resting systolic blood pressure of ≥140 mm Hg and/or diastolic blood pressure of ≥90 mm Hg. However, definitions now recognize "prehypertension" (systolic blood pressure between 120 and 139 mm Hg and/or diastolic between 80 and 89 mm Hg) as an equally important diagnosis (31). These lower blood pressure values indicate the need for early management of moderately elevated levels of blood pressure to help prevent the conversion of prehypertension to hypertension.

The Report of the Joint National Committee on Prevention, Detection, Evaluation, and Treatment of High Blood Pressure (JNC7) indicated that in people with blood pressure >115/75 mm Hg, CVD risk doubles for each increment of 20/10 mm Hg (31). Personal Trainers can make a positive impact on their clients who have hypertension or prehypertension through appropriate exercise programming as part of a comprehensive lifestyle management strategy (diet, stress reduction, smoking cessation, lower alcohol consumption, etc.) or medication regimen.

> Hypertension is often called the "silent killer" because of the lack of noticeable signs or symptoms of the disease until the development of serious problems.

## Programming Goals

General programming goals in the management of hypertension are to (7,31)

1. Lower systolic and diastolic blood pressures at rest and during exercise
2. Lower the risk of mortality from CVD (myocardial infarction, stroke, heart failure, etc.)
3. Lower the risk of other comorbidities (kidney disease, eye problems, diabetes, etc.)
4. Incorporate opportunities for clients to pursue other lifestyle changes (stress management, diet, smoking cessation, weight management, etc.)

## Aerobic Training for Clients with Hypertension

Aerobic exercise is the cornerstone activity in the total program for clients with hypertension. On average, clients may experience a decline of approximately 3–4 mm Hg for systolic blood pressure and approximately 2–3 mm Hg for diastolic blood pressure from aerobic exercise training. Greater change may be (~1 mm Hg or more) seen in those with diagnosed hypertension (48,125). Taken alone, these changes may not seem significant; however, when coupled with other treatment strategies (diet, medication, etc.), the effect will be much more appreciable. Several studies have shown that higher cardiorespiratory fitness provides a cardioprotective effect of lower mortality risk from all causes and CVD in individuals with hypertension (111). Thus, improving overall fitness in clients with hypertension may be a worthy goal to pursue, independent of the direct effects exercise may have on lowering blood pressure.

### Frequency

ACSM recommends exercise for clients with hypertension on most, if not all, days of the week. Personal Trainers should encourage their clients to participate in daily, regular exercise, as the subacute response of blood pressure following a bout of aerobic exercise is to remain below levels measured prior to exercise (7). This translates into more controlled and consistent blood pressure levels from day to day, which is ideal for clients with hypertension. In their review of past research studies, Whelton and colleagues (125) found a greater decrease in blood pressure with increased frequency of exercise (>150 min · wk$^{-1}$).

### Intensity

ACSM recommends moderate-intensity exercise, 40%–59% of $\dot{V}O_2R$ or HRR, as the primary-intensity prescription for individuals with hypertension (5,7). Personal Trainers should apply the lower end of this range for hypertensive clients who are deconditioned, older, or have comorbid conditions that can affect their risk of experiencing cardiovascular complications during exercise (diabetes, CAD, etc.).

RPE can be used to help determine intensity rather than HR in the presence of certain medications that can affect the client's HR response during exercise ($\beta$-blockers are the main culprit). An RPE range of 12–13 (on a 6–20 scale) is appropriate for these clients to achieve moderate-intensity exercise.

### Time

ACSM recommends an exercise time of 30–60 minutes of continuous or accumulated exercise per session. Exercise duration goals are to be based on individual goals and personal history (7,48,125). A caloric expenditure goal of 2,000 kcal or more per week is indicated to help treat persons with hypertension especially if weight loss is also a goal.

### Type

Clients with hypertension should primarily engage in aerobic endurance activities that involve large muscle groups and are rhythmic in nature. Avoid activities that emphasize isometric muscle contractions or that may elicit large blood pressure responses in your clients.

### Progression

The basic principle of progression generally applies to those with hypertension. Specific consideration should be given to blood pressure control, recent changes in blood pressure medications, and the other comorbidities that may be present. Progression must be gradual and avoid large increases in any of the FITT components, especially intensity for most people with hypertension.

## Resistance Training for Clients with Hypertension

Resistance training is considered a supplement to aerobic exercise and should not be prescribed as the primary form of activity for clients with hypertension (5). When supplementing with resistance training, intensity should be kept at 60%–80% 1-RM (5). Although studies have demonstrated a favorable blood pressure response to resistance training, the overall effect is not as great as the response to aerobic exercise training (74). Specific resistance training recommendations for these clients are similar to those used for apparently healthy adults. In addition, teaching clients proper exercise technique, proper breathing, and avoiding larger amounts of isometric work during resistance training will also help minimize large increase in blood pressure.

## Other Considerations for Clients with Hypertension

Hypertension is often associated with a variety of conditions that may require special attention and specific precautions during exercise.

The primary focus of these considerations is safety during and after exercise. As stated previously, hypertension is often associated with a variety of conditions that may require special attention and specific precautions during exercise. In these cases, the general exercise prescription may need to be modified to address these issues (7).

The majority of clients with hypertension are likely to be taking some form of antihypertensive medication. Although a decrease in blood pressure following exercise is to be expected, the greatest risk these medications pose is in eliciting an abnormal drop in blood pressure (hypotension) following exercise. Therefore, engaging in gradual and prolonged cool-down activities will be important in minimizing the risk for excessive postexercise hypotension. The cool-down should never be omitted for sake of time. Antihypertensive medications are diverse in their overall action and number. As stated previously, β-blockers lower the heart rate response to exercise, whereas angiotensin-converting enzyme (ACE) inhibitors lower blood pressure by preventing vasoconstriction without a significant change in heart rate. Thus, Personal Trainers are encouraged to familiarize themselves regarding the types, names, actions, and what the exercise responses are to these medications before working with hypertensive clients. The *ACSM's Guidelines for Exercise Testing and Prescription* (5) is an excellent text to use as a starting point for this information.

Lastly, Personal Trainers working with this population are encouraged to gain skill or enhance existing skills in blood pressure monitoring. Accurate measurement of blood pressure before, during, and after exercise will enhance the safety and appropriateness of the client's program. Precautions dictate that exercise be avoided if resting blood pressure exceeds 200/110 mm Hg and exercise terminated if blood pressure exceeds 220/105 mm Hg or the client experiences a 10 mm Hg or more drop in systolic blood pressure during exercise (5).

## Programming for Clients with Comorbidities

In the past century, life expectancy in the United States increased from less than 50 years to greater than 76 years. The United States Census Bureau has projected that by 2030, the number of adults 65 years of age and older will be approximately 70 million. However, current trends also show that although Americans are living longer, the number of individuals with chronic diseases continues to increase. Approximately 80% of individuals aged 65 years or older are living with at least one chronic health problem, and another 50% are living with two chronic conditions (129). Moreover, the presence of chronic conditions is linked with an even greater propensity of comorbidities. For instance, almost all individuals with diabetes have at least one other chronic condition and nearly half have three or more comorbidities (129). These facts make it increasingly likely that the Personal Trainer will be interacting with clientele that have multiple chronic conditions.

Approximately 80% of individuals aged 65 years or older are living with at least one chronic health problem, and another 50% are living with two chronic conditions (129).

A clear shortcoming of many health care models for the management of chronic conditions is that treatment has historically been approached in a singular fashion. Patients infrequently receive guidance from medical professionals on prioritizing and managing multiple chronic conditions (75). The challenge of working with individuals with comorbidities is understanding that the presence of multiple conditions may compete with a client's self-management resources, thus reducing the time and energy an individual has remaining to devote to each and every condition (30). For instance, an individual with a severe and symptomatic condition, such as heart failure, will likely have lower prioritization of other conditions (*e.g.*, Type 2 diabetes). In turn, these individuals require additional assistance and resources to ensure that their other conditions are managed effectively.

ACSM and the American Heart Association list sedentary lifestyle as a controllable risk factor for many chronic health conditions (5). Accordingly, exercise is a common therapeutic intervention strategy, and although there are exercise program guidelines for older adult and various chronic-diseased populations, these recommendations exclusively address each group separately. This section will explain critical measures that can be taken to design safe and effective exercise programs for clients with multiple chronic conditions or those with comorbidities.

## Programming Goals

General programming goals in the management of clients with comorbidities are to (7,30,31,80)

1. Lower the overall risk of mortality by identifying the condition with the highest mortality risk; prioritize exercise program design around this condition.
2. Recognize that the presence of comorbidities may serve as competing demands on client's self-management resources, thus reducing time and energy an individual has remaining to devote to each and every condition (30); these individuals will require additional guidance and resources provided by the personal trainer to ensure that all conditions are managed effectively.
3. Have realistic expectations for the expected improvement for all comorbidities; improvement is not always feasible (80), and there will be instances where maintaining functional capacity or stabilizing the disease process can, and should, be viewed as a successful outcome.

## Training for Clients with Comorbidities

Exercise training is relatively safe for the majority of clients with multiple chronic conditions provided that appropriate assessment and screening is performed prior to beginning the program (87). The likelihood of an adverse event, although not entirely preventable, can be markedly reduced with baseline assessments, risk stratification, patient education, and client adherence to established exercise recommendations. It is likely that individuals with multiple chronic conditions will be stratified into a high-risk category and therefore will require physician clearance and consent to participate in an exercise program. Clients with comorbidities require a high degree of monitoring to ensure proper adherence of the established exercise regimen and to determine that the physiological responses to each session are normal. Personal Trainers should be knowledgeable of, and able to educate clients about, the potential signs that would warrant the termination of exercise. Importantly, clients and Personal Trainers alike should consult with the medical team about any specific limitations to be aware of when designing the exercise program.

In general, the exercise prescription for individuals with comorbidities can follow the FITT-VP framework. Table 20.13 provides a summary of the basic evidence-based guidelines for common clinical populations. This resource can assist with establishing the basic parameters of the exercise prescription around the various conditions of an individual. For example, consider an individual who has arthritis, dyslipidemia, hypertension, and Type 2 diabetes. One strategy to employ, when designing the program, is to follow the specific exercise prescription for the chronic condition that poses the greatest risk of mortality for the individual. In this instance, Type 2 diabetes is generally considered to increase the risk for heart disease and all-cause mortality (14) more so than the other conditions. Other chronic conditions and specific limiting symptoms must also be carefully considered when formulating the program. In this instance, the frequency and time

| Table 20.13 | A Quick Glance at the Aerobic Exercise Prescription for Common Clinical Populations | | |
|---|---|---|---|
| Condition | Frequency (d · wk$^{-1}$) | Intensity ($\dot{V}O_2R$ or HRR) | Time (min · d$^{-1}$) |
| Arthritis | 3–5 | 40%–59% | 20–30 |
| Cardiac disease | 3–7 | 40%–80% | 20–60 |
| Dyslipidemia | ≥5 | 40%–75% | 30–60 |
| Hypertension | Most, if not all | 40%–59% | 30–60 |
| Obesity | ≥5 | 40%–59% (with potential progression to more than 60%) | 30–60 |
| Osteoporosis | 4–5 | 40%–59% | 30–60 |
| Type 2 diabetes | 3–7 | 40%–59% (60% $\dot{V}O_2R$ or HRR or higher for those already active) | 20–60 |

HRR, heart rate reserve.
Moderate intensity, resistance exercise is recommended 2–3 d · wk$^{-1}$ in addition to the amount of aerobic exercise specified above.
From American College of Sports Medicine. *ACSM's Guidelines for Exercise Testing and Prescription.* 10th ed. Philadelphia (PA): Wolters Kluwer; 2018.

parameters of the exercise prescription for each condition are comparable. Yet, there are some marked differences in the exercise intensity recommendations between conditions. Therefore, it is prudent for the exercise professional to adopt the appropriate exercise prescription for the most restrictive condition.

Occasionally, a chronic condition may become the primary focus for training rather than the comorbidity that has the highest mortality risk. For example, arthritis is characterized by periodic episodes of acute inflammation. Pain and discomfort are common throughout these flares, and without sufficient caution, exercise can actually exacerbate the symptoms (5). Under these circumstances, it would be ill-advised to pursue the exercise prescription guidelines for Type 2 diabetes despite its status as a higher risk for mortality. In this case, an exercise prescription resembling the recommendation guidelines for arthritis would be more suitable and may require consultation with the individual's health care provider.

## Other Considerations for Clients with Comorbidities

The greatest challenge for Personal Trainers in designing exercise programs for clients with comorbidities is the amount of planning required. Considerable preparation is involved in designing programs to be safe (during and after exercise) and effective. The complexity of working with clients possessing multiple chronic conditions requires a thorough preparticipation screening. Baseline assessment and screening will help identify central problems that can prove useful in designing the exercise program and recognizing limitations. For example, insulin resistance is likely to be associated with obesity, hypertension, dyslipidemia, and other metabolic disorders. Likewise, a client with Type 2 diabetes may be expected to suffer from complications of neuropathy, retinopathy, or other microvascular complications. Individuals with multiple comorbidities may also possess conditions (*e.g.*, low back pain, lupus, osteoarthritis, fibromyalgia) that fluctuate significantly within or between days in terms of severity. For example, sometimes pain levels "flare" in the early morning other times they increase just before bed. Personal Trainers must be prepared to accommodate an ever-changing chronic condition landscape with these types of clients and constantly adjust the session to best serve the client on any given day.

Although experienced Personal Trainers can work with clients with stable chronic disease who are able to exercise independently, it is important to recognize situations when consultation with medical personnel is necessary and/or when the Personal Trainer should not undertake a client.

Although experienced Personal Trainers can work with clients with stable chronic disease who are able to exercise independently, it is important to recognize situations when consultation with medical personnel is necessary and/or when the Personal Trainer should not undertake a client (*e.g.*, inappropriate changes of resting or exercise heart rate or blood pressure; new-onset discomfort in the chest, neck, shoulder, or arm; changes in pattern of discomfort during rest or exercise; shortness of breath at rest or with light exertion; fainting or dizzy spells; and claudication). Personal Trainers need to know the limits of their expertise and consider additional training and certification to work in concert with medical personal in helping clients with multiple serious or unstable comorbidities.

## SUMMARY

This chapter explored the special considerations of exercise program design for children; older adults; those with cardiac disease, pregnancy, diabetes mellitus, obesity, or hypertension; and individuals with comorbidities. Personal Trainers are ultimately responsible for designing safe and effective programs that make a positive difference in the lives of their clients. Personal Trainers are encouraged to use evidence-based practice to guide their selection and use of a specific intervention in a given situation. Evidence-based practice is the integration of best research evidence with professional expertise and client values. The rationale for basing decisions on sound evidence is clear — programs supported by research lead to an informed action plan that minimizes risk and optimizes effectiveness.

## REFERENCES

1. Aagaard P, Magnusson P, Larsson B, Kjaer M, Krustrup P. Mechanical muscle function, morphology, and fiber type in lifelong trained elderly. *Med Sci Sports Exerc.* 2007;39(11): 1989–96.
2. Adrian MJ. Flexibility in the aging adult. In: Smith EL, Serfass RC, editors. *Exercise and Aging: The Scientific Basis.* Hillside (NJ): Enslow; 1981. p. 45–57.
3. American College of Obstetricians and Gynecologists. ACOG Committee Opinion No. 650. Physical activity and exercise during pregnancy and the postpartum period. *Obstet Gynecol.* 2015;126:e135–42.
4. American College of Sports Medicine. *ACSM's Exercise Management for Persons with Chronic Diseases and Disabilities.* 4th ed. Champaign (IL): Human Kinetics; 2016. 416 p.
5. American College of Sports Medicine. *ACSM's Guidelines for Exercise Testing and Prescription.* 10th ed. Philadelphia (PA): Wolters Kluwer; 2018.
6. American College of Sports Medicine. American College of Sports Medicine position stand. Appropriate physical activity intervention strategies for weight loss and prevention of weight regain for adults. *Med Sci Sports Exerc.* 2009;41:459–71.
7. American College of Sports Medicine. American College of Sports Medicine position stand. Exercise and hypertension. *Med Sci Sports Exerc.* 2004;36:533–53.
8. American College of Sports Medicine. Exercise and type 2 diabetes: American College of Sports Medicine and the American Diabetes Association: joint position statement. *Med Sci Sports Exerc.* 2010;42:2282–303.
9. Annis AM, Caulder MS, Cook ML, Duquette D. Family history, diabetes, and other demographic and risk factors among participants of the National Health and Nutrition Examination Survey 1999–2002. *Prev Chronic Dis.* 2005;2:A19.
10. Arampatzis A, Degens H, Baltzopoulos V, Rittweger J. Why do older sprinters reach the finish line later? *Exer Sport Sci Rev.* 2011;39(1):18–22.
11. Arias E. *Changes in Life Expectancy by Race and Hispanic Origin in the United States, 2013–2014* (NCHS Data Brief No. 244) [Internet]. Hyattsville (MD): National Center for Health Statistics; [cited 2012 Jan 31]. Available from: https://www.cdc.gov/nchs/products/databriefs/db244.htm
12. Artal R, O'Toole M. Guidelines of the American College of Obstetricians and Gynecologists for exercise during pregnancy and the postpartum period. *Br J Sports Med.* 2003;37:6–12.
13. Bird M, Hill KD, Ball M, Hetherington S, Williams AD. The long-term benefits of a multi-component exercise intervention to balance and mobility in healthy older adults. *Arch Gerontol Geriatr.* 2010;52(2):211–6.

14. Blackwell DL, Lucas JW, Clarke TC. Summary health statistics for U.S. adults: National Health Interview Survey, 2012. *Vital Health Stat.* 2014;10(260);1–161.

15. Blair SN, Kampert JB, Kohl HW III, et al. Influences of cardiorespiratory fitness and other precursors on cardiovascular disease and all-cause mortality in men and women. *JAMA.* 1996;276:205–10.

16. Blair SN, Kohl HW III, Barlow CE, Paffenbarger RS Jr, Gibbons LW, Macera CA. Changes in physical fitness and all-cause mortality. *JAMA.* 1995;273:1093–8.

17. Blair SN, Kohl HW III, Paffenbarger RS Jr, Clark DG, Cooper KH, Gibbons LW. Physical fitness and all-cause mortality. A prospective study of healthy men and women. *JAMA.* 1989;262:2395–401.

18. Blair SN. Physical inactivity: the biggest public health problem of the 21st century. *Br J Sports Med.* 2009;43:1–2.

19. Blissmer B, Riebe D, Dye G, Ruggiero L, Greene G, Caldwell M. Health-related quality of life following a clinical weight loss intervention among overweight and obese adults: intervention and 24 month follow-up effects. *Health Qual Life Outcomes.* 2006;4:43.

20. Booth FW, Gordon SE, Carlson CJ, Hamilton MT. Waging war on modern chronic diseases: primary prevention through exercise biology. *J Appl Physiol.* 2000;88:774–87.

21. Boulé NG, Haddad E, Kenny GP, Wells GA, Sigal RJ. Effects of exercise on glycemic control and body mass in type 2 diabetes mellitus: a meta-analysis of controlled clinical trials. *JAMA.* 2001;286:1218–27.

22. Boulé NG, Weisnagel SJ, Lakka TA, et al. Effects of exercise training on glucose homeostasis: the HERITAGE Family Study. *Diabetes Care.* 2005;28:108–14.

23. Brooks N, Layne JE, Gordon PL, Roubenoff R, Nelson ME, Castaneda-Sceppa C. Strength training improves muscle quality and insulin sensitivity in Hispanic older adults with Type 2 diabetes. *Int J Med Sci.* 2006;4:19–27.

24. Bryner R, Ullrich I, Sauers J, et al. Effects of resistance vs. aerobic training combined with an 800 calorie liquid diet on lean body mass and resting metabolic rate. *J Am Coll Nutr.* 1999;18:115–21.

25. Burnet DL, Elliott LD, Quinn MT, Plaut AJ, Schwartz MA, Chin MH. Preventing diabetes in the clinical setting. *J Gen Intern Med.* 2006;21:84–93.

26. Caserotti P, Aagaard P, Buttrup Larsen B, Puggaard L. Explosive heavy-resistance training in old and very old adults: changes in rapid muscle force, strength and power. *Scandinavian J Med Sci Sports.* 2008;18(6):773–82.

27. Castaneda C, Layne J, Munoz-Orians L, et al. A randomized controlled trial of resistance exercise training to improve glycemic control in older adults with type 2 diabetes. *Diabetes Care.* 2002;25:2335–41.

28. Centers for Disease Control and Prevention. *Defining Obesity and Overweight* [Internet]. Atlanta (GA): Centers for Disease Control and Prevention; [cited 2008 Aug 10]. Available from: http://www.cdc.gov/nccdphp/dnpa/obesity/defining.htm

29. Centers for Disease Control and Prevention. *National Diabetes Statistics Report: Estimates of Diabetes and Its Burden in the United States, 2014* [Internet]. Atlanta (GA): U.S. Department of Health and Human Services; 2014. Available from: https://www.cdc.gov/diabetes/pubs/statsreport14/national-diabetes-report-web.pdf

30. Chernof BA, Sherman SE, Lanto AB, Lee M, Yano EM, Rubenstein LV. Health habit counseling amidst competing demands: effects of patient health habits and visit characteristics. *Med Care.* 1999;37:738–47.

31. Chobanian AV, Bakris GL, Black HR, et al. Seventh report of the Joint National Committee on Prevention, Detection Evaluation, and Treatment of High Blood Pressure. *Hypertension.* 2003;42:1206–52.

32. Chodzko-Zajko W, Proctor D, Fiatarone Singh M, et al. Exercise and physical activity for older adults. *Med Sci Sports Exer.* 2009;41(7):1510–30.

33. Church TS, LaMonte MJ, Barlow CE, Blair SN. Cardiorespiratory fitness and body mass index as predictors of cardiovascular disease mortality among men with diabetes. *Arch Intern Med.* 2005;165:2114–20.

34. Cornish AK, Broadbent S, Cheema BS. Interval training for patients with coronary artery disease: a systematic review. *Eur J Appl Physiol.* 2011;111(4):579–89.

35. Costa PB, Graves BS, Whitehurst M, Jacobs PL. The acute effects of different durations of static stretching on dynamic balance performance. *J Strength Cond Res.* 2009;23(1):141–7.

36. Cutler R, Harman S, Heward C, Gibbons M. Physical activity and aging. Longevity Health Science: the phoenix conference. *Ann N Y Acad Sci.* 2005;1005:193–206.

37. Daley MJ, Spinks WL. Exercise, mobility and aging. *Sports Med.* 2000;29(1):1–12.

38. Dempsey J, Seals D. Aging, exercise, and cardiopulmonary function. In: Lamb DR, Gisolfi CV, Nadel E, editors. *Exercise in Older Adults.* Carmel (IL): Cooper; 1995. p. 237–304.

39. Deschenes M, Carter J, Matney E, Potter M, Wilson M. Aged men experience disturbances in recovery following submaximal exercise. *J Gerontol Ser A Biol Sci Med Sci.* 2006;61(1):63–71.

40. Diabetes Prevention Program Research Group. Reduction in the incidence of type 2 diabetes with lifestyle intervention or metformin. *N Engl J Med.* 2002;346:393–403.

41. *Dietary Reference Intakes for Energy, Carbohydrate, Fiber, Fat, Fatty Acids, Cholesterol, Protein, and Amino Acids.* Washington (DC): National Academies Press; 2005. 1332 p.

42. Dishman R, Berthoud HR, Booth FW, et al. Neurobiology of exercise. *Obesity.* 2006;14(3):345–56.

43. Dunn AL, Marcus BH, Kamper JB, Garcia ME, Kohl HW III, Blair SN. Comparison of lifestyle and structured interventions to increase physical activity and cardiorespiratory fitness: a randomized trial. *JAMA.* 1999;281:327–34.

44. Dunstan D, Daly R, Owen N, Jolley D, De Courten M, Shaw J, Zimmet P. High-intensity resistance training improves glycemic control in older patients with Type 2 diabetes. *Diabetes Care.* 2002;25:1729–36.

45. Duscha BD, Slentz CA, Johnson JL, et al. Effects of exercise training amount and intensity on peak oxygen consumption in middle-age men and women at risk for cardiovascular disease. *Chest.* 2005;128:2788–93.

46. Eriksson J. Exercise and the treatment of Type 2 diabetes mellitus. An update. *Sports Med.* 1999;27:381–91.

47. Eriksson J, Taimela S, Eriksson K, Parviainen S, Peltonen J, Kujala U. Resistance training in the treatment of non-insulin-dependent diabetes mellitus. *Int J Sports Med.* 1997;18:242–6.

48. Fagard R. Exercise characteristics and the blood pressure response to dynamic physical training. *Med Sci Sports Exerc*. 2001;33:S484–92.

49. Faigenbaum AD, Kraemer WJ, Blimkie CJ, et al. Youth resistance training: updated position statement paper from the National Strength and Conditioning Association. *J Strength Cond Res*. 2009;23:S60–79.

50. Ferrari A, Radaelli A, Centola M. Invited review: aging and the cardiovascular system. *J Appl Physiol*. 2003;95:2591–7.

51. Fitzgerald MD, Tanaka H, Tran ZV, Seals DR. Age-related declines in maximal aerobic capacity in regularly exercising vs. sedentary women: a meta-analysis. *J Appl Physiol*. 1997;83:160–5.

52. Flegal KM, Carroll MD, Ogden CL, Curtin LR. Prevalence and trends in obesity among US adults, 1999–2008. *JAMA*. 2010;303:235–41.

53. Fletcher GF, Balady GJ, Amsterdam EA, et al. Exercise standards for testing and training. A statement for health care professionals from the American Heart Association. *Circulation*. 2001;104:1694–740.

54. Foster GD, Wadden TA, Phelan S, Sarwer DB, Sanderson RS. Obese patients' perceptions of treatment outcomes and the factors that influence them. *Arch Intern Med*. 2001;161:2133–9.

55. Franklin BA. Fitness: the ultimate marker for risk stratification and health outcomes? *Prev Cardiol*. 2007;10:42–6.

56. Gaesser GA, Angadi SS, Sawyer BJ. Exercise and diet, independent of weight loss, improve cardiometabolic risk profile in overweight and obese individuals. *Phys Sportsmed*. 2011;39(2):87–97.

57. Garber CE, Blissmer B, Deschenes MR, et al. American College of Sports Medicine position stand. Quantity and quality of exercise for developing and maintaining cardiorespiratory, musculoskeletal, and neuromuscular fitness in apparently healthy adults: guidance for prescribing exercise. *Med Sci Sports Exerc*. 2011;43(7):1334–59.

58. Gellish R, Goslin B, Olson R, McDonald A, Russi G, Moudgil V. Longitudinal modeling of the relationship between age and maximal heart rate. *Med Sci Sports Exer*. 2007;39(5):822–9.

59. Guidelines for the prevention of falls in older persons. American Geriatrics Society, British Geriatrics Society, and American Academy of Orthopaedic Surgeons Panel on Falls Prevention. *J Am Geriatr Soc*. 2001;49(5):664–72.

60. Hagberg JM. Physical activity, fitness, health, and aging. In: Bouchard C, Shephard RJ, Stephens T, editors. *Physical Activity, Fitness, and Health*. Champaign (IL): Human Kinetics; 1994. p. 993–1006.

61. Hare SW, Price JH, Flynn MG, King KA. Attitudes and perceptions of fitness professionals regarding obesity. *J Community Health*. 2000;25(1):5–21.

62. Harris S, Petrella R, Leadbetter W. Lifestyle interventions for Type 2 diabetes: relevance for clinical practice. *Can Fam Physician*. 2003;49:1618–25.

63. Haskell WL, Lee IM, Pate RR, et al. Physical activity and public health: updated recommendation for adults from the American College of Sports Medicine and the American Heart Association. *Med Sci Sports Exerc*. 2007;39:1423–34.

64. Heckman G, Mckelvie, R. Cardiovascular aging and exercise in healthy older adults. *Clin J Sport Med*. 2008;18(6):479–85.

65. Hollmann W, Strüder H, Tagarakis C, King G. Physical activity and the elderly. *Eur J Cardiovasc Prev Rehabil*. 2007;14(6):730–9.

66. Houmard JA, Tanner CJ, Slentz CA, Duscha BD, McCartney JS, Kraus WE. Effect of the volume and intensity of exercise training on insulin sensitivity. *J Appl Physiol*. 2004;96:101–6.

67. Howe NL, Swan, PD. Training obese clients: examining our assumptions. *ACSM's Health Fitness J*. 2003;7(6):1–4.

68. Iqbal N. The burden of type 2 diabetes: strategies to prevent or delay onset. *Vasc Health Risk Manag*. 2007;3:511–20.

69. Ishii T, Yamakita T, Sato T, Tanaka S, Fujii S. Resistance training improves insulin sensitivity in NIDDM subjects without altering maximal oxygen uptake. *Diabetes Care*. 1998;21:1353–5.

70. Jackson AS, Sui X, Hébert JR, Church TS, Blair SN. Role of lifestyle and aging on the longitudinal change in cardiorespiratory fitness. *Arch Intern Med*. 2009;169(19):1781–7.

71. Jeffery RW, Wing RR, Thorson C, Burton LR. Use of personal trainers and financial incentives to increase exercise in a behavioral weight-loss program. *J Consult Clin Psychol*. 1998;66(5):777–83.

72. Kahn B, Flier J. Obesity and insulin resistance. *J Clin Invest*. 2000;106:473–81.

73. Kara B, Pinar L, Uğur F, Oğuz M. Correlations between aerobic capacity, pulmonary and cognitive functioning in the older women. *Int J Sports Med*. 2005;26(3):220–4.

74. Kelley G, Kelley K. Progressive resistance exercise and resting blood pressure: a meta-analysis of randomized controlled trials. *Hypertension*. 2000;35:838–43.

75. Kerr EA, Heisler M, Krein SL, et al. Beyond comorbidity counts: how do comorbidity type and severity influence diabetes patients' treatment priorities and self-management? *J Gen Intern Med*. 2007;22:1635–40.

76. Klem ML, Wing RR, McGuire MT, Seagle HM, Hill JO. A descriptive study of individuals successful at long-term maintenance of substantial weight loss. *Am J Clin Nutr*. 1997;66:239–46.

77. Koopman R, van Loon L. Aging, exercise and muscle protein metabolism. *J Appl Physiol*. 2009;106(6):2040–8.

78. Kraus WE, Houmard JA, Duscha BD, et al. Effects of the amount and intensity of exercise on plasma lipoproteins. *N Engl J Med*. 2002;347:1483–92.

79. Kruk J. Physical activity in the prevention of the most frequent chronic diseases: an analysis of the recent evidence. *Asian Pac J Cancer Prev*. 2007;8(3):325–38.

80. Kujala UM. Benefits of exercise therapy for chronic diseases. *B J Sports Med*. 2006;40:3–4.

81. LaBella FS, Paul G. Structure of collagen from human tendon as influenced by age and sex. *J Gerontol*. 1965;20:54–9.

82. Lee DC, Artero EG, Sui X, Blair SN. Mortality trends in the general population: the importance of cardiorespiratory fitness. *J Psychopharmacol*. 2010;24(suppl 4):27–35.

83. Lloyd-Jones DM, Dyer AR, Wang R, Daviglus ML, Greenland P. Risk factor burden in middle age and lifetime risks for cardiovascular and non-cardiovascular death (Chicago Heart Association Detection Project in Industry). *Am J Cardiol*. 2007;99:535–40.

84. Löllgen H, Böckenhoff A, Knapp G. Physical activity and all-cause mortality: an updated meta-analysis with different intensity categories. *Int J Sports Med*. 2009;30(3):213–24.

85. Lyerly GW, Sui X, Lavie CJ, Church TS, Hand GA, Blair SN. The association between cardiorespiratory fitness and risk of all-cause mortality among women with impaired fasting glucose or undiagnosed diabetes mellitus. *Mayo Clin Proc*. 2009;84:780–6.

86. Maiorana A, O'Driscoll G, Goodman C, Taylor R, Green D. Combined aerobic and resistance exercise improves glycemic control and fitness in type 2 diabetes. *Diabetes Res Clin Pract*. 2002;56:115–23.

87. Mangani I, Cesari M, Kritchevsky SB, et al. Physical exercise and comorbidity. Results from the Fitness and Arthritis in Seniors Trial (FAST). *Aging Clin Exp Res*. 2006;18:374–80.

88. Metter E, Conwit R, Metter B, Pacheco T, Tobin J. The relationship of peripheral motor nerve conduction velocity to age-associated loss of grip strength. *Aging (Milano)*. 1998;10(6):471–8.

89. Mozaffarian D, Benjamin EJ, Go AS, et al. Heart Disease and Stroke Statistics — 2016 Update. A report from the American Heart Association. *Circulation*. 2015;133:447–54. Available from: http://circ.ahajournals.org/content/early/2015/12/16/CIR.0000000000000350

90. National Center on Health, Physical Activity and Disability. *For Fitness Professionals* [Internet]. Birmingham (AL): National Center on Health, Physical Activity and Disability; [cited 2017 Jan 31]. Available from: http://www.nchpad.org/Fitness~Professionals

91. Nelson ME, Rejeski WJ, Blair SN, et al. Physical activity and public health in older adults: recommendation for adults from the American College of Sports Medicine and the American Heart Association. *Med Sci Sports Exerc*. 2007;39:1435–45.

92. Nocon M, Hiemann T, Müller-Riemenschneider F, Thalau F, Roll S, Willich SN. Association of physical activity with all-cause and cardiovascular mortality: a systematic review and meta-analysis. *Eur J Cardiovasc Prev Rehabil*. 2008;15(3):239–46.

93. Ogden CL, Carroll MD, Fryar CD, Flegal KM. *Prevalence of Obesity Among Adults and Youth: United States, 2011–2014* (NCHS Data Brief No. 219). Hyattsville (MD): National Center for Health Statistics; 2015. 8 p.

94. Ogden CL, Carroll MD, McDowell MA, Flegal KM. *Obesity Among Adults in the United States — No Change Since 2003–2004* (NCHS Data Brief No. 1). Hyattsville (MD): National Center for Health Statistics; 2007. 8 p.

95. Park S, Park J, Kwon Y, Kim H, Yoon M, Park H. The effect of combined aerobic and resistance exercise training on abdominal fat in obese middle-aged women. *J Physiol Anthropol Appl Human Sci*. 2003;22:129–35.

96. Pate R, Pratt M, Blair SN, et al. Physical activity and public health: a recommendation from the Centers for Disease Control and Prevention and the American College of Sports Medicine. *JAMA*. 1995;273:402–7.

97. Peirce N. Diabetes and exercise. *Br J Sports Med*. 1999;33:161–73.

98. Peters A. The effects of normal aging on myelin and nerve fibers: a review. *J Neurocytol*. 2002;31(8–9):581–93.

99. Peterson M, Rhea M, Sen A, Gordon P. Resistance exercise for muscular strength in older adults: a meta-analysis. *Ageing Res Rev*. 2010;9(3):226–37.

100. Racette S, Weiss E, Hickner R, Holloszy J. Modest weight loss improves insulin action in obese African Americans. *Metabolism*. 2005;54:960–5.

101. Saris WH, Blair SN, van Baak MA, et al. How much physical activity is enough to prevent unhealthy weight gain? Outcome of the IASO 1st Stock Conference and consensus statement. *Obes Rev*. 2003;4:101–14.

102. Sequin R, Nelson M. The benefits of strength training for older adults. *Am J Prev Med*. 2003;25(suppl 2):141–9. 353 p.

103. Shephard RJ. *Physical Activity and Aging*. Chicago (IL): Yearbook Medical Publishers; 1978.

104. Shrier I. Does stretching improve performance? A systematic and critical review of the literature. *Clin J Sport Med*. 2004;14:267–73.

105. Sigal R, Kenny G, Boulé N, et al. Effects of aerobic training, resistance training, or both on glycemic control in type 2 diabetes: a randomized trial. *Ann Intern Med*. 2007;147:357–69.

106. Slentz C, Aiken L, Houmard J, et al. Inactivity, exercise, and visceral fat. STRRIDE: a randomized, controlled study of exercise intensity and amount. *J Appl Physiol*. 2005;99:1613–18.

107. Slentz CA, Duscha BD, Johnson JL, et al. Effects of the amount of exercise on body weight, body composition, and measures of central obesity: STRRIDE — a randomized controlled study. *Arch Intern Med*. 2004;164:31–9.

108. Soukup J, Maynard TS, Kovaleski JE. Resistance training guidelines for individuals with diabetes mellitus. *Diabetic Educ*. 1994;20:129–37.

109. Strasser B, Keinrad M, Haber P, Schobersberger W. Efficacy of systematic endurance and resistance training on muscle strength and endurance performance in elderly adults — a randomized controlled trial. *Wien Klin Wochenschr*. 2009;121(23–24):757–64.

110. Strotmeyer ES, de Rekeneire N, Schwartz AV, et al. Sensory and motor peripheral nerve function and lower-extremity quadriceps strength: the health, aging and body composition study. *J Am Geriatrics Soc*. 2009;57(11):2004–10.

111. Sui X, LaMonte M, Blair S. Cardiorespiratory fitness and risk of nonfatal cardiovascular disease in women and men with hypertension. *Am J Hypertens*. 2007;20:608–15.

112. Swain DP, Franklin BA. Comparison of cardioprotective benefits of vigorous versus moderate intensity aerobic exercise. *Am J Cardiol*. 2006;97:141–7.

113. Swain DP, Franklin BA. Is there a threshold intensity for aerobic training in cardiac patients? *Med Sci Sports Exerc*. 2002;34:1071–5.

114. Tanaka H, Seals DR. Endurance exercise performance in Masters athletes: age-associated changes and underlying physiological mechanisms. *J Physiol*. 2007;586(1):55–63.

115. Taylor JD. The impact of a supervised strength and aerobic training program on muscular strength and aerobic capacity in individuals with type 2 diabetes. *J Strength Cond Res*. 2007;21:824–30.

116. Teachman BA, Brownell KD. Implicit anti-fat bias among health professionals: is anyone immune? *Int J Obes Relat Metab Disord*. 2001;25(10):1525–31.

117. Thompson PD, Buchner D, Pina IL, et al. Exercise and physical activity in the prevention and treatment of

atherosclerotic cardiovascular disease: a statement from the Council on Clinical Cardiology (Subcommittee on Exercise, Rehabilitation, and Prevention) and the Council on Nutrition, Physical Activity, and Metabolism (Subcommittee on Physical Activity). *Circulation*. 2003; 107:3109–16.

118. Tokmakidis SP, Zois CE, Volaklis KA, Kotsa K, Touvra AM. The effects of a combined strength and aerobic exercise program on glucose control and insulin action in women with type 2 diabetes. *Eur J Appl Physiol*. 2004;92:437–42.

119. U.S. Department of Health and Human Services. *Physical Activity and Health: A Report of the Surgeon General*. Atlanta (GA): U.S. Department of Health and Human Services, Centers for Disease Control and Prevention, National Center for Chronic Disease and Health Promotion; 1996. 278 p.

120. U.S. Department of Health and Human Services. *The Surgeon General's Call to Action to Prevent and Decrease Overweight and Obesity* [Internet]. Atlanta (GA): U.S. Department of Health and Human Services, Office of the Surgeon General; [cited 2017 Jan 30]. Available from: http://www.surgeongeneral.gov/topics/obesity/

121. U.S. Department of Health and Human Services. *2008 Physical Activity Guidelines for Americans* [Internet]. Washington (DC): U.S. Department of Health and Human Services; [cited 2011 Mar 7]. Available from: http://www.health.gov/PAGuidelines/guidelines/default.aspx

122. Valitutto M. Common crossroads in diabetes management. *Osteo Med Prim Care*. 2008;2:4.

123. Vasan R, Beiser A, Seshadri S, et al. Residual lifetime risk for developing hypertension in middle-aged women and men: the Framingham heart study. *JAMA*. 2002;287:1003–10.

124. Warburton DER, Nicol CW, Bredin SSD. Health benefits of physical activity: the evidence. *CMAJ*. 2006;174:801–9.

125. Whelton S, Chin A, Xin X, He J. Effect of aerobic exercise on blood pressure: a meta-analysis of randomized, controlled trials. *Ann Intern Med*. 2002;136:493–503.

126. Wilborn C, Beckham J, Campbell B, et al. Obesity: prevalence, theories, medical consequences, management, and research directions. *J Int Soc Sports Nutr*. 2005;2:4–31.

127. Williams MA, Haskell WL, Ades PA, et al. Resistance exercise in individuals with and without cardiovascular disease: 2007 update. A scientific statement from the American Heart Association Council on Clinical Cardiology and Council on Nutrition, Physical Activity, and Metabolism. *Circulation*. 2007;116:572–84.

128. Wilson TM, Tanaka H. Meta-analysis of the age-associated decline in maximal aerobic capacity in men: relation to training status. *Am J Physiol Heart Circ Physiol*. 2000;278(3):H829–34.

129. Wolf JL, Starfield B, Anderson G. Prevalence, expenditures, and complications of multiple chronic conditions in the elderly. *Arch Intern Med*. 2002;162:2269–76.

130. Woo J, Derleth C, Stratton J. The influence of age, gender, and training on exercise efficiency. *J Am Coll Cardiol*. 2006;47(5):1049–57.

131. Wright V, Johns RJ. Observations on the measurement of joint stiffness. *Arch Rheum*. 1960;3:328–40.

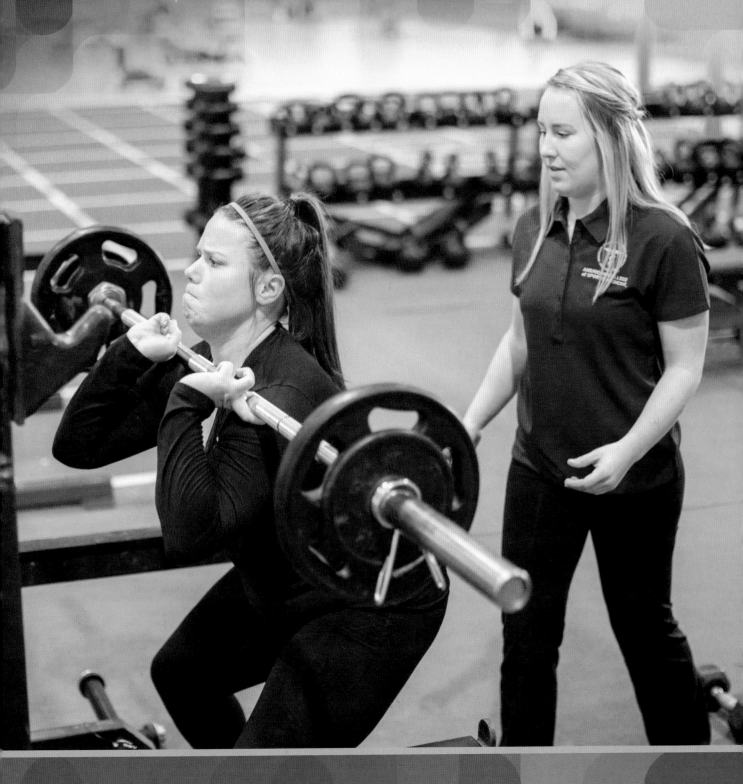

# PART VI

# The Business of Personal Training

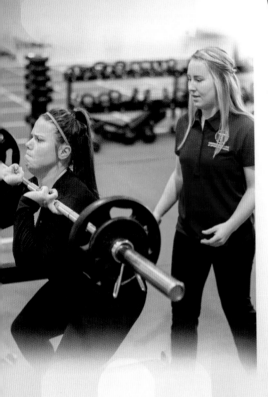

## OBJECTIVES

**Personal Trainers should be able to:**

- Learn how to sell and market training services to potential clients.

- Learn how to price training sessions.

- Learn how to maintain professional standards that will protect a business reputation.

# INTRODUCTION

A Personal Trainer may be very knowledgeable and skilled in exercise science principles and their application in a personal training session, but an understanding of the business of personal training is equally important for success. Whether working as an entrepreneur, a fitness center employee, or an independent contractor, a Personal Trainer needs business expertise in how to sell and market training services to potential clients, how to price training sessions, and how to maintain professional standards that will protect a business reputation. For success as a self-employed Personal Trainer, business planning, business models, and budgeting are also needed before a business can be started. Finally, business success will also depend on finding a work–life balance, as personal training can involve long days with numerous training sessions and interactions with many different people and their unique personalities.

> For success as a self-employed Personal Trainer, business planning, business models, and budgeting are also needed before a business can be started.

##  The Personal Trainer's Position

A Personal Trainer can work in several different and distinct settings. Some of the more common venues or "job classifications" include the solo (*i.e.*, independent) Personal Trainer, the employee or independent contractor, and the manager or personal training business owner. The independent Personal Trainer is commonly known as a Personal Trainer who is autonomous of another business entity. The Personal Trainer of this type typically markets to potential clients and schedules and delivers training sessions in the client's home, outdoors, or in the fitness facility. The employee or independent contractor is typically hired or contracted by a business owner to provide training services for the business's clients. The Personal Trainer/manager/owner typically supervises the business operations and staff management of a personal training business. Whether the Personal Trainer is a sole proprietor or an employee, success will be based on how well he or she can sell the training services. The section "Sales" in this chapter provides a comprehensive approach to selling personal training services. Although the emphasis on specific job tasks might differ from one setting to another, the goal is ultimately the same — to follow sound business practices and develop a profitable enterprise by delivering the optimal level of service to the end user, the client.

There are various compensation models (Table 21.1) for personal training programs in the fitness center setting. Some facilities compensate Personal Trainers a percentage of the revenue generated by the services they deliver, otherwise known as commission-based compensation. Other facilities hire Personal Trainers as hourly or salaried employees with designated work shifts and may pay them an additional commission for "fee for service" sessions delivered to the members. Individual salaries or commission rates for Personal Trainers typically vary based on education, certification, experience, seniority, job performance, and volume of revenue produced. Regardless of the compensation model, it is important that all program costs be considered during the business planning phase. General and administrative costs for marketing, administrative support, meetings, uniforms, payroll taxes, liability insurance, and continuing education can dramatically affect the profitability of the personal training program (3). Table 21.2 and Figure 21.1 provide employment estimates and average wage estimates for Personal Trainers according to the U.S. Bureau of Labor Statistics (9).

## Table 21.1 — Sample Compensation Models for Personal Trainers

**Sample Compensation Model for Personal Trainers Working as Independent Contractor**

| Pay/Salary | Position Perks |
|---|---|
| $42.50 per hour or session | Increase hours or sessions to make more money |

**Sample Compensation Model for Personal Trainers at Corporate Fitness Site**

| Pay/Salary | Pay by Hours Per Week | Position Perks | Limitation |
|---|---|---|---|
| $35,000 | 37.5 h on average | Benefits<br>Education fund<br>Cash incentives | Working more hours does not increase pay. |
| $15 per hour or session | $30 per week (2 sessions per week typically) | | |
| $15–$20 hourly + personal training fee split 60/40 | One-on-one training at $50 per hour:<br>Two sessions per week = $100<br>5-wk period = $500 | Increase hours to make more money or do group training | Limits to number of extra hours per week for training |
| $15–$20 hourly Plus Personal Training fee split 60/40 | Group training for 20 clients (in groups of 5) at $10 per client:<br>Two sessions per week = $400<br>5-wk period = $2,000 | | Limits to number of extra hours per week for training |

## Table 21.2 — Employment Estimate and Mean Wage Estimates for This Occupation (Fitness Trainers and Aerobics Instructors)

| Employment | Employment RSE | Mean Hourly Wage | Mean Annual Wage | Wage RSE |
|---|---|---|---|---|
| 237,760 | 1.4 % | $19.70 | $40,970 | 0.8% |

| Percentile | 10% | 25% | 50% (Median) | 75% | 90% |
|---|---|---|---|---|---|
| Hourly wage | $8.89 | $11.19 | $17.39 | $25.45 | $33.74 |
| Annual wage | $18,690 | $23,280 | $36,160 | $52,940 | $70,180 |

RSE, relative standard error.
Adapted with permission from U.S. Department of Labor, Bureau of Labor Statistics. *Occupational Employment and Wages* [Internet]. Washington (DC): Bureau of Labor Statistics; [cited 2011 Nov 21]. Available from: http://www.bls.gov/oes/current/oes399031.htm

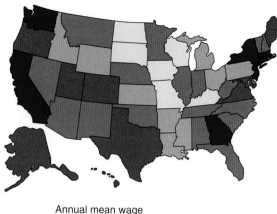

**FIGURE 21.1.** Annual mean wage of fitness trainers and aerobics instructors by state (May 2015). (Adapted with permission from U.S. Department of Labor, Bureau of Labor Statistics. *Occupational Employment and Wages* [Internet]. Washington [DC]: Bureau of Labor Statistics; [cited 2011 Nov 21]. Available from: http://www.bls.gov/oes/current /oes399031.htm)

Annual mean wage

- ☐ $20,490–$26,330
- ▨ $26,730–$28,410
- ▨ $28,800–$30,420
- ▨ $30,620–$33,390
- ▨ $35,390–$38,610
- ■ $38,870–$52,920
- ☐ No Data

## Business Success

*Long-term viability relies greatly on the ability of the Personal Trainer to establish and maintain repeat business.*

Success in the personal training business is very much dependent on the same factors affecting other service-based industries. Consequently, long-term viability relies greatly on the ability of the Personal Trainer to establish and maintain repeat business. Personal Trainers that can meld the needs of the client into a program that focuses on their goals will have an easier time retaining clients.

### Pricing Concepts

Put simply, price is the value or worth of something or some service (1). To properly understand and set your "price," answer, at a minimum, the following questions:

- Who is the buyer? Is the buyer the person using your services, or is it a spouse, significant other or someone else?
- How does the buyer decide on the worth or value of your services? Is it based on effectiveness of services; location; schedule convenience; staff qualifications and motivational capabilities; convenience of credit card processing; competitor prices; or (most likely) a combination of all of the above?
- What are your business objectives when setting prices? Do you want to maximize your profits or maximize your market share?
- Who are your competitors, and what do they offer? What are their prices, and who are their customers? Are you competing directly with another trainer or business that caters to your same clientele, or do your competitors target a different audience?
- Is the competitive environment a major, if not the primary, determinant in setting prices? Would you set your prices differently if there were no competition? How much differently?
- Who is the primary leader in establishing the customer's perception of value? Is it you or the competition? What does this do to your pricing strategy and flexibility?

### Managing a Personal Training Department

If working in a commercial fitness setting, corporate wellness facility, or a nonprofit community recreation center, a Personal Trainer may be employed to manage the personal training department while still maintaining a schedule of training clients. This added responsibility requires sound organizational skills and time management. Skills in interviewing, hiring, employee training, service pricing, marketing, sales, and policy setting are needed by the personal training manager.

## Hiring Personal Trainers

The following are important steps to follow when hiring a Personal Trainer (Box 21.1 and Case Study 21.1):

1. Résumé should be reviewed carefully for educational background, current certifications and credentials, recent training experience with a variety of clientele, and innovative training programs.
2. Applicants should be asked to bring copies of current fitness and cardiopulmonary resuscitation (CPR)-automated external defibrillator (AED)/first aid certifications to the interview appointment. This assures that the Personal Trainer's certifications are from valid agencies/organizations and have not expired.
3. The Personal Trainer/manager should create a list of standard questions to ask all personal training applicants. The questions should be practical, including scenarios that require the Personal Trainer to discuss training program options for hypothetical clients.
4. The Personal Trainer's availability and scheduling preference for appointments should be clearly assessed and agreed to at the time of the interview and prior to a job offer. If the department needs an evening Personal Trainer and the interviewee is already training elsewhere in the evening, the Personal Trainer/manager needs to know that information to effectively plan for staffing needs.
5. A practical or "hands-on" component (*i.e.*, demonstration) should be a part of the interview process. The Personal Trainer should demonstrate exercises and spotting techniques on the fitness floor.

---

**Box 21.1    Recruiting and Selecting Your Team**

**Compare Applications and Résumés to the Hiring Model**

The first step you can take when deciding who to hire is to compare every application and résumé, via a checklist, with its hiring model (job description). With this method, you can subsequently rank the applications and résumés by how closely they align with the hiring model. Performing this step will help you limit the number of candidates that graduate to the next step of the selection process.

**Use Multiple Interviews**

Every candidate should go through a series of interviews. The first interview should be conducted by the immediate supervisor and should focus on uncovering the basic values, beliefs, attitudes, and skills of the applicant. This first interview can be conducted using a structured interview format and checklist. The goal of the interview should be to evaluate the candidate against a specific model. If the candidate meets the expectations of the first interview, then a second interview should be conducted with multiple members of the team, using a structured format. The second interview should be more detailed than the first and should focus on role-play situations based on predetermined questions that are designed to be value indicators of success in the health club business. If the candidate gets through the second interview successfully, then the third interview should be conducted in a team format with several members of the team present. This interview can be more free flowing than the other two because its primary focus is to determine if an appropriate fit exists between the team and the applicant.

Adapted with permission from Tharrett SJ, Peterson JA. Recruiting and selecting your team. *IDEA Fitness Manager* [Internet]. 2008 [cited 2011 Nov 21];20(1). Available from: http://www.ideafit.com/fitness-library/recruiting-and-selecting-your-team

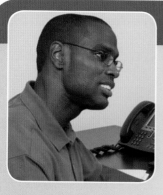

## Case Study 21.1

# Interviewing Candidates for Fitness Staff/Personal Trainer Positions

Fitness staff/personal trainers need to be knowledgeable, outgoing, motivating, able to communicate well, use active listening skills, deal with all types of clients and personalities, and handle problems immediately and effectively.

## Two-Part Interview Process

### Interview Questions

Ask common interview-type questions along with open-ended, experience-based (behavioral interview) questions. Asking candidates for specific examples of past behavior as they relate to the job requirements and problem-solving skills can provide concrete examples of what they have done in the past and can bring to your facility. The behavioral job interview is based on the logic that past behavior predicts future behavior.

Behavioral interview questions will be more pointed, more probing, and more specific than traditional interview questions. Some examples:

- Give an example of an occasion when you used logic to solve a problem.
- Give an example of a goal you reached and tell me how you achieved it.
- Describe a decision you made that was unpopular and how you handled implementing it.
- Have you gone above and beyond the call of duty? If so, how?
- What do you do when your schedule is interrupted? Give an example of how you handle it.
- Have you had to convince a team to work on a project they were not enthusiastic about? How did you do it?
- Have you ever handled a difficult situation with a coworker? If so, how was the situation handled?
- Tell me about a situation where you worked with a client who was being difficult. How did you handle it?
- Tell me about how you worked effectively under pressure.
- Tell me about a project or program you developed/conducted from which you are most proud. With this project or program, what do you feel you did best, and what could you have done better?
- Give me a 30-second elevator speech as to why I should hire you.

### Skills Assessment

Set up an interview for potential candidates where they will actually go through a typical prescreening consultation and fitness assessment by using your staff or facility members as a client. The interview candidate will conduct assessments, compare results to norms, and give results.

- Using another staff to serve as a "client" is a great way to observe the interview candidate to make sure they do know the proper protocols and can conduct the assessments correctly and efficiently. You can also observe their communication skills and see how they interact with their "client." It is best to have already tested this staff person so you know if the results are accurate.
- Provides an excellent chance to watch the interview candidate in a typical work situation. Prior to the assessment, you can brief the "client" on doing some things incorrectly to see if the candidate picks up on them and makes corrections. For example, during a submaximal bike test, the client has the opportunity to ask questions up front, so you can determine if the candidate does have actual experience in conducting these tests and is comfortable handling any situation.
- Assessments should include the initial consultation when the candidate reviews the health/history form and application with the client — you can see if the candidate has experience doing such a review, feels comfortable conducting the consultation, and is able to effectively answer the client's questions.

- Other examples of assessments can include muscular strength and endurance and cardiovascular endurance (submaximal bike or treadmill testing).
- Resting measures of blood pressure, heart rate, height, weight, body composition, flexibility can also be requested. You are looking for the following:
  - If they explain what they are doing and why
  - If they provide the results and compare to norms
  - If they act professionally and appropriately
  - If they address the client's questions and concerns
  - If they can make any necessary modifications

Someone should be designated to be a hypothetical client. The Personal Trainer/manager should observe and assess how the Personal Trainer interacts with this person.

6. A practical component consisting of fitness assessments should also be a part of the interview process. Utilizing a designated hypothetical client, the Personal Trainer should explain and demonstrate commonly used fitness assessments, such as resting blood pressure and heart rate, muscular fitness and flexibility measures, body composition, and cardiovascular endurance testing. The Personal Trainer should also be able to compare the results against norms and then provide the results to the client.

## Setting Training Standards

The Personal Training manager is ultimately responsible for the safety and customer satisfaction of every personal training client. Therefore, it is necessary to set standards for delivering personal training services in a manner that is consistent with industry standards for safety and will ensure that excellent customer service is consistently delivered. Here are some guidelines for setting the department's service standards:

1. Personal Trainers must give their undivided attention to their clients (see Chapter 10). This means that Personal Trainers must watch clients at all times and spot exercises with appropriate techniques. Policy parameters should be specific. Talking on mobile phones, talking with other Personal Trainers or other members, and watching television monitors are examples of unacceptable behaviors that would not meet training standards of practice. In addition, a Personal Trainer who spends much of the training session talking about his or her personal affairs will have difficulty focusing fully on the client's workout and exercise technique (see Chapter 1).
2. The Personal Trainer must begin training sessions on time and end training sessions on time and respect the client's time and schedule.
3. There should be a standard dress code or uniform for an organization's Personal Trainers. If possible, Personal Trainers should wear a shirt with a facility logo and the words "Personal Trainer." The shirt, along with established standards for pants and shoes, will ensure a professional look for the personal training department while also providing advertising to other members.
4. The Personal Trainer should keep written documentation of every client's workout as well as any measurements, tests, and performance tracking for that client (see Chapters 12 and 13). The personal training department manager should provide a standardized "training card" for Personal Trainers to use (Table 21.3). There should be a designated locked cabinet where the training cards are kept. With the client's written consent, the training card can be

## Table 21.3    Sample Training Card

**Sample Workout Log**

| Name: | Date: | Height: | Weight: | Goals: |
|---|---|---|---|---|
| | | | | |

**Weight Training:**

| Exercise | Sets/Reps | Sets/Reps | Sets/Reps | Sets/Reps | Sets/Reps | Sets/Reps |
|---|---|---|---|---|---|---|
| Leg press | | | | | | |
| Calf raise | | | | | | |
| Ab curl | | | | | | |
| Back extension | | | | | | |
| Lat pull-down | | | | | | |
| Asstd. chin | | | | | | |
| Chest press | | | | | | |
| Shoulder press | | | | | | |
| Upright row | | | | | | |
| Triceps extension | | | | | | |
| Biceps curl | | | | | | |

**Cardio:**

| Date | Exercise | Time (min) | Intensity | Comments |
|---|---|---|---|---|
| | Walk | 20 | 3.5 mph | Flat surface |
| | Walk/jog | 20 | Moderate | More challenging |
| | Water aerobics | 45 | | |

**Stretching:**

| Entire Body | Monday | Tuesday | Wednesday | Thursday | Friday | Saturday | Sunday |
|---|---|---|---|---|---|---|---|
| | Yes | Legs | Yes | Legs/back | Yes | No | No |

made accessible to other Personal Trainers. Another option would be a computerized program where client workouts are stored and can be accessed by the client and their Personal Trainer.

5. A client confidentiality policy should be maintained. Personal Trainers should be reminded that they should never discuss any client's personal information with others. Personal Trainers must respect their clients' privacy and be trustworthy (see Chapter 22).

6. Honesty and scope of practice standards should be emphasized (see Chapter 22). If a Personal Trainer does not know the answer to a client's health- or fitness-related question, the Personal Trainer needs to admit that he or she does not have that information but will volunteer to research the topic and provide an answer at the next training session. If the client is asking for medical advice or a diagnosis, the Personal Trainer must not overstep his or her scope of

It is necessary to set standards for delivering personal training services in a manner that is consistent with industry standards for safety and will ensure that excellent customer service is consistently delivered.

practice but should explain that the client needs to consult their physician or health care provider for that information (see Chapter 1) (6). Ideally, the Personal Trainer should establish a network of allied health care professionals through which referrals can be made to physicians, physical therapists, dietitians, psychologists, and other health care experts. See Chapter 22 for more information regarding scope of practice.

7. Personal Trainers must maintain current personal training certifications, CPR-AED/first aid certification, and liability insurance, if it is not provided by the fitness facility. Records of certification and professional liability insurance should be kept in employee files (3).

##  Training and Empowering Personal Trainers

Personal Trainers should be encouraged to continuously read, learn, and stay current on the latest industry standards and changing trends. The Personal Trainer/manager can subscribe to trade journals and publications and make them available to the Personal Trainers. Budget permitting, some Personal Trainers/managers can provide an annual educational stipend for each Personal Trainer, which will subsidize his or her participation in continuing education to maintain personal training certifications. Others provide continuing education credit (CEC) or units (CEU) approved in-house educational sessions to make it convenient and cost-effective for Personal Trainers to attend and earn credit for continuing education or for recertification. In addition, other Personal Training managers hold weekly staff meetings with Personal Trainers and have them take turns providing continuing education topics to the staff complete with handouts and group discussion time.

Managers should empower Personal Trainers by encouraging them to share training program ideas in meetings, help plan and implement new training program approaches such as small-group training or sport-specific training, and share ideas for how to increase clientele and improve sales. Attending professional conferences and workshops is a good way to earn CECs/CEUs, keep current with the latest research, learn about new programming, and to network among peers. Personal Trainers should be included in discussions about pricing of training sessions and their compensation rates. They should be treated as professionals, and their creative ideas and opinions should be valued. They should feel like an integral part of the training and business team.

## Fitness Management

A Personal Trainer may also be placed in charge of a fitness department in a commercial fitness facility, corporate fitness facility, or nonprofit community recreation center. Other Personal Trainers may also be part of this department. In addition to overseeing personal training sales and delivery, the fitness department manager may also be responsible for fitness equipment purchases, emergency drills, maintenance and repairs, special fitness programming events, health-promotion activities, and, in some cases, the group fitness program. Even with all of these responsibilities, the fitness manager may still be expected to retain personal training clients for additional department revenue and to supplement his or her income in addition to that received managing the fitness department. A checklist along with some practical guidelines may include the following:

1. Setting a schedule for available times for training and for management responsibilities
2. Using a time-management system to stay organized
3. Training exercise specialists and Personal Trainers to follow routine procedures (such as turning in time cards) that will simplify the workload
4. Handle personnel issues and problems in a timely manner

The fitness department manager may also be responsible for fitness equipment purchases, emergency drills, maintenance and repairs, special fitness programming events, health-promotion activities, American Disabilities Act (ADA) requirements, and, in some cases, the group fitness program.

5. Train staff in processes of providing quality customer service
6. Explaining tasks to other fitness staff and then delegating these tasks to those who will get them done correctly and on time (*e.g.*, assign the planning of monthly emergency drills/procedure reviews to a fitness staff member and have this person plan and execute the drills and reviews with all fitness staff, including Personal Trainers)
7. Taking time to "lead by example" for both members and fitness staff by managing a healthy lifestyle by exercising regularly and practicing good nutritional habits

 ## Starting a Business

There are six basic business models from which to choose for a personal training business: sole proprietorship, independent contractor, partnership, corporation, S corporation, and limited liability company.

Before starting a personal training business, it is important to evaluate an appropriate business model from which to operate. There are six basic business models: sole proprietorship, independent contractor, partnership, corporation, S corporation, and limited liability company (LLC).

### Sole Proprietorship

In a sole proprietorship, one person owns the business. As the simplest, least-expensive business model, often the only requirement before starting operations is a license from the state and/or local city where the business will be located. Personal income tax is paid on any business earnings. Two drawbacks to this model can be capital expenses for business start-up/expansion and personal liability for any incurred debt (4). In the eyes of the law and the U.S. Internal Revenue Service, the business and the individual are one and the same. Another point to consider as a sole proprietor is the lack of assistance with day-to-day operations when the Personal Trainer is absent from work.

### Independent Contractor

An independent contractor provides certain services for other individuals or businesses. Many Personal Trainers are independent contractors who provide personal training services to health fitness facilities; the client pays the facility for the services and the facility pays the Personal Trainer. Personal Trainers who are independent contractors often work at multiple locations, set their own schedules, are paid by the session, and often have some control over training session format and fees. However, the percentage of the training fees that the individual contractor receives is often determined by the facility's management team (4). An independent contractor is similar to a sole proprietorship except the Personal Trainer actually operates his or her own business within the health fitness facility. The primary advantage of this arrangement is the Personal Trainer's access to health fitness facility's members and equipment.

### Partnership

A business partnership is formed by two or more people, either with an informal agreement or with a formal written contract filed with local or state government. Partnerships are loosely governed by state and federal regulations and are subject to personal income tax based on each partner's ownership share. Forming a partnership allows pooled financial resources and talents, but ownership transfer among partners may be difficult, and each partner can be held liable if another partner fails to meet business-related obligations (4).

## Corporation

A corporation is a formal business entity subject to laws, regulations, and the demands of stockholders. Governed by a charter and bylaws, a corporation is a legal entity completely separate from its owners and managers and is taxed as such. The corporate profits paid as dividends are also taxed for each shareholder. Investors, whose personal risk for financial liability is limited, are often part of a corporation's start-up and growth. Corporation ownership can be more easily transferred than ownership in a sole proprietorship or partnership (4).

## S Corporation

The S corporation (or subchapter corporation), a popular alternative for small businesses, combines the advantages of the sole proprietorship, partnership, and corporation. Benefits of the S corporation include the following (4):

- Limited risk and exposure of personal assets
- No double taxation on both salary and business income
- Freedom for each partner to distribute dividends

## Limited Liability Company

A limited liability company is flexible for small- to medium-sized businesses and generally more advantageous than partnerships or S corporations. This is often the type of company organization utilized by Personal Trainers. Articles of organization must be filed with the Office of the Secretary of State and can be obtained online (5).

 # Administration

To establish and administer a business, the Personal Trainer should first develop a business plan. The business plan includes a demographic and competitor analysis, establishing a budget, developing management policies, marketing, sales, and pricing.

The first step involved in creating a solid business plan is a comprehensive demographic analysis. Acquire data about the population located in the area. Depending on the scope of the Personal Training operation, this may include individuals living in a 2- to 10-mile radius from a specified location. During this phase of the plan, one should examine the total number of people, number of households, household income, number of families, and a variety of other population characteristics. These demographic markers will provide the business operator with the preliminary information necessary to determine whether there is a chance his or her business can be successful in the chosen marketplace.

> The first step involved in creating a solid business plan is a comprehensive demographic analysis.

Once the demographic analysis has been conducted, the business operator should thoroughly evaluate the competition inside the market area (a geographic region from which one can expect the primary demand for a specific service provided at a fixed location). Virtually all fitness centers offer personal training, so these entities will represent the greatest competitive threat to the viability of the business. Other potential competitors might include gender-specific facilities, group training studios, and hospital-based wellness programs or medical fitness facilities. The strength or weakness of the competition will help determine the percentage of market share that can reasonably be expected to cultivate within the defined market.

## Establishing a Budget

A market analysis will make available valuable information useful in developing an annual operating budget (Table 21.4). It provides the baseline data to build a budget. Personal training businesses typically begin with determining sales goals. The sales goals are set by determining the projected number of training sessions over the course of a week, month, and year multiplied by the average rate per session. These totals will help determine expenses over each period of time because direct expenses correlate with sessions delivered multiplied by the cost per session (see Table 21.2). To establish a budget, the Personal Trainer should consider the following:

1. Estimate business expenses (exclusive of salary) needed to operate annually, including the following:
   a. Gas/vehicle maintenance travel allowance (an expense sometimes paid to Personal Trainers who go to homes, corporations, or other studios or facilities)
   b. Income taxes and other required national, state, or local taxes (*e.g.*, Medicare, Social Security, workers compensation, unemployment insurance)
   c. Liability insurance
   d. Telephone and technology (*e.g.*, computers, Internet, radio, television)
   e. Uniforms
   f. Professional memberships/certifications
   g. Conferences and continuing education training
   h. Business supplies (computer, office supplies, postage, printing, etc.)
   i. Fitness equipment including maintenance and cleaning costs
   j. Client gifts/awards

| Table 21.4 | Sample Budget for Personal Trainer Start-Up |
|---|---|
| **Expense** | **Estimate** |
| Trainings/CEUs | $350 |
| Equipment | $375 |
| Gas/auto | $200 |
| Professional memberships | $350 |
| Internet access/phone | $80 |
| Advertising | $175 |
| Liability insurance | $280 |
| Accounting/legal | $100 |
| Subscriptions | $75 |
| Supplies | $80 |
| **Total start-up** | **$2,065** |

CEUs, continuing education units.
Schreiber K. One-on-one: setting up a budget for a personal training business. *Strength Cond.* 1994;16(5):64–5.

    k. Accountant fees

    l. Legal fees

    m. Health/medical insurance or if self-insured, a medical savings account contribution

    n. Paid vacations, sick days, and holidays

    o. Overtime and exceptional pay (weekends, holidays, nights, etc.)

2. Determine an accurate number of training hours annually that fit into a realistic schedule (factor in vacation days, personal days for medical checkups and family emergencies, sick days, etc.).

3. Determine a dollar charge per training session to achieve a gross annual income that will cover business expenses and personal expenses and will allow some funds to be put aside for savings and/or investments (7). Consider the average price point for personal training services in the region and specifically what the competition is charging (*i.e.*, cost comparisons).

## Management and Policies

To manage a business effectively, the Personal Trainer must work from a business plan, which should include the creation of a business vision, mission statement, business values, a brief description of the business services (Box 21.2), the choice of a business model, and the listing of operational policies (8) such as the following:

- Billing (Will clients prepay for each session or will you bill them monthly?)
- Cancellation policy (How many hours of notice will you need without charging the client?)
- Late arrival policy (Will you charge for the entire session anyway?)
- Vacation policy (What will this be for both the Personal Trainer and the client?)
- Payment methods (Will the client pay by cash, check, debit/credit card, or automatic deduction?)
- "Insufficient funds" check or automatic deduction policy (Will there be a penalty and if so, what?)

---

### Box 21.2    Sample Mission Statement

**The Personal Training Academy**

**Our Vision**

- To grow profitably by delighting customers and achieving undisputed leadership in the field of personal training

**Our Mission**

- To create value for shareowners through our marketplace leadership in personal training and fitness programming that helps all of our clients achieve their goals

**Our Values**

- Integrity, honesty, and the highest ethical standards
- Mutual respect and trust in our working relationships
- Innovation and encouragement to challenge the status quo
- Communication that is open, consistent, and involves both assertive messages and active listening
- Teamwork and meeting our commitments to one another
- Continuous improvement, development, and learning in all we do
- Diversity of people, cultures, and ideas
- Performance with recognition for results

**Service Description**

- The Personal Training Academy provides personal training clients with the best possible physical and psychological advantage by improving their focus, discipline, and self-confidence. This is achieved through the most advanced state-of-the-art personal training techniques available, thus enhancing the client's ability to compete and achieve success both in fitness and in life.

# Marketing

The personal training market includes different groups of people with varying needs. A market niche represents a client group with similar needs and goals. Personal Trainers often choose to focus their marketing efforts on one or several of these groups. For example, a Personal Trainer could select a niche market based on one or more of the following:

- Client type (*e.g.*, gender, age, fitness level)
- Training needs (*e.g.*, sport-specific training, prenatal fitness, older adult fitness, group training)
- Training location (*e.g.*, in-home training, health fitness facility training, sport location training)

Personal Trainers should ask the following questions when selecting their market niches:

- What is the potential for income with this market?
- Is this market accessible in my market area?
- Does this market fit well with my training skills and interest?
- Can I feature my knowledge, services, certifications, and skills in such a way to reach this market as my clientele?

A market niche represents a client group with similar needs and goals.

One of the best ways to market personal training services is to ask for referrals from satisfied clients. Personal Trainers sometimes are hesitant to do this, but if the Personal Trainer believes that a client has benefited greatly from the training, then other potential clients may want to also receive these same benefits. Other ways of marketing personal training services include volunteering to speak at community events and organizations and networking with other business professionals in the community. Advertising on the Internet, newspapers, flyers, and by direct mail can be costly and may not provide a good return on the investment at first. Establishing a Web site and profiling the training style and qualifications, or being listed as a Certified Personal Trainer on professional organization's Web sites are other good approaches for marketing a business and staying competitive in the personal training business.

Personal training businesses use a variety of strategies to attract clients. Among the more popular strategies are as follows:

1. Client referral (the most focused strategy)
   a. The focus is on generating prospects and clients.
   b. The process involves existing clients providing the names of potential new clients.
   c. Clients are provided with referral cards to hand in the names of prospects.
   d. Incentives are typically given to clients for providing referrals.
   e. It is usually an ongoing strategy.
2. Lead boxes (provides a very low rate of return)
   a. This strategy primarily serves as a source for leads (names).
   b. The boxes are placed in business locations that tend to serve customer bases that are demographically similar to the targeted audiences.
   c. Businesses are given awards for allowing the lead boxes to be placed in their locales.
3. Advertising (most expensive and lowest rate of return on investment)
   a. In general, this strategy is designed to build brand recognition in the marketplace, enhance the image of the organization, create leads, or occasionally generate prospects.
   b. This technique is a shotgun approach to reaching clients (as opposed to more targeted methods).
   c. Cable television, radio, newspapers, billboards, and external or internal signage are examples of this method.
   d. The most effective type of advertising for generating leads or prospects provides a "Call to Action" and typically creates urgency by establishing a deadline.
   e. It is important to know the marketing target niche before the advertising medium is selected.

4. Alliances with homeowner associations (HOAs) and realtors
   a. This strategy is a good source for qualified leads and even prospects (HOAs and realtors whose customers match the organization's target market should be engaged in the process).
   b. HOAs and realtors can provide the names of new people in the area.
   c. A strategy involves providing the HOAs or realtors with a certificate or letter to give to customers that offer some complimentary service (*i.e.*, training session or preactivity screening and goals analysis).

5. Direct mail (the return rate for this technique is usually 1%–3% for mailed pieces and 7%–15% using electronic pathways)
   a. This strategy is primarily a technique for creating leads or turning leads into prospects.
   b. This method is a more focused technique than advertising.
   c. Direct mail lists from agencies should be used (targeted lists — such as ZIP codes or even specific delivery routes — can be obtained to best match the desired market area and demographics of the target audience).
   d. The piece that is mailed is typically simple, with an attention-grabbing call to action and normally incorporates an incentive to create urgency and generate an action response.

6. Community involvement (ideal for service and relationship-driven businesses such as personal training)
   a. This strategy focuses on creating relationships to uncover prospects.
   b. The technique involves creating a specific image within the community and becoming a recognized professional.
   c. An example of this approach is to become active in community organizations, such as the local chambers of commerce, the Rotary Club, church groups, and other civic organizations.
   d. Another option is hosting community events in the training facility or sponsoring community events at other locations.
   e. Volunteer as a speaker for community organizations and special events. Offer your services to provide simple screenings while advertising your services.
   f. Join small business groups and pair up with others and exchange services. For example, you can provide personal training to another small business owner in exchange for marketing services.

7. Reputation management
   a. This strategy is used to enhance the public image of the organization.
   b. Over time, this approach can be a great source for prospects.
   c. The technique involves developing a press kit on the Personal Trainer or the business as a whole (*e.g.*, a background, fact sheet).
   d. This strategy requires establishing positive relationships with the local media.
   e. The approach requires regularly issuing press releases of human interest involving the club and following up with the media.

8. Promotional materials
   a. This strategy is normally used to help convert leads to prospects or prospects to members.
   b. The materials are designed to create a positive image of the business and to help educate consumers on personal training in general, the business, and its Personal Trainers.
   c. Web sites, print brochures, and video brochures are examples of this technique.
   d. These materials are normally given to leads and more often to prospects.

9. Strategic alliances
   a. This strategy is designed to create partnerships between businesses and organizations with similar target audiences.
   b. This technique is good at bringing in leads and prospects.
   c. The approach involves cross-marketing between the businesses (*e.g.*, a Personal Trainer might partner with a home fitness equipment retailer offering equipment purchasers a

complimentary "orientation to the purchased equipment," with the objective of converting them into personal training clients; the retailer has a "value-added service" — the Personal Trainer — which might be an enticement for the customer to purchase the equipment).

d. The customers of each business become potential customers for the other partner (an alliance group) (3).

e. Exercise is Medicine™ (EIM) (www.exerciseismedicine.org) encourages health care providers to counsel patients about exercise and turns the public's focus to preventive health care through physical activity. This is a valuable and essential opportunity for Personal Trainers to contact health care providers and partner with physicians to help educate patients about physical activity. EIM encourages physicians to counsel patients about the importance of physical activity and regular exercise. The Personal Trainer can be a referral from the physician and train the patients in establishing individualized exercise programs.

## Sales

Too often, Personal Trainers focus their "sales" efforts on creating signs, flyers, and brochures, hoping that clients will flock to them for training. The mistake often made is that such efforts are "low-percentage" marketing activities that offer a low return on the investment of time, money, and effort. The Personal Trainer depends on the client to respond to the marketing piece. The key to sales success is for the Personal Trainer to use all available resources, proactively cultivate warm-market "suspects" to convert them into prospects, and finally ask the prospect for the sale.

> The key to sales success is for the Personal Trainer to use all available resources, proactively cultivate warm-market "suspects" to convert them into prospects, and finally ask the prospect for the sale.

Before going into the sales process, "sale" must first be defined. A sale is simply an agreement — a quid pro quo — between the Personal Trainer, the client, and, at times, the facility where the training sessions will take place. A sale is not an imposition on the client. All too often, a Personal Trainer is "apologetic" when asking for the sale. In actuality, every sale is a "win–win" situation because all participants position themselves to get what they want. Clients are securing the direction, expertise, or motivation they desire, and the Personal Trainer is contracting his or her professional services. The ingredient needed to fulfill the sale is commitment. The client must commit to what was agreed to at the point of sale (*i.e.*, showing up prepared for the training session at the scheduled time), and the Personal Trainer must commit to deliver on the service "promise" to the client (*i.e.*, delivering a safe, individualized, goal-oriented workout).

In the fitness center environment, the Personal Trainer's primary source of business is the membership base. This captive audience is the Personal Trainer's main resource for "prospects." It is important for the Personal Trainer to be established as an expert and to build rapport with the members. Typically a start-up has a list of between 100 and 500 names of people already known to the Personal Trainer. These are normally friends, family, and coworkers.

Before approaching members on the exercise floor, Personal Trainers should have a clear understanding of their objective and what value they bring to the potential client. It is important to be empathetic and see things through the eyes of the member. Why should the member consider personal training? What is in it for the member? The Personal Trainer should know what the benefits of personal training are to the client (Box 21.3).

The Personal Trainer needs to be aware of the prospect's questions and concerns. What are the prospect's perceptions? Will personal training help get the participant more fit? Will it help the participant look better? Will it help the participant be healthier? These are all valuable benefits and perceived outcomes for the participant, but ultimately, even a prospect who perceives these outcomes as real still might not make the commitment to purchase training sessions. Why? It is because it is all about the prospect's emotions. The Personal Trainer must consider how the

---

### Box 21.3     Benefits of Personal Training

- Client achieves results more quickly
- Reduces the risk of injury to the client
- Increases the client's motivational levels
- Provides more focused workouts for the client
- Utilizes the client's time more efficiently
- Educates the client on physical and psychological benefits of regular exercise

---

prospect feels about his or her goals and how he or she will feel when they are fulfilled (see Chapter 8).

Effective sales generation is simply a step-by-step process outlined on the following pages (and in Box 21.4), which could be used for a facility-based Personal Trainer.

### Step 1: Making Contact

*Getting a foot in the door.* A Personal Trainer needs to proactively approach a facility member or client exercising on the gym floor. The Personal Trainer should greet the member with a smile and offer his or her expertise on the basis of his or her observations of the member. Sample "openings" may include the following:

- "Hi! May I help you with your exercise program?"
- "Hey Mark, would you mind if I show you a more effective way to do this exercise?"
- "Hello Linda, I noticed you're really focusing on your lower body. Can I show you a great new combination of exercises for your hips and thighs?"

### Step 2: Building Rapport

"Trust me?" *Yes!!!* Personal Trainers must build rapport and trust so that prospects believe in them and their ability in helping the clients achieve established goals. A Personal Trainer builds trust by

---

### Box 21.4     The Fitness Facility–Based Personal Trainer's Sales Checklist

- Be proactive. Approach prospects and always remember to smile — *be positive and upbeat, no matter how bad a day you are having.*
- Top priority is to build rapport — to develop a relationship of mutual trust and confidence.
- Sell *benefits* of personal training but key into *how they will feel* when achieving those benefits.
- Be empathetic — see their world as if it was your own.
- Be genuine — exude sincerity.
- Be warm — treat prospects with respect.
- Be a good communicator and listener.
- It's a win–win!
- Clients take control of their goals by using an expert's assistance.
- Personal Trainers practice their profession, increase their earning potential, and add valuable experience, which enhances their value to the employer or facility and the fitness industry in general.
- The facility enhances the service delivered to clients by providing one-on-one management of the member.
- You must *ask* for the sale! — *It is a numbers game. The more prospects you ask, the more sales you will make.*

taking a personal interest in the prospect, making mental notes of
personal information that the prospect may share with the Personal Tr
"blurbs" include the following:

- "Hi John, it's good to see you're back on track after the holidays."
- "Hello Marie, how was your business trip?"
- "Hi Jessica, did your daughter decide between colleges?"

## Step 3: Assessing Need

*The Personal Trainer needs to "shut up and listen!"* The best salespersons are
talkers — they are usually the best active listeners. The Personal Trainer should k
it for the prospect" and focus on not just "what" the prospect wants but also learn w
wants it. Ask simple open-ended questions that encourage the prospect to share info

## Step 4: The Tease

This is how Personal Trainers continue to build trust and demonstrate and build the
The simplest way is to assist a prospect with an exercise or make program sugge
A Personal Trainer can spot the prospect as he or she is progressing through a workou
suggests a "better way." The Personal Trainer can also demonstrate a new exercise or liter
"train" the client for 5 or 10 minutes, just giving the prospect a "taste" of what it is like to wo
with him or her. This sampling of the Personal Trainer's prowess is the "tease" that should kee
the prospect wanting more.

## Step 5: Presenting a Winning Proposition

*Asking for the sale.* The Personal Trainer must present a winning solution to the prospect's need
before asking for the sale. This "frames" the pitch so that the prospect responds affirmatively when
asked for the sale.

- "With your high school reunion coming up, it's a great time to specialize your exercise program, don't you think?"
- "If I can show you how I can help you reach your goal, would that interest you?"

## Step 6: "The Close"

The Personal Trainer should give the prospect "either/or" choices, never "yes" or "no." A sample
"yes-or-no" proposal may include something like "Marie, would you like to set up a training
appointment?" A sample "either/or" proposal might be "Marie, you're usually here in the morning,
I'm available to help you any two mornings a week at 6 a.m. or 7 a.m. Which works best for you?"
Giving the prospect a choice between two "yeses" increases the likelihood that the Personal Trainer
will close the sale.

## Step 7: The Fall-Back

*Opening the backdoor — "the tickler file."* Every prospect that says "no" becomes a "future prospect." The Personal Trainer should maintain a database of contact and personal information (*e.g.*,
likes, dislikes, occupation) of these prospects for further rapport building, always looking for the
opportunity to once again ask for the sale. The Personal Trainer should continue to deliver a service
(*e.g.*, assistance on the training floor) and communicate through every available vehicle (in person,

one, e-mail, etc.), increasing his or her value as a Personal Trainer. Photocopying clips of fitness articles that prospects might be interested in and providing them to clients, e-mailing a Web-based link to a pertinent Web site, and even a press release with the Personal Trainer's own "success story" are all examples of how to effectively "drip" on prospects to build a Personal Trainer's value. Personal Trainers in a fitness center setting should also do whatever they can to keep the prospect coming in to work out, even if the prospect continues to train on his or her own; doing so helps maintain the Personal Trainer's "warm market" so that the prospect remains a prospect and is also a source of referrals to the Personal Trainer.

### Step 8: Keep in Mind

*It's a "numbers game."* An insurance company study conducted several years back showed that even the worst approach to selling can be successful if the salesperson simply goes through the numbers and "keeps asking." With this in mind, understand that a prospect is always a potential customer, so practice cautious persistence.

## ricing

Once the framework for the personal training business is complete, specific pricing and budgets can be established. Typical direct expenses include salaries, payroll taxes, and benefits. Operational expenses include marketing expenses, program materials, and facility use charges. Pricing is typically established through consideration of a number of factors. It is essential to consider the general business objectives (*e.g.*, profit, overall client retention, the projected number of clients, and average number of sessions per client per unit of time) before establishing pricing. To conduct programs within established budgetary guidelines, revenues and expenses should be reviewed regularly (3).

Ultimately, what a Personal Trainer charges for training services depends on market forces. Completing a market analysis will help determine perceived value in the marketplace and thus price point. Some key elements of a market analysis include the following:

- Demographic study: How many potential clients are there in the geographical area?
- Competitive analysis: What are other Personal Trainers charging for their services?
- Consumer survey: What is the prospective client's perceived value?
- Demand projections: How large is the market?
- Financial considerations: Based on budgetary projections, what is the required revenue per unit sale? What volume is required to meet budget?
- Focus group information: What are the perceived needs of the prospect base?
- Consider the four *E*s when considering what to charge clients (2).
    - Education
        - Bachelor's or master's degree in exercise science/physiology; level of certification (*e.g.*, ACSM Certified Personal Trainer[SM]; ACSM Certified Exercise Physiologist[SM])
    - Experience
        - Years working as a certified Personal Trainer
        - Types of training (sports specific, special medical populations)
    - Environment/location
        - Where you are physically (facility) and geographically (city, state)
        - Business or studio location (owner/operator)
    - Expenses
        - Equipment, clothing, gas (traveling trainers), personal liability insurance, advertising/marketing materials, certification/membership fees, rent/electricity/insurance, and so on

Completing a market analysis will help determine perceived value in the marketplace and thus price point.

The components under each of the four *E*s are not exhaustive, nor are they intended to be. As the Personal Training industry continues to grow, so will the needs of certified Personal Trainers and their businesses.

## Business Planning

Budgets are necessary to forecast financial expectations and goals, provide accountability, track progress of actual results versus projected results, and allow justification and scrutiny. Completing an accurate, reliable, and analyzable budget without a computer is not easy. Simple software programs like QuickBooks or MYOB (Manage Your Own Business) are available and recommended, even for the independent Personal Trainer; they will help organize business finances and make tax reporting easier (3). Software programs, such as QUICKEN and QuickBooks, are user-friendly ways to create and maintain business finance records.

Although there are many resources available for the Personal Trainer/manager/owner, it remains prudent to enlist the guidance of a legal and accounting professional.

Although there are many resources available for the Personal Trainer/manager/owner, it remains prudent to enlist the guidance of a legal and accounting professional. The U.S. Internal Revenue Service Web site is a great resource for obtaining specific tax forms and information. It is accessible at http://www.irs.gov/.

 **Professional Standards**

A code of ethics for ACSM certified and registered professionals has been established, which helps guide the ethical practice of Personal Trainers. This code (see Chapter 1) helps bring the profession of personal training in line with other professions and health care disciplines.

## SUMMARY

It is no longer true that the best "technical Personal Trainer" is the most successful. Whether the Personal Trainer is "going solo" or is a manager of a large personal training department within a fitness center, today's Personal Trainers need to be proficient in both exercise science and business management. Only by combining these varied skills can they ensure their success and that of their clients. At the conclusion of this chapter is a case study from which the various components of recruiting appropriate personnel to fill vital positions is elaborated on.

## REFERENCES

1. Alsac B. Pricing your services. *IDEA Trainer Success* [Internet]. 2008 [cited 2011 Nov 21];5(5). Available from: http://www.ideafit.com/fitness-library/pricing-your-services
2. Churilla JR. Starting a personal training business. *ACSM's Certified News.* 2008;18(2):1–7.
3. Herbert DL, Herbert WG. Legal considerations for exercise programming. In: Swain DL, editor. *ACSM's Resource Manual for Guidelines for Exercise Testing and Prescription.* 7th ed. Baltimore (MD): Wolters Kluwer Health/Lippincott Williams & Wilkins; 2014. p. 160–68.
4. Holland T. Ten important personal training guidelines. *Am Fitness.* 2001;19(1):42.
5. Horler K. Determining your corporate structure: part 1. *IDEA Trainer Success* [Internet]. 2008 [cited 2011 Nov 21];5(2).

Available from: http://www.ideafit.com/fitness-library/determining-your-corporate-structure-part-1

6. Mikeska, D. A SWOT analysis of the scope of practice for personal trainers. *Personal Trainer Quarterly* [Internet]. 2015 [cited 2016 Oct 3];2(1), 22–6. Available from: https://www.nsca.com/uploadedFiles/NSCA/Resources/PDF/Education/Articles/Assoc_Publications_PDFs/swot-analysis-of-the-scope-of-practice-for-PT.pdf

7. Miller W. One-on-one: choosing a market niche. *Strength Cond*. 1994;16(4):68–9.

8. Schreiber K. One-on-one: setting up a budget for a personal training business. *Strength Cond*. 1994;16(5):64–5.

9. U.S. Department of Labor, Bureau of Labor Statistics. Occupational employment and wages [Internet]. [cited 2016 Oct 5]. Available from: http://www.bls.gov/oes/current/oes399031.htm#st

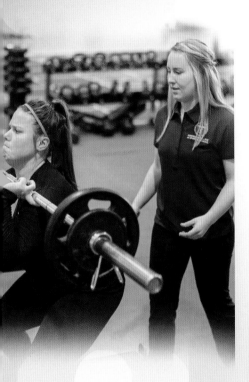

# CHAPTER 22

# Legal Issues and Responsibilities

## OBJECTIVES

**Personal Trainers should be able to:**

- Understand the primary areas of potential legal liability.

- Understand the role of industry standards and guidelines on legal liability issues.

- Learn practical strategies to manage risk.

# INTRODUCTION

A Personal Trainer must understand and appreciate the legal risks and responsibilities of the profession before undertaking the task of training any person. Awareness of potential areas of liability, coupled with conformity to professional standards, will permit the Personal Trainer to minimize these risks. The results will be decreased risk of injury to the client and an overall lessening of any legal exposure of the Personal Trainer (whether operating independently or employed with a gym, health facility, or other employer). Personal Trainers need to know what areas of potential liability affect their practice, what industry standards and guidelines direct these areas, and what measures they can take to manage risk effectively.

All physical activity holds the potential risk of injury and death in the extreme case. Working as a Personal Trainer will invariably involve exposure to some liability. To maintain professionalism and protect the longevity of a career, a Personal Trainer needs to proactively anticipate these areas of risk and manage them with common sense and an understanding of the relevant law. This knowledge of, and commitment to, safety and injury prevention not only minimizes the likelihood of professional liability but also improves quality of service and may save lives.

All physical activity involves risk of injury; accidents can and will happen. Death may happen in the extreme case. Management of these risks is key.

This chapter broadly discusses the liability related to working with clients and offering personal training services. It is structured largely to cover those topics and issues that are addressed in Domain IV (Legal, Professional, Business and Marketing) of the American College of Sports Medicine (ACSM) Certified Personal Trainer^SM performance domains (see www.acsm.org/get-certified). Local rules and regulations, definitions of standards of care, and the acceptability of waivers of liability vary from state to state, county to county, and even city to city. This chapter is not intended to be the sole source of legal advice and should not be considered a substitute for legal counsel on specific liability issues pertaining to individual situations.

> All physical activity involves risk of injury; accidents can and will happen. Death may happen in the extreme case. Management of these risks is key.

## Effectively Minimizing Risk

Although eliminating all risk is not possible, Personal Trainers can minimize risk by obtaining proper qualifications as well as by using appropriate client screening tools and documentation.

### Proper Qualifications

Without doubt, the first and most effective step that a Personal Trainer can take in minimizing risk to the client and liability for the Personal Trainer is to be properly qualified to perform the job. What constitutes proper qualifications may vary depending on the local jurisdiction or the facility employing the trainer. Regardless, the initial undertaking of the Personal Trainer should be to become aware of qualifications and/or certifications that are required. Where no specific requirements are dictated by statute or ordinance, employment policies may mandate a particular course of study or training. In many jurisdictions, there may be no formal requirements that one must meet in order to present oneself as a Personal Trainer. However, even when requirements are minimal, professional certifications and adherence to industry-recognized standards will serve to maintain professionalism, minimize liability, and offer guidance to clients as to the trainer's credentials. In addition to requirements imposed by law or policy, the representation of a facility or of a Personal Trainer regarding the qualifications of the Personal Trainer can impose heightened standards and/or qualification requirements on a Personal Trainer. Clients have filed claims after injuring themselves based on the fact that a Personal Trainer did not have the qualifications represented in a facility's advertising literature. These claims were based on a theory of breach of contract because the facility failed to provide Personal Trainers with the level of qualification that it had promised (4). The facility, through its literature, imposed a higher standard as to the level of qualification by marketing these qualifications.

> Clients have filed claims after injuring themselves based on the fact that a Personal Trainer did not have the qualifications represented in a facility's advertising literature.

The best evidence that a Personal Trainer can use to show that his or her training services meet professional standards is to maintain industry standard certification(s) and to conduct business according to the knowledge, skills, and abilities that are expected as minimum competencies by the certifying organization(s). The ACSM Certified Personal Trainer[SM] is defined as a fitness professional involved in developing and implementing an individualized approach to exercise leadership in healthy populations and/or those individuals with medical clearance to exercise. This certified professional is deemed proficient in writing appropriate exercise recommendations, leading and demonstrating safe and effective methods of exercise, and motivating individuals to begin and continue their healthy behaviors (2).

The issue of a Personal Trainer's responsibility for advising appropriate levels of training intensity is even more critical, as more people with special needs seek to work with Personal Trainers. Personal Trainers who advertise their services to targeted clientele such as older adults or people with arthritis, claiming that they are trained to serve these niche markets, need to be sure that they are sufficiently prepared to serve these clients' needs. Evidence of sufficient preparation would include additional education, training, and experience in working with people with particular needs. Personal Trainers should therefore keep written records of all certifications, continuing education, and work-related experience.

## Screening and Documentation

A preparticipation screen is used to assess a client's health and medical history. Screening is an important tool to help ensure that a Personal Trainer is well qualified to meet a particular client's needs and to develop services that are appropriate for the client. In addition, the Personal Trainer must properly interpret health risks and determine when a medical clearance is necessary. Utilizing tools such as the ACSM coronary artery disease risk factor thresholds (2), which delineate which clients are at moderate to high risk based on cardiovascular risk factors, will aid in identifying these clients. Once these precautionary steps are taken, the Personal Trainer will conduct a fitness evaluation to determine the recommended level of training that will be safe and effective to meet the particular client's needs and goals (2). A written record of these measures should be kept to document the steps taken by the Personal Trainer to create a specific exercise program (2). Documentation from the client's physician regarding medical clearance, if needed, should also be maintained.

# Scope of Practice and Professional Collaboration

Scope of practice refers to the range of permissible professional activities that a Personal Trainer may undertake, coupled with an understanding of the boundaries that serve as limits on these activities. This is an important area of potential liability for the Personal Trainer. As fitness professionals work more closely together with health care providers to deliver a continuum of care to individuals, it is important to define respective roles. According to the ACSM's Code of Ethics for Certified and Registered Professionals, "[Personal Trainers] practice within the scope of their knowledge and skills. [Personal Trainers] will not provide services that are limited by state law to provision by another health care professional only" (5). This is particularly true for Personal Trainers with advanced academic degrees or training and when working with clients who may have special exercise considerations. Both criminal and civil actions are possible for practicing medicine or some other allied health care profession without a license. An injunction against a Personal Trainer's practice is possible. An elevated standard of care is required because malpractice is certainly a viable concern.

> Personal Trainers who operate their own businesses would be wise to seek the advice of local legal counsel and to take other steps to manage risk effectively, such as maintaining certifications, obtaining releases and waivers or consents as applicable, carrying liability insurance, and keeping detailed written records.

The contemporary delivery of health care services itself is in a state of flux because of high costs and attempts to reduce costs by expanding the roles of paraprofessionals in the medical context. As a result, states vary widely on what constitutes the practice of medicine and what is appropriate behavior for a nurse, physician assistant, or other paraprofessional. According to fitness law experts David L. and William G. Herbert, many states have defined the practice of medicine broadly so that persons engaged in exercise testing and prescription activities could, under some circumstances, fall within the range of such statutes (4).

Personal Trainers, therefore, need to become familiar with the relevant guidelines for scope of practice that are established at their affiliated organizations and institutions. Personal Trainers who operate their own businesses would be wise to seek the advice of local legal counsel and to take other steps to manage risk effectively, such as maintaining certifications, obtaining releases and waivers or consents as applicable, carrying liability insurance, and keeping detailed written records.

Generally, Personal Trainers have not been considered health care providers as defined by states' medical malpractice statutes. Medical malpractice law is determined almost exclusively at the state level and will therefore vary from state to state. The relevant code sections of each state's medical malpractice act will normally define the laws to which health care providers are subjected. Typically, Personal Trainers are not placed in this category of health care providers. However, this has been tested in circumstances when a Personal Trainer's training services were delivered in a medical setting. In a 2003 Indiana case (*Community Hospital v. Avant*, 790 N.E.2d 585; Ind. App. 2003), a court held that even though a Personal Trainer was employed by a hospital and the fitness facility was owned by the hospital, the Personal Trainer was not a health care provider; thus, the case did not qualify as a medical malpractice case. The significance of this case, however, is that the client did try to sue both the fitness facility and the hospital on the basis of injuries sustained while engaged in the personal training program, and the court did examine the fact that the training occurred in a setting with a close connection to a hospital. Another court might have found that this type of training did meet the standards of health care practitioners (6,11). The Personal Trainer may be subject to different potential liability when training services are delivered in a medical setting. Generally, Personal Trainers have not been deemed health care providers and thus are not subject to medical malpractice laws.

> The Personal Trainer may be subject to different potential liability when training services are delivered in a medical setting. Generally, Personal Trainers have not been deemed health care providers and thus are not subject to medical malpractice laws.

## Medical or Dietary Advice

No cases have yet been litigated to conclusion that involved a client suing a Personal Trainer for faulty medical or dietary advice, except in the case of dietary supplements, which will be discussed later in this chapter. However, remember that health care is a highly regulated area. The consequences of stepping over the line into the protected area of a licensed health care practitioner — such as a medical doctor, physical therapist, registered dietitian, or chiropractor — vary by state. Personal Trainers are exposed to potential liability for acting outside the scope of practice if the "advice" could be interpreted as the unauthorized practice of medicine (or some other licensed profession) and if this advice results in a client injury.

Although the Personal Trainer must be cognizant of his or her scope of practice, he or she must also recognize the importance of collaborating with and referring to health care professionals. The Personal Trainer should develop a comprehensive network of allied professionals and actively refer clients who request or require specialized services to an appropriate health care provider (4). Using referrals is important both for those clients who need medical clearance prior to starting an exercise program and for existing clients who require additional assistance. Personal Trainers should maintain open lines of communication between themselves and various health care professionals to optimize client outcomes and aid in the identification of risk factors.

## Supplements

Claims related to violations of scope of practice occur most frequently in the area of supplements. A high-profile case brought against a Personal Trainer and a large fitness chain (*Capati v. Crunch Fitness Intern, Inc.*, 295 A.D.2d 181, 743 N.Y.S.2d 474; N.Y.A.D. 1 Dept 2002) involved a scenario in which a Personal Trainer sold supplements, including one that contained ephedra, to a client, who had hypertension, and died. Survivors then filed a lawsuit. In another example, a Personal Trainer sold steroids to a client, who later suffered adverse consequences and filed a claim against the Personal Trainer (6).

In another incident, a personal training company combined supplement sales with its fitness packages to increase revenue. The company eventually had a client who was allergic to an ingredient in the supplement. The problem was compounded when the client assumed that if she took more than the recommended dosage, she would see more results. She ended up in the hospital, and even though she had been a loyal client for some time, she sued the Personal Trainer and the business. The case was settled out of court, and the Personal Trainer lost his business. The problem was not that the Personal Trainer had sold the client the products, but that he had given her a written plan specifying what to eat and when to take the supplements. The fact that the client overdid it did not matter (6).

According to insurers, the problem with supplements is worsened by the fact that most supplement manufacturers do not carry any insurance coverage. Theoretically, if the manufacturers were insured, this would not only fully compensate the client for any injuries due to their products but also potentially serve to indemnify the Personal Trainer who sold the defective product. Unfortunately, because this is rarely true, there is no third-party insurance that can offer some protection when the Personal Trainer incurs liability. An ancillary consideration to this is that most of the insurance policies for fitness professionals do not include protection for product liability.

In today's market, no one, even professional registered dietitians, can be certain about the ingredients in many supplements because they are not subject to government regulation. In addition, one can never be certain regarding who may have severe allergic reactions, including the risk of death, to any particular ingredient. To proactively protect client safety and to minimize the risk of professional liability, Personal Trainers should avoid recommending and/or selling supplements.

## Development of a Comprehensive Risk Management Program

### Addressing Known Risks

Legal considerations affect many aspects of the personal training experience. Areas of potential exposure to liability include the physical setting where program activities occur; the equipment used; the nature and quality of training techniques, advice, and services rendered; the degree of emergency preparedness and responsiveness; and the method of keeping and protecting records. Although legal principles affect the training environment, as a practical matter, most cases today are settled out of court and therefore never actually create case law. To help Personal Trainers understand the practical ramifications, this chapter is organized according to the most common types of incidents likely to occur during day-to-day business. The application of legal concepts such as negligence to particular circumstances is then examined, and the role of professional standards, guidelines, position statements, and recommendations from professional organizations is considered.

The operation of a personal training facility constitutes a business/invitee relationship. The client, or invitee, has been "invited" onto the premises for the financial gain of the business. This relationship heightens the obligation of the business to the invitee. In addition to providing reasonably safe premises, the business that invites persons onto the premises of the business must also exercise reasonable care to maintain the premises in a safe condition and to regularly inspect the premises for the presence of dangerous conditions. When exercising reasonable care, it is important that the Personal Trainer (especially in the case of a self-owned facility) not only perform the regular inspections but also establish a policy or guidelines for the inspection and a method of record keeping for evidence of these inspections.

> The operation of a personal training facility is a business/invitee relationship. In these types of relationships, the obligations and duties of the business to the invitee are heightened.

### Safe Premises

Although most Personal Trainers focus on educating themselves on the latest training techniques and aspects of program design, in reality, Personal Trainers are vulnerable to professional liability for incidents that result from conditions of the physical setting where program activities occur. In general (11), any business owner who allows people to enter upon land or into a building is required to provide a reasonably safe environment under theories of tort law (Box 22.1). The area of tort law that regulates these issues is termed "premises liability." ACSM (3) has identified 34 standards for health/fitness facilities as well as 37 guidelines. These items are included in *ACSM's Health/Fitness Facility Standards and Guidelines*, 4th edition, which is a valuable resource for the Personal Trainer. Because a Personal Trainer may offer services in a variety of locations, including a health/fitness facility, the outdoors, or in a client's home, the Personal Trainer should take basic precautions to help ensure that every training setting is reasonably safe and includes an emergency action plan and an injury prevention program.

> The Personal Trainer should take basic precautions such as developing an emergency action plan and an injury prevention plan to help ensure that every training setting is reasonably safe.

### Emergency Response

Most Personal Trainer certifications require that Personal Trainers have cardiopulmonary resuscitation (CPR) training (and some require first aid training and automated external defibrillator [AED] training). As yet, no specific case has involved a claim against a Personal

| Box 22.1 | Key Terms |
| --- | --- |

*Negligence*: a failure to conform one's conduct to a generally accepted standard or duty

*Release or waiver*: an agreement by a client before beginning participation, to give up, relinquish, or waive the participant's rights to legal remedy (damages) in the event of injury, even when such injury arises as a result of provider negligence

*Risk management*: a process whereby a service or program is delivered in a manner to fully conform to the most relevant standards of practice and that uses operational strategies to ensure day-to-day fulfillment, ensure optimum achievement of desired client outcomes, and minimize risk of harm to clients

*Tort law*: body of law that regulates civil wrongdoing

Adapted from Herbert DL, Herbert WG, Herbert TG. *Legal Aspects of Preventive, Rehabilitative and Recreational Exercise Programs.* 4th ed. Canton (OH): PRC Publishing; 2002; Koeberle BE. *Legal Aspects of Personal Fitness Training.* 2nd ed. Canton (OH): PRC Publishing; 1994; American College of Sports Medicine. *ACSM's Resource Manual for Guidelines for Exercise Testing and Prescription.* 6th ed. Baltimore (MD): Wolters Kluwer/Lippincott Williams & Wilkins; 2010; Cotten DJ, Cotten MB. *Legal Aspects of Waivers in Sport, Recreation and Fitness Activities.* Canton (OH): PRC Publishing; 1997.

Trainer for wrongful death in a situation in which a client has had a sudden cardiac arrest or other medical emergency and died while under the supervision of a Personal Trainer. However, it is possible that a claim could be filed against a Personal Trainer who failed to provide an emergency response if that failure led to a death that could have otherwise been avoided. Participation in physical activity, which may be strenuous, particularly in clients who are identified as moderate or high risk based on disease-specific categories, creates a situation where there is a foreseeable risk that the administration of first aid, CPR, or other life-saving measures will be needed. In law, foreseeability is the touchstone for imposing a duty on someone to anticipate and plan for risks. In addition, numerous states have enacted legislation mandating that health/fitness facilities have at least one AED on the premises (9). Whether required by statute or by the law as it relates to foreseeability, every Personal Trainer should implement and document appropriate emergency preparedness policies and procedures. This may include, but is not limited to, CPR certification and basic first aid administration, maintaining equipment necessary for the administration of first aid, maintaining AEDs and being familiar with their use, and educating other employees about the emergency preparedness plan. In addition to these measures, which require outside training or certification, foreseeability also includes the routine implementation of policies such as when to call 911. All of these measures should be documented, and written policies should be maintained and followed. Consistency is paramount. Although drafting and utilizing emergency preparedness policies can thwart potential litigation, the failure of the Personal Trainer to abide by these policies can expose that trainer to liability. Failure to follow one's own policies and procedures may form the basis for plaintiffs asserting that the Personal Trainer breached a duty to the client.

It is possible that a claim could be filed against a Personal Trainer who failed to provide an emergency response if that failure led to a death that could have otherwise been avoided.

The ACSM and the American Heart Association (AHA) published a joint position stand in 1998 with recommendations for health/fitness facilities regarding the screening of clients for the presence of cardiovascular disease, appropriate staffing, emergency policies, equipment, and procedures relative to the client base of a given facility (7). In 2002, the ACSM and the AHA published a joint position stand to supplement the 1998 recommendations regarding the purchase and use of AEDs in health/fitness facilities (8) and supported in 2012 by the ACSM (3). These organizations agree that a comprehensive written emergency plan is essential to promote safe and effective physical activity.

The AHA, the ACSM, and the International Health, Racquet & Sportsclub Association (IHRSA) recommend that all fitness facilities have written emergency policies and procedures, which are reviewed and practiced regularly, including the use of automated defibrillators. Staff who are responsible for working directly with program participants and providing instruction and leadership in specific modes of exercise must be trained in CPR. These staff should know and practice the facility's emergency plan regularly and be able to readily handle emergencies. In addition, these organizations require health/fitness facilities to use AEDs (3,13).

As evidence of professional competency, Personal Trainers should keep CPR, first aid, and AED certifications current. Personal Trainers should proactively familiarize themselves with any affiliated organization's emergency plan and be ready to implement the plan's procedures in case of emergency. For Personal Trainers who operate a business, creating an emergency plan should be a top priority. Personal Trainers who provide training services outdoors or in a client's home should also have written emergency policies and procedures. This may include information on when to call 911, administration of CPR off-site and possibly the availability of portable AED devices as these become more readily available and their use feasible.

In addition to having an emergency plan, Personal Trainers should also document any accident or incident immediately, using an incident report form (Box 22.2). The Personal Trainer should include only the facts surrounding the incident and not any opinions regarding what may or may not have caused the incident. In addition, the names and contact information of witnesses should be included. The person who experienced the incident should sign the form. Insurers will provide incident-reporting forms, and the Personal Trainer should always carry extra forms to every training session (1,3). These forms should be kept confidential. Whether or not these become discoverable in any potential litigation will vary depending on the facts of a particular situation and on the law regarding formal litigation discovery in the particular state. As a general rule, however, documents created in anticipation of litigation will be covered under what is known as the "work product" rule and will not be available to a plaintiff in a lawsuit.

## Premise Liability

### Slip-and-Fall Injuries

The number one claim against fitness facilities and professionals is for injuries related to falls on the training premises, according to many insurance providers (6). Courts have consistently held that clients are entitled to "reasonably safe" conditions. Personal Trainers can foster reasonably safe conditions by a regular practice of inspection for, and correction and warning of, any hazards in the workout area and areas used to access the workout location (12). For example, if items that may cause a fall are on the floor, the trainer should clear these away before beginning a session. If floor surfaces are wet and incapable of correction before a session occurs, the session should be either moved or rescheduled. If safety conditions require, it is always better to be conservative and reschedule rather than to continue training in the presence of known dangers. Personal Trainers who work in aquatics facilities need to be particularly vigilant about deck conditions and pool access areas, as wet surfaces increase the likelihood of a slip-and-fall incident.

In addition to routinely inspecting locations before and during training sessions, Personal Trainers should follow a procedure of proper equipment storage when equipment is not in use (6). Regardless of the training setting, specific storage places should be designated for equipment, so items are not left where people can trip over them. Different types of equipment require different types of storage. For example, free weights require storage designed not only to accommodate their size and shape but also to support their load. Make sure to use storage practices that not only effectively store equipment out of people's way but also protect it from being used for inappropriate purposes. For example, many types of personal training equipment are attractive to young children (*i.e.,* "attractive nuisance") and may be best stored in locked cabinets if children potentially have access.

| Box 22.2 | Sample Incident Report |
| --- | --- |

**INCIDENT REPORT**

TO BE COMPLETED BY INSTRUCTOR

CONFIDENTIAL WORK—PRODUCT

Date: _____

Location/Address of Accident or Incident: _____

Name of Instructor Completing the Form: _____

Date of Accident or Incident: _____

Approximate Time of Accident or Incident: _____ : _____ am pm

Name of Injured Person: _____ Age: _____ Sex: _____

Injured Person's Address _____

City: _____ State: _____ Zip Code: _____

Home Phone #: ( ) _____ Work Phone #: ( ) _____ Cell Phone #: ( ) _____

How long has this person been under your instruction: _____

_____

Describe the accident/incident: _____

_____

_____

Describe possible injury (sprained ankle, etc.): _____

_____

_____

Describe type of equipment involved: _____

_____

List any type of treatment performed by you or by a doctor (include doctor, hospital name):

_____

_____

Were there any witnesses to the incident: yes _____ no _____

If yes, please have each witness write a brief statement about what happened.

YOUR SIGNATURE: _____

Used with permission from Jeff Frick, Fitness and Wellness Insurance Agency, 380 Stevens Avenue, Suite 206, Solana Beach, CA 92075.

Objects that are part of a facility environment but not necessarily fitness equipment can also pose risks. In one case, a client brought suit against a health club after he sustained injuries resulting from a fall that occurred as the client was reaching to adjust a television that was positioned on an overhead rack. The Personal Trainer's assessment of the fitness facility environment should include all areas and objects. Many legal tests for liability will revolve around the concept of what potential injuries are reasonably foreseeable. In the case of the television, was it foreseeable that a client reaching to adjust it would fall? If yes, then it is the duty of the business owner to accommodate this risk. This may be through signage ("Do not adjust television"), or through making remote controls available, or through repositioning the television to eliminate any awkward positioning by the client reaching to make adjustments. The important takeaway points are that business owners are obligated to identify and eliminate risks that are reasonably foreseeable and to appropriately warn patrons of any persistently hazardous conditions. In testing for these conditions, the Personal Trainer should attempt to utilize the equipment as a client would. These actual-use tests can aid in identifying risks that are not readily apparent from visual inspection alone.

Personal Trainers should also educate clients about appropriate clothing and footwear to prevent injury and to enhance training. Clothing should be comfortable, breathable, and allow movement. In particular, Personal Trainers need to check footwear and should not allow clients to train with inadequate shoes. Factors such as poor fit, excess wear, and unsuitability to the activity all increase the risk of injury. Recognition of foot and leg care issues is especially important if the Personal Trainer works with clients who have diabetes, venous insufficiency, or other medical conditions that may impact the lower extremities. An awareness of these issues will permit the Personal Trainer to make physician referrals when appropriate. Personal Trainers who work with people new to exercise may want to create a client handout that outlines appropriate exercise apparel and other exercise safety issues. If the Personal Trainer trains clients in a setting in which protection is necessary, such as a helmet for cycling or pads for inline skating, the Personal Trainer should make sure that the client wears protective equipment (12).

## Equipment Issues

According to insurance providers, the second leading reason for claims against Personal Trainers is injury resulting from the use of equipment (12). These cases are based on legal theories from tort law that a Personal Trainer's duty or standard of care is to exercise reasonable care that the client does not suffer injury (see Box 22.2). A Personal Trainer who fails to take reasonable precautions, which is determined on the basis of an evaluation of facts surrounding an incident, could be deemed negligent and therefore liable or responsible. Professional organizations such as the ACSM and National Strength and Conditioning Association (NSCA) also offer industry guidelines relating to matters of facility and equipment setup, inspection, maintenance, repair, and signage (3). Although these standards and guidelines do not have the force of law, they can be introduced as evidence via expert testimony of the Personal Trainer's duties and/or adherence to the standard of care. Keep in mind that the law does not envision that accidents never happen; laws and industry standards and guidelines exist to encourage proactive safe behavior to avoid preventable accidents.

> The law does not envision that accidents never happen; laws and industry standards and guidelines exist to encourage proactive safe behavior to avoid preventable accidents.

As a practical matter, when it comes to using equipment safely, the question then becomes, "What steps can Personal Trainers take to prevent foreseeable accidents?" Personal Trainers should always use safe, reliable, and appropriate equipment and use equipment for its intended purposes according to manufacturer guidelines (1). Whenever a Personal Trainer directs a client to use equipment, the Personal Trainer should provide proper instructions and supervision. In addition, policies and procedures for routine safety inspections, maintenance, and repair should be in place and observed systematically. Personal Trainers or facility managers should keep written records to demonstrate compliance with these policies and procedures. The importance of thorough documentation cannot be overemphasized. All of these steps are likely to minimize the risk of an accident. Then, if an accident occurs, even though everything has been done to prevent it, it is likely to be considered the type of accident that could not have been prevented by taking reasonable precautions.

Many clients will ask Personal Trainers to recommend equipment. It is important for the Personal Trainer to work only with reliable fitness equipment dealers when recommending equipment to clients. Personal Trainers who do not have a reliable vendor with whom to work should not recommend one piece of equipment over another. The topic of product liability is complex and outside the scope of this chapter. However, the Personal Trainer should be warned that equipment product manufacturers are now pursuing clubs and Personal Trainers for improper installation and maintenance in cases that the manufacturers face due to theories of product liability.

### FREE WEIGHTS

For a concrete example of potential liability for client injury from equipment use, consider the common scenario that involves an experienced Personal Trainer supervising an apparently healthy client who is performing a squat or similar exercise with free weights. The Personal Trainer encourages the client to use a heavier weight and perform more repetitions even though the client complains of fatigue. The client suffers a debilitating back injury and sues the Personal Trainer and fitness facility.

Under theories of negligence, the Personal Trainer owes this client a duty to exercise reasonable care to prevent injury. Reasonable steps that a Personal Trainer can take to avoid this type of incident include fostering open communications with the client to encourage feedback and listening when the client communicates that he or she is reaching fatigue. Personal Trainers should know how to spot signs of fatigue and be conservative when implementing program progressions. Injuries are not uncommonly sustained by clients who are new to exercise. In one instance (*Lumpkin v. Fitness Together I, Inc., et al.*, Jefferson County Circuit Court Case Number CV-2005-6512, Jefferson County, Alabama), a client filed suit alleging that he was pushed too aggressively by a Personal Trainer to continue squats after he reported severe muscle fatigue and pain with accompanying physical symptoms of trembling and an inability to stand. The client subsequently developed rhabdomyolysis (*i.e.*, a condition that occurs when muscle fibers release myoglobin into the bloodstream; in worst-case scenarios, the kidneys can't filter effectively and kidney damage occurs) and required hospitalization. Although such an outcome is not always predictable, strong lines of communication increase the likelihood that the attuned Personal Trainer will recognize and can appropriately respond to feedback provided by the client.

Another step that a Personal Trainer could take is to keep detailed records of numbers of repetitions, sets, and weight loads on specific training days. In this manner, a client can follow a reasonable plan of progression that minimizes injury risk. Before implementing progression in a program, Personal Trainers can discuss the client's feeling of readiness to increase intensity and further evaluate whether the timing is appropriate for such a change. If specific records are maintained, the Personal Trainer is also in a position to evaluate whether or not a client's response to a particular exercise session is abnormal and requires referral to a physician (2).

### WEIGHT MACHINES

Even though machines carry a reduced risk of injury because the client's body is more stable and movement is more restricted than with free weights, injuries still occur. Most injuries happen when a client is encouraged to handle a weight that is too heavy, a weight plate slips and falls because a pin was not properly inserted, or a cable breaks. Weight plates have fallen and crushed ankles and feet or hit people in the head. In turn, clients suffer physical injuries and sue the Personal Trainer, fitness facility, and equipment manufacturer.

Here again, to ensure that the client does not suffer this type of injury, a Personal Trainer can exercise reasonable care through a consistent practice of regular inspections and correction of any known hazards such as worn or faultily maintained equipment; through keeping records of what weight the client has been able to lift, the number of repetitions, and sets; and through following a conservative plan to increase intensity in close communication with the client. When working with weight training equipment, the Personal Trainer can develop a procedure of instruction and supervision for each exercise that includes an equipment and body scan to check for proper equipment setup and body alignment. Creating this type of instructional technique so that an inspection becomes a routine part of each and every exercise can go a long way toward preventing accidents.

Factors that courts have examined in equipment-related cases include whether or not the equipment has been maintained appropriately and used for its intended purpose per specific manufacturer guidelines. In particular, courts examined whether or not parts had been replaced in a timely manner and whether or not facility owners had ensured that routine inspections and maintenance were conducted and documented (6). Regardless of the setting, a Personal Trainer should be proactive in learning about equipment safety inspections, maintenance, and record-keeping policies as well as the procedures for reporting the need for repairs. Before putting a client on any piece of equipment, the Personal Trainer should have firsthand knowledge of its readiness for use.

> Before putting a client on any piece of equipment, the Personal Trainer should have firsthand knowledge of its readiness for use.

Keep in mind that courts also examine appropriateness of use. In one case (*Nelson v. Sheraton Operating Corp.*, 87 Wash. App. 1038, Not Reported in P.2d, 1997 WL 524034; Wash. App. Div. 1, 1997), hotel management had placed equipment in a hotel gym that was intended for private home use. The court found the hotel liable for injuries suffered by the client. A training facility should provide commercial grade equipment; manufacturers do not design home equipment to withstand the wear and tear of frequent use by multiple users. A Personal Trainer who owns or manages a training studio should use professional equipment.

### CARDIOVASCULAR MACHINES

Treadmills are currently among the most popular form of exercise equipment in fitness facilities; however, it is imperative that their popularity not lead the Personal Trainer to assume that clients will be familiar with their use. Numerous cases feature instances in which a client loses control and falls from a treadmill. These cases often involve middle-aged or older adult clients who are unfamiliar with the machine's workings and unable to keep up with the movement speed. In one instance (*Corrigan v. Musclemakers, Inc.*, 258 A.D.2d 861, 686 N.Y.S.2d 143; N.Y.A.D.; 3 Dept 1999), a 49-year-old client who had never patronized a gym and who had never been on a treadmill was placed on one by a Personal Trainer. The Personal Trainer provided no instruction on the use of the machine, including no instruction on how to adjust the speed, stop the belt, or operate the controls. The client, being thrown from the machine, suffered a broken ankle. Subsequently, a lawsuit concerning the injury was filed. This case is consistent with others that show that the consequences from falls include back, neck, shoulder, and other joint injuries, broken bones, and even death. Clients (or their survivors) sue the Personal Trainer, fitness facility, and equipment manufacturer under theories of either negligent instruction or defective product (6).

Of course, these examples should not discourage a Personal Trainer from using equipment to train clients. Equipment is an essential part of creating effective training programs. These incidents simply underscore that whenever equipment is being used, Personal Trainers must remain alert to the special risks presented and take proactive steps to manage and minimize these risks. Furthermore, Personal Trainers should maintain detailed records to document the preventive steps that have been taken (12).

> Personal Trainers must remain alert to the special risks presented and take proactive steps to manage and minimize these risks.

## Claims of Sexual Harassment

Sexual harassment claims represent a third area of potential liability for Personal Trainers according to insurance providers (6). Because the personal training relationship can seem "intimate," it lends itself to creating more opportunity for abusive conduct on the part of the Personal Trainer or for a misinterpretation of actions on the part of the client. Numerous cases involve a male Personal Trainer and a female client. The female client believes that inappropriate touching has occurred and that she has been violated. Or, a personal relationship develops between the Personal Trainer and the client who then raises questions about the legitimacy of the business services rendered. The client believes that undue influence was used to create an exploitive situation.

One strategy to protect against a claim of inappropriate touching is to always ask a client for permission to use tactile spotting and to avoid it unless absolutely necessary.

Sexual harassment is difficult to prove and often rests on credibility. Personal Trainers, therefore, should be vigilant and act professionally at all times. One strategy to protect against a claim of inappropriate touching is to always ask a client for permission to use tactile spotting and to avoid it unless absolutely necessary. Some Personal Trainers do not touch clients directly, but spot them through the use of another prop, such as a ball. Also, situations behind closed doors where no one else is present should be avoided. For example, if skinfold body composition assessments are offered, the procedure should be conducted in a room with other Personal Trainers, perhaps behind a folding screen, or with another Personal Trainer or staff member present. If a personal relationship develops with a client, the professional relationship should be discontinued and the client should be referred to another Personal Trainer.

## Continuing Education and Adherence to Ethical Guidelines

In evaluating negligence claims, there are four elements that a plaintiff must prove in order to prevail in a lawsuit. These are duty, breach of duty, proximate cause, and damages. The imposition of a duty may be determined by specific circumstances. Broadly, one general duty is to provide a safe premise for invitees of a business. This means that there should be no unnecessarily dangerous conditions present in the physical space utilized for training. Another generally recognized duty for the Personal Trainer is to conform one's activities to the standard of care (*i.e.*, degree of care that a reasonable or prudent Personal Trainer would utilize under similar circumstances). This standard will vary by jurisdiction and the setting in which training sessions are offered. Other legal duties may be self-imposed by certain conduct or by contract. For example, by advertising certain credentials or guaranteeing outcomes, a Personal Trainer may create duties or legal obligations, which would not otherwise be present under the law. The breach of duty element in negligence law is frequently examined based on whether the person deviated from the standard of care. In establishing what the standard of care is for a Personal Trainer, there are usually no statutory guidelines that prescribe a particular standard. Instead, courts will normally turn to an industry standard — what is customary in the particular industry. Although the customs and norms will vary by locale, there are national entities, which provide initial certification and ongoing and continuing education. Demonstrating adherence to the standard of care then, can be best accomplished by closely following and maintaining these professional certifications and continuing education credits as well as operating in accordance to industry standards/guidelines and position stands. In doing so, the Personal Trainer reflects professionalism and commitment to the integrity of the field. In addition to the obligation the Personal Trainer has to stay abreast of new knowledge and skills through education, the Personal Trainer should also select activities that are permitted within the scope of practice and adhere to the ethical guidelines as defined by the certifying organization. In the setting of a lawsuit for negligence, even when duty and breach can be proven, a plaintiff must additionally prove damages (some injury or legal harm) and proximate causation that the alleged breach actually led to the injury. Absent evidence of all four of these elements, a plaintiff cannot prevail on a claim for negligence.

## Development of a Business Plan

The structure of the Personal Trainer's business model will vary according to each individual's needs and objectives, as well as the laws regarding business organizations by state. There are, however, some overall principles that are broadly relevant. Personal Trainers may be employees of an existing business. Most people are familiar with an employer–employee relationship. This model, although affording many benefits (such as predictable income stream, possibly insurance and other employment-related benefits, etc.), will limit the autonomy of the Personal Trainer.

Alternatively, a Personal Trainer may choose to operate independently or establish a business. Independent operation as a sole proprietor normally does not afford the trainer any protection of personal assets. Most states permit individuals to form business entities, such as a corporation or limited liability company, which will shield personal assets in the event of legal liability, and permit only those assets of the business to be available in the event of claim or judgment. If a trainer chooses to form a business entity (rather than a sole proprietorship or "doing business as"), an attorney and/or a tax professional should be consulted for advice on particular business structures and the tax implications. Operating outside an employer–employee relationship will necessitate research regarding start-up costs, budgeting, purchasing or leasing space, licensing, advertising costs, and many other issues. Proper planning and seeking advice from other professionals will promote a smooth transition into business ownership.

In the event the Personal Trainer is entering into a partnership or business with others, it will be critical to plan for any eventual dissolution through a buy–sale agreement or other operational/organizational contingency plan, which will govern dissolving a business. This may incorporate noncompete agreements and other restrictive language on the trainer's ability to practice. The enforceability of these agreements varies widely by jurisdiction, so include this consideration in discussions with counsel.

## Risk-Management Strategies

Personal Trainers should manage risk exposure with a multilayered approach that incorporates a number of important strategies. As the first line of defense, Personal Trainers should create written policies, procedures, and forms that meet industry standards and guidelines and maintain detailed written records that document compliance with these policies. This strategy minimizes the likelihood that the Personal Trainer would fail to demonstrate that he or she exercised reasonable care under the circumstances. In other words, the Personal Trainer should make every effort not to be negligent.

The second strategy involves using a release, waiver, or informed consent, depending on which legal document is recognized under the laws of the place where the Personal Trainer conducts business (10). The purpose of these documents is either (a) to demonstrate that the Personal Trainer fully informed the client of all of the potential risks of physical activity and the client decided to undertake the activity and waive the Personal Trainer's responsibility or (b) to demonstrate that the client knowingly waived his or her right to file a claim against the Personal Trainer even if the Personal Trainer

> As the first line of defense, Personal Trainers should create written policies, procedures, and forms that meet industry standards and guidelines and maintain detailed written records that document compliance with these policies.

is negligent. Courts have consistently held that in order for a release to operate as an effective bar to liability, the release should be clear and unambiguous and should refer specifically to the negligence of the party seeking the release. The Personal Trainer should keep these records indefinitely and in a safe place. Consent forms are not infinity contracts so provisions should also be made for an annual signing of these important documents. Each state has its own statutes of limitations on waivers and consent forms. The Personal Trainer is advised to check with legal authorities within their jurisdiction.

The third strategy is to carry professional liability insurance (4,12). This transfers the risk to the insurer. In that instance, even if the Personal Trainer is negligent, the insurance company assumes responsibility for resolving any claims. Most insurers of Personal Trainers provide coverage for certified professionals. The fourth strategy is to incorporate the business to protect personal assets from any potential claims. The fifth strategy is to cultivate strong relationships with clients and colleagues. Clients are much less likely to sue if they perceive a Personal Trainer as caring, responsible, and responsive to their needs. The final strategy is to consult local legal counsel to ensure that business practices meet the requirements of the specific location (6).

##  Written Policies, Procedures, and Forms

> Personal Trainers should conduct their business according to written policies, procedures, and forms that ensure that their business practices conform to the standards set by professional organizations.

Personal Trainers should conduct their business according to written policies, procedures, and forms that ensure that their business practices conform to the standards set by professional organizations (1,2–4,6,11,12). In addition to policies discussed in the business practices chapter, every Personal Trainer should also have risk management policies that include a written emergency plan and a preparticipation screening procedure.

The most important forms for a Personal Trainer include the following:

1. Preparticipation screening form such as a Physical Activity Readiness Questionnaire (PAR-Q)
2. Health history questionnaire
3. Physician's statement and medical clearance
4. Fitness assessment or evaluation form
5. Client progress notes
6. Incident Reports

As important as *having* these forms is *using* these forms. The Personal Trainer should complete all portions of the forms. A form that is only partially completed is often the source of more questions than answers and may imply that the Personal Trainer was not thorough in their use. When utilizing these forms, blank spaces are unacceptable.

In the event that a Personal Trainer is encouraging a client to train independently on equipment in a particular fitness facility, an equipment orientation form for the client to sign indicates that he or she has received instruction on the proper setup and use of weight training equipment and would be useful to document equipment instruction.

##  Informed Consent, Release, or Waiver

In numerous states, courts are holding up waivers more and more as valid means of protection against litigation. In 2001, a California case (*Bendek v. PLC Santa Monica, LLC*, 104 Cal.App.4th 1351, 129 Cal.Rptr. 197; Cal.App.2 Dist 2002) was dismissed after a court held that the waiver form signed by a facility member when she joined protected the facility and its owners from liability when the member filed a lawsuit claiming that she slipped and injured herself. This case is

| Box 22.3 | **Sample of Informed Consent Form for a Symptom-Limited Exercise Test** |
|---|---|

1. **Purpose and Explanation of the Test**

   You will perform an exercise test on a cycle ergometer or a motor-driven treadmill. The exercise intensity will begin at a low level and will be advanced in stages, depending on your fitness level. We may stop the test at any time because of signs of fatigue or changes in your heart rate, electrocardiogram, or blood pressure, or symptoms you may experience. It is important for you to realize that you may stop when you wish because of feelings of fatigue or any other discomfort.

2. **Attendant Risks and Discomforts**

   There exists the possibility of certain changes occurring during the test. These include abnormal blood pressure, fainting, irregular, fast or slow heartbeat, and in rare instances, heart attack, stroke, or death. Every effort will be made to minimize these risks by evaluation of preliminary information relating to your health and fitness and by careful observations during testing. Emergency equipment and trained personnel are available to deal with unusual situations that may arise.

3. **Responsibilities of the Participant**

   Information you possess about your health status or previous experiences of heart-related symptoms (*e.g.*, shortness of breath with low-level activity, pain, pressure, tightness, heaviness in the chest, neck, jaw, back, and/or arms) with physical effort may affect the safety of your exercise test. Your prompt reporting of these and any other unusual feelings with effort during the exercise test itself is very important. You are responsible for fully disclosing your medical history as well as symptoms that may occur during the test. You are also expected to report all medications (including nonprescription) taken recently and, in particular, those taken today, to the testing staff.

4. **Benefits to Be Expected**

   The results obtained from the exercise test may assist in diagnosing your illness, in evaluating the effect of your medications, or in evaluating what type of physical activities you might do with low risk.

5. **Inquiries**

   Any questions about the procedures used in the exercise test or the results of your test are encouraged. If you have any concerns or questions, please ask us for further explanations.

6. **Use of Medical Records**

   The information that is obtained during exercise testing will be treated as privileged and confidential as described in the Health Insurance Portability and Accountability Act of 1996. It is not to be released or revealed to any person except your referring physician without your written consent. However, the information obtained may be used for statistical analysis or scientific purposes with your right to privacy retained.

7. **Freedom of Consent**

   I hereby consent to voluntarily engage in an exercise test to determine my exercise capacity and state of cardiovascular health. My permission to perform this exercise test is given voluntarily. I understand that I am free to stop the test at any point if I so desire.

I have read this form, and I understand the test procedures that I will perform and the attendant risks and discomforts. Knowing these risks and discomforts, and having had an opportunity to ask questions that have been answered to my satisfaction, I consent to participate in this test.

_____     _____
Date                        Signature of patient

_____     _____
Date                        Signature of witness

_____     _____
Date                        Signature of physician or authorized delegate

Reprinted with permission from American College of Sports Medicine. *ACSM's Guidelines for Exercise Testing and Prescription*. 10th ed. Philadelphia (PA): Wolters Kluwer; 2018.

consistent with other California cases (6). Depending on where a Personal Trainer lives, he or she may need to have a document entitled one of the following:

- Express assumption of the risk
- Informed consent
- Release or waiver of liability

An assumption of the risk or informed consent document (Box 22.3) essentially explains the risks of participating in physical activity to a prospective client. The client then agrees that he or she knowingly understands these risks, appreciates these risks, and voluntarily assumes responsibility for taking these risks. These documents help strengthen the assumption of risk defense for the Personal Trainer when inherent injuries occur but do not provide protection for negligence.

A waiver or release of liability (Box 22.4) document states that the client knowingly waives or releases the Personal Trainer from liability for any acts of negligence on the part of the Personal Trainer (3). In other words, the prospective client waives his or her right to sue the Personal Trainer, even if the Personal Trainer is negligent (13). A Personal Trainer needs to consult with an attorney in his or her location to determine which type of document is the standard practice for his or her state. For additional forms, please refer to *ACSM's Health/Fitness Facility Standards and Guidelines*, 4th edition (3).

---

| **Box 22.4** | **Sample Agreement and Release of Liability Form** |

I, _____, the undersigned, wish to participate in a fitness evaluation, which consists of a submaximal cardiovascular assessment (bike or treadmill), body fat analysis by skinfold, strength, and flexibility assessments, muscular endurance assessment and individualized exercise program at the *<name of facility>* in *<city, state>*, which is to be conducted on this _____ day of _____, 20_____. The evaluation will be conducted under the direction of a Personal Trainer. I understand and acknowledge that participation in the fitness evaluation activities involves an inherent risk of physical injury and I assume all such risks. I understand that I will participate in all fitness exercises in said fitness evaluation. I assume all risks of damage or injury, including death, that may be sustained by me while participating in the fitness evaluation test.

For and in consideration of *<name of facility>* allowing me to take the fitness evaluation, I hereby release and covenant not to sue *<name of facility>*, the officers, agents, members, and employees of each, from any and from all claims or actions, including those of negligence, which might arise as a result of any personal injury, including death, or property damage which I might suffer as a result of my participation in the fitness evaluation on the date set forth above.

By signing this document, I hereby acknowledge that I am at least 18 years of age and have read the above carefully before signing, and agree with all of its provisions this _____ day of _____, 20_____.

_____          _____
Signature of Participant                        Witness

Note: This form is presented for information purposes only and should be not considered legal advice or used as such. The use of this form in specific situations requires substantive legal judgments and a licensed attorney should be consulted before using the form.

# Professional Liability Insurance

In today's litigious environment, for the most protection, a Personal Trainer should carry professional liability insurance ($2 million per occurrence is the current recommended amount), even when working in a business as an employee, where the Personal Trainer may be covered under the business owner's policy. The reason for this is that it is not unusual for a single claim to result in a million dollar judgment. Purchasing the best protection enables the Personal Trainer to practice responsibly and feel confident that his or her business will not be destroyed by one situation. ACSM Certified Personal Trainers can purchase professional liability insurance through the ACSM. For more information, go to http://www.acsm.org/Content/Navigation Menu/MemberServices/MemberResources/AccessBenefitsOnline/Access_online_benefi.htm. This content is restricted to members only.

Professional liability insurance provides a broad spectrum of protection from claims such as those arising from negligence, breach of contract, or even sexual harassment, and it can provide coverage for both injuries to a person or to property. Another potential consideration is to ensure that policies cover one outside a fitness facility if working with clients outdoors and particularly in challenging environments (*e.g.*, mountain biking, kayaking, rollerblading).

> Professional liability insurance provides a broad spectrum of protection from claims such as those arising from negligence, breach of contract, or even sexual harassment, and it can provide coverage for both injuries to a person or to property.

Insurance professionals are expert at handling claims and will take care of all of the details, enabling the Personal Trainer to continue to operate his or her business (6). This includes, when necessary, providing the defense to a lawsuit. Frequently, this duty to provide a legal defense for the Personal Trainer is as valuable to the insured as is the duty of the insurance company to pay for covered claims brought against the Personal Trainer.

# Client Confidentiality

The failure to protect client confidentiality is another emerging area of potential liability for a Personal Trainer. It is important to protect confidentiality to prevent potential harm to a client's reputation. The Personal Trainer must keep detailed written records from the first client prescreening to notes documenting each training session. These records provide critical evidence that can document that the Personal Trainer exercised reasonable care in performing his or her professional duties. At the same time, the Personal Trainer must exercise care to protect this information. A system should be in place that provides for and protects the complete confidentiality of all user records and meetings. User records should be released only with an individual's signed authorization. Before a Personal Trainer discloses any personal information, even for marketing purposes, such as a client testimonial or "before and after" photos, the Personal Trainer should obtain and store a signed release form. A law passed by the U.S. Congress requires health care professionals to have strict policies regarding the safety and security of private records (the Health Insurance Portability and Accountability Act [HIPAA] of 1996, Public Law 104-191, which amends the Internal Revenue Service Code of 1986, also known as the Kennedy-Kassebaum Act) and came into effect on April 14, 2003. Although it is still un-

> For liability protection, the Personal Trainer must keep detailed written records from the first client prescreening to notes documenting each training session.

clear whether HIPAA extends to Personal Trainers, it is wise to become familiar with this law and how it may affect the release of any personal information to a third party. It is clear that when a Personal Trainer works under the auspices of a "covered health care provider" as defined by HIPAA (*e.g.*, a hospital, physician office), this law will govern the release of client information.

## SUMMARY

The personal training industry is in a rapid state of growth and redefinition, as more health care providers acknowledge the need for exercise training as part of a program of preventive health care. In addition, the wellness trend is fueling more and more individuals to assume responsibility for their personal health and to consult with experts such as Personal Trainers to provide training services that enhance the quality of their daily lives. Personal Trainers have great opportunities to work in a variety of settings and make a powerful difference in the lives of their clients.

More professional opportunities, however, increase expectations of responsible professional conduct. More professional responsibility means more potential exposure to liability for failing to act responsibly. Today's Personal Trainer must understand these potential areas of risk exposure and the legal issues and industry standards and guidelines that surround these issues to deliver services confidently and to proactively manage risk. This professionalism in all aspects of doing business not only increases the personal and professional rewards of life as a Personal Trainer but also ensures lasting business success amid the growing complexity of our modern legal environment. Ultimately, the purpose of liability is to protect individuals. The most successful Personal Trainers will always keep in mind that the core of personal training is ultimately personal: to protect the best interests of the client at all times and in all ways. To this end, the ACSM has developed a code of ethics for ACSM certified and registered professionals (see Chapter 1) that will help establish the Personal Trainer profession.

## REFERENCES

1. American College of Sports Medicine. *ACSM's Certification Review*. 4th ed. Baltimore (MD): Lippincott Williams & Wilkins; 2013. 320 p.

2. American College of Sports Medicine. *ACSM's Guidelines for Exercise Testing and Prescription*. 10th ed. Philadelphia (PA): Wolters Kluwer; 2018.

3. American College of Sports Medicine. *ACSM's Health/Fitness Facility Standards and Guidelines*. 4th ed. Champaign (IL): Human Kinetics; 2012. 256 p.

4. American College of Sports Medicine. *ACSM's Resource Manual for Guidelines for Exercise Testing and Prescription*. 7th ed. Baltimore (MD): Lippincott Williams & Wilkins; 2013. 896 p.

5. American College of Sports Medicine. *Code of Ethics for ACSM Certified and Registered Professionals* [Internet]. Indianapolis (IN): American College of Sports Medicine; [cited 2016 Jul 8]. Available from: http://certification.acsm.org/faq28-codeofethics

6. Archer S. Reward carries risk: a liability update. *IDEA Personal Trainer*. 2004;15(4):30–4.

7. Balady GJ, Chaitman B, Driscoll D, et al. Recommendations for cardiovascular screening, staffing and emergency policies at health/fitness facilities. *Circulation*. 1998;97(22):2283–93.

8. Balady GJ, Chaitman B, Foster C, et al. Automated external defibrillators in health/fitness facilities: supplement to the AHA/ACSM recommendations for cardiovascular screening, staffing and emergency policies at health/fitness facilities. *Circulation*. 2002;105(9):1147–50.

9. Connaughton JO, Spangler JO, Zhang J. An analysis of automated external defibrillator implementation and related risk management practices in health/fitness clubs. *J Legal Aspects Sport*. 2007;17(1):101–26.

10. Cotten DJ, Cotten MB. *Legal Aspects of Waivers in Sport, Recreation and Fitness Activities*. Canton (OH): PRC Publishing; 1997. 206 p.

11. Herbert DL, Herbert WG. *Legal Aspects of Preventive, Rehabilitative and Recreational Exercise Programs*. 4th ed. Canton (OH): PRC Publishing; 2002. 508 p.

12. Koeberle BE. *Legal Aspects of Personal Fitness Training*. 2nd ed. Canton (OH): PRC Publishing; 1994. 199 p.

13. McInnis K, Herbert W, Herbert D, Herbert J, Ribisl P, Franklin B. Low compliance with national standards for cardiovascular emergency preparedness at health clubs. *Chest*. 2001;120(1):283–8.

# Editors from the Previous Two Editions of *ACSM's Resources for the Personal Trainer*

## FOURTH EDITION

### SENIOR EDITOR

**Barbara A. Bushman, PhD, FACSM, ACSM-PD, ACSM-CES, ACSM-HFS, ACSM-CPT**
Professor
Department of Kinesiology
Missouri State University
Springfield, Missouri

### ASSOCIATE EDITORS

**Rebecca Battista, PhD**
Associate Professor
Department of Health, Leisure, and Exercise Science
Appalachian State University
Boone, North Carolina

**Lynda Ransdell, PhD, FACSM**
Dean
College of Education, Health, and Human Development
Montana State University
Bozeman, Montana

**Pamela Swan, PhD, FACSM, ACSM-CES**
Associate Professor
Healthy Lifestyle Research Center, School of Nutrition and Health Promotion
Arizona State University
Phoenix, Arizona

**Walter R. Thompson, PhD, FACSM, ACSM-PD, ACSM-RCEP**
Regents' Professor
Department of Kinesiology and Health (College of Education) and Division of Nutrition, School of Health Professions, College of Health and Human Sciences
Georgia State University
Atlanta, Georgia

## THIRD EDITION

### SENIOR EDITOR

**Walter R. Thompson, PhD, FACSM**
Regents' Professor
Department of Kinesiology and Health (College of Education) and Division of Nutrition, School of Health Professions, College of Health and Human Sciences
Georgia State University
Atlanta, Georgia

### ASSOCIATE EDITORS

**Barbara A. Bushman, PhD, FACSM**
Professor
Department of Health, Physical Education, and Recreation
Missouri State University
Springfield, Missouri

**Julie Desch, MD**
Founder
New Day Wellness
Palo Alto, California

**Len Kravitz, PhD**
Associate Professor and Coordinator of Exercise Science
Department of Health, Exercise, and Sports Sciences
University of New Mexico
Albuquerque, New Mexico

# Contributors from the Previous Two Editions of *ACSM's Resources for the Personal Trainer*

## FOURTH EDITION

**Brent A. Alvar, PhD, FACSM**
Rocky Mountain University of Health Professions
Provo, Utah

**Dan Benardot, PhD, DHC, RD, FACSM**
Georgia State University
Atlanta, Georgia

**Barbara A. Bushman, PhD, FACSM, ACSM-PD, ACSM-CES, ACSM-HFS, ACSM-CPT**
Missouri State University
Springfield, Missouri

**Kathy Campbell, EdD, FACSM**
Arizona State University
Phoenix, Arizona

**Marissa E. Carraway, MA**
East Carolina University
Greenville, North Carolina

**Carol N. Cole, MS, ACSM-HF/D**
Sinclair Community College
Dayton, Ohio

**Dino Costanzo, MA, FACSM, ACSM-RCEP, ACSM-PD, ACSM-ETT**
The Hospital of Central Connecticut
New Britain, Connecticut

**Lance Dalleck, PhD, ACSM-RCEP**
The University of Auckland
Auckland, New Zealand

**Emily K. Di Natale, MA**
East Carolina University
Greenville, North Carolina

**Danae Dinkel, MS, ACSM-HFS**
University of Nebraska Medical Center
Omaha, Nebraska

**Ayla Donlin, MS, ACSM-CPT**
California State University
Long Beach, California

**Julie J. Downing, PhD, FACSM, ACSM-HF/D, ACSM-CPT**
Central Oregon Community College
Bend, Oregon

**Diane Ehlers, MS**
Arizona State University
Phoenix, Arizona

**Yuri Feito, PhD, MPH, ACSM-RCEP, ACSM-CES**
Kennesaw State University
Kennesaw, Georgia

**Brian Goslin, PhD**
Oakland University
Rochester, Michigan

**B. Sue Graves, EdD, FACSM**
Florida Atlantic University
Boca Raton, Florida

**Trent Hargens, PhD, ACSM-CES**
James Madison University
Harrisonburg, Virginia

**Andy Hayes, MS, ACSM-HFS**
Missouri State University
Springfield, Missouri

**Jennifer Huberty, PhD, ACSM-HFS**
Arizona State University
Phoenix, Arizona

**Jeffrey M. Janot, PhD, ACSM-CES**
University of Wisconsin–Eau Claire
Eau Claire, Wisconsin

**Alexandra Jurasin, MS**
Plus One Health Management, Inc.
New York, New York

**NiCole R. Keith, PhD, FACSM**
Indiana University–Purdue University Indianapolis
Indianapolis, Indiana

**Jim Lewis, PT, DPT, ATC**
Georgia State University
Atlanta, Georgia

**Lesley Lutes, PhD**
East Carolina University
Greenville, North Carolina

**Mike Motta, MS**
Plus One Health Management, Inc.
New York, New York

**Nicholas Ratamess, Jr., PhD**
The College of New Jersey
Ewing, New Jersey

**Jan Schroeder, PhD**
California State University
Long Beach, California

**Deon L. Thompson, PhD, ACSM-PD**
Georgia State University
Atlanta, Georgia

**Walter R. Thompson, PhD, FACSM, ACSM-PD, ACSM-RCEP**
Georgia State University
Atlanta, Georgia

**Anita Tougas, MS**
North Dakota State University
Fargo, North Dakota

**Jacquelyn Wesson, JD, RN**
Wesson & Wesson, LLC
Warrior, Alabama

**Daniel Wilson, PhD**
Missouri State University
Springfield, Missouri

**Mary Yoke, MA, MM**
Indiana University
Bloomington, Indiana

## THIRD EDITION

**Laura Alderman, MEd**
MeritCare Medical Center
Fargo, North Dakota

**William R. Barfield, PhD, FACSM**
College of Charleston & Medical University of
    South Carolina
Charleston, South Carolina

**Dan Benardot, PhD, DHC, RD, FACSM**
Georgia State University
Atlanta, Georgia

**Christopher Berger, PhD**
University of Kentucky
Lexington, Kentucky

**Barbara A. Bushman, PhD, FACSM**
Missouri State University
Springfield, Missouri

**Nikki Carosone, MS**
Plus One Health Management, Inc.
New York, New York

**Carol N. Cole, MS**
Sinclair Community College
Dayton, Ohio

**Richard T. Cotton, MA**
American College of Sports Medicine
Indianapolis, Indiana

**Lance C. Dalleck, PhD**
Minnesota State University
Mankato, Minnesota

**Shala E. Davis, PhD, FACSM**
East Stroudsburg University of Pennsylvania
East Stroudsburg, Pennsylvania

**Julie Desch, MD**
New Day Wellness
Palo Alto, California

**Julie J. Downing, PhD, FACSM**
Central Oregon Community College
Bend, Oregon

**Heidi Duskey, MA**
Zest! Coaching
Medford, Massachusetts

**Gregory B. Dwyer, PhD, FACSM**
East Stroudsburg University of Pennsylvania
East Stroudsburg, Pennsylvania

**Rebecca Ellis, PhD**
Georgia State University
Atlanta, Georgia

**Maren S. Fragala, MS**
University of Connecticut
Storrs, Connecticut

**Ellen G. Goldman, MEd**
EnerG Coaching
Livingston, New Jersey

**B. Sue Graves, EdD, FACSM**
Florida Atlantic University
Davie, Florida

**Billie Jo Hance, BS**
Take Care Health Systems
Sunnyvale, California

**Disa L. Hatfield, PhD**
University of Rhode Island
Kingston, Rhode Island

**Stanley Sai-chuen Hui, PhD, FACSM, FAAHPERD**
The Chinese University of Hong Kong
Shatin, N.T., Hong Kong

**Jeffrey M. Janot, PhD**
University of Wisconsin–Eau Claire
Eau Claire, Wisconsin

**Alexandra Jurasin, MS**
Plus One Health Management, Inc.
New York, New York

**William J. Kraemer, PhD, FACSM**
University of Connecticut
Storrs, Connecticut

**Len Kravitz, PhD**
University of New Mexico
Albuquerque, New Mexico

**Mike Motta, MS**
Plus One Health Management, Inc.
New York, New York

**Cynthia Pavell, MS**
Fitness + Wellness
Springfield, Virginia

**Neil I. Pire, MA, FACSM**
InsPIRE Training Systems
Ridgewood, New Jersey

**Kathleen Querner, MA**
Sinclair Community College
Dayton, Ohio

**Stacey Scarmack, MS**
Retrofit_U
Lancaster, Ohio

**Jan Schroeder, PhD**
California State University Long Beach
Long Beach, California

**Barry A. Spiering, PhD**
Wyle Laboratories
Houston, Texas

**Gwendolyn A. Thomas, MA**
University of Connecticut
Storrs, Connecticut

**Deon L. Thompson, PhD, FAACVPR**
Georgia State University
Atlanta, Georgia

**Walter R. Thompson, PhD, FACSM, FAACVPR**
Georgia State University
Atlanta, Georgia

**Jakob L. Vingren, PhD**
University of North Texas
Denton, Texas

**Jacquelyn Wesson, JD, RN**
Wesson & Wesson, LLC
Warrior, Alabama

# Index

Page numbers in *italics* designate figures; page numbers followed by the letter "t" designate tables; page numbers followed by the letter "b" designate text boxes; (*see also*) designates related topics or more detailed subtopics.

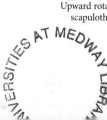